Vibrant and Healthy Kids

ALIGNING SCIENCE, PRACTICE, AND POLICY
TO ADVANCE HEALTH EQUITY

Committee on Applying Neurobiological and
Socio-Behavioral Sciences from Prenatal Through Early
Childhood Development: A Health Equity Approach

Jennifer E. DeVoe, Amy Geller, and Yamrot Negussie, *Editors*

Board on Population Health and Public Health Practice

Health and Medicine Division

A Consensus Study Report of

The National Academies of
SCIENCES · ENGINEERING · MEDICINE

THE NATIONAL ACADEMIES PRESS
Washington, DC
www.nap.edu

THE NATIONAL ACADEMIES PRESS   500 Fifth Street, NW   Washington, DC 20001

This activity was supported by a contract between the National Academy of Sciences and the Robert Wood Johnson Foundation (#72444). Any opinions, findings, conclusions, or recommendations expressed in this publication do not necessarily reflect the views of any organization or agency that provided support for the project.

International Standard Book Number-13:   978-0-309-49338-3
International Standard Book Number-10:   0-309-49338-2
Digital Object Identifier: https://doi.org/10.17226/25466
Library of Congress Control Number: 2019948065

Additional copies of this publication are available from the National Academies Press, 500 Fifth Street, NW, Keck 360, Washington, DC 20001; (800) 624-6242 or (202) 334-3313; http://www.nap.edu.

Printed in the United States of America

Suggested citation: National Academies of Sciences, Engineering, and Medicine. 2019. *Vibrant and healthy kids: Aligning science, practice, and policy to advance health equity.* Washington, DC: The National Academies Press. https://doi.org/10.17226/25466.

The National Academies of
SCIENCES · ENGINEERING · MEDICINE

The **National Academy of Sciences** was established in 1863 by an Act of Congress, signed by President Lincoln, as a private, nongovernmental institution to advise the nation on issues related to science and technology. Members are elected by their peers for outstanding contributions to research. Dr. Marcia McNutt is president.

The **National Academy of Engineering** was established in 1964 under the charter of the National Academy of Sciences to bring the practices of engineering to advising the nation. Members are elected by their peers for extraordinary contributions to engineering. Dr. John L. Anderson is president.

The **National Academy of Medicine** (formerly the Institute of Medicine) was established in 1970 under the charter of the National Academy of Sciences to advise the nation on medical and health issues. Members are elected by their peers for distinguished contributions to medicine and health. Dr. Victor J. Dzau is president.

The three Academies work together as the **National Academies of Sciences, Engineering, and Medicine** to provide independent, objective analysis and advice to the nation and conduct other activities to solve complex problems and inform public policy decisions. The National Academies also encourage education and research, recognize outstanding contributions to knowledge, and increase public understanding in matters of science, engineering, and medicine.

Learn more about the National Academies of Sciences, Engineering, and Medicine at **www.nationalacademies.org**.

The National Academies of
SCIENCES · ENGINEERING · MEDICINE

Consensus Study Reports published by the National Academies of Sciences, Engineering, and Medicine document the evidence-based consensus on the study's statement of task by an authoring committee of experts. Reports typically include findings, conclusions, and recommendations based on information gathered by the committee and the committee's deliberations. Each report has been subjected to a rigorous and independent peer-review process and it represents the position of the National Academies on the statement of task.

Proceedings published by the National Academies of Sciences, Engineering, and Medicine chronicle the presentations and discussions at a workshop, symposium, or other event convened by the National Academies. The statements and opinions contained in proceedings are those of the participants and are not endorsed by other participants, the planning committee, or the National Academies.

For information about other products and activities of the National Academies, please visit www.nationalacademies.org/about/whatwedo.

COMMITTEE ON APPLYING NEUROBIOLOGICAL AND SOCIO-BEHAVIORAL SCIENCES FROM PRENATAL THROUGH EARLY CHILDHOOD DEVELOPMENT: A HEALTH EQUITY APPROACH

JENNIFER E. DeVOE (*Chair*), Professor and Chair, Department of Family Medicine, Oregon Health & Science University

CYNTHIA GARCÍA COLL, Adjunct Professor, Department of Pediatrics, University of Puerto Rico Medical School; Charles Pitts Robinson and John Palmer Barstow Professor Emerita, Brown University

ELIZABETH E. DAVIS, Professor, Department of Applied Economics, University of Minnesota

NADINE BURKE HARRIS, Surgeon General, State of California (*since February 2019*); Chief Executive Officer, Center for Youth Wellness, California (*until February 2019*)

IHEOMA U. IRUKA, Chief Research Innovation Officer, Director, Center for Early Education Evaluation, HighScope Educational Research Foundation

PAT R. LEVITT, Chief Scientific Officer, Vice President, and Director, Saban Research Institute, Simms/Mann Chair in Developmental Neurogenetics, Children's Hospital Los Angeles; W.M. Keck Provost Professor of Neurogenetics, Keck School of Medicine, University of Southern California

MICHAEL C. LU, Professor and Senior Associate Dean, Academic, Student, and Faculty Affairs, The George Washington University

SUNIYA S. LUTHAR, Foundation Professor of Psychology, Department of Psychology, Arizona State University; Professor Emerita, Teachers College, Columbia University

AMY ROHLING McGEE, President, Health Policy Institute of Ohio

MYRA PARKER, Assistant Professor, Center for the Study of Health and Risk Behaviors, University of Washington

JAMES M. PERRIN, Professor of Pediatrics, Harvard Medical School; Pediatrician, MassGeneral Hospital for Children

NATALIE SLOPEN, Assistant Professor, Epidemiology and Biostatistics, University of Maryland School of Public Health

ALBERT WAT, Senior Policy Director, Alliance for Early Success

BILL J. WRIGHT, Director, Providence Health System, Center for Outcomes Research and Education

National Academy of Medicine Norman F. Gant/American Board of Obstetrics and Gynecology Fellow

EBONY BOYCE CARTER, Assistant Professor, Washington University School of Medicine in St. Louis

v

Study Staff

AMY GELLER, Study Director
YAMROT NEGUSSIE, Associate Program Officer
SOPHIE YANG, Research Associate
ANNA MARTIN, Administrative Assistant
PAMELA McCRAY, Senior Program Assistant (*from April 2019*)
ROSE MARIE MARTINEZ, Senior Board Director, Board on Population
    Health and Public Health Practice
DANIEL BEARSS, Senior Research Librarian
MARY JANE PORZENHEIM, Intern (*from June to August 2018*)
MISRAK DABI, Financial Associate
TASHA BIGELOW, Editor

Title: Chasing Sunshine
Artist: Stephanie Kohli (Weston, Wisconsin)
Year: 2017
Medium: Mixed Media

Artist statement:

This piece is based off of my daughter running in our garden. Feeding children the best quality food and letting them explore nature in community gardens is a beautiful way to help them shine.

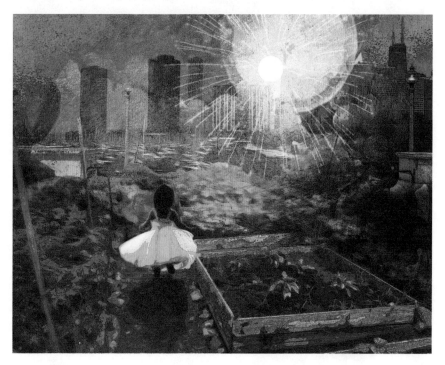

This artwork was submitted as part of the National Academy of Medicine's Visualize Health Equity Community Art Project nationwide call for art. This call for art encouraged artists of all kinds to illustrate what health equity looks, sounds, and feels like to them. More information on this project can be found at nam.edu/VisualizeHealthEquity.

Reviewers

This Consensus Study Report was reviewed in draft form by individuals chosen for their diverse perspectives and technical expertise. The purpose of this independent review is to provide candid and critical comments that will assist the National Academies of Sciences, Engineering, and Medicine in making each published report as sound as possible and to ensure that it meets the institutional standards for quality, objectivity, evidence, and responsiveness to the study charge. The review comments and draft manuscript remain confidential to protect the integrity of the deliberative process.

We thank the following individuals for their review of this report:

JEANNE BROOKS-GUNN, Columbia University
ALISON EVANS CUELLAR, George Mason University
KENNETH A. DODGE, Duke University
ROBERT A. HAHN, Centers for Disease Control and Prevention
MAXINE HAYES, University of Washington
MILTON KOTELCHUCK, Harvard University
MARVA L. LEWIS, Tulane University
APARNA MATHUR, American Enterprise Institute
HANNAH MATTHEWS, Center for Law and Social Policy
BRUCE S. McEWEN, The Rockefeller University
JACK P. SHONKOFF, Harvard University
PAUL G. SPICER, The University of Oklahoma

Although the reviewers listed above provided many constructive comments and suggestions, they were not asked to endorse the conclusions or recommendations of this report, nor did they see the final draft before its release. The review of this report was overseen by **ROBERT M. KAPLAN,** Stanford University, and **BOBBIE BERKOWITZ,** University of Washington. They were responsible for making certain that an independent examination of this report was carried out in accordance with the standards of the National Academies and that all review comments were carefully considered. Responsibility for the final content rests entirely with the authoring committee and the National Academies.

Contents

Preface

All children deserve the opportunity to meet their full health potential and lead fulfilling lives. Our nation's future depends on it. Yet, there are millions of children in the United States who are not afforded this opportunity today. While spending a record amount of money on health care services, the United States has the worst infant mortality rate among 19 similar wealthy nations, and the U.S. maternal mortality rate in 2018 was our highest since 2000. Although the United States is one of the richest nations in the world, in 2015 more than 9.6 million children lived in families with annual incomes below the poverty line (based on the Supplemental Poverty Measure), with approximately 2.1 million living in deep poverty. The highest rates of poverty were found among Hispanic, African American, and American Indian/Alaska Native families. This is deeply concerning because poverty during pregnancy and childhood is directly tied to poor health and developmental outcomes. Our nation's health disparities, of which there are many, are directly linked to what happens in early childhood and prenatally (and even earlier). For all children to lead fulfilling lives, we need to first achieve health equity as a nation, and to do so, we must focus on the youngest, and most vulnerable, in our nation. We also need to look beyond health care for solutions; while health care is necessary to improve health outcomes, fixing health care alone will not address health inequities.

A multitude of factors, from the macro to the micro levels, contribute to the divergent health trajectories that children experience. A child's health ecosystem is influenced by social, economic, cultural, and environmental factors that impact healthy development and well-being. These influences start before birth and have an impact throughout an individual's life and across generations. Exposure to positive influences consistently and longitudinally increases the likelihood of health production, while exposure to negative influences decreases opportunities to be healthy. The timing of these exposures in life also matters—the prenatal to early childhood period is one of the most sensitive times for children to get on the right track to meet their full health potential. Lifelong and multigenerational health disparities are a result of children in this critical age group lacking access to positive opportunities (such as high-quality early care and education, stable and safe housing, and healthy foods) that promote health combined with a preponderance of negative influences that harm health trajectories. Children's health is inextricably linked to family health and community health. For many communities, population health disparity gaps are widening. Persistent, additive disadvantages and early adversity are significant contributors to the widening gaps. Past historical injustices, such as segregated schooling laws, redlining, and assimilation policies, continue to impact children due to structural injustices put in place in the past that persevere today and continue to create barriers to health for those who live in contexts that undermine their opportunity to reach their health potential. This has led to persistent childhood (and lifelong) health disparities. Communities of color have much higher rates of preterm birth, infant mortality, chronic disease (e.g., diabetes), and exposure to adverse childhood experiences, to name just a few.

In preparing this report, the committee took seriously its charge to review the ways in which early life stress affects health, the pathways by which health disparities develop and persist, and the roadmap needed to get all children on positive health trajectories. Scientific discoveries have built a solid base of evidence about what impacts children's health trajectories positively and negatively—now is the time to apply and advance science to chart a course of action to get all children back on track for health. During the committee's time reviewing the scientific evidence for how to translate the best science into action to positively impact health during early childhood, we strove to close the disconnect between evidence and practice in the nation today. While some scientific evidence has laid the groundwork for actionable practice, policy, and systems solutions, other emerging scientific findings are ripe for further research and inquiry. The committee also acknowledged that achieving and sustaining health equity is a long-term goal with many interrelated strategies and tactics. Thus, we included some recommendations that can be feasibly implemented more quickly by a focused group of actions, while other recommendations may take longer and will require broad support from many different actors at all levels of society.

This report details the latest scientific information about factors impacting health and how to achieve equitable promotion of health for all children. Multilevel and multipronged strategies focused on prevention, early detection and referral, and mitigation are needed to gain momentum toward achieving health equity. These strategies involve intervening at the policy, system, and program levels—this will ultimately require a concerted effort from the nation to distribute resources where they are needed and change policies to better align with the science and evidence. With this in mind, where possible, the committee sought to leverage existing resources or systems that serve children as platforms by which to improve and scale services for children. Furthermore, intentional strategies to understand and reduce inequitable outcomes, access, and experiences across communities of different races, linguistic backgrounds, income groups, genders, and geography are needed. Taking action requires a life course lens, multisector collaboration, and ongoing measurement of outcomes that can be assessed longitudinally and across multiple generations. What science teaches us about sensitive periods and the plasticity of the brain and body provides a clear path for action—if we follow that path regarding prevention and mitigation of adversity during this crucial life period, we can turn the tide for our nation's children. This report provides a roadmap for doing so.

The committee is grateful to the Robert Wood Johnson Foundation for appreciating the need for this work and for supporting putting science into action. The committee welcomed this unique opportunity to shine a brighter spotlight on cutting-edge developmental science about how children develop and grow. Furthermore, we appreciated the opportunity to deepen our understanding about how the key principles and tenets of this critical scientific evidence base on optimal development can be made more accessible to prime the public, practitioners, and policy makers for action. It is the committee's hope that this report's bold recommendations will move our nation to practices and policies that center this science, hand in hand with equity, to advance health and well-being for all.

Jennifer E. DeVoe, *Chair*
Committee on Applying Neurobiological and Socio-Behavioral
Sciences from Prenatal Through Early Childhood Development:
A Health Equity Approach

Acknowledgments

The committee wishes to thank and acknowledge the many individuals and organizations that contributed to the study process and development of this report. To begin, the committee would like to thank the Robert Wood Johnson Foundation—the study sponsor—for its support of this work.

The committee found the perspectives of multiple individuals and groups immensely helpful in informing its deliberations through presentations and discussions that took place at the committee's public meetings. Speakers provided presentations on the state of the science in several domains and offered promising models for action, which informed the committee's work; these include (in order of appearance) Dwayne Proctor, Paula Braveman, Fernando Martinez, Phil Fisher, Sarah Barclay Hoffman, Robert Kahn, Suzanne C. Brundage, Megan Smith, Lee Beers, Neal Halfon, Milton Kotelchuck, Ron Haskins, Greg Miller, Greg Duncan, Jessica Pizarek, Helena Sabala, Anne Mauricio, and Elisa Nicholas. The committee also heard policy perspectives from state Representative Ruth Kagi, state Senator Elizabeth Steiner Hayward, Bobby Cagle, and state Senator David Wilson—the committee greatly appreciates the perspectives they brought to the discussions.

The committee's work was enhanced by the technical expertise and support provided by Marisa Gerstein Pineau, Petra Jerman, and Nat Kendall-Taylor, who served as consultants. The committee expresses its gratitude to Angela Diaz, who shared her time as a liaison from the Committee on the Neurobiological and Socio-Behavioral Science of Adolescent Development and Its Applications.

Importantly, the committee heard from a number of caregivers who shared their personal stories and experiences with the committee. These discussions helped ground the committee in the lived experiences of the complex issues that the committee needed to tackle in this report, and the committee is incredibly grateful for their bravery in sharing their experiences in a public forum. Thank you to Abraham Gomez, Shalice Gosey, Lori Hernandez, Ana De Jesus, Yesenia Manzo-Meda, Maria Rodgers, and discussants Alexa Bach, Jennifer Eich, Patricia McKenna, and Reggie Van Appelen.

The committee thanks the National Academies of Sciences, Engineering, and Medicine staff who contributed to the production of this report, including study staff Amy Geller, Yamrot Negussie, Sophie Yang, Anna Martin, Pamela McCray, and Rose Marie Martinez. Thanks go to Mary Jane Porzenheim, summer intern, and other staff in the Health and Medicine Division who provided additional support, including Carla Alvarado, Alina Baciu, Aimee Mead, Andrew Merluzzi, Cyndi Trang, Alexis Wojtowicz, and Hayat Yusuf. The committee thanks the Health and Medicine Division communications staff, including Jeanay Butler, Greta Gorman, Nicole Joy, Sarah Kelley, and Tina Seliber. This project received valuable assistance from Stephanie Miceli (Office of News and Public Information); Misrak Dabi (Office of Financial Administration); and Clyde Behney, Lauren Shern, and Taryn Young (Health and Medicine Division Executive Office). The committee also appreciated the collaboration with the study staff for the concurrent study on adolescence; thanks to Emily Backes, Dara Shefska, and Liz Townsend. Appreciation also goes to the National Academy of Medicine (NAM) Culture of Health Program team for their collaboration and support: Charlee Alexander, Kyra Cappelucci, and Ivory Clarke. The committee was also fortunate to have support from Ebony Carter (NAM Norman F. Gant/American Board of Obstetrics and Gynecology Fellow), who contributed her time and expertise throughout the report's development.

The committee received valuable research assistance from Daniel Bearss, Senior Research Librarian (National Academies Research Center). At the end of the report process, Daniel Bearss passed away. Daniel was a dedicated, meticulous, and respected colleague, and he will be missed by the study team, who are incredibly grateful for his contributions to this report and the National Academies.

Finally, the National Academies staff offers additional thanks to the executive assistants and support staff of committee members, without whom scheduling the multiple committee meetings and conference calls would have been nearly impossible: Iris An, Gatanya Arnic, Mai Castillo, Saúl Cruz, Dhiana Dhahrulsalam, Justin Farmer, Lynne Lathbury, Suzanne Lee, Lauren Oujiri, Kathy Rentie, Katie Rivers, and Lorena Segarra.

Acronyms and Abbreviations

ABC	Attachment and Biobehavioral Catch-Up Intervention
ACE	adverse childhood experience
ACH	Accountable Communities of Health
ADHD	attention-deficit/hyperactivity disorder
AI/AN	American Indian/Alaska Native
ASD	autism spectrum disorder
BPA	bisphenol A
BRFSS	Behavioral Risk Factor Surveillance System
CDC	U.S. Centers for Disease Control and Prevention
CHIP	Children's Health Insurance Program
CPS	Child Protective Services
CRH	corticotropin-releasing hormone
CVD	cardiovascular disease
DLL	dual-language learner
ECE	early care and education
ECHO	Environmental influences on Child Health Outcomes
ED	emergency department
EEG	electroencephalogram
EHB	essential health benefit
EITC	Earned Income Tax Credit

HAS	high-achieving school
HHS	U.S. Department of Health and Human Services
HomVEE	Home Visiting Evidence of Effectiveness
HPA	hypothalamic-pituitary-adrenal
HUD	U.S. Department of Housing and Urban Development
IOM	Institute of Medicine
IPV	intimate partner violence
IUGR	intrauterine growth restriction
LBW	low birth weight
MBH	mental and behavioral health
MIECHV	Maternal, Infant, and Early Child Home Visiting Program
MLP	Medical-Legal Partnership
NFP	Nurse-Family Partnership
NHANES	National Health and Nutrition Examination Survey
NICU	neonatal intensive care unit
NRC	National Research Council
OECD	Organisation for Economic Co-operation and Development
PTSD	posttraumatic stress disorder
RCT	randomized controlled trial
SDOH	social determinants of health
SES	socioeconomic status
SNAP	Supplemental Nutrition Assistance Program
SPM	Supplemental Poverty Measure
SSA	U.S. Social Security Administration
SSI	Supplemental Security Income
TANF	Temporary Assistance for Needy Families
TIC	trauma-informed care
WIC	Special Supplemental Nutrition Program for Women, Infants, and Children

Summary

ABSTRACT

Health inequities have persisted in the United States, and the factors that drive these inequities from preconception through early childhood are complex, interconnected, and systemic; they result from exposures and experiences that children and families encounter throughout their lives and across multiple generations. These exposures accumulate over the life course to exert a cumulative effect on health that is probabilistic, not deterministic. That is, the odds of good health are never fixed; individual exposures, experiences, and choices help set and adjust them over time. Specific subgroups of the population have varying rates of exposure to positive and negative experiences that shape choices and opportunities throughout the life course; therefore, from the very beginning, certain groups have different odds for good or poor health outcomes. Among the factors that may buffer negative outcomes in the early childhood period, supportive relationships between children and the adults in their lives are essential. Furthermore, reducing health disparities by addressing root causes, such as poverty and racism, is foundational to advance health equity.

Biologically, a number of critical systems develop in the prenatal through early childhood periods, and neurobiological development is extremely responsive to environmental influences during these stages. This report provides an overview of the core concepts of brain development and other body systems relevant to understanding the impact of early life adversity, including the mechanisms that link early life experiences to later outcomes. This information can be used by the public and policy makers to better inform effective actions for advancing health equity.

1

The committee provides both short- and long-term recommendations in several key areas that can be leveraged to improve health outcomes for children and families. Recommendations aimed at supporting caregivers include implementing paid parental leave and strengthening and expanding home visiting programs. Recommendations for creating supportive and stable early living conditions include improving economic security through increases in resources available to families to meet their basic needs; increasing the supply of high-quality affordable housing; and supporting and enforcing efforts to prevent and mitigate the impact of environmental toxicants. To maximize the potential of early care and education (ECE) to promote better health outcomes, the committee recommends developing a comprehensive approach to school readiness that explicitly incorporates health outcomes, developing and strengthening curricula that focus on key competencies of educators, and improving the quality of ECE programs and expanding access to comprehensive high-quality and affordable ECE programs. The committee recommends leveraging the health care system to make care in the preconception through early childhood periods more continuous, equitable, integrative, and comprehensive by transforming services to apply a life course perspective and address the social, economic, cultural, and environmental determinants of health. To mitigate the early life drivers of health inequities, there is no one-sector solution—the complex and interconnected root causes call for coordination across multiple sectors. Therefore, the committee provides recommendations for sector alignment and collaboration, as well as the need for child- and family-serving sectors to enhance detection of early life adversity, improve response systems, and develop trauma-informed approaches.

The committee identifies knowledge gaps and recommends multidisciplinary research efforts to bring new ideas and practical approaches to advance efforts to achieve health equity. However, substantial advances in knowledge in the past 20 years make it clear that policy makers, health providers, business leaders, and others in the public and private sectors do not need to wait any longer to take action.

Health inequities by race, ethnicity, socioeconomic status, geography, and other important demographic characteristics have persisted in the United States despite increasing evidence about their contributions to poor health. Research shows that exposures to factors that shape health trajectories can start early and are multigenerational; thus, the preconception, prenatal, and early childhood periods are critical to setting the odds for lifelong health. Importantly, science can inform actions in policy and practice to advance health equity[1] and reduce health disparities.

---

[1] Health equity is the state in which everyone has the opportunity to attain full health potential and no one is disadvantaged from achieving this potential because of social position or any other socially defined circumstance.

Neurobiological and socio-behavioral research indicate that early life experiences shape prenatal and early childhood development, and these experiences have a powerful impact on the developing brain and peripheral organ systems that impact health outcomes across the life course.

When different groups vary in their exposures to key experiences (both positive and negative), their odds for positive health diverge systematically over time, producing disparities in health outcomes across the life-span and across generations. These exposures accumulate over the life course to exert a cumulative effect on health that is probabilistic, not deterministic. That is, the odds of positive or negative health are never fixed; individual exposures, experiences, resilience, and choices help set and adjust them over time. Individuals' distinct contexts also shape their choices and opportunities, and thus they have different odds of experiencing positive or negative health outcomes over time. Because the odds of these exposures are affected by policies and systems, advancing health equity will require more than individual-level interventions. It will necessitate systems-level changes, including changes to laws and policies and investment of resources, to improve the odds of positive experiences and reduce the odds of adverse exposures for all populations, especially those experiencing the most adversity.

Scientific evidence shows that prevention and early intervention are effective for children on at-risk developmental trajectories. Recent advances in science, technology, data sharing, and cross-disciplinary collaboration present opportunities to apply this emerging knowledge systematically to practice, policy, and systems changes. Given the burgeoning science available to advance health equity during early development, the Robert Wood Johnson Foundation, as part of its Culture of Health Initiative, asked the Health and Medicine Division of the National Academies of Sciences, Engineering, and Medicine to

1. Provide a brief overview of stressors that affect prenatal through early childhood development and health;
2. Identify promising models and opportunities for translation of the science to action;
3. Identify outcome measures to enable subgroup analyses;
4. Develop a roadmap to apply the science to tailored interventions (i.e., policies, programs, or system changes) based on biological, social, environmental, economic, and cultural needs; and
5. Provide recommendations in these areas, including how systems can better align to advance health equity.

To respond to this charge, the Committee on Applying Neurobiological and Socio-Behavioral Sciences from Prenatal Through Early Childhood

Development: A Health Equity Approach was formed. The committee applied a health equity frame and built on the concepts of the 2017 report *Communities in Action: Pathways to Health Equity*. As identified in the 2000 National Research Council and Institute of Medicine report *From Neurons to Neighborhoods: The Science of Early Childhood Development*, prenatal through early childhood are critical phases of development that have lifelong impacts on health and well-being. This report reviews the science that has emerged since that landmark report.

The health of both men and women before they have children is important for not only pregnancy outcomes, but also the lifelong health of their children; thus, the committee included the preconception period as an important focus of the report. The committee also adopted the life course approach to its work because an individual's health status and outcomes reflect the accumulation of experiences over the life-span. This approach takes into account an individual's larger social, economic, and cultural context and acknowledges that the life trajectory may be changed, negatively or positively, through interactions between the brain, body, and environment. Protective factors (such as stable, high-quality caregiver relationships and economic security) support positive, or flourishing, trajectories; risk factors (such as exposure to abuse, neglect, or racism) exacerbate the likelihood of poor trajectories.

Children in the United States may be perceived to be healthier now than in the past because they are much less likely to encounter the major infections and debilitating diseases of past generations and are typically able to recover fully from "acute" childhood illnesses. However, ailments of the past have been supplanted with chronic physical (e.g., diabetes, asthma, obesity) and socio-emotional (e.g., depression, anxiety) conditions, with large subsets of U.S. children facing barriers to positive mental and physical health and well-being as a result of poverty, food insecurity, unsafe or unstable housing, neighborhood segregation, and other substantial adversities (such as adverse childhood experiences) in the first few years of life.

Children who are born and raised in poverty are at particularly high risk for poor health outcomes, more problems in early development (e.g., lack of readiness for school at age 5, diagnoses of developmental delays and/or disorders), and higher rates of most childhood chronic conditions (such as mental illness, developmental disabilities, obesity, and asthma). Early adverse experiences may have intermediate effects on school readiness, weight, and physical and/or mental well-being and contribute to chronic disease and poor functioning in adulthood. In fact, these impacts are cumulative, and adults who experience adversity in childhood have substantially higher rates of heart disease, lung disease, metabolic syndrome, and other costly health conditions.

CONCEPTUAL MODEL

The committee's conceptual model (see Figure S-1) served as a unifying framework for its approach to this report. It is important to note that risk and protective factors can be transferred intergenerationally, which makes parents and other family and community primary caregivers a central focus of interventions to improve child health. Within the context of the life course, the diagram's nested circles illustrate the complex sociocultural environment that shapes development at the individual level and the opportunities for interventions to improve individual health and developmental outcomes, as well as population health, well-being, and health equity. Individual social and biological mechanisms and culture operate and interact within and across the three levels.

Structural inequities operate at the outer level, the "socioeconomic and political drivers." Structural inequities are deeply embedded in policies, laws, governance, and culture; they organize the distribution of power and resources differentially across individual and group characteristics (i.e., race, ethnicity, sex, gender identity, class, sexual orientation, gender expression, and others). The next level represents social, economic, cultural, and environmental states (i.e., the social determinants of health [SDOH]). In the model, these interdependent factors are

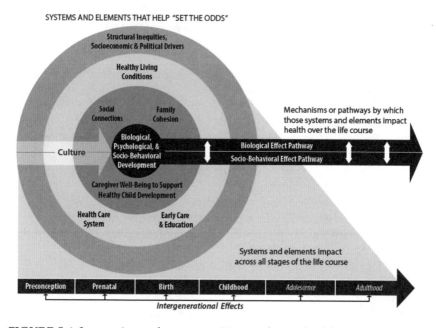

FIGURE S-1 Leveraging early opportunities to advance health equity across the life course: A conceptual framework.

grouped into three domains—healthy living conditions, health care, and education. These domains were identified by the committee based on the available evidence and existing resources as important for targeting prenatal and early childhood interventions and are the primary foci of Chapters 5–7. The next level represents the factors that most directly and proximally shape children's daily experiences and routine patterns: family cohesion and social connections, which also affect access to critical resources for health, well-being, and development in early life (see Chapter 4). The innermost circle and crosscutting arrows—biological, psychological, and socio-behavioral development—are the focus of Chapters 2 and 3.

THE SCIENCE OF EARLY DEVELOPMENT: CORE CONCEPTS

Based on its review of the science, the committee updated and adapted the core concepts from the 2000 report *From Neurons to Neighborhoods* and identified 12 core concepts of early development, with a focus on health equity. The evidence underlying these concepts is described in Chapters 2–4, and this evidence guided the committee in its development of recommendations that apply the science of early development. In brief, these concepts include the following (see Chapter 1 for more detailed descriptions of each concept):

1. Biology–environment interaction impacts health and development.
2. Brain development proceeds in well-defined but continuous steps.
3. Major physiological systems develop rapidly during pregnancy and early childhood.
4. The early caregiving environment is crucial for long-term development.
5. The developing child plays an important role in interactions and development.
6. The development of executive functions is a key aspect of early childhood development.
7. Trajectories—positive or negative—are not immutable.
8. There is variability in individual and group development.
9. Experiences across environmental contexts play a significant role in early development.
10. Disparities in access to critical resources matter.
11. Health outcomes are the result of experiences across the life course.
12. Early interventions matter and are more cost effective than later ones.

A large body of recent research provides insights into the mechanisms by which early adversity in the lives of young children and their families can change the timing of sensitive periods of brain and other organ system development and impact the "plasticity"[2] of developmental processes. In the past two decades, there has been a convergence of research that has led to many of the advances described in this report. First, a wave of neurobiological studies in model systems and humans found that responses to pre- and postnatal early life stress are rooted in genetic and environmental interactions that can result in altered molecular and cellular development that impacts the assembly of circuits during sensitive periods of development. The demonstration that certain systems involved in cognitive and emotional development are more sensitive to early disturbances that activate stress response networks, such as the frontal cortex, hippocampus, amygdala, and the hypothalamic-pituitary-adrenal axis, provided a basis for both short- and long-term functional consequences of early life stress.

Many of the new scientific advances in neuroscience are still in development, and more research is needed to apply these new findings in clinical and public health practice and to use them to inform policies. In particular, greater effort and support are needed to develop, implement, and evaluate programs based on scientific discoveries regarding the optimal timing for interventions. However, new research has clarified that altered nutrition, exposure to environmental chemicals, and chronic stress during specific times of development can lead to functional biological changes that predispose individuals to manifest diseases and/or experience altered physical, socio-emotional, and cognitive functions later in life. The committee provides information about major biological responses to stressors and new discoveries that have contributed to advancing knowledge about how and when to intervene to improve health outcomes for children.

ROADMAP FOR APPLYING AND ADVANCING
THE SCIENCE OF EARLY DEVELOPMENT

With the goal of decreasing health inequities, the broad question this report addresses is, "For those children who are placed at risk for negative outcomes, what can be done—guided by science-based evidence—to expediently and effectively move each of them toward positive developmental health trajectories?" In this report, the committee provides

---

[2] The process by which neurons within the brain change their gene expression, cellular architecture and connections with other neurons, and function in response to experiences and changes in the environment (i.e., change over time).

recommendations for practice, policy, and systems changes to achieve this goal. The roadmap the committee has put forth includes a suite of key strategies to advance health equity[3]:

- **Intervene early**—In most cases, early intervention programs are easier to implement, more effective, and less costly.
- **Support caregivers**—This includes both primary caregivers and caregivers in systems who frequently interact with children and their families.
- **Reform health care system services to promote healthy development**—Redesign the content of preconception, prenatal, postpartum, and pediatric care while ensuring ongoing access, quality, and coordination.
- **Create supportive and stable early living conditions:**
  o **Reduce child poverty and address economic and food security,**
  o **Provide stable and safe housing, and**
  o **Eliminate exposure to environmental toxicants.**
- **Maximize the potential of early care and education to promote health outcomes.**
- **Implement initiatives across systems to support children, families, other caregivers, and communities**—Ensure trauma-informed systems, build a diverse and supported workforce, and align strategies that work across sectors.
- **Integrate and coordinate resources across the education, social services, criminal justice, and health care systems, and make them available to translate science to action.**

In this report, the committee provides a range of recommendations for practice, policy, and systems changes, including recommendations that will take time and sustained commitment to achieve and recommendations that could be implemented immediately or in the near term. Some of the committee's recommendations will be difficult to implement; however, the degree of difficulty in implementing any given recommendation does not determine the value of pursuing it. Where possible, the committee also recommends or highlights ways to leverage existing programs that either embrace the core scientific principles laid out above or have a strong basic structure from which to build.

---

[3] Note that recommendations are not always presented in numerical order, as the summary has grouped them by topic in some cases; however, all report recommendations are presented.

Supporting Family Cohesion and Social Connections

The construct of resilience[4] from developmental science is important, as it implies the ability to correct what otherwise might have been negative trajectories, given major life stressors. To set the foundation for the committee's considerations on the topic of supporting family systems, the committee discusses universal principles of human development pertaining to the broad domain encompassing children's psychological and behavioral adjustment (see Chapter 4). For example, for children, the single most important factor in promoting positive psychosocial, emotional, and behavioral well-being is having a strong, secure attachment to their primary caregivers—usually their mothers. Strong attachment presupposes effective parenting behaviors in everyday life, and "effective parenting" changes in complexity with development over time.

There is an urgent need to develop preventive interventions well suited for fathers and other male caregivers; existing approaches that are developed for and tested with women cannot be assumed to generalize to other caregivers with equal effectiveness (e.g., in the successful recruitment, retention, and support of men and fathers who take care of young children).

> **Recommendation 4-1: Federal, state, and local agencies, along with private foundations and philanthropies that invest in research, should include in their portfolios research on the development of preventive interventions that target fathers and other male caregivers. Special attention should be given to the recruitment, retention, and support of men and fathers parenting young children from underserved populations.**

Specific subgroups of children have unique needs and challenges when adjusting to adversity. Careful attention to potent subculture-specific processes needs to be paid in working with subgroups well known to face serious inequities in relation to mental health—including families experiencing chronic poverty; immigrants; lesbian, gay, bisexual, transgender, and queer (LGBTQ) children; LGBTQ parents; children who are separated from parents due to incarceration, foster care, or other reasons; and children exposed to high achievement pressures, usually in relatively affluent communities.

---

[4] There are two essential conditions that make up resilience: (1) exposure to significant threat or severe adversity, and (2) achievement of positive adaptation despite major assaults on the developmental process.

Recommendation 4-2: Federal, state, local, tribal, and territorial agencies, along with private foundations and philanthropies that invest in research, should include in their portfolios research on the development of interventions that are culturally sensitive and tailored to meet the needs of subgroups of children known to be vulnerable, such as those living in chronic poverty, children from immigrant backgrounds, children in foster care, and children with incarcerated parents.

In addition to addressing major goals relevant for children in general (e.g., fostering caregiver well-being and minimizing maltreatment), programs need to include components that specifically address unique risk and protective processes within these subgroups of children.

A growing body of evidence suggests that home visiting by a nurse, a social worker, or an early educator during pregnancy and as needed in the first years of a child's life improves a wide range of child and family outcomes, including promotion of maternal and child health, prevention of child abuse and neglect, positive parenting, child development, and school readiness. These positive effects continue well into adolescence and early adulthood. Researchers, program leaders, and policy makers need to focus on expanding the concept of tailored home visiting to advance knowledge on which programs and activities are best for which family, in which communities, and for what outcomes.

Recommendation 4-3: To strengthen and expand the impact of evidence-based home visiting programs,

- **Federal policy makers should expand the Maternal, Infant, and Early Childhood Home Visiting Program.**
- **The Health Resources and Services Administration (HRSA) and the Administration for Children and Families (ACF) should work with program developers to increase flexibility for states and communities, to tailor the program to the needs and/or assets of the community or population being served.**
- **Federal, state, local, tribal, and territorial agencies overseeing program implementation should continue to strengthen programmatic coordination and policy alignment between home visiting, other early care and education programs, and medical homes.**

State policy makers should further expand support for evidence-based home visiting services through the use of general funds, Medicaid, and a combination of multiple funding streams. HRSA and ACF should support research to continue to ensure program effectiveness and accountability of the expanded program. Expansion of home visiting programs should be done in conjunction with the expansion of other public investments and services.

Intervention trials have shown strong benefits of relational interventions, such as interventions to foster strong attachments, and group-based supports in communities for caregivers and their families. The core components of several effective interventions suggest that in addition to providing particular skills, improving the overall well-being of caregivers (especially mothers) is the most critical "engine" of change.

> **Recommendation 4-4: Policy makers at the federal, state, local, territorial, and tribal levels and philanthropic organizations should support the creation and implementation of programs that ensure families have access to high-quality, cost-effective, local community-based programs that support the psychosocial well-being of the primary adult caregivers and contribute to building resilience and reducing family stress.**

It is necessary to consider measures that should be included in evaluating results of large-scale preventive interventions targeting young children and their mothers. Given the need to identify individuals at risk for early adversity and the toxic stress response, regular brief assessments of the mothers' depressive symptoms, stress, feelings of rejection to the child, any involvement with child protective services, and the degree to which they have positive, buffering relationships in their lives should occur routinely.

> **Recommendation 4-5: Health care providers who care for pregnant women and children should routinely track levels of individual health and social risk among mothers and children over time, using periodic assessments via a short set of scientifically validated measures.**

Leveraging the Health Care System to Promote Health Equity

The health care system can serve as a platform, along with public health and other sectors, to address the social determinants that underlie many health inequities. However, the current health care system focuses mainly on clinical goals and addresses other determinants of health in fragmented and highly variable ways. U.S. health care provides only limited attention to integration of health care for the whole family, health care across the life course, or integration of mental and behavioral health into clinical care. Recognizing that preconception through early childhood are sensitive and important life periods to optimize health outcomes, care during these periods needs to become more continuous (access), equitable (quality), integrative (delivery), and comprehensive (content); therefore, the committee offers the following recommendations:

Improving Access to Health Care

Recommendation 5-1: The U.S. Department of Health and Human Services, state, tribal, and territorial Medicaid agencies, public and private payers, and state and federal policy makers should adopt policies and practices that ensure universal access to high-quality health care across the life course. This includes

- **Increasing access to patient- and family-centered care,**
- **Ensuring access to preventive services and essential health benefits, and**
- **Increasing culturally and linguistically appropriate outreach and services.**

Achieving this recommendation will require actively promoting inclusion in coverage and care.

Improving Quality of Care

Recommendation 5-2: To expand accountability and improve the quality of preconception, prenatal, postpartum, and pediatric care,

- **Public and private payers should include new metrics of child and family health and well-being that assess quality using a holistic view of health and health equity. Federal, state, and other agencies, along with private foundations and philanthropies that invest in research, should support the development and implementation of new measures of accountability, including key drivers of health, such as social determinants, along with measuring variations by key subgroups to determine disparities;**
- **Public and private payers, including the Health Resources and Services Administration's (HRSA's) Bureau of Primary Care and Maternal and Child Health Bureau, Centers for Disease Control and Prevention, Centers for Medicare & Medicaid Services (CMS), and perinatal and pediatric quality collaboratives, should expand the use of continuous quality improvement, learning communities, payment for**

performance, and other strategies to enhance accountability; and

- Health care–related workforce development entities should expand efforts to increase diversity, inclusion, and equity in the health care workforce, including diversity-intensive outreach, mentoring, networking, and leadership development for underrepresented faculty and trainees.

Needed metrics include social determinants and social risk measures; cross-sector developmental measures that move beyond common indicators of child development, including mental and behavioral health; and disparities as explicit measurement domains that hold providers accountable for not just delivering services but also improving outcomes. Workforce development (as noted in bullet 3) will need to be addressed by several entities, including the Accreditation Council for Graduate Medical Education and specialty boards, professional schools, training programs, teaching hospitals, including children's hospitals, and funders of graduate education in health professions (CMS, HRSA, and others).

Organization and Integration of Health Care Services

Recommendation 5-3: The U.S. Department of Health and Human Services, state, tribal, and territorial government Medicaid agencies, health systems leaders, and state and federal policy makers should adopt policies and practices that improve the organization and integration of care systems, including promoting multidisciplinary team-based care models that focus on integrating preconception, prenatal, and postpartum care with a whole-family focus, development of new practice and payment models that incentivize health creation and improve service delivery, and structures that more tangibly connect health care delivery systems to other partners outside of the health care sector.

Achieving this recommendation will require disseminating multidisciplinary team-based care models in community settings; developing integrated models for preconception, prenatal, postpartum, and pediatric care delivery modes; adopting and spreading integrated, whole-family and family-centered care models; developing and using new technologies that improve care and improve accessibility; aligning payment reform with health creation rather than service delivery; and developing systemic and cross-sector collaboration.

Transforming the Content of Care

> **Recommendation 5-4: Transform preconception, prenatal, post-partum, and pediatric care to address the root causes of poor health and well-being—the social, economic, environmental, and cultural determinants of health and early adversity—and to align with the work of other sectors addressing health equity.**
>
> **The U.S. Department of Health and Human Services should convene an expert panel to reconceptualize the content and delivery of care, identify the specific changes needed, develop a blueprint for this transformation, and implement a plan to monitor and revise the blueprint over time. Implementation of this recommendation will require**
>
> - **An update of clinical care guidelines and standards by the Women's Preventive Services Initiative, Bright Futures, American College of Obstetricians and Gynecologists, American Academy of Pediatrics, American Academy of Family Physicians, and others actively developing clinical care guidelines and standards to include this new content of care;**
> - **Medical accreditation bodies, relevant programs, and agencies to develop performance monitoring and quality improvement based on this new content of care;**
> - **Clinical care educational authorities, such as the Accreditation Council for Graduate Medical Education, to develop curricula, training, experiences, and competencies based on the updated guidelines; and**
> - **Public and private payers to cover services reflecting this new content of care.**

This work should take place in a larger framework of social and reproductive justice and include more diverse voices, especially from communities most affected by adverse birth and child health outcomes. Such a shift will require that the health care system recognize the impact of both adverse and enriching experiences across the life course and cumulative effects on health and well-being by the health care system. It will also require integrating attention to social and environmental determinants as well as trauma assessment and response into clinical practice.

Although health care plays an integral role in advancing health equity, health care alone cannot meaningfully address health inequities, nor is it the primary actor or leader. Cross-sectoral and multidisciplinary collaboration is essential for decreasing health inequities.

Creating Healthy Living Conditions for Early Development

Reducing or managing caregiver stress is key to giving caregivers the capacity, supports, and resources to care for their children and serve as buffers against adversity. Addressing the primary needs of families and children is critical to achieving this goal. The committee identified four areas of fundamental needs that, if met, would have an impact on health inequities: (1) food security, (2) safe and stable housing, (3) economic stability and security, and (4) safe physical environments.

Food Security

Given the importance of good nutrition for brain growth and development (during the preconception, prenatal, and early childhood periods), the committee concludes that providing resources to ensure families have access to sufficient and healthy foods can improve birth and child health outcomes. Because safety net programs such as WIC and SNAP have been shown to improve birth and child (and adult) health outcomes and to reduce food insecurity, the committee recommends:

Recommendation 6-2: Federal, state, local, territorial, and tribal agencies should reduce barriers to participation in the Special Supplemental Nutrition Program for Women, Infants, and Children (WIC) and Supplemental Nutrition Assistance Program (SNAP) benefits. Receipt of WIC and SNAP benefits should not be tied to parent employment for families with young children or for pregnant women, as work requirements are likely to reduce participation rates.

Safe and Stable Housing

Evidence suggests that lack of affordable or quality housing, housing instability, and overcrowding have significantly detrimental effects on the health, well-being, and development of infants, children, and families. Housing affordability and quality is an acute problem that disproportionately affects people of color and contributes to health inequities among children. Over half of black and Hispanic renters live in unaffordable housing, and health issues related to poor-quality housing, such as elevated blood lead levels and asthma, are more prevalent among these renters. Current federal housing programs are not adequately funded, and there are not enough safe, affordable housing units in high-opportunity areas. Additional funding for programs can move families out of poverty and allow them to reallocate money for other basic needs that support child health and development. Incentives and/or regulations, along with enhanced programming, can increase the supply of affordable housing. Recognizing the centrality of housing to health and healthy child development, the committee recommends:

> **Recommendation 6-3: The U.S. Department of Housing and Urban Development, states, and local, territorial, and tribal public housing authorities should increase the supply of high-quality affordable housing that is available to families, especially those with young children.**

> **Recommendation 6-4: The Secretary of the U.S. Department of Health and Human Services, in collaboration with the U.S. Department of Housing and Urban Development and other relevant agencies, should lead the development of a comprehensive plan to ensure access to stable, affordable, and safe housing in the prenatal through early childhood period. This strategy should particularly focus on priority populations who are disproportionately impacted by housing challenges and experience poor health outcomes.**

> **Recommendation 6-5: The Center for Medicare & Medicaid Innovation should partner with states to test new Medicaid payment models that engage providers and other community organizations in addressing housing safety concerns, especially focused on young children. These demonstrations should evaluate impact on health, health disparities, and total cost of care.**

Economic Stability and Security

Children's well-being and life course outcomes are strongly related to family income. Given the strong evidence that economic security matters, an important factor in reducing health disparities in early childhood is to ensure that families with young children have adequate resources. The committee concludes that public programs that provide resources to families in the form of cash, tax credits, or in-kind benefits improve childhood well-being and life course outcomes and that these effects are long lasting. Furthermore, while income support programs that are contingent on employment status or based on earned income have positive benefits for families, they should avoid regulations and policies that might have unintended consequences for childhood outcomes through negative effects on family relationships and attachments, breastfeeding, and caregiver stress.

Additional income support for families with young children through paid parental leave would recognize the special needs of infants and their caregivers. Unpaid parental leave through the Family and Medical Leave

Act does not cover all employees, and most families with low incomes cannot afford to take an unpaid leave.

> **Recommendation 6-1: Federal, state, local, tribal, and territorial policy makers should implement paid parental leave. In partnership with researchers, policy makers should model variations in the level of benefits, length of leave, and funding mechanisms to determine alternatives that will have the largest impacts on improving child health outcomes and reducing health disparities.**

> **Recommendation 6-6: Federal, state, tribal, and territorial policy makers should address the critical gaps between family resources and family needs through a combination of benefits that have the best evidence of advancing health equity, such as increased Supplemental Nutrition Assistance Program benefits, increased housing assistance, and a basic income allowance for young children.**

This recommendation focuses on strategies that are likely to have particularly important impacts on health outcomes for young children. A child allowance would fill in some of the gaps in the current safety net and particularly benefit the lowest-income children and those most at risk of poor health outcomes. The key advantage of a child allowance (over, for example, tax credits) is that funds are available to families on an ongoing monthly basis rather than once per year. In addition, under the current structure of the child and working-family tax credits, the lowest-income families receive few benefits. Children whose parents are in unstable employment or not employed suffer the short- and long-term health consequences of living in poverty. Reducing health disparities requires reaching these children during their earliest years, regardless of parental employment. Increased SNAP benefits and housing allowances would address current inadequacies in both of these programs and provide targeted support for the critical food and housing needs of young children.

Environmental Exposures and Exposure to Toxicants

There are numerous potential environmental toxicants that may be transmitted through the air, water, soil, and consumer products with which food and water come into contact. Many of these occur naturally in the environment (e.g., arsenic, radon, etc.), and many more are released through human-based processes (e.g., heavy metals, chemicals from plastic production and degradation, and particulates). The embryonic, fetal, and early childhood periods represent greater risk than adulthood for adverse mental and physical health outcomes from environmental exposures due to children's smaller size, proportionally large intake of food, air, and water to body weight, and rapid developmental processes that may be influenced and disrupted by chemicals and toxicants. As a result of toxicant exposures, children may suffer from a variety of developmental problems, chronic conditions, and even premature death. Poverty, substandard and/or unstable housing, minority racial/ethnic status, and proximity to known sources of pollutants heighten children's risk of exposure and poor health and developmental outcomes. The committee identified three areas where current efforts could be improved to prevent and mitigate the impact of environmental toxicants in the prenatal through early childhood periods:

> **Recommendation 6-7: The Administration for Children and Families, Maternal and Child Health Bureau, and federal and state regulators should strengthen environmental protection in early care and education settings through expanded workforce training, program monitoring, and regulations.**

> **Recommendation 6-8: Professional societies, training programs, and accrediting bodies should support expanded or innovative models for training of prenatal and childhood health care providers on screening, counseling, and interventions to prevent or mitigate toxic environmental exposures.**

> **Recommendation 6-9: Federal, state, local, tribal, and territorial governments should support and enforce efforts to prevent and mitigate the impact of environmental toxicants during the preconception through early childhood period. This strategy should particularly focus on priority populations who are disproportionately impacted by harmful environmental exposures. This includes**

>   - **The U.S. Environmental Protection Agency (EPA) fully exercising the authorities provided by Congress to safeguard children's environmental health under the Toxic Substances Control Act as amended by the Frank R. Lautenberg Chemical Safety for the 21st Century Act.**
>   - **Continued allocation of resources and technical assistance from the federal government through the Centers for Disease Control and Prevention, EPA, U.S. Food and Drug Administration, and the U.S. Consumer Product Safety Commission to translate existing data and research findings into actionable policies and practices.**
>   - **Ongoing review and updating of environmental exposure levels by federal agencies to reflect health and safety standards specific to the unique vulnerability of children (from fetal development through early development).**

In Chapter 6, the committee also discusses the role of civil rights strategies to promote healthy communities for developing children.

Promoting Health Equity Through Early Care and Education

While most of the attention on early care and education (ECE)[5] has focused on whether it improves children's cognitive and socio-emotional development and academic readiness, research shows that ECE affects various other child health outcomes, including children's physical, emotional, and mental health. ECE programs increase children's cognitive, social, and health outcomes through enhancing their motivation for school and readiness to learn and the early identification and intervention of problems that impede learning. This, in turn, helps children improve their cognitive ability and social and emotional competence, while increasing their access to and use of preventive health care. Access to ECE may lead to lower risk of dropping out of school, greater school engagement, and subsequently better educational attainment, which lead to increased income and decreased social and health risks, resulting in greater health equity.

Allocation of Adequate Resources to Support ECE Programs and Educators

Intentional policies and allocation of adequate resources to support these programs and educators are needed for ECE programs to contribute significantly to a health promotion and equity strategy.

> **Recommendation 7-1: The committee recommends that early care and education (ECE) systems and programs, including home visiting, adopt a comprehensive approach to school readiness. This approach should explicitly incorporate health promotion and health equity as core goals. Implementing this approach would require the following actions:**
>
> - **Federal, state, local, tribal, and territorial governments and other public agencies (e.g., school districts, city governments, public–private partnerships) that have decision-making power over ECE programs should establish program standards and accountability systems, such as a quality rating and improvement system, linked with better school readiness and health outcomes and provide adequate funding and resources to implement and sustain these standards effectively.**

---

[5] ECE can be defined as nonparental care that occurs outside of the child's home. ECE services may be delivered in center-, school-, or home-based settings.

- The Office of Child Care and the Office of Head Start at the federal level, along with state, local, tribal, and territorial early care and other education agencies, should assess the full cost of implementing standards that promote health outcomes and equity as described above, including supporting educators' own health and well-being, and work with Congress to align funding levels of the major federal ECE programs—child care subsidy and Head Start—accordingly.
- Health and human service entities, the federal Early Learning Interagency Policy Board, state Early Childhood Advisory Councils, and federal, state, local, tribal, and territorial agencies that oversee home visiting and ECE programs should ensure greater programmatic coordination and policy alignment to ensure effective allocation of resources.
- The Office of Planning, Research & Evaluation in the Administration for Children and Families, along with the U.S. Department of Education, should examine the feasibility and seek resources to conduct (a) an implementation study to examine the design and implementation of this comprehensive ECE approach that incorporates health standards and (b) an outcomes study that examines the impact on children's school readiness and achievement, and health outcomes, with particular attention to eliminating disparities and gaps prior to school entry.

Health-Focused Competencies of the ECE Workforce

Policies and systems that prepare and support early childhood educators and program leaders, including those in public schools, need to incorporate the latest evidence about how to support children's school readiness and success by fostering their health and well-being. This would entail providing comprehensive supports and resources to degree granting institutions and preparation programs, including the development of curricula, textbooks, practicum experiences, toolkits, and fact sheets.

> **Recommendation 7-2: Building off the 2015 Institute of Medicine and the National Research Council report *Transforming the Workforce for Children Birth Through Age 8*, the committee recommends that degree granting institutions, professional preparation programs, and providers of ongoing professional learning opportunities develop or strengthen coursework or practicums that focus on competencies of educators, principals, and early care and education program directors that are critical to children's health, school readiness, and life success.**

Access and Affordability to ECE Programs

Maximizing the impact of ECE on positive early childhood development and health and well-being at the community or population level will require increasing public funds for ECE programs. Currently, eligibility for ECE programs is limited, and among eligible families, access is low due to lack of funding and availability of programs and services. Therefore, even if existing publicly funded programs have the resources to provide robust supports that improve young children's health and well-being, these will not reach most children, especially those who live in low-income households or confront adverse experiences and toxic stress.

Recommendation 7-3: Federal, state, local, tribal, and territorial policy makers should work with the U.S. Department of Health and Human Services (HHS), the Office of Head Start, and the Office of Child Care to develop and implement a plan to

a. **Improve the quality of early care and education (ECE) programs by adopting the health-promoting standards discussed in Recommendation 7-1, such as building on the performance standards of Early Head Start and Head Start, and**
b. **Within 10 years, expand access to such comprehensive, high-quality, and affordable ECE programs across multiple settings to all eligible children. Disproportionately underserved populations should be prioritized.**

The Secretary of HHS should conduct a process evaluation to inform the expansion effort and, once implemented, conduct rigorous and comparative outcomes studies to ensure that the expansion is having the intended impacts on children and families, with particular attention on what group(s) may be benefiting.

The strategic plan should be modeled after and build on the relevant performance standards of Early Head Start and Head Start, which emphasize mixed settings, the whole child, family and community engagement, transition between home and school, and continuous quality improvement. It should also strengthen those program components discussed in Chapter 7 that lead to stronger school readiness and health outcomes, including mitigation of the impact of adverse experiences and toxic stress for children, families, teachers, and staff. Critical components include a comprehensive social-emotional strategy that encompasses both the classroom (curriculum, teacher training and support) and program/school (leadership, culture and climate) levels and educators who have competencies described in Recommendation 7-2.

Systems Approach

Advancing health equity in the preconception through early childhood periods cannot be achieved by any one sector alone—it will take action, collaboration, and alignment across all sectors that frequently interact with children, families, and the professionals who serve them. Systems are a collection of interacting, interdependent parts that function as a whole. For the purposes of this report, most of the systems are social constructs and are organized around a key functional area (e.g., education, health care, housing). Systems change is not an easy strategy, it seldom yields speedy returns, and it may not be sufficient without an investment of resources designed to take advantage of new and better aligned approaches. However, given that disparities are systematically generated, it is likely a necessary precursor to real and widespread advances in health equity. The committee identified eight crosscutting recommendation areas where multiple sectors need to take action, based on review of the evidence in Chapters 1–7 and the committee's collective expertise. In brief (additional details available in Chapter 8), the committee recommends:

Policy makers and leaders in the health care, public health, social service, criminal justice, early care and education/ education, and other sectors should

- **Recommendation 8-1: Support and invest in cross-sector initiatives that align strategies and operate community programs and interventions that work across sectors to address the root causes of poor health outcomes. This includes addressing structural and policy barriers to data integration and cross-sector financing and other challenges to cross-sector collaboration.**
- **Recommendation 8-2: Adopt and implement screening for trauma and adversities early in life to increase the likelihood of early detection. This should include creating rapid response and referral systems that can quickly bring protective resources to bear when early life adversities are detected, through the coordination of cross-sector expertise, as covered in Recommendation 8-1.**
- **Recommendation 8-3: Adopt best practices and implement training for trauma-informed care and service delivery. Sector leadership should implement trauma-informed systems that are structured to minimize implicit bias and stigma and prevent retraumatization. Standards for trauma-informed practice exist in a variety of service sectors, including health care**

and social services; those standards should be replicated and implemented across systems.

- Recommendation 8-4: Develop a transdisciplinary and diverse workforce to implement culturally competent service delivery models. The workforce should reflect the diversity of populations who will engage in sector services.
- Recommendation 8-5: Improve access to programs or policies that explicitly provide parental or caregiver supports and help build or promote family attachments and functioning by engaging with the families as a cohesive unit. For families with intensive support needs, develop programs or initiatives designed to provide comprehensive wraparound supports along a number of dimensions, such as health care, education, and social services, designed to address needs related to the social determinants of health that are integrated and community based.
- Recommendation 8-6: Integrate care and services across the health continuum, including the adoption of models that provide comprehensive support for the whole person in a contextually informed manner, leveraging and connecting existing community resources wherever possible, with a focus on prevention.
- Recommendation 8-7: Invest in programs that improve population health and in upstream programs that decrease long-term risk and poor health outcomes. These changes should be accompanied by accountability metrics to ensure that the spending is tangibly and demonstrably in service to the goals behind the original funding, but offer more flexibility in how those goals are achieved.

Crosscutting Research Needs

A tremendous amount is known about what works to advance health equity in early development (and the lifelong benefits of doing so), and efforts to translate this science into action and to scale up effective interventions needs to be accelerated. Many interventions have shown promising results at a small scale but have not been fully tested across multiple settings or in diverse communities and populations. Others have promising preliminary data but require more evidence. In addition, the evidence around systems and policy changes—the work needed to address inequities with a multisector and systems-based approach—remains less certain than programmatic evidence in many cases precisely because it is complex and set in shifting environments that make confident attribution of effects challenging. In Chapter 8, the committee recommends newly designed and adapted research strategies to help translate science to action across sectors, including needed data to inform subgroup analyses and elucidate the complex causality related to health inequities to better design interventions across sectors.

An important caution, however, is that although targeted research is needed to address population heterogeneity with more precision, enough is already known to act now to advance health equity in the prenatal and early childhood periods. The research recommended below is important to continually improve efforts and increase impact but should not impede action. Here the committee provides guidance on charting the course for future research to better meet the health and social needs of the nation's children in the future and, specifically, to advance health equity.

Recommendation 8-8: The National Institutes of Health, Agency for Healthcare Research and Quality, Centers for Disease Control and Prevention, Health Resources and Services Administration, Centers for Medicare & Medicaid Services, U.S. Department of Education, philanthropies, and other funders should support research that advances the state of the science in several critical ways to advance health equity. Specific actions and research to support include the following:

- **Explore alternative methods to address complex causality.**
- **Expand research into individual differences (heterogeneity) in response to adversity and treatment.**
- **Promote scientific research that includes individuals and families from underrepresented communities.**
- **Promote research that explicitly seeks to understand the interconnected mechanisms of health inequities.**
- **Support research that addresses discrimination and structural racism.**
- **Support research for trauma-informed care and implicit bias training.**
- **Support systematic dissemination and implementation research.**
- **The National Institutes of Health and other relevant research entities should support the development of public–private partnerships, or other innovative collaborations, to**
  - **Build multidisciplinary teams, including but not limited to researchers in neuroscience, endocrinology, immunology, physiology, metabolism, behavior, psychology, and primary care to identify the most relevant factors in a child's complex environment that promote resilience and promote outcomes related to physical and mental health.**

    o **Conduct research that measures the impact of chronic stress on all relevant organ systems and determines the specific molecular and biological pathways of interaction during the pre- and postnatal periods, which are directly relevant to potential interventions to address health disparities.[6]**

Many of the items in this recommendation will require recruiting diverse populations, with explicit attention to addressing racial/ethnic and socioeconomic inequities in developmental outcomes.

Measuring Success

The committee has identified a number of measures and indicators that can currently be measured and are important for tracking progress within each of the systems that act as key leverage points for early childhood development discussed in this report. For example, for caregivers, the committee proposes measuring maternal depression and stress, feelings of rejection or hostility to the child, available support for mothers, and any contact with child protective services. However, other measures will be needed. To further the ability for subgroup and other analyses and continuous data collection on both successes and failures, the following are needed (see Chapter 8 for more detail):

Understanding and measuring cumulative exposure. A number of factors impact early life development, ranging from influences in the microsocial or family environment, such as attachment, nurturing, and maternal well-being, to institutional levers, such as access to prenatal care or effective responses to trauma exposure, to macrosocial forces, such as racism and poverty. Effective tools already exist to measure exposure to some of these factors but there are few methods for empirically understanding how exposures to risks or protective factors accumulate and combine over time to establish a cumulative overall risk profile.

Understanding the interaction among developmental pathways. There are few frameworks for understanding the multidirectional relationship between the biological, social-behavioral, and psychological development of young children. In particular, understanding how these interactions may vary across the life course in response to changing plasticity of biological systems, different stages of personal and cognitive development,

---

[6] For reference, this is Recommendation 2-1 in this report.

and different life conditions and accumulated experiences is critical to building a health equity strategy.

Measuring interactions between systems. Models that can estimate "integrated risk" by combining key data from across the sectors where people live their lives are needed. Similarly, measures that examine results from cross-sector collaboration can help in documentation and accountability.

Improving methods to assess complex causality. Perhaps the biggest challenge facing health equity research is complex causality. Many of the preferred tools of science, such as randomized controlled trials, are designed to control for and isolate single causes rather than embrace complex, interrelated causality that may include multilevel, multidirectional, and nested effects—for which a larger toolbox of strategies is needed. For example, there needs to be greater exploration of effective community-based intervention approaches that use existing resources (e.g., as in "natural experiments").

CONCLUSION

The advances in the science of early development are ready to be acted on—there is no reason to wait for this additional science before taking action. Long-term psychological, behavioral, and physical health is shaped by biological and environmental factors, including their interactions, before conception and throughout the life course. This interplay necessitates action at the practice, policy, and systems levels that takes into account the full range of factors that shape health and well-being. These actions need to be taken before insults to early development occur. The science of plasticity shows that it is never too late to intervene but that early identification and intervention are generally more effective and cost-saving and require less effort. (See Box S-1 for a high-level overview of the report's findings and Table 9-1 for a summary of recommended actions in this report.) Furthermore, these actions need to take a life course, multigenerational approach to decrease health inequity, as children's well-being depends on the well-being of the primary caregivers and the quality of their relationship. Progress toward health equity can be achieved through multipronged, cross-sector interventions that focus on prevention, early detection, and mitigation and that work at the practice, policy, and systems levels to address the SDOH. The committee hopes that the roadmap laid out in this report will catalyze the steps that need to be taken across systems to close the health equity gap and improve the lives of our nation's children.

BOX S-1
Chapter Key Messages

A. **Lessons from the science of early development are clear and actionable.** A tremendous amount is known about how development occurs in the prenatal and early childhood periods. When the science of early development is coupled with a health equity approach to inform decision making, it provides an opportunity to improve outcomes for children and families. (Chapters 1 and 2)

B. **Over time, biological and social-psychological development interact to shape the way health develops over the life course.** Neither is deterministic—health outcomes are never set in stone. Rather, they are probabilistic—together, they cumulatively "set the odds" for good health. (Chapter 2)

C. **Biology and environment work together to affect children's growth and development.** Intervening early—to both prevent and mitigate adverse outcomes—is crucial. During the prenatal and early life periods, critical biological systems that will help shape health across the life course are developed and affected by the early environment. Intervening early, when the plasticity of these systems is at its greatest, is the best way to improve chances of developing in ways that optimize health outcomes. (Chapters 2 and 3)

D. **Ensuring the well-being of caregivers by supporting and caring for them is critical for healthy child development.** Reducing children's exposure to maltreatment is a critical lever, as is promoting nurturing behaviors, fostering self-regulation, and developing coping skills for caregivers and children. (Chapter 4)

E. **Preconception, prenatal, postpartum, and pediatric care needs to be reconceptualized** to address the root causes of health inequities and to better meet the developing health and health care needs of children and their families. Content, quality, and access to care are critical components of change. (Chapter 5)

F. **Families need adequate resources available for meeting basic needs, especially when children are young.** Bolstering resources should not come at the expense of attachment or caregiver well-being, so programs such as paid parental leave, basic support, and housing stability are needed. (Chapter 6)

G. **Early care and education (ECE) can be a platform for delivering or supporting services and interventions to advance health equity.** However, increasing the capacity and resources for ECE professionals is needed. (Chapter 7)

H. **To advance health equity and meet the developmental needs of children, a systems approach, including collaboration and alignment across sectors, is needed,** such as workforce support and training, trauma-informed systems and care, enhanced detection of early life adversity and improved response systems, and integration of care and services across all dimensions of health. (Chapter 8)

1

The Need to Intervene Early to Advance Health Equity for Children and Families

INTRODUCTION

Neurobiological and socio-behavioral research indicate that early life conditions, including social supports (e.g., supportive relationships) and adversity (e.g., chronic or severe stress), shape prenatal and early childhood health and development. These experiences have a powerful impact on developing biological systems that impact physical and mental health outcomes throughout life and are further influenced by the social determinants of health (SDOH) (e.g., education, housing, physical and social environment). Despite increasing evidence about what contributes to poor health, these health inequities have persisted, and for some populations and outcomes, they are worsening. Scientific evidence can be used to better inform efforts to advance health equity; this report uses that evidence to support policy actions, program development, practice changes, systems reform, and research priorities. (See Box 1-1 for a high-level overview of this chapter.)

THE PROBLEM

The United States spends much more on health care than any other Organisation for Economic Co-operation and Development (OECD) nation, yet it ranks poorly on most measures of population health (NRC and IOM, 2013; OECD, 2017). Significant, long-standing disparities exist in most health outcomes by education, income, race, ethnicity, geography, gender, neighborhood, disability status, sexual orientation, and citizenship

BOX 1-1
Chapter in Brief: The Need to Intervene Early

Health disparities during the prenatal through early childhood periods:

- Significant, long-standing disparities exist for many health outcomes by education, income, race, ethnicity, geography, gender, neighborhood, disability status, and citizenship status. These disparities put children on a course for poor health outcomes throughout the life-span.
- These health disparities are evident in the rates of infant and maternal mortality, low birth weight, and chronic childhood diseases (such as diabetes, asthma, obesity, depression, and anxiety).
- Clinical care is necessary but not sufficient to address health inequities. To advance health equity, the root causes of poor health and chronic adversity—the social, economic, environmental, and cultural determinants of health—need to be addressed.

Scientific advances in the neurobiological and socio-behavioral sciences:

- The importance of the environment on biological processes (i.e., the complex interplay of biology and environment), including the impact of early adversity, poverty, and racism on lifelong health outcomes, is now well understood.
- While more research is needed to develop a better understanding of tailoring interventions to address heterogeneity, research has advanced dramatically to apply new and more effective interventions.
- Evidence shows that prevention and early intervention for children on at-risk trajectories works, and it is generally more effective and less costly than intervening later in life.
- Negative and positive exposures accumulate over the life course to exert a cumulative effect on health that is probabilistic, not deterministic. That is, the odds of positive or negative health are never fixed; individual exposures, experiences, resilience, and choices help set and adjust these odds over time.

The committee's approach:

- This report takes a life course approach, which emphasizes that a temporal and social perspective—looking across an individual's life experiences or across generations—to gain a better understanding of health outcomes is needed. This approach takes into account an individual's larger social, economic, and cultural context and that the trajectory of an individual's life may be changed, negatively or positively, through interactions among the brain, body, and environment throughout the life-span.
- Achieving health equity for children will require attention and commitment from a range of sectors. Although there are many barriers, this report identifies many opportunities to make long-lasting reductions in long-standing and persistent health inequities.
- Building off 12 core concepts of early development, the committee used scientific evidence to guide its recommendations.

This report provides a range of recommendations for practice, policy, and systems changes, including recommendations that will take time and sustained commitment to dismantle structural barriers, and recommendations that could be implemented immediately or in the near term.

status (NASEM, 2017). Notably, the past few decades have marked a troubling rise in U.S. maternal mortality rates, including black-white disparities, while maternal mortality rates have declined globally (WHO, 2015). Similarly, disparities in infant mortality rates persist, where non-Hispanic black, American Indian/Alaska Native (AI/AN), and Hispanic babies experience higher rates of mortality before their first birthdays compared to non-Hispanic white and Asian and Pacific Islander babies (CDC, 2019b). Children in the United States rank behind their peers in most OECD nations in health status and key determinants of health, and they experience growing disparities on multiple measures of child well-being (OECD, 2009; Seith and Isakson, 2011) (see Box 1-2). For children living in both urban and rural communities, lack of access to critical resources is a major driver of increasing disparities, and this is compounded for economically disadvantaged groups. These disparities put children on a course for poor health outcomes later in life. For more information on maternal and child health disparities, see the section on Early Childhood and Maternal Health Disparities in the United States on page 41.

Many families in the United States do not receive health care when needed, receive it too late, and/or experience problems in quality; however, pathways to better health do not depend on health care alone. For example, children in relatively affluent communities, who ostensibly have easy access to the best mental health services, also show elevated distress compared to national norms—as do their low socioeconomic status (SES) counterparts, but due to a different set of life stressors (Korous et al., 2018). The factors that ultimately contribute to good health (such

---

BOX 1-2
United States Compared to Other OECD Countries
on Key Health Indicators and Outcomes

Compared with other OECD countries, the United States has

- Higher infant mortality
- Higher child mortality
- Higher poverty
- Higher gun violence and death
- Higher rates of hunger
- Higher rates of obesity
- Much higher rates of incarceration of young adults
- Lower secondary school graduation

SOURCES: Grinshteyn and Hemenway, 2016; OECD, 2014, 2017; Walmsley, n.d.

as nutrition, stress, exposure to environmental toxicants) are on multiple interrelated causal pathways along the life-span (NASEM, 2017).

Over the past 100 years, there has been a strong trend toward the conflation of "health" and "health care," where the health of an individual is considered only through a biomedical lens, not taking into account the multiple social and developmental determinants that drive health (Lantz, 2018). Instead, health has been erroneously equated with health care and health disparities erroneously equated with health care disparities. The result is a narrow policy focus on health care interventions to improve health. More recently, research and practice has shifted away from this prevailing paradigm to one that targets upstream factors that shape health (Hahn, 2019; NASEM, 2017).

The 2017 National Academies of Sciences, Engineering, and Medicine (the National Academies) report *Communities in Action: Pathways to Health Equity* reviewed the root causes of health disparities and concluded that health inequity arises from root causes that could be organized in two clusters:

1. Intrapersonal, interpersonal, institutional, and systemic mechanisms (also referred to as "structural inequities") that organize the distribution of power, and access to critical resources, differentially across lines of race, gender, social class, sexual orientation, gender expression, and other dimensions of individual and group identity, and
2. Unequal allocation of and access to power and resources—including goods, services, and societal attention—which manifests itself in unequal social, economic, and environmental conditions, also called the "determinants of health" (NASEM, 2017, p. 7).

Therefore, health inequities are the result of more than individual choice or random occurrence. They are the result of the historical and ongoing interplay of inequitable structures, policies, and norms that shape lives. Interventions targeting the above factors hold the greatest promise for advancing health equity and promoting positive health outcomes at the population level.

Furthermore, the report concluded that

Health equity is crucial. Health equity is fundamental to the idea of living a good life and building a vibrant society because of its practical, economic, and civic implications. Promoting health equity could afford considerable economic, national security, social, and other benefits. Yet, recent research demonstrates that worsening social, economic, and environmental factors are affecting the public's health in serious ways that compromise opportunity for all (NASEM, 2017, Summary).

Health inequity is costly. Beyond significant costs in direct health care expenditures, health inequity has consequences for the U.S. economy, national security, business viability, and public finances considering the impact of poor health and disability on one's ability to participate in the workforce, military service, or society. Addressing health inequities is a critical need that requires this issue to be among our nation's foremost priorities (NASEM, 2017, Summary).

Given these findings, it is critical to address health disparities (differences in health outcomes) with a comprehensive approach—by treating all of the factors that impact individual health, such as education, employment, health systems and services, family, community, housing, income and wealth, physical and social environments, public safety, and transportation (SDOH), in addition to racism, discrimination, segregation, and poverty. To achieve equitable health outcomes in the prenatal through early childhood periods and throughout the life course, all of these contexts need to be addressed.

Health inequities are systemic challenges, and chronic childhood adversities have biological implications and affect childhood development, with lifelong impacts on health and well-being. When exposures to key experiences (both positive and negative) differ for specific groups (e.g., black/African American, AI/AN, Hispanic), their odds for good health diverge systematically over time, producing disparities in outcomes. Because the odds of these exposures are impacted by systems, advancing health equity will require more than individual-level interventions. It will require systems to change in ways that improve the odds of good experiences and reduce the odds of adverse exposures for specific populations.

The focus of this report is on how to best maximize well-being among all young children and families, especially those who are vulnerable at the outset—because life circumstances have rendered them statistically more likely to be on negative adjustment trajectories from early life onward. "Inequities" are operationally defined for the purpose of this report, in part, as the unequal likelihood of thriving or attaining positive adjustment outcomes over time because of differences in opportunity that lead to unfair and avoidable differences in health outcomes.

OPPORTUNITIES

Failing to address the context in which children live, grow, and learn undermines the potential of so many children. Evidence shows that prevention and early intervention for children on at-risk trajectories works and is generally more effective and less costly than later intervention. Luckily, a great deal is known about the science of prenatal and childhood development and the biological mechanisms and effects of chronic adversity and adverse childhood experiences (ACEs) (see Chapters 2 and 3). Recent advances in science—especially around epigenetics,[1] technology and data sharing, and cross-disciplinary collaboration—present an opportunity to systematically apply this knowledge to practice, policy, and systems changes. A large body of research now explicates the mechanisms by which early adversity can change the timing of sensitive periods of brain and other organ systems development, impacting the "plasticity"[2] of developmental processes that are driven by experiences in the life of the young child and his or her family. It is now known that what takes place in early development has lifelong impacts—both positive and negative—on health and well-being. While diseases may appear clinically throughout the life-span, it is known that many diseases originate during early development (Gluckman et al., 2007; Heindel and Vandenberg, 2015). For example, altered nutrition, exposure to environmental chemicals, or stress during specific times of development can lead to functional biological changes, predisposing individuals to diseases that manifest later in life and affecting physical, mental, and cognitive functions.

This report employs the science of early development to inform multidisciplinary and developmentally appropriate systems to support optimal health and well-being for all children throughout their life-spans. The tremendous advances in the theoretical and empirical science in the past 30 years position practitioners and policy makers to take informed action to improve child health outcomes. There is now a firm understanding of the importance of the environment—the constant interplay of nurture–nature and biology–environment—on biological processes, including the impact of early adversity, poverty, and racism on lifelong health outcomes. While there is more to be discovered that will lead to a better understanding of best practices and address challenges of heterogeneity, research has advanced dramatically to apply new and more effective interventions now than ever before.

Given these advances and the understanding of how science can be used to advance health equity during early development, the Robert Wood Johnson Foundation (RWJF), as part of its Culture of Health Initiative,

---

[1] The study of how genes are expressed due to changes in the environment and how these biological changes can be passed down from one generation to the next.

[2] The process by which neurons within the brain change their gene expression, cellular architecture, connections with other neurons, and function in response to experiences and changes in the environment (i.e., change over time).

BOX 1-3
Committee on Applying Neurobiological and Socio-Behavioral Sciences from Prenatal Through Early Childhood Development: A Health Equity Approach Statement of Task

Building on the science base described in the 2000 NRC and IOM report *From Neurons to Neighborhoods: The Science of Early Childhood Development* and the concepts in the 2017 National Academies of Sciences, Engineering, and Medicine report *Communities in Action: Pathways to Health Equity*, and drawing on new insights from 21st-century science in the neurobiological and socio-behavioral fields in the prenatal to early childhood period, an ad hoc committee will

1. Provide a brief overview of
   - the key stressors that affect brain development and health outcomes during this period (e.g., structural inequities, income, housing, employment, access to health care, transportation, and others) and
   - the biological and environmental factors that lead to disparities in health and disease outcomes for subgroups of individuals and the pathways by which biological factors interact with and are influenced by sociocultural factors.
2. Identify promising models and opportunities for translation of the science to action and the intervention points during the prenatal and early childhood periods that will yield the greatest impact, with a focus on practice-based changes and the goal of facilitating broader systems change and alignment based on the science. The committee will draw from international examples as appropriate.
3. Identify the specific outcome measures needed to enable subgroup analyses based on the biological dynamics of the social determinants of health, and identify methods to continuously collect data on both successes and failures to enhance the knowledge base in the future.
4. Based on its review of the evidence and committee expertise, develop a roadmap to systematically apply the science to inform tailored interventions (i.e., policies, programs, or system changes) based on biological, social, environmental, economic, and cultural needs. The roadmap will identify pathways to implement the science in practice and policy.
5. Provide recommendations in the areas above as well as recommendations on how systems can better align to advance health equity and identify specific research needs, as deemed appropriate based on its review of the evidence and its collective expertise.

NOTE: IOM = Institute of Medicine; NRC = National Research Council.

asked the Health and Medicine Division of the National Academies to (see Box 1-3 for the full Statement of Task)

1. Provide a brief overview of stressors that affect prenatal through early childhood development and health;

2. Identify promising models and opportunities for translation of the science to action;
3. Identify outcome measures to enable subgroup analyses;
4. Develop a roadmap to apply the science to tailored interventions (i.e., policies, programs, or system changes) based on biological, social, environmental, economic, and cultural needs; and
5. Provide recommendations in these areas, including how systems can better align to advance health equity.

To respond to this charge, the Committee on Applying Neurobiological and Socio-Behavioral Sciences from Prenatal Through Early Childhood Development: A Health Equity Approach was formed. The committee applied a health equity frame and builds on the 2017 National Academies report *Communities in Action: Pathways to Health Equity*. As identified in the 2000 National Research Council and Institute of Medicine (NRC and IOM) report *From Neurons to Neighborhoods: The Science of Early Childhood Development*, prenatal through early childhood are critical phases of development for the production of health. This report reviews the science that has been developed since *From Neurons to Neighborhoods*.

The committee also adopted the life course approach to its work, which emphasizes a temporal and social perspective, while looking back across an individual's life experiences—or across generations—to gain a better understanding of health outcomes (Braveman and Barclay, 2009). This approach takes into account an individual's larger social, economic, and cultural context and that the trajectory of that individual's life may be changed, negatively or positively, through interactions between the brain, body, and environment throughout the life-span. An individual's health status and outcomes reflect the accumulation of experiences over the life course. Protective factors support positive, or flourishing, trajectories, while risk factors exacerbate the likelihood of poor trajectories (see Figure 1-1).

In line with the life course approach, the committee included the preconception period as an important focus of the report. The health of men and women before conception is important for pregnancy outcomes and the lifelong health of their children. During the preconception period, parents may be exposed to several types of stressors (e.g., chronic stress, environmental toxicants, poverty) that could have repercussions for the health of their future children even into adulthood.

For the purpose of this report, early childhood refers to birth through the onset of puberty and the beginning of adolescence (approximately 8 years of age). The committee uses the terms "preconception," "prenatal," "postpartum," and "early childhood" to refer to the various periods of development. The committee uses the term "early development" to refer to the preconception through early childhood periods.

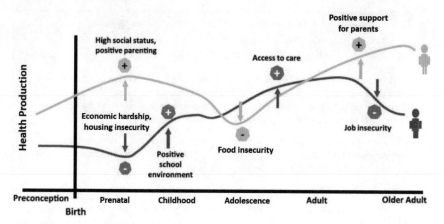

FIGURE 1-1 Variable health trajectories: Life course approach.
NOTE: This figure includes several examples; however, there are many other variables that impact health trajectories (see Chapter 3).
SOURCE: Adapted from Halfon et al., 2014.

Another National Academies study that was under way during the course of this study—also looking at the neurobiological and closed-behavioral sciences—covered adolescence (NASEM, 2019a).

The outcomes that the committee seeks to improve across the life course fall into four categories, adapted from the 2016 National Academies report *Parenting Matters: Supporting Parents of Children Ages 0–8*:

1. Physical health and safety,
2. Emotional and behavioral competence,
3. Social competence, and
4. Cognitive competence.

See Box 1-4 for definitions of key terms used in this report.

WHY INVEST IN EARLY INTERVENTION AND PREVENTION?

There are many reasons to intervene in the prenatal through early childhood periods to prevent and mitigate adverse health outcomes both in early life and over the life course. First, preventing or reducing poor outcomes in the prenatal through early childhood periods generally leads to improved health outcomes later on and therefore can yield health care savings in the long term. For example, in 2007, the IOM reported that the cost associated with premature birth in the United States was $26.2 billion each year (IOM, 2007), and the Centers for Disease Control

BOX 1-4
Key Terms as Used in This Report

Child health: The extent to which individual children or groups of children are able or enabled to (a) develop and realize their potential, (b) satisfy their needs, and (c) develop the capacities that allow them to interact successfully with their biological, physical, and social environments (NRC and IOM, 2004).

Early childhood: A time of tremendous physical, emotional, behavioral, social, and cognitive development. For the purpose of this report, early childhood encompasses from birth to approximately 8 years of age.

Early development: The period from preconception through early childhood.

Health disparities: Differences that exist among specific population groups in the United States in the attainment of full health potential that can be measured by differences in incidence, prevalence, mortality, burden of disease, and other adverse health conditions (NASEM, 2017).

Health equity: The state in which everyone has the opportunity to attain full health potential and no one is disadvantaged from achieving this potential because of social position or any other socially defined circumstance (Center on the Developing Child at Harvard University, n.d.).

Health inequities: Systematic differences in the opportunities that groups have to achieve optimal health, leading to unfair and avoidable differences in health outcomes (NASEM, 2017).

Social determinants of health: The conditions in the environments in which people live, learn, work, play, worship, and age that affect a wide range of health, functioning, and quality-of-life outcomes and risks. These include education, employment, health systems and services, housing, income and wealth, the physical environment, public safety, the social environment (including structures, institutions, and policies), and transportation (Center on the Developing Child at Harvard University, n.d.).

Structural inequities: Personal, interpersonal, institutional, and systemic drivers—such as racism, sexism, classism, ableism, xenophobia, and homophobia—that make those identities salient to the fair distribution of health opportunities and outcomes. For example, policies that foster inequities at all levels (from organization to community to county, state, and nation) are critical drivers of structural inequities (NASEM, 2017).

Toxic stress response: Prolonged activation of the stress response systems that can disrupt the development of brain architecture and other organ systems, and increase the risk for stress-related disease and cognitive impairment, well into the adult years. The toxic stress response can occur when a child experiences strong, frequent, and/or prolonged adversity—such as physical or emotional abuse, chronic neglect, caregiver substance abuse or mental illness, exposure to violence, and/or the accumulated burdens of family economic hardship—without adequate adult support (Center on the Developing Child at Harvard University, n.d.). Toxic stress is the maladaptive and chronically dysregulated stress response that occurs in relation to prolonged or severe early life adversity. For children, the result is the disruption of the development of brain architecture and other organ systems and an increase in lifelong risk for physical and mental disorders.

and Prevention reported that the United States spends $147 billion in obesity-related health care costs each year (CDC, 2019a). Health care savings are also seen when preventing lead poisoning (Gould, 2009) and some childhood diseases. McLaughlin and Rank (2018) estimate that childhood poverty results in $192.1 billion in aggregate health costs (with another $96.9 billion due to child homelessness and $40.5 billion due to maltreatment). Furthermore, inequity is costly. As noted in *Communities in Action* (NASEM, 2017), advancing progress toward health equity (across the life course) could produce economic, national security, and other benefits for the nation. The report made the case that beyond the dollar cost of health care services (which itself is significant at $3.5 trillion in 2017, accounting for 17.9 percent of the nation's gross domestic product [GDP]; CMS, 2017; Martin et al., 2018a), health inequities contribute to overall poor health for the nation and therefore have consequences for the U.S. economy, including diminished productivity in the business sector. In 2009, the Urban Institute projected that from 2009 to 2018, racial disparities in health will cost U.S. health insurers approximately $337 billion in total (Waidmann and Urban, 2009). Furthermore, the rising cost of health insurance and medical care for workers cuts into companies' ability to make a profit and stay competitive (IOM, 2015; Shak et al., 2013).

Investing in early development through prevention and early intervention yields cost savings because the investment costs are often less than the downstream costs of poor health and development. For example, investing in high-quality early care and education (ECE) is one way to improve outcomes related to child health. Not only do early childhood intervention programs yield benefits in academic achievement, behavior, educational progression and attainment, and labor market success, among other domains, but well-designed early childhood interventions have been found to generate a return to society (Karoly et al., 2005).[3] Garcia et al. (2017) found a 13.7 percent return on investment for comprehensive, high-quality, birth-to-5 early education.[4] From a public health perspective, a 2017 systematic review by Masters and colleagues found that national and public health interventions are highly cost-saving for interventions ranging from vaccination to larger determinants of health, though those focusing on the latter had a lower return on investment because they are more complex, resource intensive, and sustained.[5]

---

[3] Studies looking at cost-effectiveness often rely on different underlying assumptions, limiting comparisons across studies and programs. However, overall studies have shown that investments in early childhood appear to save money in the longer term.

[4] The study analyzed a wide variety of life outcomes, such as health, crime, income, IQ, schooling, and the increase in a mother's income after returning to work due to child care.

[5] The review included studies from Australia, Canada, Japan, New Zealand, the United Kingdom, the United States, and Western Europe.

Child maltreatment is costly to the nation as well. The total lifetime economic burden in the United States in 2008 resulting from new cases of fatal and nonfatal child maltreatment was approximately $124 billion (Fang et al., 2012). Furthermore, Bellis and colleagues (2017) found that disproportionate health expenditure in later life might be reduced through childhood interventions to prevent ACEs, showing the long-lasting costs of early adversity.

While the primary beneficiaries of prevention and early intervention efforts are children and their families, the nation as a whole also benefits through cost savings, a healthier and more productive workforce, and strengthened national security (NASEM, 2017).

CURRENT STATE OF CHILDREN'S HEALTH

Overall Well-Being of Children and Families in the United States

This section begins with a broad overview of the current state of child health in the United States, followed by a summary of key health disparities in child and maternal health in the country. Child health is the extent to which individual children or groups of children are able or enabled to (a) develop and realize their potential, (b) satisfy their needs, and (c) develop the capacities that allow them to interact successfully with their biological, physical, and social environments (NRC and IOM, 2004). Children in the United States are generally perceived to be healthier now than in the past because they are much less likely to encounter the major infections or debilitating diseases of past generations and are typically able to recover fully from "acute" childhood illnesses. However, ailments of the past have been replaced with chronic conditions (such as diabetes, asthma, obesity, depression, and anxiety), with large segments of U.S. children facing barriers to good health and well-being as a result of poverty, food insecurity, unsafe or unstable housing, and substantial adversity (such as ACEs) in the first few years of life.

Children who are born and raised in poverty are at particularly high risk for poor health outcomes, more problems in early development (e.g., lack of readiness for school at age 5, diagnoses of developmental delays and/or disorders), and higher rates of most childhood chronic conditions. Early adverse experiences have intermediate effects on physical and/or mental well-being and contribute to chronic disease and poor functioning in adulthood (Hughes et al., 2017; Shonkoff et al., 2012). In fact, these impacts are cumulative, and adults who experience adversity in childhood have substantially higher rates of heart disease, lung disease, metabolic syndrome, and other costly health conditions (see Chapters 2 and 3 for more information). Many of these health disparities are rooted in historical practices and policies (such as segregation and redlining), and this historical legacy continues to shape the development of children today. (See Chapter 3 for a discussion on historical trauma and NASEM [2017] for an overview of historical injustices that impact health outcomes.)

Early Childhood and Maternal Health Disparities in the United States

This section provides a brief overview of child and maternal health disparities and indicators of health in the United States. It is not a comprehensive overview but rather highlights some of the key health disparities. The most recent data available are presented. Chapter 3 provides a detailed overview of health disparities and critical influences or factors that can either promote or hinder healthy development, with a focus on factors that shape inequities at the child/family level and the community and population levels.

Infant Mortality Rates

In 2015, infant mortality rates per 1,000 live births by race and ethnicity were as follows: non-Hispanic black (11.3), AI/AN (8.3), Hispanic (5.0), non-Hispanic white (4.9), and Asian/Pacific Islander (4.2) (CDC, 2019b) (see Figure 1-2). In 2014, infant mortality in rural counties was 6.55 deaths per 1,000 births, 6 percent higher than in small and medium

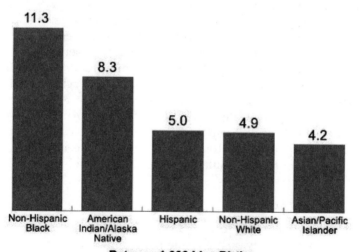

FIGURE 1-2 Infant mortality rates by race and ethnicity, 2015.
SOURCE: CDC, 2019b.

urban counties and 20 percent higher than in large urban counties (Ely et al., 2017). Neonatal mortality was 8 percent higher in both rural (4.11 per 1,000 births) and small and medium urban counties compared with large urban counties (Ely et al., 2017).

Mortality for infants of non-Hispanic white mothers in rural counties (5.95 per 1,000) was 41 percent higher than in large urban counties and 13 percent higher than in small and medium urban counties (Ely et al., 2017). For infants of non-Hispanic black mothers, mortality was 15 percent higher in small and medium urban counties and 16 percent higher in rural counties (12.08) compared with large urban counties (Ely et al., 2017).

Low Birth Weight

Low birth weight (LBW; less than 5.5 pounds at birth) babies are more at risk for many short- and long-term health problems, such as infections, delayed motor and social development, and learning disabilities (CDC, 2016). Causes of LBW include maternal smoking, use of alcohol, or lack of weight gain and social and economic factors, such as low income, low parental educational level, maternal stress, and domestic violence or other abuse (CDC, 2016).

LBW levels among race and Hispanic-origin groups in 2016 ranged from 6.97 percent for births to non-Hispanic white women to 13.68 percent for births to non-Hispanic black women. Rates among Hispanic subgroups ranged from 6.9 percent for births to Mexican women to 9.5 percent for births to Puerto Rican women (Martin et al., 2018b). In 2016, 14 percent of black infants were LBW, compared with 8 percent of Asian and Pacific Islander, 8 percent of AI/AN, 7 percent of white, and 7 percent of Hispanic infants. Among those of Hispanic origin in 2016, Puerto Rican infants were the most likely to be LBW (9 percent) (Child Trends, 2018b). In 2013, the most recent year that information for Asian and Pacific Islander subgroups was available, Asian Indian infants were the most likely to be LBW (11 percent), followed by Filipinos (9 percent). Black infants are also more than twice as likely as other infants to be very LBW—less than 3 pounds 5 ounces—at 2.9 percent in 2016, compared with between 1.1 and 1.2 percent for white and Hispanic infants, respectively (Child Trends, 2016b).

Chronic Childhood Diseases

Conditions that rarely lead to death in children and youth are now more prevalent: obesity, asthma, mental health conditions (especially attention-deficit/hyperactivity disorder, depression, and anxiety), and neurodevelopmental conditions (including autism spectrum disorders) (Perrin et al., 2007, 2014; Van Cleave et al., 2010). For example, in children less than 18 years of age, asthma was prevalent among 8.1 percent of white non-Hispanic children, 12.6 percent of black non-Hispanic children, 8.2 percent of other non-Hispanic children, and 7.7 percent of Hispanic children. Among Hispanic children, 11.3 percent of Puerto Rican children and 6.2 percent of Mexican/Mexican American children had asthma (CDC, 2019c). During 2016, asthma affected children living in families with incomes of less than 100 percent of the federal poverty level (FPL) (10.5 percent) more than those living in families with incomes of ≥250 percent of the FPL (250 to <450 percent FPL: 6.9 percent; ≥450 percent FPL: 6.7 percent) (Zahran et al., 2018).

Mental and Behavioral Conditions

Particularly noteworthy is the growth of mental and behavioral conditions among children and youth. Recent work has documented their (a) high prevalence, (b) major impact on youth well-being and functioning, (c) common association with other chronic conditions, (d) high costs, and (e) complication of the course, treatment, and outcomes of most other conditions (Ghandour et al., 2012; Houtrow et al., 2014; Perrin et al., 2018). Importantly, most of these high-prevalence conditions occur at higher rates and usually higher severity among low-income children, even though the rate of growth has increased in all SES levels (Houtrow et al., 2014). Although all of these conditions have genetic components, they also often reflect the consequences of early childhood experiences and their influence through epigenetics and other physiological mechanisms. Furthermore, less than optimal access to and use of health care in early years can negatively affect these conditions over time.

Early Life Adversity

The impacts of early life adversity and disparities are discussed in detail in Chapters 2 and 3; however, a highlight of a few disparities is provided here. ACEs (including physical, emotional and sexual abuse, physical and emotional neglect, and household stressors, including parental mental illness, substance use or incarceration, parental separation or divorce, and domestic violence) are highly prevalent in all racial and socioeconomic groups. Almost 50 percent of children and adolescents (age 0–17) have experienced at least one category of ACE according to national population-based studies (Bethell et al., 2014), and black, Hispanic, and poorer children are exposed to more ACEs relative to white or wealthier children (Slopen et al., 2016).[6] Foster care children are at

---

[6] ACEs are discussed in detail in Chapter 3.

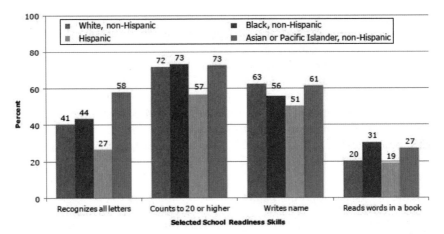

FIGURE 1-3 Percentage of children ages 3–6 with selected school readiness skills, by race and Hispanic origin, 2012.
NOTES: Data represent parent reports of specific cognitive and literacy skills. Data are sourced from Child Trends' analysis of the National Household Education Survey.
SOURCE: Child Trends, 2015.

between 1.5 and 7 times greater odds of having experienced any 1 of the 10 traditional ACEs compared to children not placed in foster care, even after controlling for race and ethnicity, parent education and employment, welfare services, and poverty status (Turney and Wildeman, 2017).

School Readiness

School readiness[7] is an important indicator for future child well-being, and there are deep disparities across race and ethnicity (see Chapter 7 for a detailed overview of the importance of ECE). Figure 1-3 provides examples of important measures of school readiness by race and Hispanic origin. Using 2016 National Survey of Children's Health data, Ghandour et al. (2018) found that only 41.8 percent of 3- to 5-year-olds in the United States were estimated to be on track in all four domains of school readiness. Overall, Hispanic children are less likely to show cognitive/literacy readiness skills than are white, black, or Asian/Pacific Islander children.

---

[7] That is, children possessing the skills, knowledge, and attitudes necessary for success in school and for later learning and life. The concept of "school readiness" is broader than cognitive or pre-academic skills, such as early literacy and math. However, comparable data across communities or states are limited mostly to such outcomes, which are what is presented here. All states have developed some form of school readiness assessment, and most of them focus on children's social-emotional development, approaches to learning, and physical health and development, as well as cognitive abilities (Daily et al., 2010).

In 2012, 27 percent of Hispanic 3- to 6-year-olds could recognize all 26 letters of the alphabet, compared with 41 and 44 percent, respectively, of white and black children. Asian/Pacific Islander children had the highest rate of recognizing all of the letters, at 58 percent. A similar pattern in the ability to count to 20 and write their name was seen by race, although Asian/Pacific Islander children were similar to their white and black counterparts (Child Trends, 2015). Young pre-K children living in poverty are much less likely to have cognitive and early literacy readiness skills than are children living above the poverty threshold. Disparities in all measures of early school readiness by income level were greatest in 1999, but these narrowed in 2007 (Child Trends, 2015).

Poverty

Poverty affects large numbers of U.S. children. A 2019 National Academies report, *A Roadmap to Reducing Child Poverty*, estimated that in 2015, more than 9.6 million children under 18 years of age lived in poverty, as measured by the Supplemental Poverty Measure (SPM) (NASEM, 2019b). Thus, 13 percent of the child population lived in households with annual incomes ranging from $22,000 to $26,000 for a family of four. Moreover, of those 9.6 million children, 2.1 million lived in "deep poverty," defined as having family resources below half of the poverty line—$11,000 to $13,000 annual income. An additional 22 percent of U.S. children live in "near poverty" households, defined as between 100 and 150 percent of the SPM poverty line. These 16.7 million children live in households that frequently pay more in taxes than they receive in tax credits, reducing their net incomes (NASEM, 2019b). Many U.S. families with children face persistent problems related to poverty, including inadequate housing, clothing, and food for their children, and health problems accompany those deficits.

Health Insurance Coverage

From 2008 to 2016, the rate of uninsured children steadily decreased from 9.7 to 4.7 percent. However, the percentage of uninsured children increased to 5 percent in 2017 (Alker and Pham, 2018). See Figure 1-4 for the rate of uninsured children from 2008 through 2017.

For the percentage breakdown of the number of uninsured children by race and ethnicity in 2016 and 2017, see Figure 1-5. As the figure shows, for black, white, Asian/Native Hawaiian/Pacific Islander, and Hispanic children, the rate of children without insurance increased from 2016 to 2017. In the same 2-year period, the rate of children without insurance decreased for AI/AN children by 0.2 percent. However, the rate of children without insurance for this group is far higher than for other racial

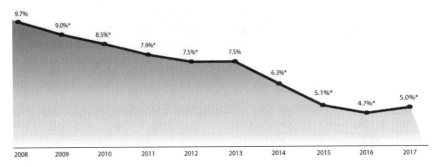

FIGURE 1-4 Rate of uninsured children, 2008–2017.
NOTES: * Change is significant at the 90 percent confidence level. Significance is relative to the prior year. 2013 was the only year that did not show a significant 1-year increase or decrease in the national rate of uninsured children. The Census began collecting data for the health insurance series in 2008; therefore, there is no significance available for 2008. Data are sourced from Table HIC-5, Health Insurance Coverage Status and Type of Coverage by State—Children Under 19: 2008 to 2017, Health Insurance Historical Tables, U.S. Census Bureau American Community Survey.
SOURCE: Alker and Pham, 2018.

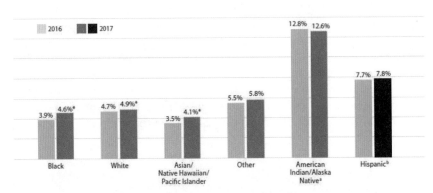

FIGURE 1-5 Children's uninsured rate by race and ethnicity, 2016–2017.
   * Change is significant at the 90% confidence level.
   [a] Indian Health Service is not considered insurance coverage by the Census Bureau. See the methodology section for more information.
   [b] Hispanic refers to a person's ethnicity, and these children may be of any race. See the methodology section for more information.
SOURCE: Alker and Pham, 2018.

and ethnic groups at 12.8 percent in 2016 and 12.6 percent in 2017 (Alker and Pham, 2018). In 2017, 27 states and Washington, DC, had significantly lower rates of children without insurance than the national rate of 5.0 percent, and 11 states had no statistically significant difference from the national rate. However, 12 states had significantly higher rates, with the highest rates of children without insurance in Texas (10.7 percent), Alaska (9.6 percent), and Wyoming (9.5 percent).

MATERNAL HEALTH IN THE UNITED STATES

Women in other high-income countries fare better in terms of access to health care and health status than women in the United States. U.S. women in have the highest rate of maternal mortality because of complications from pregnancy or childbirth and among the highest rates of cesarean sections, and maternal mortality rates are rising for them while declining in other countries (see Figure 1-6). For the past six decades, black women have died at a rate that ranges from three to four times that of white women, with 38.9 deaths per 100,000 live births among black women versus 12 deaths per 100,000 live births among white women as of 2010 (Creanga et al., 2015; MHTF, n.d.). AI/AN women also fare worse than white women, with approximately twice as many pregnancy-related deaths per 100,000 live births. Some researchers point to structural drivers of maternal mortality disparities in the United States, such as racism

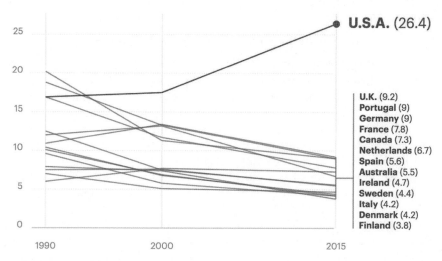

FIGURE 1-6 Global, regional, and national levels of maternal mortality, 1990–2015.
NOTE: Data from GBD 2015 Maternal Mortality Collaborators, 2016.
SOURCES: Martin and Montagne, 2017. Courtesy of Propublica.

and discrimination (ACOG, n.d.) and adverse changes in chronic diseases and insufficient health care access (Nelson et al., 2018). See Chapter 5 for a detailed overview of preconception through postpartum care.

Prenatal Care

Access to prenatal care varies across race and ethnicity groups. In 2016, about 77 percent of women who gave birth initiated prenatal care in the first trimester. However, only 66.5 percent of black, 72.0 percent of Hispanic, 63.0 percent of AI/AN, and 55.9 percent of Native Hawaiian or other Pacific Islander women received it, whereas 82.3 percent of non-Hispanic white women did (Osterman and Martin, 2018). People of color are much more likely to be affected by late initiation of prenatal care, which is most common in Pacific Islanders at 18.4 percent, with non-Hispanic white women at 3.3 percent. AI/AN women have a 9.2 percent chance of late prenatal care initiation, and black women have a 7.0 percent chance (Osterman and Martin, 2018). (See Chapter 5 for more statistics and information on prenatal care.)

CURRENT ENVIRONMENT FOR CHILDREN AND FAMILIES

In the past 20 years, much has changed in the landscape in which prenatal to childhood development takes place in the policy and funding environment and the social, economic, and cultural context. The following section outlines some of these important changes.

Changes in the Funding and Policy Environment

Federal spending (not including tax reductions) on children under 18 increased from $210 billion in 2000 to $375 billion in 2017, driven largely by increased health spending on Medicaid, which nearly tripled between 2000 and 2017, and the Children's Health Insurance Program (CHIP) (Isaacs et al., 2018) (see Table 1-1). Federal spending on nutrition, income security, ECE, and housing also increased substantially between 2000 and 2010, though many programs have seen a decline in federal support since 2010. Approximately 61 percent of federal expenditures in 2017 served children in low-income families through means-tested programs and tax provisions (Isaacs et al., 2018).

Altogether, federal spending on children in 2017 accounted for 9.4 percent of total federal outlays (see Figure 1-7), and it is projected to fall to 6.9 percent. In contrast, federal spending on adults through Social Security, Medicare, and Medicaid accounted for 45 percent of total federal outlays, which is projected to grow to 50 percent by 2028 (Isaacs et al., 2018). It should also be noted that federal spending on children

TABLE 1-1 Federal Expenditures on Children by Program, Selected Years 1960–2017

	1960	1980	2000	2010	2017
1. Health	0.2	7.6	36.8	95.1	111.9
Medicaid	—	6.9	32.8	80.7	89.9
CHIP	—	—	1.7	8.5	15.4
Vaccines for children	—	—	0.7	4.0	4.4
Other health	0.2	0.8	1.6	1.9	2.1
2. Nutrition	1.5	22.5	30.9	60.8	58.0
SNAP (food stamps)	—	11.7	13.4	36.1	30.6
Child nutrition	1.5	9.1	12.7	18.3	22.3
Special Supplemental food (WIC)	—	1.6	4.8	6.4	5.0
3. Income Security	14.6	33.6	46.4	58.0	54.3
Social Security	7.0	17.7	18.6	22.3	20.8
Temporary Assistance for Needy Families	4.8	11.0	15.9	17.2	12.8
Supplemental Security Income	—	0.9	6.7	11.0	10.5
Veterans benefits	2.5	3.5	2.1	3.5	6.8
Child support enforcement	—	0.9	4.4	4.9	4.1
Other income security	0.3	−0.4	−1.3	−1.0	−0.6
4. Education	3.0	18.7	30.3	76.1	41.6
Education for the Disadvantaged (Title I, Part A)	—	8.3	11.8	21.9	16.2
Special education/IDEA	—	2.1	6.9	19.4	12.7
School improvement	—	2.0	3.5	6.0	4.4
Innovation and improvement	—	—	—	1.1	1.3
Impact Aid	1.7	1.8	1.2	1.4	1.5
Dependents' schools abroad	0.2	0.9	1.3	1.3	1.2
Other education	0.1	2.5	3.9	25.1	4.3
5. Early Education and Care	--	2.1	10.8	15.5	14.9
Head Start (including Early Head Start)	—	2.1	6.2	9.0	8.9
Child Care and Development Fund	—	—	4.6	6.6	5.7
Other early education and care	—	—	—	—	0.3
6. Social Services	—	4.6	10.7	11.2	10.1
Foster care	—	0.8	6.0	4.9	4.9
Adoption assistance	—	—	0.2	2.6	2.5

continued

TABLE 1-1 Continued

	1960	1980	2000	2010	2017
Other social services	—	3.9	4.5	3.6	2.7
7. Housing	—	2.8	8.3	10.7	9.5
Section 8 low-income housing assistance	—	1.4	6.5	8.0	7.7
Low-rent public housing	—	0.6	1.1	1.3	1.0
Other housing	—	0.8	0.8	1.4	0.7
8. Training	—	6.4	1.5	2.2	1.2
9. Refundable Portions of Tax Credits	—	3.1	34.5	81.8	74.0
Earned income tax credit	—	3.1	33.3	54.8	53.1
Child tax credit	—	—	1.1	25.4	19.4
Premium tax credit	—	—	—	—	0.6
Other refundable tax credits	—	—	—	1.6	0.8
10. Tax Reductions	41.2	50.1	93.1	105.1	106.2
Dependent exemption	40.6	42.3	39.7	36.0	37.8
Exclusion for employer-sponsored health insurance	NA	4.1	13.7	21.5	22.9
Child tax credit (nonrefundable portion)	—	—	26.8	33.4	29.9
Earned income tax credit (nonrefundable portion)	—	1.8	5.9	5.3	7.0
Dependent care credit	—	—	3.2	3.8	3.3
Other tax reductions	0.7	1.9	3.7	5.1	5.3
TOTAL EXPENDITURES ON CHILDREN	**60.5**	**151.5**	**303.2**	**516.4**	**481.5**
OUTLAYS SUBTOTAL (1–9)	**19.3**	**101.4**	**210.1**	**411.3**	**375.3**

NOTES: Numbers in billions of 2017 U.S. dollars. CHIP = Children's Health Insurance Program; IDEA = Individuals with Disabilities Education Act; SNAP = Supplemental Nutrition Assistance Program; WIC = Special Supplemental Nutrition Program for Women, Infants, and Children.
SOURCE: Isaacs et al., 2018.

(which accounted for 34 percent of total public spending on children) in 2017 represented only 2 percent of the GDP in the United States, which is well below that of other developed nations. An international comparison of public spending on children from 1985 to 2000 ranked U.S. spending (2.4 percent of GDP) as the second lowest among 20 OECD countries, much less than the 9.6 percent median across OECD countries (Lynch, 2006).

One of the most important changes in the policy landscape over the past 20 years has been the Patient Protection and Affordable Care

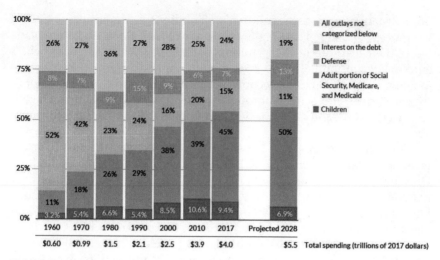

FIGURE 1-7 Share of federal budget outlays on children and other items, selected years, 1960–2028.
NOTES: Authors' estimates based primarily on Congressional Budget Office, The Budget and Economic Outlook: 2018 to 2028 (Washington, DC: Congressional Budget Office, 2018), and Office of Management and Budget, Budget of the United States Government, Fiscal Year 2019 (Washington, DC: U.S. Government Printing Office, 2018) and past years. For more source information, see the appendix in Isaacs et al., 2018. Numbers may not sum to totals because of rounding.
SOURCE: Isaacs et al., 2018. Republished with permission of Urban Institute, from Kid's Share 2018, Isaacs et al., 2018; permission conveyed through Copyright Clearance Center, Inc.

Act (ACA), which expanded health care access for children and families through a combination of Medicaid expansions, private insurance reforms, and premium tax credits (Kaiser Family Foundation, 2019). The uninsured rate among women ages 19–34 decreased from 25 percent in 2010 to 14 percent in 2016 (Gunja et al., 2017), which has significant implications for preconception and prenatal health. The ACA requires coverage for women's preventive services at no cost-sharing, including well-woman visits, and eliminates exclusions for preexisting conditions (e.g., pregnancy and depression), which improves access for women with chronic conditions (Gunja et al., 2017). The ACA mandates coverage for essential health benefits (EHBs), which include maternity care and mental health services. For children, the ACA requires coverage for preventive services at no cost-sharing and EHBs, eliminated exclusions for preexisting conditions, and prohibits lifetime dollar limits, which improves access for children with special health care needs (National MCH Workforce Development Center, 2015). Even though the ACA did not substantially increase children's eligibility for Medicaid (or CHIP), the process of parents seeking enrollment in Medicaid or exchange plans led to their learning of their children's eligibility, which increased child enrollment substantially. Presently, it is unclear how recent policy changes to deregulate consumer protections under the ACA and to restrict eligibility, enrollment, and benefits through Medicaid waivers will impact health care access and equity for children and families. (See Chapter 5 for more about the ACA.)

Federal funding for ECE has steadily increased over the past 10 years; however, total spending on ECE in the United States remains limited. Only 0.5 percent of the U.S. GDP is spent on ECE, whereas other peer nations spend 1 percent or more (OECD, 2019). Recent increases include lawmakers approving an $890 million increase for Early Head Start and Head Start, including $170 million for Early Head Start—Child Care Partnerships, from fiscal year (FY) 2016 levels to FY 2019 levels (FFYF, 2018; see Chapter 7 for more on these programs). In addition, in response to decades of early childhood and brain development research, policy makers, advocates, program administrators, and other leaders in the child care community have advanced a number of policies and initiatives that recognize child care programs as opportunities to improve children's development rather than solely as work-support programs. As a result, for example, the most recent reauthorization of the Child Care Development Block Grant[8] provides for more continuity of care by allowing parents to receive subsidies for 1 year, even if their income, work, or education status changes during that period. There has also been more attention paid to increased compensation for the workforce. For example, states and local communities have developed a number of strategies to enhance compensation for early childhood educators, including tax credits, wage supplements (often tied to attaining higher education or credentials), targeted increases for child care subsidy rates, salary scales, provision of benefits, and parity with K–12 teachers. More recently, there has been greater recognition from policy makers, advocates, and ECE practitioners of the importance of ECE program leaders (including elementary school principals).

CHANGES IN THE ECONOMIC, SOCIAL, AND CULTURAL ENVIRONMENT

Income inequality has been growing—the income gap between higher- and lower-income individuals has increased substantially over the past

---

[8] See https://www.acf.hhs.gov/occ/ccdf-reauthorization (accessed July 29, 2019).

30 years (NASEM, 2017).[9] Those with incomes in the top 10 percent average 9 times the income of those in the bottom 90 percent, and those with incomes in the top 0.1 percent have more than 188 times the income of the bottom 90 percent (Inequality.org, n.d.). Lasting effects of the 2008 recession include displacement of vulnerable populations, which exacerbated the impact on both their health and their economic well-being and resulted in greater income inequality and wealth inequality (Smeeding, 2012).

People of color continue to face structural barriers when it comes to securing quality housing, health care, employment, and education (NASEM, 2017; Pager and Shepherd, 2008). For example, data suggest that schools are becoming increasingly segregated by poverty and race, which has implications for which communities have access to high-quality, well-funded education (Boschma and Brownstein, 2016; Darling-Hammond, 1998). Racism also continues to be a pressing problem, and it is built into systems, as seen by racial profiling by law enforcement officers, disproportionate suspension and expulsion rates of young boys of color (see Chapter 7), and the difficulty that some subgroups have in breaking the cycle of poverty (see Chapter 6). Chapter 3 expands on these issues and the impact they have on the health of children and families.

In terms of family structure, American families have changed, with a Pew Research Center (2015b) survey finding that there is no longer one dominant family type in the United States today (as compared to 1980, where 61 percent of children were living with married parents in their first marriage—today, that number is 46 percent) (see Figure 1-8). Pew also found, for example, that two-parent households are no longer the norm as rates of divorce, remarriage, and cohabitation have increased. This decline has been offset by an almost threefold increase in those living with just one parent—typically the mother (10.5 percent of children age 18 or younger lived with only a mother in 2018, compared to 2.4 percent living with the father only [U.S. Census, 2018]). Women who are single or living with a nonmarital partner account for 4 in 10 births in the United States. Single-parent families are more than 4 times more likely to be poor than are two-parent families (Pascoe et al., 2016), and this can affect their ability to invest time and resources in their children, which would have longer-term implications for the persistence of poverty across generations. More mothers (of children 18 or younger) have also entered the workforce (70 percent), with 40 percent of them being the primary earner (Pew Research Center, 2015a).

---

[9] There are several different ways to measure income inequality, including the use of different datasets, that lead to different results (with no single source that illustrates all of the major trends in inequality) (CBPP, 2018). However, regardless of the method or data used, results consistently show an increase in income inequality in the past three decades. See a draft paper by Auten and Splinter (2018) for additional analysis that argues that income inequality has not grown as much as others have estimated.

% of children living with ...

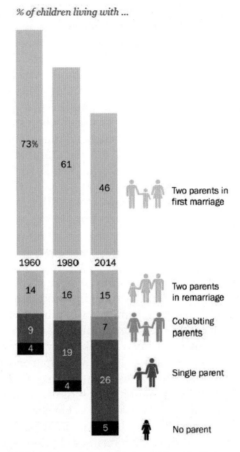

FIGURE 1-8 For children, growing diversity in family living arrangements.
NOTES: Based on children under 18. Data regarding cohabitation are not available
for 1960 and 1980; in those years, children with cohabiting parents are included
in "one parent." For 2014, the total share of children living with two married
parents is 62 percent after rounding. Figures do not add up to 100 percent due to
rounding. Data are sourced from Pew Research Center's analysis of 1960 and 1980
decennial census and 2014 American Community Survey.
SOURCE: Pew Research Center, 2015b.

The makeup of children in the United States has changed as well.
In 2000, 61 percent of all U.S. children were non-Hispanic white; in 2016
that number was 51 percent, with the proportion of children with Hispanic origins growing from 17 to 25 percent between 2000 and 2016.
The percentage of non-Hispanic black children has stayed relatively
constant since 1980 (14 to 15 percent) (Child Trends, 2018c). From 1994

to 2017, the population of children of immigrants[10] grew by 51 percent, from 18 to 27 percent (Child Trends, 2018a). These children are mainly second-generation immigrants (16.7 million), with first-generation immigrants making up a much smaller number (2.9 million, which is 3 to 5 percent of all children). In 2016, 33 percent of U.S. children lived in a household where more than one language is spoken (dual-language learners), with Spanish being the most common other language for these children (Child Trends, 2016).

Evidence shows that populations from immigrant backgrounds and ethnic and racial enclaves might bring or develop particular child-rearing practices that lead to strengths and weaknesses in their children's adaptations and success in other environments. For example, Galindo and Fuller (2010) have shown that Latino children have higher social-emotional skills in preschool but some of the academic skills of low-income Latino children lag beyond other groups. School success as measured by grades is associated with different family constellations and practices in immigrant populations, such as Cambodian, Dominican, and Portuguese populations (García Coll and Kerivan Marks, 2009). When examining cultural variation, no particular parenting or household composition is associated with success across all domains of child outcomes, aside from preventing extreme neglect, abuse, or lack of stimulation.

A more general cultural shift has been the increase in personal-use technology (e.g., computers, tablets, mobile phones), which has advanced at a rapid pace in the past 20 years. The divide in access to digital devices has decreased significantly, with more families having access to smartphones across socioeconomic lines. Access to other devices, however, continues to create a digital divide that children in non-mainstream populations have to surpass. School districts across the country are integrating technology into the classroom. The health care field has advanced in the area of telehealth, providing greater remote access to health care providers. This access can have positive and negative effects, and it can even increase inequities when not used properly.

ABOUT THIS REPORT

Report Conceptual Model

The committee's conceptual model (see Figure 1-9) served as a unifying framework for the committee's approach to the report, aiming to improve prenatal through early childhood development with a health equity approach. The model adapts elements and concepts from the

---

[10] Immigrant children are defined here as those who have at least one foreign-born parent.

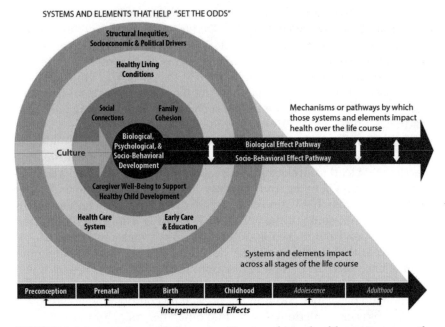

FIGURE 1-9 Leveraging early opportunities to achieve health equity across the life course: A conceptual framework.
NOTE: The elements and systems included in the nested circles impact every stage of the life course.

World Health Organization (WHO) Commission on Social Determinants of Health conceptual framework (WHO, 2010), the socio-ecological model (Bronfenbrenner, 1979; McLeroy et al., 1988; NASEM, 2017; Velez-Agosto et al., 2017), a model of children's health and its influences (NRC and IOM, 2004), and the life course health development model (Halfon et al., 2014).

Building on the life course model, this figure shows early development within the context of the life course stages, beginning with preconception and ending with adulthood along the bottom. It is important to note that risk and protective factors can be transferred intergenerationally, which makes the parent or primary caregiver and/or the parent–child dyad a central focus of intervention. With the necessary supports and conditions, healthy biological, socio-emotional, cognitive, and socio-behavioral development increase across the life course.

Within the context of the life course, the diagram's nested circles illustrate the complex sociocultural environment that shapes development at the individual level and the opportunities for interventions to improve individual health and developmental outcomes and population health, well-being, and health equity. The context and conditions here continue to play an important role in health and well-being throughout the life course. Individual social and biological mechanisms operate and interact within and across the three levels.

The outer level, "socioeconomic and political drivers," is adapted from the WHO social determinants framework and represents the level at which structural inequities operate. These structural inequities are deeply embedded into policies, laws, governance, and culture; they organize the distribution of power and resources differentially across characteristics of identity (i.e., race, ethnicity, gender, class, sexual orientation, and others) (NASEM, 2017; WHO, 2010).

The next level represents social, economic, and environmental conditions (i.e., the SDOH): education, employment, health systems and services, housing, income and wealth, physical environment, transportation, public safety, and social environment. In the model, these nine interdependent factors are grouped into three domains that the committee has identified, based on the available evidence and existing resources, as important for targeting prenatal and early childhood interventions: healthy living conditions, ECE, and health systems and services. These domains in the gray and light blue circles are the primary foci of Chapters 5–7, and each is discussed in terms of evidence-based solutions, opportunities for intervention, barriers, promising models, and research needs.

The next level represents the factors that most directly and proximally shape children's daily experiences and routine patterns; these include caregiver well-being and support and attachment and family cohesion, which affect social connections in early life.

Culture, according to Velez-Agosto and colleagues (2017), operates at various levels, including all of the levels in the committee's conceptual model. Systems, such as ECE and health care, have cultures and also enact in their daily operations ways of conceptualizing the child's development, how to promote it, and what resources have to be accessed in order to correct illness and developmental problems. Cultures can also be sources of strength, providing support for coping with life demands and toxic stress (García Coll et al., 1996). Families and communities also have cultures that are similarly enacted in daily routines and in developmental goals and expectations. Inequities might arise from lack of understanding of normative cultural frameworks between any of these levels, lack of respect and acceptance for different ways of being that are considered normative in other settings, and lack of access to critical resources, such as high-quality ECE and health care, due to racism and discrimination (García Coll et al., 1996).

Types of Interventions

The committee deployed lessons from the latest insights in neurobiological and closed-behavioral sciences that define how early childhood experiences translate into health outcomes and inequities across the life course in order to offer promising practices or transformational levers that might help move the needle in a positive direction. In its Statement of Task (see Box 1-3), the committee was asked to look at interventions defined as policies, programs, or system changes. What is meant by each of these is briefly described below (see Box 1-5 for examples).

Systems

Systems are a collection of interacting, interdependent parts that function as a whole. For the purposes of this report, most of the systems are social constructs and are organized around a key functional area (education, health care, criminal justice). Systems have existing patterns and

---

BOX 1-5
Example of Systems, Policy, and Programmatic Changes

Conceptual Example: How do we build more integrated care that helps support people in both the clinical and social drivers of poor health outcomes?

Systems Change: Altering the basic or fundamental structures or patterns by which information, money, people, or other resources flow through or between systems.

- Example: A health care system implements standardized social determinants screening (e.g., asking questions at medical appointments about housing and food security) for all patients and builds out a standard referral system to community agencies.

Policy Change: Altering the overarching legal or regulatory structure that governs how systems operate or interact with each other.

- Example: Data and privacy regulations are changed to allow partners in other sectors to see and share important information on their mutual clientele.

Programmatic Change: Creating specific alternative structures or patterns that alter the default experience for targeted subsets of a population.

- Example: A system builds an enhanced model of intensive case management for its clients with the most intensive needs. These clients receive extra supports, but the experiences of others remain mostly unchanged.

structures that define how people tend to move through them. A few essential features that define a system include

- **Structures:** The essential organizational components of a system, including how it is governed.
- **Flows:** How information, money, or people move through and are configured in relation to each other.
- **Goals:** The actions the system is trying to accomplish—its purpose or function.
- **Rules and Norms:** How a system is organized and what can and cannot happen within it.
- **Paradigms:** Assumptions that system makes that inform how things are organized and flow within it.

These features could be thought about in the context of a single system or considered through a social ecosystem lens and applied to how systems interact with each other.

Programs

A program is a targeted or specialized pathway by which a specific group of people move through a system or between a set of systems—a change in the system's structures or flows for certain kinds of clients. It is often driven by a recognition that the standard approaches are not achieving the system's goals for some people. Programs usually do not change the goals or rules or the system itself; rather, they generally offer a new way to achieve improved outcomes within the current system's structures (such as a support group for new mothers offered in a primary care setting).

Policy

Policy is a shift in the overarching legal or regulatory structure that governs how systems operate or interact with one another. Policies usually set the rules, goals, norms, or paradigms within which systems establish structures and flows, and they may also set the limits on the types of exceptions or changes that systems can put in place. Some policies can impact large swathes of the population, such as laws, regulations, court rulings, administrative rules, or executive orders, and often have consequences when not followed. Some policies have a smaller scope, such as guidelines issued by professional organizations, recommendations of expert panels, or local programs.

In general, policies, systems, and programs can be thought of as nested within each other. The impact profile of efforts at any given level may be constrained by what is happening in the others—promising programs that do not consider the potential limitations that the policy environment places on potential adoption and spread will not be as useful as those that do.

Committee's Methodology

As discussed above, an intervention could consist of policies, programs, or system changes, or a combination of those approaches. The literature on the effectiveness and applicability of interventions provides important information for assessing which interventions are most effective and suitable for a general or more specific population. However, many interventions have not been adequately evaluated for their effectiveness—in general, for a specific outcome, or when brought to scale. In addition, studies vary in dimensions such as appropriateness of design and setting, quality of execution, interactions with other interventions, and consideration of economic consequences.

With the above in mind, the committee examined the available literature, conducting a comprehensive review from the peer-reviewed and gray literature.[11] This entailed a systematic search of academic and governmental databases and websites for studies that evaluated or assessed the effects of interventions. Where possible, the committee relied on existing systematic reviews and meta-analyses with strong methodologies and existing comprehensive reviews.

Comparisons across studies are needed to better assess intervention opportunities; however, such comparisons are often not available or difficult to interpret due to methodological strengths and limitations relating to the nature of the study design and the data collected. For example, what is considered the gold standard research design to show that a program does in fact lead to the results it is trying to achieve—the randomized controlled trial (RCT)—may not always be feasible. This is because RCTs are not appropriate in all settings, particularly not to study community-level interventions, and for some interventions, randomization can be considered ethically objectionable if it denies a service or treatment known to be beneficial (Center on the Developing Child at Harvard University, 2016). While large-scale, multiyear RCTs will continue to be

---

[11] The date range for the search was 2013–2019. Search terms included the following categories: prenatal and early childhood, neurobiological, socio-behavioral, biology/biomarkers, health indicators/outcomes, structural inequities, social determinants of health, and model/intervention.

important to demonstrate program impacts, there is also an important role for short-term, flexible study methodologies to test program components and subgroup variability and allow for mid-course corrections and enhancements (such corrections are not possible in traditional RCTs) (Center on the Developing Child at Harvard University, 2016). While there is nothing fundamental in the design of an RCT that precludes investigating heterogeneous effects in different populations, to do so requires careful consideration of the sample size and identification of subgroups of interest prior to the randomization. As a result, many RCTs have not been able to answer important questions about variability in effects across subpopulations or which components of an intervention are driving the results. While RCTs can be used to study the effect of separate program components, it is difficult to use RCTs to examine complex programs with multiple dimensions (or for community-level interventions). RCTs remain a critical tool for studying the effectiveness of programs, but it is important to note their limitations as well. (See Chapter 8 for a research recommendation on this topic.)

Because of the limitations of RCTs in some contexts, and limitations of observational studies that are correlational in nature, researchers have increasingly used "natural experiments" to estimate causal effects. Such studies harness changes in state and local policies that generate plausibly random or quasi-random variation in exposure to a given service or treatment to estimate its causal effect on outcomes of interest (see Angrist and Pischke, 2009, for an overview of these methods). Despite the limitations of estimation based on observational data, careful use of observational data has many advantages. First, it is very useful for identifying associations that can be more rigorously studied using other approaches. Second, in some cases, careful use of natural experiments or other research designs can minimize the bias from confounding. Finally, some questions are, by their nature, not amenable to randomized trials and so can only be studied using observational data. The way data are gathered across study designs also varies, as data collection may occur for different outcomes at different points in time, so the data may be incomplete and therefore hard to compare.

When reviewing the science on a certain intervention or policy, there may be cases with strong evidence for one or more important outcomes and weaker (or mixed, or null) evidence for one or more other outcomes. This does not mean that the intervention or policy should not be considered or implemented. If there is a strong theoretical basis for making the change (e.g., from a biological pathway or development standpoint) and strong evidence for one or more salient health outcomes that is being targeted and has a large population health impact, the intervention or policy could be deemed appropriate despite its limitations. This is true for several interventions and policies recommended in this report.

About the Report Recommendations

The committee provides a range of recommendations for practice, policy, and systems change, including recommendations that will take time and sustained commitment to achieve and recommendations that could be implemented immediately or in the near term. Some of the committee's recommendations will be difficult to implement; however, the degree of difficulty in implementing any given recommendation does not mean it is not worth pursuing. Achieving health equity for children will require attention and commitment from a range of sectors. For example, in Chapter 8, the committee discusses the need for better alignment among the many children- and family-serving sectors in the United States. Although there are many barriers to achieving alignment, there is also great opportunity to make long-lasting reductions in long-standing and persistent inequities. Furthermore, inequities that originate at the system and institutional levels will require solutions that target policy and structures. Given this understanding, the committee provides the recommendations with the long-term outcomes in mind and the goal of both improving the current state and making strides today to establish systems where inequities will no longer be the status quo. Where possible, the committee also recommends or highlights ways to leverage existing programs that either embrace the core scientific principles laid out in this report (see the Core Concepts below and Chapter 2) or have a strong basic structure from which to build (e.g., home visiting). Therefore, the committee makes some recommendations for improving programs that are not optimally or extensively implemented but have the potential to be updated, scaled, or better used to promote related services that advance health equity.

Given the fragmented nature of many systems in the United States (e.g., the health care system has both public and private payers and multiple entities that set guidelines for care and accountability), many of the committee's recommendations are directed to multiple actors with varying roles and responsibilities, each of whom is important to advancing child and family outcomes. Furthermore, as a matter of jurisdiction, some recommendations are better targeted to varying levels of government (e.g., local, state, tribal, and territorial). To address deeply rooted inequities, which play out across multiple sectors, some recommendations entail a comprehensive approach that requires partnerships across sectors and levels of government—this is consistent with *Communities in Action* (NASEM, 2017), which identifies cross-sector collaboration as a key element for promoting health equity in communities.

Resources Resources will be needed to implement many of the recommendations in this report. The root causes of structural inequities are found in differential access by virtue of race or ethnicity to resources for some groups, due in part to certain laws and policies (NASEM, 2017; see also Chapter 3). Calling for change of any kind to advance health equity will require changes to laws, policies, and other sources of inequity so as not to perpetuate structural racism and discrimination. Decision makers and leaders can coordinate, integrate services, and educate on all of these issues, but if the resources are not there to back the needed changes, the change likely will not occur. The committee was asked by RWJF to identify *what* practice, policy, and systems changes need to be implemented, based on what is known from developmental science; however, the committee was not tasked to identify the sources or mechanisms for funding those changes. In a few instances, the committee was able to provide estimates of the potential costs for implementing its recommendations using existing estimates. Doing so, however, was complicated when those estimates did not include cost savings from improved health outcomes resulting from the intervention, producing a one-sided picture.

Although the committee was not asked to identify the mechanisms and sources for implementing the report recommendations, there are many extant mechanisms and proposals for funding various public or population health activities. For example, taxes on tobacco, alcohol, and other products (such as sugary beverages) have been used to channel resources and shape economic incentives (NASEM, 2018b). An IOM (2012) committee proposed establishing a tax on medical care transactions to provide a long-term financing structure to cover public health services. Other mechanisms—both within and outside the health sector—include federal or state Wellness Trusts (Prevention Institute, 2015), hospital community benefit expenditures (Rosenbaum et al., 2015), community wealth building (including the role of anchor institutions; see Porter et al., 2019), and Children's Services Councils.[12] (A National Academies Proceedings of a Workshop—in Brief [NASEM, 2018b] provides an overview of several of these options and others.) Each of these financing mechanisms has advantages and disadvantages that would need to be weighed for the specific intervention or program for which it is considered.

Promising Models

In its Statement of Task, the committee was asked to identify promising examples of models that apply the science of early development to health equity. The committee adapted the selection criteria used in the *Communities in Action: Pathways to Health Equity* (NASEM, 2017) report

---

[12] See, for example, http://flchildrenscouncil.org/about-cscs/overview (accessed June 17, 2019).

to guide this process.[13] The committee used the three sets of criteria from the 2017 National Academies report (see Appendix A for a list of all of the selection criteria), which were informed by research and practice-based evidence and the expertise of the committee members. The committee made a few additions based on the focus of this report (the prenatal through early childhood period) and removed those not relevant to this study. The first set consists of six core criteria, which need to be met by all of the promising models. These core criteria ensure that the examples chosen are substantively significant. The committee used these promising models as examples throughout the report to highlight bright spots that have been able to use what is known from the science to advance health equity in the preconception through early childhood periods. Furthermore, "promising" does not imply that the model is new but rather that it is a program or intervention that met the committee's core criteria, and each promising model has a unique approach and is at a different phase of development: some have been around for more than 30 years and have changed based on evaluations or input from users, while others have emerged in the past few years. In Chapters 4–7, three promising models were identified for each chapter (each model is summarized in a box). These examples are not blueprints, and exact replicas might not work with all populations or locations; however, the lessons learned and approaches used prove valuable to those working to create positive change toward health equity during the preconception through early childhood periods. Note that throughout the report, the committee cites many other examples of current practices and programs that illustrate the topic being discussed; however, those examples may not meet all of the committee's criteria (and are not labeled as promising models).

The first core criterion requires that the model's main focus be during the prenatal and/or early childhood period, as that is the focus of this report; this inevitably involves the mother (or other primary caregiver). The second notes that the intervention is informed by findings from the neurobiological, socio-behavioral, and/or biological sciences—also a focus of this report.

The third core criterion is that the model addresses at least one (preferably more) of the nine SDOH identified by the 2017 National Academies report: education, employment, health systems and services, housing, income and wealth, the physical environment, public safety, the social environment, and transportation. "This criterion was informed by the wealth of literature suggesting the importance of targeting the social and economic conditions that affect health, especially at the community

---

[13] The original criteria from the 2017 National Academies report are available at https://www.nap.edu/read/24624/chapter/7#323 (accessed July 29, 2019).

level" (Bradley et al., 2016; Galea et al., 2011; Heiman and Artiga, 2015; Hood et al., 2016; NASEM, 2017; Wenger, 2012). Furthermore, this criterion is basic to the committee's charge, which posits that the SDOH need to be addressed to reduce health inequities. The fourth criterion is that the model is designed to have or has evidence of having an impact on a group or population that experiences health inequities.

The fifth core criterion "states that the solution needs to be multisectoral, meaning that it engages one or more sectors" (ideally, at least one "nontraditional" sector, meaning other than public health or health care). Multisector collaboration is a powerful lever for addressing health inequities and building a culture of health (APHA, 2015; Danaher, 2011; Davis et al., 2016; Kottke et al., 2016; Mattessich and Rausch, 2014). Engaging stakeholders across multiple sectors provides the opportunity for innovative and cost-effective methods to sustain solutions at the community level (NASEM, 2017).

The sixth core criterion requires the solution to be evidence informed.

This entails an assessment of evidence or the best available information to identify a problem and develop a solution that has a measurable outcome. Here, there is considerable flexibility in terms of the type of evidence that will qualify. This flexibility is based on the understanding that low-resource communities that suffer from health inequities often do not have the infrastructure, personnel, or financial resources to provide the highest standard of evidence. (NASEM, 2017, p. 326)

The sixth core criterion is that there needs to be an evaluation plan with identified outcome measures to track the impact of the intervention.

The second set of criteria—aspirational criteria—reflects the elements, processes, and outcomes of interventions that the committee identified as valuable for promoting health equity. This set of criteria highlights important features of interventions, such as nontraditional partners or nonhealth domains (e.g., community organizers, public libraries, Parent Teacher Association groups) and an intervention being interdisciplinary and/or multilevel (the intervention has multiple levels of influence, such as individual, family, organizational/institutional, or governmental).

THE SCIENCE OF EARLY DEVELOPMENT: CORE CONCEPTS

Based on its review of the science, the committee updated the core concepts from the 2000 NRC and IOM report *From Neurons to Neighborhoods* and identified 12 core concepts of early development, with a focus on equity. The evidence behind these concepts is described in Chapters 2–4, and this evidence guided the committee in developing recommendations that are responsive to the science of early development.

1. **Biology–environment interaction impacts health and development:** Human long-term social, emotional, behavioral, cognitive, and physical health is shaped by genetic, epigenetic, and environmental factors that integrate biological information at the level of molecular, cellular, and organ systems with the family, neighborhood, and culture in which the individual is embedded. These developmental processes start before conception through a dynamic and continuous interaction between biology and aspects of the environment and extend throughout the life-span.

2. **Brain development proceeds in well-defined but continuous steps:** Human developmental processes are now conceptualized as continuous, rather than occurring in discrete stages as was originally thought. A sequence of temporally well-defined sensitive periods (sometimes referred to as *"critical periods"*) of brain maturation—in tandem with environmental influences—lead to the acquisition of social, emotional, and cognitive skills. During these sensitive periods, early adverse experiences influence brain development and can alter the trajectories of development in each of these functional domains, impacting long-term well-being.

3. **Major physiological systems develop rapidly in pregnancy and early childhood:** It is now known that physiological systems other than the brain, such as the immune system, microbiome, and endocrine system, can also be influenced preconceptionally. Like the brain, these systems begin to develop prenatally, with early sensitive pre- and postnatal periods that can be disrupted by early adversity. These early influences can have long-term consequences for mental and physical health.

4. **The early caregiving environment is crucial for long-term development:** The family and community caregiving professionals have a central role in early childhood development, indicating the need for a multigenerational approach to ensuring optimal growth and development. The child thrives in healthy relationships throughout childhood, but relationships with parents are the building blocks for subsequent relationships and child outcomes. For example, maternal–child interactions impact the well-being of both mother and child, where a positive mother–child relationship rests on good maternal well-being (whereas prolonged maternal distress impairs parenting and the quality of attachment).

5. **The developing child plays an important role in interactions and development:** Children are active participants in their own development, reflecting the intrinsic human drive to explore and master one's environment. Early experiences create biological

structures, and shape psychological and behavioral adjustment, in ways that influence how the child will react and act in response to later environmental demands.

6. **The development of executive functions[14] is a key aspect of early childhood development:** The emergence and maturation of executive functions (inhibitory control, mental flexibility, and working memory) are a cornerstone of early childhood development. Executive function maturation continues through early adulthood and contributes to the health, well-being, and productivity of adults.

7. **Trajectories—positive or negative—are not immutable:** The developing child remains vulnerable to risks and open to protective influences through adolescence and young adulthood, although early life represents the stage at which interventions are most effective in positively influencing a child's development.

8. **There is variability of individual and group development:** Individual children demonstrate significant variability in these sensitive periods of brain development and in response to interventions. This variability often makes it difficult to distinguish among typical development, maturational delays, transient disorders, and persistent impairments or to predict response to treatment. Understanding this heterogeneity of development and individual differences in access and responsiveness to interventions is a major goal.

9. **Experiences across environmental contexts play a significant role in early development:** Children can be more or less sensitive to experiences due in part to their biological makeup, but this is impacted powerfully by multiple family and community factors. These include family interactions and adversity, accessibility to community programs and interventions, and environmental factors, such as quality and stability of housing, toxic environmental exposures, food accessibility, early childhood education, family support, and culture. Effective interventions can alter the course of development throughout childhood by changing the balance between risk and protective processes, leading to more adaptive outcomes.

---

[14] Executive function (and self-regulation) skills "are the mental processes that enable us to plan, focus attention, remember instructions, and juggle multiple tasks successfully. Just as an air traffic control system at a busy airport safely manages the arrivals and departures of many aircraft on multiple runways, the brain needs this skill set to filter distractions, prioritize tasks, set and achieve goals, and control impulses" (Center for the Developing Child at Harvard University, see https://developingchild.harvard.edu/science/key-concepts/executive-function [accessed June 17, 2019]).

10. **Disparities in access to critical resources matter:** Disparities in health and developmental outcomes result from not only health care disparities but also disparities and inequities in family and community factors. Achieving equity in health and developmental outcomes in young children requires addressing health care disparities and also ensuring those family and neighborhood conditions in which all children and families can be healthy and thriving.

11. **Health outcomes are the result of experiences across the life course:** Birth and early developmental outcomes are influenced by the health of the mother and father not only during pregnancy but also before and between pregnancies and across the life course, starting with their own prenatal and early life experiences. Disparities in the child's birth and early developmental outcomes are therefore the consequences of not only differential exposures during pregnancy and early childhood but of differential parental life course trajectories set forth by early programming mechanisms and influenced by cumulative life adversity.

12. **Early interventions matter and are generally more cost effective than later ones:** Family-based interventions that consider both risk and resilience and are informed by or sensitive to the mores and values of the target population can potentially positively change developmental pathways. The integration of various levels of services that are community based and have supportive policies in place tends to be more effective.

OVERVIEW OF THE STUDY PROCESS AND REPORT

To address its charge, the committee gathered information through a variety of means. It held two information-gathering meetings that were webcast live, in August and October 2018 (the meeting agendas are listed in Appendix B). The committee also held deliberative meetings throughout the study process. The committee received public submissions of materials for its consideration throughout the course of the study.[15] The committee's online activity page provided information to the public about its work and facilitated communication with the public.[16]

Throughout this report, the committee provides conclusions and recommendations. Chapter 2 provides an overview of healthy development from conception through early childhood, including what is new in the science of development since the publication of *From Neurons to Neighborhoods* (NRC and IOM, 2000). It aims to demystify the "black box"

---

[15] Public access materials can be requested from paro@nas.edu.

[16] See nationalacademies.org/earlydevelopment (accessed July 29, 2019).

of development for the public, practitioners that work with children, and policy makers and to convey that we know enough about early development to act now to advance health equity for children and families. Chapter 3 provides an overview of the critical influences or factors that can either promote or hinder healthy development, with a focus on factors that shape inequities at the child/family level and the community and population levels across the SDOH. Chapter 4 focuses on how to best foster children's healthy psychosocial development, emotional adjustment, and physical health using what science has shown about risk and resilience and the importance of healthy relationships among children and families in high-risk contexts. Chapter 5 explores the role of the health care system in advancing health equity and what the system would need to look like from preconception through early childhood to meet the developmental needs of children. Chapter 6 provides recommendations on how to better meet the fundamental needs of families and children through economic security, stable and safe housing, and protection from environmental toxicants. Chapter 7 discusses the critical role of ECE and how it can serve as a platform for advancing health equity for children and families. Chapter 8 addresses needed systems changes and summarizes the opportunities to overcome barriers to strengthen a systems approach, the key stakeholders who need to be involved, and necessary alignment, measures, and research based on the committee's assessment of the literature in Chapters 2–7. Finally, Chapter 9 highlights the main findings and concepts discussed throughout this report and summarizes the report recommendations, laying out a roadmap for applying and advancing the science of early development.

CONCLUDING OBSERVATIONS

The science of early development is clear. Long-term physical health and emotional, behavioral, social, and cognitive competence is shaped by genetic, epigenetic, and environmental factors, including their interactions, before conception and through the life-span. There are risk factors that necessitate action at the practice, policy, and systems levels that take into account the full range of factors that impact health and well-being. These actions need to be taken before insults to early development occur; however, the science of plasticity indicates that it is never too late to intervene. These actions need to take a life course, multigenerational approach to make progress on health inequity, because the well-being of a child depends on the well-being of a parent/caregiver. Multipronged, cross-sector interventions, focused on prevention, early detection, and mitigation and working at the policy, system, and program levels, are needed to move toward health equity.

REFERENCES

ACOG (American College of Obstetricians and Gynecologists). n.d. *Racial disparities in maternal mortality in the United States: The postpartum period is a missed opportunity for action.* https://www.acog.org/-/media/Departments/Toolkits-for-Health-Care-Providers/Postpartum-Toolkit/ppt-racial.pdf?dmc=1&ts=20190716T2208336641 (accessed July 16, 2019).

Alker, J., and O. Pham. 2018. *Nation's progress on children's health coverage reverses course.* Washington, DC: Georgetown University Health Policy Institute, Center for Children and Families.

Angrist, J. D., and J. Pischke. 2009. *Mostly harmless econometrics: An empiricist's companion.* Princeton, NJ: Princeton University Press.

APHA (American Public Health Association). 2015. *Opportunities for health collaboration: Leveraging community development investments to improve health in low-income neighborhoods.* Washington, DC: American Public Health Association.

Auten, G., and D. Splinter. 2018. *Income inequality in the United States: Using tax data to measure long-term trends.* http://davidsplinter.com/AutenSplinter-Tax_Data_and_Inequality.pdf (accessed August 12, 2019).

Bellis, M., K. Hughes, K. Hardcastle, K. Ashton, K. Ford, Z. Quigg, and A. Davies. 2017. The impact of adverse childhood experiences on health service use across the life course using a retrospective cohort study. *Journal of Health Services Research & Policy* 22(3):168–177.

Bethell, C. D., P. Newacheck, E. Hawes, and N. Halfon. 2014. Adverse childhood experiences: Assessing the impact on health and school engagement and the mitigating role of resilience. *Health Affairs* 33(12):2106–2115.

Boschma, J., and R. Brownstein. 2016. *The concentration of poverty in American schools.* https://www.theatlantic.com/education/archive/2016/02/concentration-poverty-american-schools/471414 (accessed July 13, 2019).

Bradley, E. H., M. Canavan, E. Rogan, K. Talbert-Slagle, C. Ndumele, L. Taylor, and L. A. Curry. 2016. Variation in health outcomes: The role of spending on social services, public health, and health care, 2000–09. *Health Affairs (Project Hope)* 35(5):760–768.

Braveman, P., and C. Barclay. 2009. Health disparities beginning in childhood: A life-course perspective. *Pediatrics* 124(Suppl 3):S163–S175.

Bronfenbrenner, U. 1979. *The ecology of human development: Experiments by nature and design.* London: Harvard University Press.

Campbell, F., G. Conti, J. J. Heckman, S. H. Moon, R. Pinto, E. Pungello, and Y. Pan. 2014. Early childhood investments substantially boost adult health. *Science* 343(6178):1478–1485.

CBPP (Center on Budget and Policy Priorities). 2018. *A guide to statistics on historical trends in income inequality.* https://www.cbpp.org/research/poverty-and-inequality/a-guide-to-statistics-on-historical-trends-in-income-inequality (accessed July 13, 2019).

CDC (Centers for Disease Control and Prevention). 2016. *Reproductive and birth outcomes.* https://ephtracking.cdc.gov/showRbLBWGrowthRetardationEnv.action (accessed April 17, 2019).

CDC. 2019a. *Division of nutrition, physical activity and obesity at a glance.* https://www.cdc.gov/chronicdisease/resources/publications/aag/dnpao.htm (accessed July 13, 2019).

CDC. 2019b. *Infant mortality.* https://www.cdc.gov/reproductivehealth/maternalinfanthealth/infantmortality.htm (accessed July 15, 2019).

CDC. 2019c. *Most recent asthma data.* https://www.cdc.gov/asthma/most_recent_data.htm (accessed July 16, 2019).

Center on the Developing Child at Harvard University. 2016. *From best practices to breakthrough impacts: A science-based approach to building a more promising future for young children and families.* Cambridge, MA: Harvard University.

Center on the Developing Child at Harvard University. n.d. *Toxic stress.* https://developingchild.harvard.edu/science/key-concepts/toxic-stress (accessed July 13, 2019).

Child Trends. 2015. *Early school readiness.* https://www.childtrends.org/wp-content/uploads/2016/03/indicator_1457981601.385.pdf (accessed July 16, 2019).

Child Trends. 2016. *Dual language learners.* https://www.childtrends.org/indicators/dual-language-learners (accessed July 13, 2019).

Child Trends. 2018a. *Immigrant children.* https://www.childtrends.org/indicators/immigrant-children (accessed July 13, 2019).

Child Trends. 2018b. *Low and very low birthweight infants.* https://www.childtrends.org/indicators/low-and-very-low-birthweight-infants (accessed July 5, 2019).

Child Trends. 2018c. *Racial and ethnic composition of the child population.* https://www.childtrends.org/indicators/racial-and-ethnic-composition-of-the-child-population (accessed July 13, 2019).

CMS (Centers for Medicare & Medicaid Services). 2017. *National health expenditures 2017 highlights.* https://www.cms.gov/Research-Statistics-Data-and-Systems/Statistics-Trends-and-Reports/NationalHealthExpendData/Downloads/highlights.pdf (accessed July 16, 2019).

Creanga, A. A., C. J. Berg, C. Syverson, K. Seed, F. C. Bruce, and W. M. Callaghan. 2015. Pregnancy-related mortality in the United States, 2006–2010. *Obstetrics & Gynecology* 125(1):5–12.

Daily, S., S. Burkhauser, and T. Halle. 2010. A review of school readiness practices in the States: Early learning guidelines and assessments. *Child Trends: Early Childhood Highlights* 1(3):1–12.

Danaher, A. 2011. *Reducing health inequities: Enablers and barriers to inter-sectoral collaboration.* Ontario, Canada: Wellesley Institute.

Darling-Hammond, L. 1998. *Unequal opportunity: Race and education.* Washington, DC: The Brookings Institution.

Davis, R., S. Savannah, M. Harding, A. Macaysa, and L. F. Parks. 2016. *Countering the production of inequities: An emerging systems framework to achieve an equitable culture of health.* Oakland, CA: Prevention Institute.

Ely, D. M., A. K. Driscoll, and T. J. Mathews. 2017. *Infant mortality rates in rural and urban areas in the United States, 2014. NCHS data brief no. 285.* Hyattsville, MD: National Center for Health Statistics.

Fang, X., D. S. Brown, C. S. Florence, and J. A. Mercy. 2012. The economic burden of child maltreatment in the United States and implications for prevention. *Child Abuse and Neglect* 36(2):156–165.

FFYF (First Five Years Fund). 2018. *After recent historic progress, early childhood education could be a unifying issue for a divided Congress.* https://www.ffyf.org/after-recent-historic-progress-early-childhood-education-could-be-a-unifying-issue-for-a-divided-congress (accessed July 13, 2019).

Galea, S., M. Tracy, K. J. Hoggatt, C. Dimaggio, and A. Karpati. 2011. Estimated deaths attributable to social factors in the United States. *American Journal of Public Health* 101(8):1456–1465.

Galindo, C., and B. Fuller. 2010. The social competence of Latino kindergartners and growth in mathematical understanding. *Developmental Psychology* 46(3):579–592.

Garcia, J. L., J. J. Heckman, D. E. Leaf, and M. J. Prados. 2017. *Quantifying the life-cycle benefits of a prototypical early childhood program.* NBER Working Papers from National Bureau of Economic Research, No. 23479.

García Coll, C., and A. Kerivan Marks. 2009. *Immigrant stories: Ethnicity and academics in middle childhood.* New York: Oxford University Press.

García Coll, C., K. Crnic, G. Lamberty, B. H. Wasik, R. Jenkins, H. V. Garcia, and H. P. McAdoo. 1996. An integrative model for the study of developmental competencies in minority children. *Child Development* 67(5):1891–1914.

GBD (Global Burden of Diseases, Injuries, and Risk Factors) 2015 Maternal Mortality Collaborators. 2016. Global, regional, and national levels of maternal mortality, 1990–2015: A systematic analysis for the Global Burden of Disease Study 2015. *Lancet* 338:1775–1812.

Ghandour, R. M., M. D. Kogan, S. J. Blumberg, J. R. Jones, and J. M. Perrin. 2012. Mental health conditions among school-aged children: Geographic and sociodemographic patterns in prevalence and treatment. *Journal of Developmental and Behavioral Pediatrics* 33(1):42–54.

Ghandour, R. M., K. Anderson Moore, K. Murphy, C. Bethell, J. Jones, R. Harwood, J. Buerlein, M. Kogan, and M. Lu. 2018. School readiness among U.S. children: Development of a pilot measure. *Child Indicators Research* 1–23.

Gluckman, P. D., M. A. Hanson, and A. S. Beedle. 2007. Early life events and their consequences for later disease: A life history and evolutionary perspective. *American Journal of Human Biology* 19(1):1–19.

Gould, E. 2009. Childhood lead poisoning: Conservative estimates of the social and economic benefits of lead hazard control. *Environmental Health Perspectives* 117(7):1162–1167.

Grinshteyn, E., and D. Hemenway. 2016. Violent death rates: The US compared with other high-income OECD countries, 2010. *American Journal of Medicine* 129(3):266–273.

Gunja, M., S. Collins, M. Doty, and S. Beutel. 2017. *How the Affordable Care Act has helped women gain insurance and improved their ability to get health care: Findings from the Commonwealth Fund Biennial Health Insurance Survey, 2016*. https://www.commonwealthfund.org/publications/issue-briefs/2017/aug/how-affordable-care-act-has-helped-women-gain-insurance-and (accessed July 16, 2019).

Hahn, R. A. 2019. Two paths to health in all policies: The traditional public health path and the path of social determinants. *American Journal of Public Health* 109(2):253–254.

Halfon, N., K. Larson, M. Lu, E. Tullis, and S. Russ. 2014. Lifecourse health development: Past, present and future. *Maternal and Child Health Journal* 18(2):344–365.

Heckman, J. J., J. E. Humphries, and G. Veramendi. 2018. Returns to education: The causal effects of education on earnings, health, and smoking. *Journal of Political Economy* 126(Suppl 1):S197–S246.

Heiman, H., and S. Artiga. 2015. *Beyond health care: The role of social determinants in promoting health and health equity*. Washington, DC: Kaiser Family Foundation.

Heindel, J. J., and L. N. Vandenberg. 2015. Developmental origins of health and disease: A paradigm for understanding disease cause and prevention. *Current Opinion in Pediatrics* 27(2):248–253.

Hood, C. M., K. P. Gennuso, G. R. Swain, and B. B. Catlin. 2016. County health rankings: Relationships between determinant factors and health outcomes. *American Journal of Preventive Medicine* 50(2):129–135.

Houtrow, A. J., K. Larson, L. M. Olson, P. W. Newacheck, and N. Halfon. 2014. Changing trends of childhood disability, 2001–2011. *Pediatrics* 134(3):530–538.

Hughes, K., M. A. Bellis, K. A. Hardcastle, D. Sethi, A. Butchart, C. Mikton, L. Jones, and M. P. Dunne. 2017. The effect of multiple adverse childhood experiences on health: A systematic review and meta-analysis. *Lancet Public Health* 2(8):e356–e366.

Inequality.org. n.d. *Income inequality in the United States*. https://inequality.org/facts/income-inequality (accessed July 16, 2019).

IOM (Institute of Medicine). 2007. *Preterm birth: Causes, consequences, and prevention*. Washington, DC: The National Academies Press.

IOM. 2012. *For the public's health: Investing in a healthier future*. Washington, DC: The National Academies Press.

IOM. 2015. *Business engagement in building healthy communities: Workshop summary.* Washington, DC: The National Academies Press.

Isaacs, J. B., C. Lou, H. Hahn, A. Hong, C. Quakenbush, and C. E. Steuerle. 2018. *Kids' share 2018: Report on federal expenditures on children through 2017 and future projections.* Washington, DC: The Urban Institute.

Kaiser Family Foundation. 2019. *The uninsured and the ACA: A primer—key facts about health insurance and the uninsured amidst changes to the Affordable Care Act.* https://www.kff.org/report-section/the-uninsured-and-the-aca-a-primer-key-facts-about-health-insurance-and-the-uninsured-amidst-changes-to-the-affordable-care-act-how-have-health-insurance-coverage-options-and-availability-changed (accessed July 16, 2019).

Karoly, L. A., M. R. Kilburn, and J. S. Cannon. 2005. *Early childhood interventions: Proven results, future promise.* Santa Monica, CA: RAND.

Korous, K., J. Causadias, R. H. Bradley, and S. Luthar. 2018. Unpacking the link between socioeconomic status and behavior problems: A second-order meta-analysis. *Development and Psychopathology* 30(5):1889–1906.

Kottke, T. E., M. Stiefel, and N. P. Pronk. 2016. "Well-being in all policies": Promoting cross-sectoral collaboration to improve people's lives. *Preventing Chronic Disease* 13:160155.

Lantz, P. 2018. The medicalization of population health: Who will stay upstream? *The Milbank Quarterly* 97(1):36–39.

Lynch, J. 2006. *Age in the welfare state.* London: Cambridge University Press.

Martin, A., M. Hartman, B. Washington, A. Catlin, and the National Health Expenditure Accounts Team. 2018a. National health care spending in 2017: Growth slows to post–great recession rates; share of GDP stabilizes. *Health Affairs* 38(1):96–106.

Martin, J. A., B. E. Hamilton, M. J. K. Osterman, A. K. Driscoll, and P. Drake. 2018b. Births: Final data for 2016. *National Vital Statistics Reports* 67(1). https://www.cdc.gov/nchs/data/nvsr/nvsr67/nvsr67_01.pdf (accessed August 12, 2019).

Martin, N., and R. Montagne. 2017. *U.S. has the worst rate of maternal deaths in the developed world.* https://www.npr.org/2017/05/12/528098789/u-s-has-the-worst-rate-of-maternal-deaths-in-the-developed-world (accessed June 25, 2019).

Masters, R., E. Anwar, B. Collins, R. Cookson, and S. Capewell. 2017. Return on investment of public health interventions: A systematic review. *Journal of Epidemiology and Community Health* 71(8):827–834.

Mattessich, P. W., and E. J. Rausch. 2014. Cross-sector collaboration to improve community health: A view of the current landscape. *Health Affairs (Project Hope)* 33(11):1968–1974.

McFarlane, A. C. 2010. The long-term costs of traumatic stress: Intertwined physical and psychological consequences. *World psychiatry: Official Journal of the World Psychiatric Association (WPA)* 9(1):3–10.

McLaughlin, M., and M. R. Rank. 2018. Estimating the economic cost of childhood poverty in the United States. *Social Work Research* 42(2):73–83.

McLeroy, K. R., D. Bibeau, A. Steckler, and K. Glanz. 1988. An ecological perspective on health promotion programs. *Health Education Quarterly* 15(4):351–377.

MHTF (Maternal Health Task Force). n.d. *Maternal health in the United States* https://www.mhtf.org/topics/maternal-health-in-the-united-states (accessed July 16, 2019).

Muennig, P., D. Robertson, G. Johnson, F. Campbell, E. P. Pungello, and M. Neidell. 2011. The effect of an early education program on adult health: The Carolina Abecedarian project randomized controlled trial. *American Journal of Public Health* 101(3):512–516.

NASEM (National Academies of Sciences, Engineering, and Medicine). 2016. *Parenting matters: Supporting parents of children ages 0–8.* Washington, DC: The National Academies Press.

NASEM. 2017. *Communities in action: Pathways to health equity.* Washington, DC: The National Academies Press.

NASEM. 2018a. *Building sustainable financing structures for population health: Insights from non-health sectors: Proceedings of a workshop.* Washington, DC: The National Academies Press.

NASEM. 2018b. *Exploring tax policy to advance population health, health equity, and economic prosperity: Proceedings of a workshop—in brief.* Washington, DC: The National Academies Press.

NASEM. 2019a. *The promise of adolescence: Realizing opportunity for all youth.* Washington, DC: The National Academies Press.

NASEM. 2019b. *A roadmap to reducing child poverty.* Washington, DC: The National Academies Press.

National MCH Workforce Development Center. 2015. *The Affordable Care Act: A working guide for MCH professionals.* http://www.amchp.org/Transformation-Station/Transformation_Station_Documents/ACA-guide.pdf (accessed June 18, 2019).

Nelson, D., M. Moniz, and M. Davis. 2018. Population-level factors associated with maternal mortality in the United States, 1997–2012. *BMC Public Health* 18:1007.

NRC and IOM (National Research Council and Institute of Medicine). 2004. *Children's health, the nation's wealth: Assessing and improving child health.* Washington, DC: The National Academies Press.

NRC and IOM. 2013. *Health in international perspective: Shorter lives, poorer health.* Washington, DC: The National Academies Press.

OECD (Organisation for Economic Co-operation and Development). 2009. *United States country highlights—doing better for children.* https://www.oecd.org/unitedstates/43590390.pdf (accessed June 25, 2019).

OECD. 2014. *Society at a glance 2014: OECD social indicators.* http://www.oecd.org/els/soc/OECD2014-SocietyAtAGlance2014.pdf (accessed June 18, 2019).

OECD. 2017. *Health at a glance 2017—OECD indicators.* https://read.oecd-ilibrary.org/social-issues-migration-health/health-at-a-glance-2017_health_glance-2017-en#page1 (accessed July 13, 2019).

OECD. 2019. *PF3.1: Public spending on childcare and early education.* http://www.oecd.org/els/soc/PF3_1_Public_spending_on_childcare_and_early_education.pdf (accessed July 13, 2019).

Osterman, M. J. K., and J. A. Martin. 2018. Timing and adequacy of prenatal care in the United States, 2016. *National Vital Statistics Reports* 67(3):1–14.

Pager, D., and H. Shepherd. 2008. The sociology of discrimination: Racial discrimination in employment, housing, credit, and consumer markets. *Annual Review of Sociology* 34:181–209.

Pascoe, J. M., D. L. Wood, J. H. Duffee, and A. Kuo. 2016. Mediators and adverse effects of child poverty in the United States. *Pediatrics* 137(4).

Perrin, J. M., S. R. Bloom, and S. L. Gortmaker. 2007. The increase of childhood chronic conditions in the United States. *JAMA* 297(24):2755–2759.

Perrin, J. M., L. E. Anderson, and J. Van Cleave. 2014. The rise in chronic conditions among infants, children, and youth can be met with continued health system innovations. *Health Affairs* 33(12):2099–2105.

Perrin, J. M., J. R. Asarnow, T. Stancin, S. P. Melek, and G. K. Fritz. 2018. Mental health conditions and health care payments for children with chronic medical conditions. *Academic Pediatrics* 19(1):44–50.

Pew Research Center. 2015a. *The American family today.* https://www.pewsocialtrends.org/2015/12/17/1-the-american-family-today (accessed July 16, 2019).

Pew Research Center. 2015b. *Parenting in America: Outlook, worries, aspirations are strongly linked to financial situation.* Washington, DC: Pew Research Center.

Porter, J., D. Fisher-Bruns, and B. H. Pham. 2019. *Anchor collaboratives: Building bridges with place-based partnerships and anchor institutions.* Washington, DC: Democracy Collaborative.

Prevention Institute. 2015. *Sustainable investments in health: Prevention and wellness funds.* Oakland, CA: Blue Shield of California Foundation, The Kresge Foundation, and The California Endowment.

Rosenbaum, S., D. A. Kindig, J. Bao, M. K. Byrnes, and C. O'Laughlin. 2015. The value of the nonprofit hospital tax exemption was $24.6 billion in 2011. *Health Affairs* 34(7):1225–1233.

Seith, D., and E. Isakson. 2011. *Who are America's children: Examining health disparities among children in the U.S.* New York: National Center for Children in Poverty.

Shak, L., L. Mikkelsen, R. Gratz-Lazarus, and N. Schneider. 2013. *What's good for health is good for business: Engaging the business community in prevention efforts.* Oakland, CA: Prevention Institute.

Shonkoff, J. P., A. S. Garner, American Academy of Pediatrics Committee on Psychosocial Aspects of Child and Family Health, Committee on Early Childhood, Adoption, and Dependent Care, Section on Developmental and Behavioral Pediatrics. The lifelong effects of early childhood adversity and toxic stress. *Pediatrics* 129(1):e232–e246.

Slopen, N., J. P. Shonkoff, M. A. Albert, H. Yoshikawa, A. Jacobs, R. Stoltz, and D. R. Williams. 2016. Racial disparities in child adversity in the U.S.: Interactions with family immigration history and income. *American Journal of Preventive Medicine* 50(1):47–56.

Smeeding, T. 2012. *Income, wealth, and debt and the great recession.* Stanford, CA: Stanford Center on Poverty and Inequality.

Turney, K., and C. Wildeman. 2017. Adverse childhood experiences among children placed in and adopted from foster care: Evidence from a nationally representative survey. *Child Abuse and Neglect* 64:117–129.

U.S. Census. 2018. *Table FG10, family groups 2018.* https://www2.census.gov/programs-surveys/cps/techdocs/cpsmar18.pdf (accessed July 16, 2019).

Van Cleave, J., S. L. Gortmaker, and J. M. Perrin. 2010. Dynamics of obesity and chronic health conditions among children and youth. *JAMA* 303(7):623–630.

Velez-Agosto, N. M., J. G. Soto-Crespo, M. Vizcarrondo-Oppenheimer, S. Vega-Molina, and C. García Coll. 2017. Bronfenbrenner's bioecological theory revision: Moving culture from the macro into the micro. *Perspectives on Psychological Science* 12(5):900–910.

Waidmann, T., and Urban Institute. 2009. *Estimating the cost of racial and ethnic health disparities.* Washington, DC: Urban Institute. http://www.urban.org/UploadedPDF/411962_health_disparities.pdf (accessed July 13, 2019).

Walmsley, R. n.d. *World prison population list.* London: International Centre for Prison Studies King's College London School of Law.

Wenger, M. 2012. *Place matters: Ensuring opportunities for good health for all.* Washington, DC: Joint Center for Political and Economic Studies.

WHO (World Health Organization). 2010. *A conceptual framework for action on the social determinants of health. Social determinants of health discussion paper 2.* Geneva, Switzerland: World Health Organization.

WHO, UNFPA (United Nations Population Fund), World Bank Group, United Nations Population Division. 2015. *Trends in maternal mortality: 1990 to 2015: Estimates by WHO, UNICEF, UNFPA, World Bank Group and the United Nations Population Division.* https://www.who.int/reproductivehealth/publications/monitoring/maternal-mortality-2015/en (accessed August 12, 2019).

Zahran, H. S., C. M. Bailey, S. A. Damon, P. L. Garbe, and P. N. Breysse. 2018. Vital signs: Asthma in children—United States, 2001–2016. *Morbidity and Mortality Weekly Report* 67(5):149–155.

2

Healthy Development from Conception Through Early Childhood

INTRODUCTION TO THE SCIENCE FROM PRENATAL THROUGH EARLY CHILDHOOD

Fetal and early child development are often conceptualized as a "black box," in which children simply learn by soaking up information, much like a sponge and water. Developmental science has demonstrated that development is, in fact, an active process and that it starts early. Thus, understanding early development, when biological systems and functions are coming "online," is essential for ensuring that prevention, interventions, policies, and systems are responsive to the needs of children. This will provide children with the best opportunity for healthy outcomes. When the science of early development is coupled with a health equity approach to inform decision making, it provides an opportunity to improve outcomes for children and families in at-risk contexts. The goal of this chapter is to reveal core concepts of brain development and other systems relevant to understanding the impact of disparities on cognitive, social-emotional, and physical health and to describe new scientific advances in this area over the past 20 years. This information can be used by the public and policy makers to better inform effective actions for promoting healthy outcomes. (See Box 2-1 for an overview of this chapter.)

Early understanding of children's development, as postulated by Piaget and many others in the 20th century, consisted of age-specific stages, ruled primarily by maturation and biology (Flavell, 1963). This characterization has undergone profound revisions. The 2000 publication by the National Research Council and the Institute of Medicine,

BOX 2-1
Chapter in Brief: Healthy Development

There are theoretical, technical, and scientific advances over the past 20 years that have been instrumental in rapidly advancing the science of child development. This chapter highlights those advances and provides an overview of the core concepts of brain development and other body systems relevant to understanding the impact of early life adversity on cognitive, social-emotional, and physical health, including the mechanisms that link early life experiences to later outcomes. This information can be used by the public and policy makers to better inform effective actions for advancing health equity.

Scientific advances in the past 20–30 years include the following:

• Early experiences are essential for building brain connections that underlie biobehavioral health, and current understanding of whole-child development relies on an interplay of organ systems with each other and the environment.
• Responses to pre- and postnatal early adversity, such as poverty or maltreatment, are rooted in gene–environment interactions that can result in altered molecular and cellular development during sensitive periods of development.
• Chronic early adversity has negative impacts on the assembly of certain brain circuits and emotional control, cognitive growth, and stress responsiveness.
• Certain body systems involved in cognitive and emotional development are more sensitive to early disturbances that activate stress response networks and provide a basis for both short- and long-term functional consequences of early life stress.
• Early adversity can change the timing of critical periods of brain development, impacting the "plasticity" of developmental processes that are driven by experiences in the life of the young child and the family.
• Deciphering the mechanisms through which adversity disrupts foundational developmental processes of the whole child and the long-term impact on

From Neurons to Neighborhoods: The Science of Early Childhood Development, provided a transformational synthesis of existing research to reveal a complexity of factors that influence development beyond previous simplified models. This landmark report integrated a wealth of scientific knowledge on early childhood development to emphasize the continuous, dynamic interaction between the environment and the biological systems of each individual across the life course. The report offered clear recommendations for policy and the future of developmental science that were organized around core principles of child development that remain accurate to this day (NRC and IOM, 2000). The report inspired new science and novel ways to communicate the science to the public, service providers, and policy makers. *From Neurons to Neighborhoods*

health, wellness, personal and community relationships, and life-span productivity is being achieved through multidisciplinary, longitudinally designed research that has incorporated principles of human development, including individual differences and differential sensitivity to context.

Chapter conclusions in brief:

- Healthy development of the child begins in the preconception period and is dependent on a strong foundation built prenatally.
- Among all of the factors that may serve to buffer negative outcomes produced by toxic stress, supportive relationships between the child and the adults in life are essential.
- When considering the entire life course, it is early experiences, pre- and postnatally, that are the most powerful in working together with individual genetic makeup to influence the physical, mental, and cognitive development of the child.
- Science shows that maternal health and well-being is a major contributing factor to the development of the fetus and establishes a foundation for positive or negative child health outcomes.
- Based on the abundant science, the influence of access to basic resources prenatally, particularly nutritional, psychosocial, and health care components, is powerful. Resources to help families limit chronic stress may reduce risk for disrupted development and help close disparities based on race, ethnicity, and socioeconomic status.
- New data, combined with previous studies, provide a compelling demonstration that toxic stress substantially increases later-life risk for lower educational achievement and physical illnesses, including obesity and type 2 diabetes, cardiovascular disease, substance abuse, mental illness, cancer, and infectious disease. In addition to the adverse effects of toxic stress on the brain and nervous system, it also affects every other organ system in the child's body, impacting short- and long-term health.

spurred research to refine the fields' understanding of how environmental influences shape child development, even at a molecular resolution. The report motivated research to understand how health-promoting environments and responsive relationships enable a strong foundation for healthy child development (i.e., learning, adaptive behaviors, and optimal health), while chronic adversity in the absence of supporting caregivers can lead to increased risk for negative learning and health outcomes, both in childhood and well into adulthood.

In the two decades since the publication of the report, there has been a convergence of activities that led to many of the advances that will be described in this chapter. First, a wave of neurobiological studies in model systems and in humans underscored that responses to pre- and postnatal early life stress are rooted in genetic and environmental interactions that can result in altered molecular and cellular development that impacts the assembly of circuits during sensitive periods of development (Cameron et al., 2017; McEwen and Morrison, 2013; Shonkoff and Levitt, 2010). The demonstration that certain systems involved in cognitive and emotional development are more sensitive to early disturbances that activate stress response networks, such as the frontal cortex, hippocampus, amygdala, and hypothalamic-pituitary-adrenal (HPA) axis, provided a basis for both short- and long-term functional consequences of early life stress (Chen and Baram, 2016; Shonkoff et al., 2012). Second, life course theory (Ben-Shlomo et al., 2014; Kuh et al., 2003) and the developmental origins of an adult health and disease framework (Gluckman et al., 2007; Halfon et al., 2014) have become more widely adopted. Third, a key policy statement from the American Academy of Pediatrics in 2012 emphasized the important life-span health implications of the impact of early adversity, declaring a "need for the entire medical community to focus more attention on the roots of adult diseases that originate during the prenatal and early childhood periods" (Shonkoff et al., 2012, p. e233).

Numerous research teams have clearly documented the effects and some mechanisms through which early childhood adversity affects development. Early adversity, such as maltreatment (Cicchetti, 1996; Teicher et al., 2016) and poverty (Cicchetti and Curtis, 2006; Council on Community Pediatrics, 2016; Gabrieli and Bunge, 2017; Johnson et al., 2016; McEwen and McEwen, 2017), has negative impacts on selective brain circuits and emotional control, cognitive growth, and stress responsiveness. A new discovery from multiple animal studies shows that early adversity can change the timing of critical periods of brain development (Bath et al., 2016; Cameron et al., 2017; Hensch, 2016a; Heun-Johnson and Levitt, 2018), impacting the "plasticity" of developmental processes that are driven by experiences in the life of the young child and their family (Cicchetti, 2015a,b; Cicchetti and Blender, 2006; Pollak et al., 1997) (see Box 2-2). The extensions of the original retrospective Adverse Childhood Experiences (ACEs) Study by the Centers for Disease Control and Prevention and Kaiser Permanente fostered sustained scientific interest in the long-term implications of early childhood adversity (see Chapter 3 for more information). In addition, the prospective Dunedin Multidisciplinary Health and Development (Poulton et al., 2015), the Perry Preschool longitudinal study, and the Abecedarian studies (see Chapter 7 for more information on the Perry Preschool and Abecedarian projects) added to a growing body of scientific evidence that early experiences, positive or negative, have profound long-term effects on physical, mental, and cognitive functions. The U.S. Department of Health and Human Services introduced Healthy People 2020—and, subsequently, Healthy People 2030—which elevated the importance of research on strategies to intervene in health disparities, including among pregnant women and children, by declaring "the elimination of health disparities" as a national goal.[1]

Taken together, these research endeavors have generated many new questions about *when* and *how* early childhood adversity is incorporated biologically to influence long-term outcomes and about optimal approaches to address early adversity and racial/ethnic and socioeconomic health disparities. These activities, and others, have pioneered and proliferated a new field of research on the importance of prenatal and early childhood experiences for health across generations.

Beyond scientific advances, *From Neurons to Neighborhoods* can also be credited as the impetus for the establishment of the National Scientific Council on the Developing Child in 2003, which uses science to catalyze public and private activities to promote the healthy development of children (Center on the Developing Child at Harvard University, 2014) to "close the gaps" between what the science says and which actions will promote child well-being. Composed of subsets of members of the *From Neurons to Neighborhoods* committee and the MacArthur Foundation Research Network on Early Experience and Brain Development, the Council has a central objective of communicating the science to the public and policy makers. Through an ongoing collaboration with the FrameWorks Institute on applying qualitative and quantitative research on communicating the science of brain and child development, a suite of effective "explanatory metaphors" has been developed, including a taxonomy of the stress response: positive, tolerable, and toxic stress (National Scientific Council on the Developing Child, 2014; Shonkoff and Bales, 2011). The term "toxic stress" was proposed to describe "excessive or prolonged activation of the stress response systems" in the absence of buffering protection from adult caregivers (National Scientific Council on the Developing Child, 2014). Unlike positive or tolerable stress, "toxic stress" refers to biological changes in the child that can result in disruption of developing brain architecture and other maturing organs, dysregulation of metabolic processes, and excessive stress system activation. These responses can lead to increased risk for chronic diseases later in life (Shonkoff et al., 2009). These explanatory metaphors have been adopted by the American Academy of Pediatrics (Garner et al., 2012; Shonkoff and Garner, 2012) and helped the science of child development be incorporated into federal and state legislation that generated evidence-based policies (Center on the Developing Child at Harvard University, 2014; Thompson, 2016).

This chapter highlights a selection of important scientific advances since *From Neurons to Neighborhoods* (NRC and IOM, 2000). Next, key

---

[1] For more information, see https://www.cdc.gov/dhdsp/hp2020.htm (accessed June 17, 2019).

BOX 2-2
Chapter 2 Key Terms

- **Adaptive immune system:** A portion of the immune system that uses highly specialized cells to eliminate foreign pathogens in the body and that, through exposure to certain pathogens, is able to eliminate those pathogens again in future infections.
- **Allostasis:** The process by which the body responds to internal or external stressors to return to homeostasis, or balance.
- **Amygdala:** A brain structure that is responsible for detecting threats in the environment and preparing the individual for emergency events.
- **Autonomic nervous system:** A network of nerves and ganglia that uses specific neurotransmitters (see below) to regulate internal organ function. The autonomic nervous system has two complementary components:
  - ○ **Parasympathetic nervous system:** Often referred to as the "rest and digest" system, the parasympathetic nervous system activates the digestive system, slows breathing, and decreases heart rate.
  - ○ **Sympathetic nervous system:** Often referred to as the "fight or flight" system, the sympathetic nervous system prepares the organism for action by propelling blood to the brain and limbs to provide increased oxygen and glucose for energy, slowing digestion, and increasing attentiveness.
- **Axon:** A main component of neurons; relatively long, extended structures that conduct a signal down the length of the neuron and play a key role in how neurons communicate with each other.
- **Brain plasticity:** The process by which neurons within the brain change their gene expression, function, cellular architecture, and connections with other neurons in response to experiences and changes in the environment.
- **Cellular homeostasis:** The notion that, when perturbed by some internal or external stimulus, cells react via feedback loops to achieve physiological balance with their immediate environment.
- **Chemical signature:** A general term used to highlight how epigenetics results in changes to DNA by placing chemical marks to modify how genes are expressed.
- **Connectome:** A general term for the amalgamation of connections between different parts of the brain.
- **Cortex:** The outermost region of the brain that exhibits the greatest expansion in evolution, where billions of neurons reside, trillions of connections are made, and much of the brain's most complex computational activity takes place.
- **Cortisol:** A key hormone involved in the physiological stress response. It elevates cell metabolism by binding to receptors in all organs to influence how they function during a "flight or fight" response. In the human brain, specific brain circuits express high levels of the glucocorticoid receptor. When cortisol activates the receptor, this impacts mood, motivation, and threat detection. Cortisol also helps to restore physiological balance after stress and regulates how the body uses carbohydrates, fats, and proteins; inflammation; blood pressure and blood sugar; and the sleep/wake cycle. Excessive exposure to cortisol prenatally also impacts development.

- **Endogenous versus exogenous:** Endogenous materials are produced within an organism or cell (e.g., hormone or neurotransmitter), whereas exogenous materials are introduced from the outside environment (e.g., medication or environmental toxicant).
- **Epigenetics:** The study of how genes are expressed or suppressed based on chemical changes to cells' DNA due to biological factors that come from changes in the environment, including how these biological factors can be passed down from one generation to the next.
- **Gene expression:** The mechanism by which DNA (composed of individual genes) is read and then turned into proteins that perform various functions throughout the body.
- **Genome:** An organism's complete set of DNA, including all of its genes. In humans, all cells that have a nucleus contain a copy of the genome, which consists of a highly organized arrangement of more than 3 million DNA base pairs.
- **Genome sequencing:** The scientific technique of identifying the genes that are present in a genome. This can be a sequence of either an organism's entire genome or certain parts of it.
- **Genomics:** The study of the structure, expression, and function of specific genes and of the entire collection of genes (genome).
- **Germ cells:** Embryonic cells that contain half the genetic material (chromosomes) necessary to form a complete organism. In men, they produce sperm, and in women, they produce eggs/ova.
- **Glia:** A category of cells within the brain that do not make connections (synapses) like neurons but do perform many important functions, including supporting neuronal metabolic health, contributing to the integrity of the blood–brain barrier to mediate access by blood-borne substances, viruses, and bacteria, controlling access by neurons to chemical neurotransmitters that are released by other neurons, aiding in the conduction of electrical signals, and removing cellular debris.
- **Innate immune system:** A portion of the immune system that removes foreign substances in tissues throughout the body and acts as a physical or chemical inflammatory barrier to infections but is not highly adaptable to a wide variety of infections.
- **Intergenerational transmission of risk:** The concept that epigenetic changes from certain behaviors in a parent may be transmitted from one generation to the next, separate and apart from the genes that are passed down through reproduction.
- **Lymphatic system:** The network of vessels through which waste products and toxins from tissues are drained for removal from the body.
- **Microbiome:** The collection of bacteria that comprise the microbial communities that exist on and within human beings.
- **Myelination:** The process by which oligodendrocytes (a type of glial cell in the brain) and Schwann cells (a type of glial cell outside of the brain) wrap axons with myelin, a protein- and fat-rich insulation substance that increases the speed of information conduction between neurons.

continued

BOX 2-2 Continued

- **Neuroimaging:** A technique that provides structural, functional, or metabolic information and images from living human beings within a brain scanner.
- **Neurons:** Cells within the brain that communicate with each other via chemical signaling and underlie consciousness, sociability, emotion, motivation and reward, and cognition.
- **Neurotransmitters:** Substances synthesized and released by neurons to excite or inhibit other neurons at their points of connection—synapses.
- **Oligodendrocyte:** A glial cell responsible for wrapping the axons of neurons in myelin sheaths in order to aid the speed of electrical conduction between neurons.
- **Sensitive period:** A time in development in which the developing organism is especially likely to undergo change (either positive or negative) in response to some experience or environmental change (e.g., an environmental toxicant, intervention training, or certain nutrients). Sensitive periods for certain functions can extend into adulthood.
- **Synapse:** The connection between neurons, separated by a small gap, in which neurotransmitters and other chemicals are released by one neuron to influence the activity of other neurons with which they connect. This forms the basic unit of communication, resulting in the activation of circuits that process information and leading to a specific functional readout.
- **Transcriptomics:** The scientific field aimed at understanding how and when certain genes are expressed or suppressed.

---

processes of healthy development from conception through early childhood are described, and some of the major biological responses to stressors are summarized. The chapter concludes with a discussion of individual differences in responsiveness and susceptibility. Throughout, the chapter identifies key points in development where disparities in health by race/ethnicity or socioeconomic status (SES) can emerge, which could inform strategies for prevention-oriented interventions.

The goal of this chapter is to provide essential information about the state of the science on human development from preconception through early childhood and some of the exciting findings in the past two decades within the fields of neurobiology, social psychology, epidemiology, and others that have contributed to advancing knowledge about how and when to intervene to improve outcomes for children. All of this information needs to be read through the lens of life course theory (Ben-Shlomo and Kuh, 2002), which recognizes that early experiences influence health outcomes within and across generations. It is also important to keep in mind the interconnectedness of brain and body health, as brain activity controls peripheral systems, which in turn affect brain structure and function. The committee provides this evidence to help "bridge the gap" between what science tells us and what actions need to be taken—by policy makers, health care providers, educators, religious leaders, parents, and others—to close disparities and improve outcomes for all children in the United States. At present, many of the new scientific advances in neuroscience are still in development, and more study is needed to apply these new findings in clinical and public health practice and to use them to inform policies. In particular, greater effort and more support is needed to develop, implement, and evaluate programs based on scientific discoveries regarding the optimal timing for interventions. The committee could not be comprehensive with regard to coverage of all scientific advances, biological processes of healthy development, biological responses to stressors, and factors associated with individual differences, as each is a complex and active area of research.

SCIENTIFIC AND TECHNOLOGICAL ADVANCEMENTS SINCE *FROM NEURONS TO NEIGHBORHOODS*

The big questions driving research on child development and interventions to improve well-being are the same today as they have been for decades. "What are the influences of genes and experience on child health and development?" "To what degree does the brain exhibit **plasticity** (i.e., change over time)?" "What are the brain circuits that control specific kinds of behaviors, and how can their functioning be influenced through experience-based interventions and/or medications?" "Why does early experience have lasting disease risk and functional effects into adulthood?" "How does a child's environment impact development of the brain, immune system, endocrine, metabolism, and cardiovascular systems, as well as physical and mental health?" (See Box 2-3 for highlights of applications of neurobiological research in practice.)

Much more is known today than two decades ago about the process of child development, and the explosion of research reports on child development since the publication of *From Neurons to Neighborhoods* (NRC and IOM, 2000) is remarkable. A PubMed search using just the term "early adversity" generated a list of 2,047 research articles,[2] 96 percent of which were published since 2001. Advances in several related fields of study have developed simultaneously to refine understanding of child health and development and the responses that each child may have to early adverse experiences. The following section outlines a selection of major developments, including genetics, transcriptomics, epigenetics, neuroimaging, computational modeling, maternal–fetal interactions, advances

---

[2] Accessed November 12, 2018.

BOX 2-3
To What End—Examples of Application of
Neurobiological Research in Practice

1. The discovery of molecules responsible for putting the "brakes" on critical period timing have led to clinical studies that manipulate the function of certain brakes in order to demonstrate that critical periods can be reopened far later in life than previously believed.
2. Eye tracking, coupled with machine learning and neural network algorithms, has been used to discover patterns of scene viewing that serve as a sensitive and specific signature to identify children who have normal facial morphology but were exposed to alcohol during fetal development and exhibit cognitive difficulties.
3. Neuroimaging and behavioral data were combined to demonstrate continued maturation of executive functions. These studies clarified the component skills and have led to a flurry of intervention strategies to train working memory, mental flexibility, and inhibitory control in toddlers, children, adolescents, and young adults.
4. The neurobiology of early adversity led to discoveries of genetic variants that increase vulnerability in the response to adverse childhood experiences (ACEs). HSP-90 and FKBP5 were discovered as partner regulators of the hormonal response to stress by controlling glucocorticoid receptor signaling, and sequence single nucleotide polymorphisms predict response to early environmental stressors, which can increase the risk for adult depression and anxiety disorders. To support preventative efforts, current research studies in clinical settings are under way to determine the effectiveness of genetic screening, combined with history of ACEs, to identify those individuals at greatest risk for recurring and treatment-resistant depression.
5. The advances in the neurobiology of sociability and the burgeoning research area of infant–mother and infant–father synchrony have led to foundational discoveries about the importance of a child's environment of relationships. There are many more studies and direct community applications of targeting both child and caregiver in interventions—for example, multidimensional therapeutic foster care or coaching to promote healthy caregiver–infant bidirectional, responsive interactions.

in longitudinal research, and the study of social interactions and physical environments. Refer to Box 2-2 for definitions of the key terms in bold below.

Genetics

Technological advances have led to cost-effective methods for capturing whole **genome sequences**. This has been completed for tens of thousands of human genomes, highlighting remarkable genetic variation among all individuals. **Genome sequencing** also has revealed a small but consistent set of genes, including HSP-90 and FKBP5, both of which are involved in regulating responses to stress activation through the HPA axis. Genome sequencing led to the discovery of specific sequence variations, some of which alter gene expression and are correlated with specific psychiatric disorders and stress lability. The variations in these genes contribute to individual differences in vulnerability and heterogeneity in response to early adverse experiences (Criado-Marrero et al., 2018). For complex outcomes, such as psychopathology, researchers are increasingly exploring polygenic risk (i.e., the combined contribution of many genes that influence brain development and function) rather than single gene variants that have very small contributions to risk. One idea being tested is that polygenic risk "scores" may better predict an individual's likelihood of a given outcome (Brikell et al., 2018). **Genomics** has developed in tandem with experimental animal models and clinical discoveries in humans to provide opportunities to study (1) genes that control the formation and physiological maturation of neural connections; (2) the molecules responsible for the onset and termination of **sensitive periods**; (3) the molecular basis for experience-driven **synapse** formation, elimination (pruning), and stabilization; (4) regulation of inflammatory responses; and (5) regulation of hormonal activation and feedback of the stress response (Bae et al., 2015; Geschwind and Rakic, 2013; Hensch, 2016b; Sudhof, 2018; Sudhof and Malenka, 2008).

Epigenetics[3]

Genomics discoveries were followed rapidly by advanced methods to identify the consequences of differences in how, where, and when specific genes are expressed—that is, the epigenetic ("above the genome") profile of specific cells (Waddington, 1942, 1957). Initial discoveries recognized that epigenetic changes are **chemical signatures** (National Scientific Council on the Developing Child, 2010) placed on an individual's inherited DNA due to environmental experiences and related contributing factors (e.g., nutrition, mental and physical stressors, immune activation, environmental toxicants, enriched environments) (Goldberg et al., 2007). Once thought to be limited in scope and immutable, there are millions of sites on DNA that can be chemically modified epigenetically, and the

---

[3] For a more in-depth discussion on epigenetics and how the environment gets under the skin, see Chapter 3 of the 2019 National Academies report *The Promise of Adolescence: Realizing Opportunity for All Youth* by the Committee on the Neurobiological and Socio-Behavioral Science of Adolescent Development and Its Applications (NASEM, 2019).

modifications at these sites can be gained and lost rapidly, or, in many instances, remain stable over the lifetime (Goll and Bestor, 2005). Recent studies have shown that environmental experience influences the genome with specific molecular changes, such as DNA methylation and modifications to chromatin (Goldberg et al., 2007; Heim and Binder, 2012; Kalish et al., 2014; Kumsta, 2019; Miguel et al., 2019). While evidence of these molecular changes has been observed in many studies, the process by which these changes are controlled is complex and not completely understood. Exposures and experiences can result in profound epigenetic modifications that alter the timing and location of expressed or suppressed genes (McEwen, 2017; Miguel et al., 2019). For instance, epigenetics is one mechanism that results in identical twins exhibiting distinct physical and mental traits. Preliminary data suggest that epigenetic changes may explain how early experiences get "under the skin" of individuals for whom physical and brain-related disruptions and disease risk can last a lifetime (McEwen, 2017; Miguel et al., 2019). Research shows that epigenetic changes that alter the DNA chemistry in **germ cells** of adult humans may be one way that experiences are passed on to the next generation through their children (Donkin et al., 2016). However, the best evidence for such intergenerational transmission comes from animal studies. Epigenetic changes occurring during preconception or during pregnancy can impact the germ cells of the offspring and result in intergenerational transmission of the parental experiences (Weber-Stadlbauer, 2017). Moreover, it has been hypothesized that germ cells of the fetus may be altered during pregnancy, meaning that the mother, and even the child when that child is grown and has children of his or her own, can pass on influences that occurred several generations previously (Bale, 2015; Rodgers et al., 2015; Rowold et al., 2017).

Transcriptomics

Keeping in mind that one's entire genome is in every cell of the body, the study of **transcriptomics** uses methods to identify how particular genes are expressed over time, in specific types of cells, and under specific circumstances (Li et al., 2018). New methods facilitated the organization of a research consortium that led to a remarkably detailed, open-access atlas[4] of gene expression in 16 different human brain areas during pre- and postnatal development and into adulthood, building a unique bridge between human and model system brain research (Carlyle et al., 2017; Enoch et al., 2014; Li et al., 2018; Vied et al., 2014). For example, the expression of genes responsible for producing the thousands of neuron types

---

[4] For more information, see http://www.brainspan.org (accessed June 16, 2019).

in the brain is enriched during the first trimester of pregnancy. As development continues, many of those genes are turned off because neuron production ceases, and other genes are newly expressed that control the initial wiring and building of the unique architecture of the brain. After birth, genes are turned on to cause the rapid formation of synapses, pruning, and the signaling between neurons to process more and more complex information. The ability to relate specific events in development to the changing transcriptome has been accomplished by creating enormous databases of gene expression in the pre- and postnatal human brain and in experimental animal models. These new data offer a detailed directory of **gene expression** in space and time in the complex and rapidly changing developing brain, thereby providing the framework for ongoing research to determine how the interplay of genetic and environmental factors and experience alters the gene expression that contributes to typical or atypical developmental maturation.

Neuroimaging

Human and animal **neuroimaging** have provided the basis for a new understanding of the brain **connectome,** which defines the breadth and complexity of circuits that relay information between ensembles of neurons. New technologies provide unprecedented resolution of the organization of the connectome in humans, painting a far more complex picture that begins prenatally as early as the third trimester of pregnancy (Kostović et al., 2014; Krsnik et al., 2017) and continues in infancy and toddlerhood as remarkable periods of growth for the brain. Functional maturation of circuits continues throughout childhood, but connectome research, combined with genomics, has identified adolescence as a second period of dynamic changes in brain wiring.[5] In humans, it is now understood that while classic diagrams of brain development present a well-delineated blueprint, there is far more variability in infants and toddlers than expected in the timing and extent of development of connectivity within the standard connectome blueprint. This basic neuroimaging research in humans has provided a foundation for determining the impact of disparities resulting from poverty and other social factors on the trajectory of brain growth and development of circuitry (Gabrieli and Bunge, 2017; Hanson et al., 2013; Johnson et al., 2016; Luby et al., 2012). Given the vast heterogeneity between individuals in terms of brain development, drawing generalizations about the overall connectome and its influence on social, emotional, and cognitive maturation remains a key research challenge.

---

[5] For a comprehensive discussion of the developing adolescent brain, see NASEM, 2019.

Maternal and Fetal/Infant Interactions

Prenatal development is marked by a unique relationship between the mother, the fetus, and a transient organ, the placenta. Once thought of as a filtration system of cells contributed mostly by the fetus and blood vessels from both mother and fetus to control the passage of nutrients and other substances, the placenta has been shown by current genomic, cell biological, and physiological evidence to be an active partner in fetal development and influenced by maternal health. For example, maternal immune activation or persistent stress during pregnancy can alter placental cell gene expression and function (Hoffman, 2016). Depending on the stage, the placenta expresses 40 to 60 percent of the human genome and produces cytokines, hormones, **neurotransmitters,** and growth factors that are necessary for healthy fetal development (Gonzalez et al., 2018; Jones, 2019; Paquette et al., 2018; Zhao et al., 2019). These genes are subject to environmentally regulated epigenetic changes; exposure to toxicants, nutrient status, high stress, or infection can result in altered gene expression through epigenetic changes (Bale, 2015). Thus, while the organ clearly is involved in regulating transport of maternally produced substances, the placenta also serves as a critical resource for organ development and maturation of functions to ready the fetus for birth (Bonnin and Levitt, 2011; Bonnin et al., 2011; Goeden et al., 2016; Nugent and Bale, 2015). Developmentally, the maternal–placental–fetal relationship begins between the third and fourth week postconception through a complex process of extraembryonic cell differentiation and vascularization that results in implantation in the maternal uterus. Given that the main functional cell of the placenta, the trophoblast, is embryonic in origin and that there are thousands of genes expressed in the placenta, any gene mutation that could functionally disrupt the embryo also can impact placental function (McKay, 2011).

Intergenerational Transmission of Risk

Evidence from both animals and humans indicates that adverse social/psychological and physical exposures in one generation can alter risks for psychopathology, maladaptive behavior, and chronic disease in the next generation (i.e., the children of individuals who endured severe threat have elevated rates for psychiatric disorders and dysregulated physiology, despite an absence of direct exposure) (Boyce and Kobor, 2015; Burton and Metcalfe, 2014; Franklin et al., 2010; Matthews and Phillips, 2012; Santavirta et al., 2018; Yehuda and Bierer, 2007; Yehuda et al., 2014). For example, research has documented that (1) adolescents born to women who experienced severe child abuse are at higher risk of smoking and overweight/obesity (Roberts et al., 2014), (2) there is altered **cortisol** expression among children who were in utero at the time of the 2001 World Trade Center attack in New York City (Yehuda et al., 2005), and (3) there are differences in stress reactivity in children of women affected by the Dutch Hunger Winter (Painter et al., 2006). These excess risks may emerge through a variety of mechanisms that are not mutually exclusive, such as altered parenting behaviors, lower socioeconomic position, epigenetic pathways (described above), or an altered fetal environment.

Adverse experiences before and during pregnancy can influence maternal stress-related physiology, including immune activation and endocrine disruptions (Entringer, 2013; Entringer et al., 2010, 2015; Hantsoo et al., 2019; Howerton and Bale, 2012). Increasing evidence suggests that maternal immune and endocrine activity during pregnancy (including the under- or overproduction of cortisol and levels of pro- or anti-inflammatory cytokines) are associated with adverse birth outcomes (Bastek et al., 2011; Wadhwa et al., 2011), the child's brain (Buss et al., 2017) and cognitive development (Gilman et al., 2017; Rudolph et al., 2018), and future risk for chronic disease (Entringer et al., 2013, 2015), providing support for embryonic and fetal life as sensitive periods for the intergenerational transmission of adverse maternal experiences (Buss et al., 2017; Entringer et al., 2010; Meaney, 2001). Much of this work is preliminary, and further research needs to be conducted before drawing concrete conclusions about **intergenerational transmission of risk.** At present, there is a limited understanding of how plastic or modifiable these intergenerational risk factors are and why some individuals are resilient to intergenerational risks whereas others are not. This is an area of active research that has elevated the importance of applying the life course approach to health and development, and by further understanding the pathways of both risk and resilience, scientists may uncover social, behavioral, or pharmacologic interventions that can interrupt the intergenerational transmission of the effects of stress on the developing embryo and fetus. Later in the chapter, the section on Biological Mechanisms of Healthy Development presents a more extensive discussion on the role of the placenta and how it can be influenced by social experiences.

Computational Methods

There has been a rapid increase in the capacity to collect and analyze enormous datasets with social and biological information. These datasets may be developed through research consortia that can involve dozens of investigators from around the world or from the linkage of administrative files, de-identified electronic health records (McGregor et al., 2013; Roden et al., 2008), and other sources (McCarty et al., 2011). In parallel, engineers and computer scientists have advanced sophisticated computational methods, including signal processing and machine learning, to extract predictable patterns that relate to outcomes of interest (Krishnan et al., 2017; Tseng et al., 2013; Van Essen et al., 2013). For example, connectomics and genomics have depended heavily on these methods, and the rapid advances in collecting physiological data from children (electroencephalogram [EEG], eye tracking, wearable devices to monitor physical activity, sleep habits, stress, and metabolic activity) also have benefited from the advanced analytical methods that help identify patterns of maturation of brain architecture and function (Bagot et al., 2018; Frazier et al., 2018; Hosseini et al., 2016; Medland et al., 2014; O'Driscoll et al., 2013; Wee et al., 2017). These measures have been used to predict risk for behavioral and cognitive disturbances later in development. Relatedly, there is growing interest in using machine learning and predictive risk modeling methods to identify children in adverse environments and predict risk or resilience (Amrit et al., 2017; Gillingham, 2016; Schwartz et al., 2017). For example, advanced analytical methods have been applied to produce highly sensitive and specific metrics for the prospective diagnosis of fetal alcohol spectrum disorder (Zhang et al., 2019). However, there is still much more research needed to determine how well these methods may be applied to determine underlying causal mechanisms. Finally, meta-analytic approaches are using new analytical methods to synthesize the results of multiple independent studies and are now widely employed to inform evidence-based recommendations, policies, and programs for children. For example, meta-analyses have been used to summarize the effects of center-based early education (Grindal et al., 2016; Schindler et al., 2015) and parenting programs (Casillas et al., 2016; Chen and Chan, 2016).

Advances in Longitudinal Research

Investments by the National Institutes of Health, the U.S. Department of Education, numerous private foundations, and other agencies have resulted in a substantial growth in child development research using longitudinal data from prospective cohort studies with large subgroups of racial/ethnic minority children and stratified-probability samples. These studies have documented more extensively the pervasiveness of health disparities in these populations and the mechanisms by which these disparities arise. For example, the Eunice Kennedy Shriver National Institute of Child Health and Human Development supports the Fragile Families & Child Wellbeing Study, a birth cohort of nearly 5,000 children in 20 large U.S. cities that used a stratified random sample with an oversample of nonmarital births (McLanahan et al., 2003). Baseline interviews for this study occurred between 1998 and 2000, and follow-up is still ongoing. The Institute of Education Sciences, an independent evaluation arm of

the U.S. Department of Education, conducts the Early Childhood Longitudinal Study program, which has generated large representative cohorts
for studies of child development for the United States, from birth onward
(Tourangeau et al., 2009).

Longitudinal studies are critical to understanding both normative
developmental processes and those involving deviations from the norm.
These studies facilitate examination of changes across development within
individuals and subgroup differences in within-person changes over time
(Lerner et al., 2009). Prospective studies are critical for documenting what
changes—in brain, behavior, or health—are due to normal developmental progression and what changes are caused by chronic family-level
stressors, structural inequalities, and/or positive environmental stimuli.
Longitudinal data, combined with advances in statistical methods for
identifying underlying pathways, have made it possible to show the
lasting impact of early adverse experiences and to ask questions about
mediating processes that underlie the association between early childhood adversity and poor health or educational outcomes (Danese et al.,
2009; Iacono et al., 2008; Poulton et al., 2015). In parallel, longitudinal data
have shown that for children who have been exposed to severe adversity,
such as maltreatment, providing appropriate care can reverse early damage, even to biological systems, such as brain functioning (Cicchetti and
Curtis, 2006; Cicchetti and Handley, 2017).

In spite of these advances, it is important to note that U.S. investment
in large birth cohort studies lags severely behind European countries.
One new study, launched in 2016, is the Environmental influences on
Child Health Outcomes (ECHO) program. It is a 7-year research initiative focused on understanding the effects of environmental exposures
on child health and development, and it draws on existing U.S. cohorts.
The cohort studies that compose ECHO collectively include approximately 50,000 children and will address environmental exposures in relation to four pediatric outcomes with high relevance to public health:
pre-, peri-, and postnatal outcomes, neurodevelopment (i.e., cognition,
emotion, and behavior), upper- and lower-airway function, and obesity.

Of note, many longitudinal studies of child development have been
the product of interdisciplinary collaborations, which have become
increasingly common. An example is the long-term follow-up of the
Perry Preschool[6] project, which started in the 1960s (Gramlich, 1986;
Schweinhart et al., 1985). This longitudinal study of the effects of a randomized controlled trial is the result of a long-term collaboration between
educational researchers and practitioners, developmental psychologists,

---

[6] For more information, see https://highscope.org/perry-preschool-project (accessed
March 29, 2019).

and economists. The latest follow-up of the intervention administered at 3 and 4 years of age still yields positive results on the life trajectory of its participants at age 40, including more positive health outcomes, improved employment trajectory, and less crime involvement (Belfield et al., 2006; Social Programs That Work, 2017). Consistent with these findings, the Carolina Abecedarian Project—a randomized study of an early childhood intervention for economically disadvantaged children with long-term follow-up—found that children randomly assigned to the early intervention displayed lower cardiovascular and metabolic risk factors in their mid-30s, with effects most pronounced for men (Campbell et al., 2014). Baby's First Years,[7] launched in 2018 and funded by both private and public grants, is a new longitudinal study that seeks to establish causal links between parental income level and brain development in very young children.

Advances in the Study of Social Interactions

Since the publication of *From Neurons to Neighborhoods*, researchers have introduced a number of novel topics and measurement approaches that have advanced the understanding of early development and consequences for later physical and mental health outcomes. In particular, there has been a shift of focus to the well-being of salient caregivers as "a dependent variable" in research and associated interventions. In other words, rather than continuing to report (as psychologists had over decades) that a good relationship with the primary caregiver is the single most important protective process in promoting resilience among children whose life circumstances render them at risk, there is now explicit focus on the question of what it is that helps parents maintain good parenting when they are struggling with high ongoing stress. How can we promote resilience among the adults primarily responsible for raising children in stressful life circumstances? (For reviews, see Luthar et al., 2015, and Luthar and Eisenberg, 2017.) Relatedly, intervention approaches are going beyond simply teaching parents what they should and should not do in didactic parenting classes or even imparting approaches to regulate their own affect (via mindfulness or trying to cope effectively with their own ongoing life stressors). Increasingly, programs are also seeking to provide the support that parents need to successfully negotiate the many challenges in sustaining good parenting behaviors with multiple children and across multiple decades (for examples of such programs, see Corso et al., 2015; Kaminski et al., 2013; Luthar et al., 2007, 2017).

---

[7] For more information, see https://www.babysfirstyears.com (accessed April 18, 2019).

An emerging field of research suggests that there is a biological basis to healthy caregiver–child relationships and that caregiver–child synchrony in biological processes such as EEG or heart rate variability can help children to develop control of their behavior and emotions. The science of caregiver–child synchrony advances previous views that a child's central nervous system is primarily responsible for developing self-regulation (Welch, 2016). This research suggests that children display dysregulated behavior due to deficient coregulation from nonoptimal caregiver relationships and that coregulation can be improved via interventions, such as the Family Nurture Intervention, developed by Martha Welch and colleagues (2014, 2015). Although there are a number of neuroendocrine changes that occur during the process of parenting, a substantial amount of this research has focused on oxytocin measures in the infant and caregiver. In addition to oxytocin's roles in the birthing process, lactation, and maternal care in mammals, studies have demonstrated that oxytocin (and its close neuropeptide relative vasopressin) facilitates affiliative social behavior through modulation of the activity of specific forebrain circuits (Feldman and Bakermans-Kranenburg, 2017; Hammock et al., 2005; Insel, 2010b; King et al., 2016; Numan and Young, 2016). Both observational and experimental research studies suggest that oxytocin influences the synchrony between caregivers and children, and it is also associated with sensitivity of caregiving and amount of contact (Feldman and Bakermans-Kranenburg, 2017). Researchers are exploring how specific caregiver health conditions (e.g., postpartum depression) or social experiences (e.g., traumatic experiences in early childhood) influence oxytocin, other neuroendocrine hormones related to nurturing behaviors, and caregiver–infant synchrony and how interventions may target these processes to improve caregiver–child relationships.

Another major advancement is that there has been a growing appreciation for the role of culture for the development of children (Coll et al., 1996). In a study of children and families in the United States outside of the white middle class (i.e., minority families based on race/ethnicity, immigrant status, sexual orientation, and others at both SES extremes) there has been a growing emphasis on potent culturally specific risk and protective factors and processes (see Velez-Agosto et al., 2017), especially those that can be harnessed in beneficial interventions. As an example, *American Psychologist* devoted a special issue to marginalization, defined "as a multidimensional, dynamic, context-dependent, and diverse web of processes, rooted in power imbalance and systematically directed toward specific groups and individuals, with probabilistic implications for development" (Causadias and Umaña-Taylor, 2018). The special section contains a rich collection of articles addressing issues related to various marginalized groups, including recent immigrants and youth from different ethnic and racial minority groups. In another recent special section in *Research in Human Development*, Cunningham (2019) compiled papers addressing "myths and realities associated with human development research and theorizing" encompassing

> diverse perspectives on sexual minority youth, resilience and risk for youth in high-achieving schools (HASs), a reconceptualization of hostility in African American parenting styles, a critical examination of diversity and contact for students attending racial/ethnically diverse schools, and a thoughtful consideration of contextual factors associated with aggressive attitudes and prosocial behaviors in African American males. (Cunningham, 2019, p. 1)

Many of these studies move the conceptualization of "children or family at risk" to "children and family living in at-risk conditions." The "problem" to be "fixed" is not the child and/or family but the at-risk conditions within which they live, an important paradigm shift for early identification and prevention. (On a related topic, there have also been advances in connecting racism to child and adult health outcomes; see Box 2-4.)

Advances in the Study of Physical Environments

Although the family remains a major determinant of the child's outcomes, studies following more comprehensive theoretical models (e.g., Bronfenbrenner, 1979; Bronfenbrenner and Evans, 2000; Ferguson et al., 2013) have documented the importance of neighborhood contexts on family interactions and child development. Neighborhood context can be characterized as positive and negative, and it can reflect the physical or built environment and psychosocial characteristics. It has become increasingly common for researchers to link measures of neighborhood social and structural environments to individual-level data on children. As long as families are willing to share an address, researchers are able to draw on information from the Census and other free and proprietary data sources in order to characterize a child's social and physical environment. When this field of research began, most studies focused on neighborhood SES (e.g., the proportion of the population in the Census tract that is below the federal poverty line), as this measure is associated with the physical infrastructure of the community, noise and pollution, amenities such as parks and groceries, and availability of health centers and early childhood education (Evans, 2004; Evans et al., 2010). However, use of neighborhood SES as a proxy for neighborhood quality and conditions does not provide sufficient information about the mechanisms of action—that is, the specific pathway through which neighborhoods influence child health. The majority of research on neighborhood SES and health is observational, but

BOX 2-4
Racism and Child Health

Another major scientific advancement in the science of health disparities since *From Neurons to Neighborhoods* is the research linking racism to child and adult health outcomes (Pachter and Coll, 2009; Paradies et al., 2015; Priest et al., 2013; Williams and Mohammed, 2013). Much of the impetus for the work on the effects of racism on children's development stemmed from the critical analyses of the prevalent use of the deficits model to understand health disparities in minority children (García Coll, 1990; McLoyd, 1990; Ogbu, 1981; Spencer and Markstrom-Adams, 1990).

Beginning in the 1990s, several theoretical models and empirical work started to place the burden on the social and environmental conditions where the majority of the minority populations in the United States lived (Coll and Szalacha, 2004; García Coll et al., 1996; Stein et al., 2016). McLoyd's work showed that the stress associated with poverty explained harsh parenting among African American families. These segregated communities had a majority of families living below the poverty line, with schools, health care, recreation, housing, and transportation facilities below standards or with fewer resources than where predominantly white, middle-class populations lived. Health disparities were now considered a function of these environmental conditions and not the parents and children themselves. Most of these social and environmental conditions are now seen as a function of pervasive institutional and interpersonal racism (Pager and Shepherd, 2008). Similarly, scientists have denounced the use of race and ethnicity as variables in biological research (Collins, 2004; Foster and Sharp, 2004), noting that "historical racial categories that are treated as natural and infused with notions of superiority and inferiority have no place in biology" (Yudell et al., 2016, p. 565).

A large body of scientific evidence has documented that both institutional racism and interpersonal experiences of discrimination can influence the health and well-being of both children and adults in multiple ways, including reducing access to material resources and services that promote long-term health and development and acting as a psychosocial stressor that can lead to worse outcomes over time (Priest et al., 2013; Williams and Mohammed, 2009). Studies of children and adolescents indicate that experiences of discrimination are positively associated with depression and anxiety and negatively associated with positive mental health outcomes, such as self-esteem and resilience (Priest et al., 2013). Research also suggests that parental experiences of discrimination are associated with child and adolescent mental health and socio-emotional outcomes (Heard-Garris et al., 2018; Tran, 2014), as well as some indicators of physical health (Priest et al., 2012; Slopen et al., 2019). There are also a diverse set of health outcomes in adults resulting from racism (Williams et al., 2019).

Measures for experiences of racism and discrimination in children have relied mostly on parent- or self-reported answers to survey questions (Fisher et al., 2000; Pachter et al., 2010; Williams et al., 1997). These instruments are subjected to social desirability, recall biases, and other potential issues associated with self-reports. Some research in adults has begun to combine traditional measures of racial discrimination with implicit measures, in order to advance understanding of how conscious and unconscious experiences of racism influence outcomes (Krieger, 2012; Krieger et al., 2010). Future research is needed to examine whether similar approaches are useful for children and adolescents.

there are a few exceptions, including the Moving to Opportunity study (Chetty et al., 2016; Ludwig et al., 2011).

The Project on Human Development in Chicago Neighborhoods (PHDCN)—an interdisciplinary study that began in 1995 and aimed to explore how families, schools, and neighborhoods influence child and adolescent development—was among the first to provide an intensive investigation of neighborhood conditions related to economic, social, organizational, political, and cultural structures and how communities change over time. The investigators conducted systematic social observations by videotaping one side of each block within the selected 80 Chicago neighborhood clusters, and they maintained observer logs about the activities of residents and the presence of detracting elements (e.g., garbage, abandoned cars). This study identified neighborhood collective efficacy and social capital as important aspects of neighborhood social organization for child and adolescent outcomes (Sampson and Raudenbush, 1997, 1999; Sampson et al., 1999).

Since PHDCN, researchers have begun to characterize neighborhood social and physical information for health research using Google Street View (Rundle et al., 2011; Rzotkiewicz et al., 2018), which has the benefits of being lower cost and more efficient, although it can be limited by resolution and availability for a given temporal period. There has also been a substantial amount of research to examine child health in relation to neighborhood violence or crime, which can be derived from police crime reports (Beck et al., 2016; Goldman-Mellor et al., 2016; McCoy et al., 2015). Some studies use surveys to assess parental perceptions of neighborhood safety (Christian et al., 2015). Other research has focused on the physical neighborhood environment, such as opportunities for physical activity, access to healthy food, density of fast food, air quality, and presence of natural environments (e.g., green space) (Gascon et al., 2016; Gorski Findling et al., 2018; McCracken et al., 2016; Sallis et al., 2018). While some studies use single measures of neighborhood context, other studies rely on more complex indexes, such as the Child Opportunity Index (Acevedo-Garcia et al., 2014, 2016). This measure—developed by diversitydatakids.org and the Kirwan Institute for the Study of Race and Ethnicity—combines 19 component indicators related to education, health and environment, and social and economic context to rank neighborhoods (defined by Census tract) to other neighborhoods within the metropolitan area (Acevedo-Garcia et al., 2014; Beck et al., 2017a,b).

BIOLOGICAL MECHANISMS OF HEALTHY DEVELOPMENT

Introduction

Development is an interplay between biology and the profound impact that experiences have on biological systems. There are basic biologically driven mechanics that involve the production and specialization of cells that serve as the ingredients to build different organ systems, such as the brain, heart, digestive system, and kidneys. These systems are ultimately responsible for performing specific functions and become specialized over different periods of developmental time. This developmental process begins prenatally, and for the most complex organ—the brain—it extends into young adulthood. The developmental process is designed to promote maximal functioning and survival of the individual. The challenges an individual faces from infancy to adulthood are numerous and varied, and through the powerful biology–experience relations, development establishes both functional and adaptive capacities in order to adjust to the environment and to future experiences. Optimal functioning and robust adaptability to the environment are signatures of healthy development. No matter which organ system or cell type is considered, a core principle of development involves the regulation of the expression of the 23,000 genes in each person's genome at specific times, and in specific combinations, in order to achieve optimal functioning of each organ system.

It is important to re-emphasize here that the genome is composed mostly of regions of DNA that do not code for proteins but rather are responsible for using information from experiences and the environment to regulate gene expression. Gene expression is the first step toward producing proteins, which are the primary functional units of specialized cells that characterize each organ system. Thus, while all cells contain identical genetic material (DNA code), gene expression and production of proteins varies greatly between types of cells, which specialize during development to perform specific functions. Because the brain is massively complex, with billions of **neurons** and trillions of connections, at least 85 percent of the genome is expressed at various times and locations during development (Negi and Guda, 2017), whereas other organ systems may express far fewer genes in order to perform their functions. This orchestrated temporal and spatial expression of genes depends on maintaining healthy **cellular homeostasis** and accessing nutrients that serve as the building blocks for proteins and eventually organ systems. Research has shown that regulation of fundamental metabolic processes, including mitochondrial function in the brain and periphery, is essential for cellular adaptations to developmental psychosocial stress that can impact mental and physical health (Eisner et al., 2018; Picard and McEwen, 2018). The most productive means to facilitate early healthy development include providing access to healthy nutrition, avoiding factors that can be detrimental to nutritional status for mother and fetus over the course of pregnancy, limiting chronic stress, and offering access to quality health care. Proper nutrition is needed postnatally through childhood as well. Moreover, disrupting the fetal–placental–maternal biological relationship through infection, toxicants, alcohol, nicotine, or poor diet increases risk for altering a typical, healthy developmental trajectory. Thus, improving physical environments to limit exposure risk and providing access to high-quality maternal health care during pregnancy is an additional essential ingredient for healthy development. These well-researched factors make up a strategy for viewing early development through a "prevention lens" that ultimately leads to reduced risk for later physical, mental, and cognitive disorders.

Recent studies, mostly in animal models, indicate that the developmental process starts even prior to conception (Chan et al., 2018). Certain stressors, including psychosocial factors, toxicants, or drug exposure, can impact reproductive cells through an epigenetic process that ultimately may alter the expression of the genes that are inherited by the embryo. This suggests that parental behavior may impact how a child's genes are ultimately expressed and therefore what the child's biology and behavior will be. This transgenerational impact on development requires studies in humans before firm conclusions are made, but the research indicates that maternal and paternal experiences prior to conception may be an important factor to consider for programs that promote family health and welfare.

The following sections outline how several biological systems, those most relevant to this committee's report, develop between gestation and puberty and serve as a baseline for understanding how early environmental stressors and adversity affect child development and the emergence of health disparities: maternal physiological adaptations during pregnancy and the nervous, immune, endocrine, and reproductive systems. Note that in addition to psychosocial stressors in the environment of a developing child, adversity may include limited or no physical activity; exposure to toxicants, including alcohol and nicotine; and chronic disruption of bodily physiological functions, such as sleep (Feldman et al., 2014; Jones et al., 2019; McEwen and Getz, 2013; Thompson et al., 2009). Each of the following sections describes typical processes from the prenatal period through early childhood and how the system may be impacted by experiences that disrupt typical development.

Maternal Physiological Adaptations During Pregnancy

Remarkable changes take place in women during pregnancy to accommodate the needs of the developing fetus. A woman's heart pumps out 30 to 50 percent more blood every minute, while her lungs take in more air with each deep breath, in order to deliver oxygen and nutrients to the baby (Cheung, 2013; Costantine, 2014). Her kidney functions also improve by 50 percent to filter out more waste products and toxins from the blood (Cheung and Lafayette, 2013). Her immune system is dampened to avoid rejection of the fetus, and she becomes progressively insulin resistant, which allows an increasing amount of blood glucose to stay in the bloodstream to nourish the growing fetus.

A comprehensive review of maternal adaptations is beyond the scope of this report, but it is important to note that how well a woman's body can adapt to these physiological changes during pregnancy is closely related to her overall health going into the pregnancy. For example, a healthy heart can readily adjust to the increased workload, but a diseased heart will have a much more difficult time; heart disease is a leading cause of maternal death in the United States. Pregnancy predisposes blood to clotting, but the risk of severe complications from thromboembolism and pulmonary embolus is substantially increased in women with preexisting conditions, such as hypertension, diabetes, or obesity. Pregnancy causes a physiological anemia, which can be exacerbated by ongoing iron deficiency, thereby increasing the risk of having a low birth weight baby. The insulin resistance in pregnancy is made worse if a woman enters pregnancy overweight, obese, or with preexisting diabetes mellitus; fetal exposure to excess blood glucose has been associated with adverse birth outcomes and obesity and diabetes later in life (Garcia-Vargas et al., 2012). As we will discuss in Chapter 5, advancing health equity in birth and child health outcomes first requires improving preconception health for all women.

One of the most important adaptations during pregnancy is the formation of the placenta, an organ that is responsible for controlling access of maternal-derived factors to the fetus and also serves as a source of growth factors and other molecules that support healthy fetal development. The placenta begins to form very early in pregnancy, and disruption of this process has been associated with pregnancy complications, such as intrauterine growth restriction and preeclampsia (Sharma and Sharma, 2016). At term, approximately 600–700 milliliters of blood flows through the placenta, delivering oxygen and nutrients to the baby (Wang and Zhao, 2010). The placenta also acts as a critical regulator of maternal–fetal interactions and resource allocation. For example, if a pregnant woman experiences acute stress, the placenta shields the fetus from overexposure to maternal cortisol by turning up the activity and expression of a placental enzyme called 11β-hydroxysteroid dehydrogenase type-2 (HSD11B2), which inactivates cortisol as it passes through the placenta. However, chronic stress has been found to be associated with reduced activity and expression of placental HSD11B2, suggesting that the placenta's built-in ability to limit fetal exposure to maternal cortisol may be diminished in the face of chronic stress (Cuffe et al., 2012; O'Donnell et al., 2012; Welberg et al., 2005).

Nervous System Development

The neurobiological processes that build the brain share some common elements with other organ systems, such as producing specialized cells (e.g., neurons and **glia**) with functions specific to that organ system. However, understanding of neurodevelopment lags behind the understanding of other organ systems, in large part because the brain is extraordinarily complex. Experimental studies in model systems have identified basic mechanisms and the genes that are involved in specializing areas of the developing brain into what will make up function regions, the production of a diversity of neuron types, and the initial wiring of circuits that occurs prenatally (Kast and Levitt, 2019; Kolodkin and Tessier-Lavigne, 2011). Identification of mutations in some of these same genes in humans has validated the highly conserved nature of the ingredients that are responsible for the initial brain blueprint (Doan et al., 2018; Geschwind and Rakic, 2013; Jayaraman et al., 2018; Rubenstein and Rakic, 2013). Genes and their protein products involved in later events, including the extended period of synaptogenesis (the formation of synapses), have been identified and studied experimentally (Akins and Biederer, 2006; Favuzzi and Rico, 2018; Sudhof, 2018). For all of the advances in the basic understanding of neurodevelopment, there is a knowledge gap in determining the many ways in which the environment and experience are woven into the developmental process. Figure 2-1 is a diagram showing development from the first trimester to puberty, with respect to both neurodevelopment and the development of other biological systems.

Within a few weeks of conception in the first trimester, neurons begin to be produced. By 10–12 weeks gestation, most of the neurons that make up the brain are generated (Bystron et al., 2008; Stiles, 2008). Specific types of neurons in structures like the cerebellum, hippocampus, and olfactory bulb continue to be produced prenatally. Unlike many other types of cells in the human body, once formed, neurons lose the capacity to renew themselves, even if injured (a small number of neurons in the olfactory bulb and hippocampus represent limited exceptions). Because the neurons are "born" at sites in the developing brain that are different from their final position, all neurons migrate using a combination of mechanical guides,

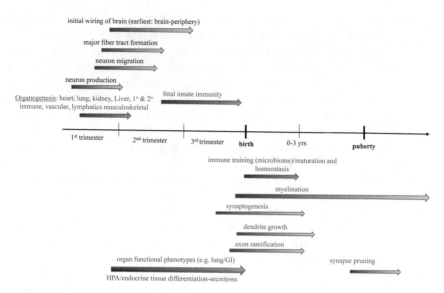

FIGURE 2-1 Human development of the brain and other organ systems from prenatal to pubertal periods.
NOTES: Arrows represent time frames of approximate onset (darker shading) and completion (lighter shading) of specific developmental events for neural (green) and nonneural (blue) systems. For the neural components, above the line represents events that occur within the prenatal period, and below the line represents events that extend into postnatal periods. GI = gastrointestinal; HPA = hypothalamic-pituitary-adrenal axis.

the extended processes of radial glial cells, and molecules that serve as guidance cues. This migration process begins as soon as neurons are produced, and as the brain grows through the second trimester, the later-produced neurons take longer to reach their final position. This developmental process is further complicated because newly formed neurons not only migrate but simultaneously extend a long process—the **axon**—that will connect each neuron to its appropriate target. At the same time, the receiving end of the neuron—the dendrite—develops but takes much longer to reach maturity, in sync with the formation of individual neural connections—the synapses. Throughout each of these developmental stages, additional sets of genes are expressed that drive a specific process to completion. Many of the earliest born neurons will regulate peripheral organ function (e.g., heart, lungs, gastrointestinal tract). Connections are formed between these neurons and their targets in the first trimester as the targets continue to develop. By the beginning of the second trimester, long connections from the hypothalamus to the autonomic brain stem are formed, providing the capacity for top-down regulation of what are called the **sympathetic** and **parasympathetic nervous systems**—in essence, the systems that control the "fight or flight" and "rest and digest" responses.

By the second and third trimesters, sensory systems are connected from the periphery to the brain's cerebral **cortex**—the most complex part of the brain with the greatest neuronal diversity, which processes complex information from all of the senses. Toward the end of fetal development in the third trimester, the basic blueprint of neuronal connections is initiated, during a temporally extended process of synapse formation that continues through 2–3 years postnatally (Levitt and Eagleson, 2018; Silbereis, 2016). The human neocortex contains approximately 20 billion neurons, each with an average of several thousand synapses and connected with thousands of kilometers of dendrites and axons (Tang et al., 2001).

By birth, sensory systems are sufficiently wired to be able to take in information from the infant's environment and begin to process the most salient stimuli (e.g., visual, tactile, and auditory stimuli of the primary caregiver that are experienced in temporal lockstep with satisfying the hunger, thirst, and warmth needs). The nervous system continues to build by adding more synapses, ultimately reaching its greatest synapse density during toddlerhood. Experimental studies in animals show that experiences can influence the initial organization and sheer number of synapses (Berbari et al., 2005; Turner and Greenough, 1985). In early human infant development, differences in growth parameters of gray and white matter have been shown to be influenced by experience in the human cerebral cortex (Brito and Noble, 2014; Hair et al., 2015), which assumes synaptogenesis changes due to experience. In humans, more than 1 million synapses are added per second for this 2–3-year period (Center on the Developing Child at Harvard University, n.d.-a). During early childhood, and as an individual approaches the onset of puberty, the number of synapses remains relatively stable, but this does not imply that no developmental activity is taking place. Instead, experience-driven processes impact maturation by influencing which specific genes are expressed and therefore how synapses process information. Over time, synapses that become activated more frequently and in concert with other synapses processing the same information become more stable and better at processing; those that are used less, on the other hand, are eliminated (Katz and Shatz, 1996). Remarkably, both early spontaneous and patterned activity (from sensory stimuli in the environment) influence synapse formation and stabilization (Leighton and Lohmann, 2016). In all mammalian species examined, including humans, synapse pruning (i.e., the controlled elimination of certain synapses) in the cerebral cortex begins before puberty, with a reduction of approximately 40 percent by the end of adolescence (Bourgeois, 1997). A core concept that has emerged from decades of neurobiological studies of the development and reorganization of connectivity is that environmental factors, which include fetal, postnatal, and child experiences, regulate the expression of genetic predispositions, and these experiences can dramatically change outcomes. This underlies the mechanism through which early exposure to chronic stressors and trauma so powerfully influences developmental processes in the brain and periphery. The research also makes clear that brain development and maturation depends on experience—what Greenough labeled "experience-expectant" development (Greenough et al., 1987).

Myelination is an often overlooked developmental process. Myelination entails forming the insulation around axons and is essential for increasing the capacity for rapid and efficient transmission of information in neural circuits (Bercury and Macklin, 2015). During the entire postnatal period discussed above (Gogtay et al., 2004), the glial cells responsible for myelination (Miller et al., 2012)—the **oligodendrocytes** in the brain and Schwann cells in the periphery—become the most active, forming the sheath around axons that promotes more rapid signaling between neurons. Myelin is composed mostly of protein and lipids (i.e., fats) to form the ensheathing membranes; myelination is highly dependent on nutritional status, experience, and other environmental factors (McLaughlin et al., 2017). Neurons are among the most metabolically active cells in the body, so they too are highly dependent on nutritional status. Myelination begins and ends in different regions of the nervous system at different times postnatally (Yeung et al., 2014), with the axon tracts beneath the frontal lobes taking the longest; myelination in this region can extend into the third decade of life (Miller et al., 2012). The timing of myelination completion corresponds to the reduction or ending of sensory critical periods, suggesting that myelin not only facilitates improved information processing but also participates in the maturation of synapse networks. This correlation has been tested experimentally by reversing myelination, resulting in reopening the critical period (McGee et al., 2005). This suggests that for human brain regions that have long periods of circuit myelination (such as frontal-lobe-associated circuits, in which executive functions continue to develop into young adulthood), extended periods of plasticity continue (Diamond, 2013).

Plasticity

The circuits of the brain undergo initial construction prenatally and remain relatively immature until postnatal periods, when experience drives remarkable growth that is reflected in formation of extensive connections (synapses) that form at a rate of at least 1 million per second during the first 2 years (Center on the Developing Child at Harvard University, n.d.-b,c). The role of experience in the development of functional circuits was established half a century ago in landmark studies of the visual system (reviewed by Hensch, 2016b; Hensch and Bilimoria, 2012). Binocular vision requires the use of both eyes by the infant to form an accurate representation of the visual world. This occurs during a sensitive or critical period, when there is heightened plasticity for changes in the fine details of circuits that will establish functioning for a lifetime. Since that time, neuroscience research has shown that all sensory and motor circuits, as well as those involved in social and emotional behaviors, cognition, motivation and reward, executive functioning, and even stress responsiveness, develop through experience-dependent mechanisms that involve heightened plasticity. Moreover, circuits remain open to change for different periods of time—sensory functions that are essential for the infant and toddler to perceive and respond to the environment are built first, followed by gross and fine motor and basic cognitive functions that provide the baby with opportunities to respond in more complex ways to experiences that provide input to the brain. This concept reflects the basic developmental rule that simple skills beget more complex skills, the paramount exemplar being language: from phoneme discrimination, to motor imitation, to making sounds that become part of a repertoire in which sounds become associated with objects, to objects becoming associated with words as the child begins the process of integrating language with more complex cognitive skills. It is important to emphasize that certain experiences, including physical exercise, are not necessarily limited in impact within certain periods and can be drivers of brain plasticity across the life-span. The evidence in basic and clinical research is compelling, showing effects on both physical well-being and cognitive and social-emotional capacities (Khan and Hillman, 2014; McEwen and Getz, 2013).

For all of these steps, there are heightened sensitive periods when experiences that occur over and over are the most potent. Periods have a beginning, a peak of varying length, and then a stretch of reduced plasticity when change can occur but in a far more limited fashion and with much greater effort. Think about learning a second language for the first time as an adolescent or adult. For all circuits that will be responsive to either positive or negative experiences, critical period shifts can occur that result in more rapid maturation or longer times of remaining open. Neither outcome of changes in plastic periods is beneficial. Note that genetic factors can also change circuit maturation (Heun-Johnson and Levitt, 2018), which then causes a different response to early experience, as if events were occurring in an older individual. In a model of early adversity (Bath et al., 2016), precocious maturation of molecular and behavioral measures was induced by early adversity. Disrupting neuronal metabolism in certain types of neurons prolongs the visual system's critical period plasticity (Morishita et al., 2015). All of these experimental studies mean that the normal periods of heightened plasticity are out of sync with the timing of when normal experiences are supposed to have optimal impact on circuit development. In humans, early adversity affects circuits that underlie specific functions in different ways (Nelson et al., 2014), with the timing of interventions (e.g., the Bucharest Early Intervention Project, which has done extensive research on the timing of placement in quality foster care after experiencing neglect in an orphanage) (Almas et al., 2018; Nelson et al., 2007; Wade et al., 2018; Zeanah et al., 2003) having a lasting effect on the quality of executive functioning, stress responsiveness, and attachment-related behaviors. Here, the impact on critical periods can only be hypothesized, but based on measures taken years later, it is likely that the timing of optimal sensitivity to experiences is changed in relation to specific functional domains.

The concept that altered neural development through genetic and experience-dependent mechanisms establishes different sensitivity to later-life adversity has been suggested for postadolescent onset psychiatric disorders (Keshavan et al., 2014) and more recently for ACEs (Danese et al., 2009; Loria et al., 2014; Morrison et al., 2017; Shalev and Belsky, 2016). The second adversity may be related to normal challenges or other life experiences that all of us endure and to which those without early adverse experiences are able to adapt. The mechanisms through which this vulnerability is read out have recently been addressed in a new set of animal studies (Peña et al., 2017). These demonstrate that there are early molecular changes in specific brain reward circuits due to early life stress that are responsible for the negative impact of later-endured juvenile social defeat (bullying) to produce depressive-like symptoms. For both human and animal studies, it is important to note that while early adverse experiences can have both acute and long-term impacts on mental and physical health, men and women may express these changes in different ways (e.g., externalizing or internalizing behaviors, respectively), which need to be accounted for in any intervention programs.

Immune System Development

The newborn immune system is shaped largely by the gut **microbiome,** which is initially primed by the vaginal or skin maternal microbiome during childbirth (depending on birth process) and early life, such as through breastfeeding (Miller, 2017). The gut microbiome refers to the vast collection of microbes that populate the gastrointestinal system and contribute to whole-body physiology. Molecules produced by the immune system impact various aspects of brain development, with strong evidence for mediating the formation and molecular adaptation of neural connections. The immune system also plays a role in the response of the brain and body to early life stress. In addition to the development of neurons and their connections with the periphery, the fetus' immune system undergoes rapid development in the first years of life and is yet another system that may be impacted by early adversity and stress (Simon et al., 2015). The **innate immune system**—which includes specialized cells, such as resident neutrophils, macrophages, and monocytes—develops in the fetal stage, though it is not robust enough to ward off most external pathogens. Of course, this lack of strong innate immunity may also provide the substrate for healthy microbiota to develop symbiotically with the newborn infant; the bacteria colonizing the gut, skin, and mucosa, for instance, assist in digestion and protection from other pathogens. Children's **adaptive immune systems**—governed by the **lymphatic system**—are relatively undeveloped at the time of birth, rendering them prone to bacterial, viral, and fungal infections soon after birth. At this time, the fetal adaptive immune system is prepared for "training" by the maternal microbiome, which occurs rapidly after birth via vaginal, skin, or mammary exposure (Lynch and Pedersen, 2016). Throughout childhood, children are exposed to countless microbes that are either summarily dismissed by the immune system without notice or produce a robust immune response that primes the immune system to protect the body against similar pathogens in the future.

The immune system can be trained to cope with certain challenges. For example, the "hygiene hypothesis" suggests that the prevalence of asthma has increased dramatically in certain parts of the world where children are no longer exposed to microbes that can train the immune system (Harding, 2006). In the face of other challenges, the nervous system activates the HPA axis, which can lead to suppressed immune functioning and thus increased susceptibility to infections (Cohen et al., 2007; Thompson, 2014). When children experience sustained exposure to challenges (e.g., chronic stressors, such as poverty or maltreatment), HPA axis activity may become blunted, which can reduce inhibition of inflammation and lead to elevated levels of chronic low-grade inflammation (Koss and Gunnar, 2018; Miller et al., 2011). In the past two decades, researchers have attempted to clarify (1) the relationship between social stressors and inflammation and other immune markers in children (Slopen et al., 2012), and (2) the role of the immune system in the development of neurodevelopmental (Entringer et al., 2015; Gilman et al., 2017) and psychiatric disorders (Danese and Baldwin, 2017; O'Connor et al., 2014) and the cardiovascular and atherosclerotic disease process (Hansson and Hermansson, 2011; Pearson et al., 2003). There is now evidence from longitudinal research that inflammation tracks from childhood to adulthood (Juonala et al., 2006) and that chronic inflammation is a risk factor for a wide range of diseases, including cardiovascular diseases and depression (Dantzer et al., 2008; Libby et al., 2002).

Endocrine System Development

The endocrine system is composed of several glands that secrete hormones—signaling molecules—that reach their target organs through the circulatory system to modulate every physiological function, such as growth and development, reproduction, stress responses, and metabolism. A key characteristic of the endocrine system is that it operates on feedback loops to allow the hormones to perform a function (e.g., the "fight or flight" stress response) and then resets to be ready for the next event that may trigger an endocrine response. In all mammals, including humans, the hypothalamus and pituitary are the center of control for the endocrine system. Because they impact many stages of development, the organs of the endocrine system themselves develop early on, in the first trimester of gestation. Moreover, early in the first trimester, the placenta produces the same releasing factor proteins that are synthesized in the hypothalamus of nonpregnant women. These proteins control the production and release of hormones from the pituitary and peripheral tissues in the mother and the fetus.

Neuroendocrine hormone markers are evident by the second trimester. The endocrine systems work in concert with the **autonomic nervous system** to regulate organ function. Autonomic regulation can be measured in the late second trimester and throughout the third trimester and is intact and operational at the time of birth (DiPietro, 2015). The **autonomic neurotransmitters** norepinephrine, epinephrine, and acetylcholine and the endocrine hormones reach their targets via body circulation. Thus, they affect metabolic processes through binding to membrane protein receptors that are expressed by target cells in the brain and other organs as early as the second trimester. Related to the stress response via cortisol production, activation of the glucocorticoid receptors in the hippocampus and hypothalamus serve as classic feedback loops to reduce hormone production in order to reset the stress response capacity.

Research in humans and animals shows that overexposure to stress hormones and autonomic neurotransmitters during prenatal or early postnatal development can result in a fetal programming response, which includes epigenetic changes in the genes that encode the stress hormone receptors. This process produces long-term changes in receptor expression and less robust negative feedback to limit stress hormones' chronic effects (for examples, see Maternal and Fetal/Infant Interactions section) (Meaney and Ferguson-Smith, 2010). In contrast, high levels of maternal care documented in animal studies show that the stress response system is capable of better management of later-life stress (Meaney, 2001; Plotsky and Meaney, 1993; Plotsky et al., 2005).

Reproductive System Development

The development of the reproductive system also begins early in gestation, in the first trimester. In the first 2 months of pregnancy, differentiation between male and female gonadal development occurs, which continues into the second and third trimesters. As noted above, animal studies show that intergenerational transmission of the impact of adversity during pregnancy can influence the mother, the fetus, and, if the developing gonads are affected, the offspring of the fetus when he or she matures into a reproductive adult. Sexual differentiation is controlled primarily by levels of testosterone, estrogen, and androgen, a process that can be influenced by **exogenous** chemicals similar in structure to these hormones. Among women, the ovarian follicle pool develops during the prenatal period; therefore, in-utero exposures may impact the size and quality of the follicle pool and influence the timing of ovarian loss and menopause (Bleil et al., 2018). For example, studies show that in-utero cigarette smoking exposure (Strohsnitter et al., 2008), famine (Yarde et al., 2013), and extremes of birth weight (Tom et al., 2010) are associated with earlier menopause. There is also evidence to suggest that maternal metabolic factors during pregnancy, including obesity and pregnancy hyperglycemia, are also associated with the timing of puberty (Kubo et al., 2018).

There has been a trend toward an earlier age of puberty for boys and girls in the United States that is not yet fully understood, and currently 9 years of age is within the normal range for onset of puberty (Herman-Giddens et al., 1997, 2012). Adverse social experiences in early and middle childhood—including socioeconomic adversity (Hiatt et al., 2017; Kelly et al., 2017; Sun et al., 2017) and child maltreatment (Mendle et al., 2016; Noll et al., 2017), as well as exposure to endocrine-disrupting chemicals (Buttke et al., 2012)—are associated with earlier pubertal development (Ellis and Giudice, 2019). In the United States and elsewhere, the age of puberty is earlier among racial/ethnic minority children (Herman-Giddens et al., 1997, 2012; Kelly et al., 2017; Reagan et al., 2012). These patterns by early childhood adversity and race/ethnicity may have implications for health disparities into adulthood (Bleil et al., 2017; Golub et al., 2008), as earlier puberty is associated with increased risk for depression (Wang et al., 2016) and substance use (Cance et al., 2013) during adolescence and numerous chronic disease outcomes in adulthood, including diabetes, cardiovascular diseases, and cancer (Canoy et al., 2015; Day et al., 2015; Elks et al., 2013).

Conclusion 2-1: Scientific research demonstrates healthy development of the child begins at preconception and is dependent on a strong foundation built prenatally. Therefore, access for the family to high-quality resources to limit chronic stress reduces risk for disrupted development and has the potential to close disparities based on race/ethnicity and socioeconomic status. Research findings show that specific types of resources are key to best outcomes, including healthy food, standard of care with a woman's health professional, maternal stress-reducing strategies, parenting education, and coaching. Research also has revealed that supportive relationships after birth are major contributors to healthy child development and building resilience.

BIOLOGICAL MECHANISMS OF STRESS

When the brain perceives a stressor, it induces a response that calls on multiple biological systems that, in the short term, are critical for adaptation and survival—sometimes defined as the "fight or flight" response. This stress response is a normal and healthy part of human biology. The spectrum of the stress response includes positive, tolerable, and toxic stress (Center on the Developing Child at Harvard University, 2005) and is governed by a complex interplay between the severity and duration of the stressor, individual genetic differences, gene–environment interaction, family environmental factors, developmental experiences, and the availability of buffering and coping strategies and resources. Positive and tolerable stress responses are characterized by a return to homeostasis, while the toxic stress response may induce lasting changes in brain architecture and function and in organ system development. Specific endocrine, immune, and brain cell populations produce bioactive chemicals that signal through their receptor proteins, which are present on cells throughout the body. These signals control cellular metabolism and physiological activity, which, in the short term, is a positive adaptation to the stressor.

Chronic activation of the stress response system can lead to risk for short- and long-term poor health outcomes beyond the early childhood period, including dysregulation of neuroendocrine and immune system development, altered cardiovascular functioning, metabolic dysregulation related to obesity and type 2 diabetes, changes to the gut microbiome, and epigenetic modifications that alter gene expression (Black, 2003; Campbell et al., 2014; Dinan and Cryan, 2012; Taylor et al., 2011; Vaiserman, 2015). There are individual differences in risk caused by chronically activated stress response systems, due in part to variation in the intrinsic sensitivity of the child, and physiological adaptive capacities that can be impacted by supportive environments (as discussed in greater detail below).

Activation of the stress response involves circuits in the brain that are essential for threat detection (**amygdala**), emotional regulation (frontal cortex), neuroendocrine regulation to produce cortisol (HPA axis), feedback to shut down the stress response (hippocampus), and the vagal complex in the brain stem that sends information to peripheral organs, such as the heart, lungs, and gastrointestinal systems (Cameron, 2009;

Dedovic et al., 2009; Forsythe et al., 2014; Goodman et al., 2013). The sympatho-adreno-medullary (SAM) axis responds to stress by producing and secreting adrenaline and noradrenaline through the vascular system. Adaptive responses of the SAM axis include increased arousal, alertness, and vigilance, improved cognition, focused attention, enhanced analgesia, and inhibition of appetite, feeding, digestion, growth, reproduction, and immunity (Chrousos, 2009). Adaptive responses of the HPA axis include regulation of cognitive, behavioral, affective, cardiovascular, and immune system functioning (Kudielka and Kirschbaum, 2005; McEwen et al., 2015). See Figure 2-2 for a diagram illustrating the stress response pathway.

Dysregulation of the Stress Response

Severe or chronic activation of the stress response, in the absence of adequate caregivers who serve as buffers to the stress activation, can lead to disruption of homeostatic mechanisms and long-term changes to brain architecture and organ systems (the toxic stress response) (Shonkoff et al., 2012). Early life stress can also result in epigenetic changes that can sensitize the individual to stress and adversity, alter the development of many organ systems, and impact the response to subsequent stressors later in the life course (see Epigenetics section) (National Scientific Council on the Developing Child, 2014). Exposure to high levels of adversity in early childhood is associated with the following multisystemic disruptions, with some of these changes occurring as early as infancy (e.g., changes to brain structure), while others are not evident until later in life (e.g., hypertension):

- Neurologic: There are structural and functional changes to stress-sensitive regions of the brain (McEwen and Morrison, 2013; National Scientific Council on the Developing Child, 2014).
- Endocrine: There is excessive activation of both the SAM and HPA axes, associated with loss of feedback inhibition of the HPA axis, increased levels of corticotropin-releasing hormone, and disruption of the daily cortisol pattern, leading to abnormally lower morning cortisol levels, elevated afternoon cortisol levels, and an overall increase in cortisol exposure. Over time, excess HPA activation may recede, leading to low or deficient HPA axis response. HPA axis overactivity is associated with suppression of thyroid function. High doses of early adversity are associated with changes in reproductive function through the HPA axis' effect on gonadotropins and/or cytokine suppression of reproductive function (Dedovic et al., 2009; Kudielka and Kirschbaum, 2005; Slopen et al., 2014).
- Immune function: There is dysregulation of neuro-endocrine-immune relations, leading to increased pro-inflammatory

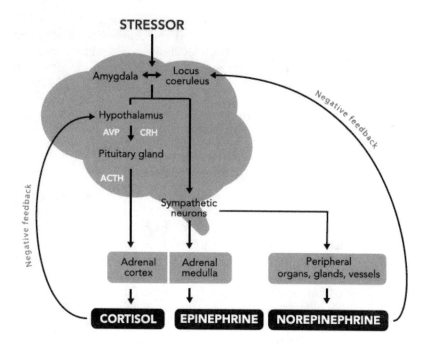

The HPA axis controls the body's response to stress and is a complex interplay of direct interactions. The HPA axis is composed of:

1. The **hypothalamus** which releases AVP and CRH to the pituitary gland

2. The **pituitary gland** which secretes ACTH when stimulated by AVP and CRH

3. The **adrenal cortex** which secretes glucocorticoids (cortisol) when stimulated by ACTH

The SAM axis mediates a rapid response to stress through interconnected neurons and regulates autonomic functions in multiple organ systems. The SAM axis is composed of:

1. The **sympathetic neurons** which release epinephrine and norepinephrine and activate the body's "fight or flight" response

2. The **parasympathetic neurons** which withdraw the activity of the sympathetic neurons and promote the body's "rest and digest" response

3. The **adrenal medulla** which when triggered by the sympathetic neurons secretes circulating epinephrine and activate the body's "fight or flight" response

FIGURE 2-2 Stress response pathway.
NOTE: ACTH = adrenocorticotropin hormone; AVP = arginine vasopressin; CRH = corticotropin-releasing hormone; HPA axis = hypothalamic-pituitary-adrenal axis; SAM axis = sympatho-adreno-medullary axis.
SOURCE: Bucci et al., 2016. Reprinted from Advances in Pediatrics, 63/1, Bucci et al. Toxic Stress in Children and Adolescents, 403–428, Copyright (2016), with permission from Elsevier.

cytokines and inhibition of anti-inflammatory pathways. In addition, humoral (antibody production) and cell-mediated acquired immunity can be impaired. High levels of early adversity in childhood are associated with increased risk of autoimmune disease in adulthood (Nusslock and Miller, 2016; Padgett and Glaser, 2003).

- Cardiometabolic: There is insulin resistance, obesity, glucose intolerance, reduced control over blood lipid levels, and hypertension (Non et al., 2014; Woo Baidal et al., 2016).

Buffering the Stress Response

From a population health perspective, ameliorating the toxic stress response and understanding the biological mechanisms by which toxic stress can be prevented or mitigated is of high priority. Importantly, research suggests several mechanisms to buffer against toxic stress. One mechanism—studied in depth in animal models—is social relationships (Gunnar and Fisher, 2006). Research on resilience has clearly demonstrated that the single most important protective factor for children facing adversity is a strong, secure relationship with at least one parent; this helps foster positive outcomes across domains ranging from psychological adjustment to positive peer relationships (Cicchetti, 2013; Luthar et al., 2015; Masten, 2018; Sroufe, 2005). Moreover, a child who is securely attached to a primary caregiver is more likely to have high self-esteem, emotion regulation skills, and a positive outlook later in life (Sroufe, 2005). It also has been demonstrated that supportive relationships early in life play an important role in buffering stress responses, thereby allowing children to more easily confront stressful situations (Hostinar et al., 2014). (See Chapter 4 for an in-depth discussion on caregiver and social connections.) Some studies have shown an effect of social buffering on regulating the HPA axis, autonomic nervous system, and immune functioning, though more research is needed for more in-depth assessment of neuro-endocrine-immune, metabolic, and genetic regulatory functions (Hennessy et al., 2009; Hostinar et al., 2014; Kikusui et al., 2006).

While the mechanisms through which nurturing relationships buffer against toxic stress are likely to be complex, some studies have shown that the neuropeptide hormones oxytocin and vasopressin play important roles in affiliative social behavior (Bartz et al., 2011; Gunnar and Hostinar, 2015; Ross and Young, 2009; Ross et al., 2009a,b), though experimental work in social neuroscience is challenging (Insel, 2010a). Studies in animals and humans have shown that oxytocin and/or vasopressin play a role in social memory, pair bonding, empathy, altruism, emotion regulation, and trust (De Dreu and Kret, 2016; Donaldson and Young, 2008; Hostinar et al., 2014; Israel et al., 2012; Quirin et al., 2011; Rodrigues et al., 2009; Snowdon et al., 2010). It is thought that increased oxytocin counteracts the biological underpinnings of toxic stress, including increased inflammation, cardio-vascular dysfunction, oxidative stress, and alterations in brain structure and function (Detillion et al., 2004; Donaldson and Young, 2008; Heinrichs et al., 2003; Hostinar et al., 2014; Mantella et al., 2004). Social buffering to toxic stress, and its action through oxytocin and vasopressin (Gobrogge and Wang, 2015), is still an ongoing area of research, as is intergenerational transmission of trauma and trauma-related stress (Kim and Strathearn, 2017). For example, how such mechanisms change with development still remains to be determined (Gunnar and Hostinar, 2015). Still, this evidence suggests that interventions to create strong social relationships may ward against the long-term impacts of ACEs and other chronic adversity over the course of child development and into adulthood. More research is needed to understand other buffers against toxic stress (e.g., sleep, exercise, nutrition) and the biological mechanisms through which they operate; prefrontal cortex plasticity is one such mechanism (McEwen and Morrison, 2013).

Conclusion 2-2: Among all of the factors that may serve to buffer negative outcomes produced by toxic stress, supportive relationships between the child and the adults in his or her life are essential.

Biological Measures of Stress in Children

In the decades since *From Neurons to Neighborhoods*, there have been substantial efforts to understand the biological changes that occur in response to early adversity (Danese and McEwen, 2012; NRC and IOM, 2000), at least in part inspired by the goal of developing valid, minimally invasive, low-burden measures of biological stress and neurobiological functioning in children that can be used to identify individuals at risk for poor long-term outcomes and, importantly, the impact of early life intervention (Shonkoff, 2010; Shonkoff et al., 2009). An increasing number of developmental studies with children now collect biological measures of stress, aiming to study how social experiences relate to changes in the biology of the child that may not cause immediate, gross disturbances (i.e., biological alterations that increase risk for subsequent chronic diseases) but rather set up the brain and peripheral systems for later emergence of physical and mental health problems over time. This research shows that traumatic experiences (such as child maltreatment) or prolonged exposure to chronic stress (such as poverty) can result in a chronically activated physiological stress response, which has a host of downstream consequences across biological systems. Some of this research has applied the concept of "**allostasis**" or "allostatic load," which provides a method to evaluate the cumulative biological impact, or "wear and tear," on the body as the result of a given social exposure (Danese and McEwen, 2012; McEwen, 1998). As noted in previous sections of this chapter, both animal and human research has demonstrated that early life stress contributes to altered brain development (i.e., structure and function) and therefore to allostatic load.

Synthesis

Advances in science technologies, big data collection and information technology, and new strategies for analyzing complex data have been instrumental in rapidly advancing the science of brain and child development over the nearly 20 years since *From Neurons to Neighborhoods* was released to the public (NRC and IOM, 2000). Research findings have revealed the details of how early experiences are essential for building brain connections that underlie biobehavioral health, the role of genetics in development, and a new understanding of whole-child development that relies on organ systems interacting with each other and the environment to establish health and biobehavioral fitness or risk due to early influences of adversity.

Conclusion 2-3: Research has changed the discourse to include scientific facts in child development that have determined that when considering the entire life course, it is early experiences, pre- and postnatally, that are the most powerful in working together with an individual's genetic makeup to influence the physical, mental, and cognitive development of the child. Science also shows that maternal health and well-being is a major contributing factor to the development of the fetus and establishes a foundation for positive or negative child health outcomes.

Conclusion 2-4: Based on the abundant science, the influence of access to basic resources prenatally, particularly nutritional, psychosocial, and health care components, is powerful. The new understanding defines three interrelated parts:

1. *Chronic activation of the stress response system of primary caregivers, and in the infant and toddler, can occur due to a large number of factors in the environment of the family, including lack of access to quality health care, child care, economic security, community support programs, transportation, stable housing, and healthy nutritional sources; institutional and individual racism and sexism; and community violence;*
2. *Sustained stress activation can produce a response in the child known as toxic stress, which affects the development of the structural organization and functioning of brain circuits that impact the quality of cognition and social and emotional regulation, including the child's own stress response, reward, and motivation. The toxic stress response therefore directly impacts the behavioral and psychological well-being of the child; and*

3. *New data from longitudinal studies, combined with previous work from retrospective analyses of the early life experiences of adults, provides a compelling demonstration that toxic stress response substantially increases later-life risk for physical illnesses, including obesity and type 2 diabetes, cardiovascular disease, substance abuse, mental illness, lower educational achievement, cancer, and infectious disease. In addition to the adverse effects of toxic stress on the brain and nervous system, it also affects every other organ system in the child's body, impacting short- and long-term health.*

Individual Differences in Responsiveness and Susceptibility

Research over the past two decades clearly shows that what were previously considered to be universal developmental processes (see Chapter 4) do not occur uniformly. Relevant to the focus of this chapter, this can be due in part to variation in the development trajectory of stress-sensitive brain circuits in infancy, as well as the interplay between genes and environments that mediates the neurobiological and physical impact of positive or negative early life experiences. Thus, heterogeneity with substantial variations is often observed, such as across groups that differ by SES or ethnicity. Diversity brought about by individual and subgroup differences, based on factors such as personal experiences, individual temperament, culture, and the family and community context, can alter the pace and trajectories of developmental, biological, and psychological processes. For example, humans are predisposed to become attached to our main caregivers, but the quality of interactions between caregiver and child and other environmental conditions can contribute to the development of various types of infant attachment. To consider another example, a rich literature supports the notion that children differ in their temperament: behavioral predispositions can permeate how children react to and process environmental input. From conception, children bring differential responsiveness to—and processing of—their physical and relational context. Infants are described as difficult, inhibited or uninhibited, shy or slow to warm up (Conture et al., 2013). These dispositions carry consequences for adaptability to new environments, relational difficulties, and even long-term mental health problems (Clauss et al., 2015). One research notion from the temperament literature proposes that there are behavioral predispositions that are normative variations across individuals (Durbin and Hicks, 2014). Another theory sees the origin of these individual differences as consequences of exposure to early stress, whereby stress experienced by the mother and fetus before birth conditions the nervous system to respond, perhaps in an exaggerated way, to neutral or mild environmental input (Miller et al., 2011).

Recently, there has been an emphasis on elucidating the mechanisms underlying the differential susceptibility to the environment hypothesis. Work by both Belsky and Boyce has advanced understanding of how individual differences in how children process and react to the environment contribute to individual risk and resilience (Boyce, 2019; Bush and Boyce, 2016). Behavioral genetics research defined the contributions of both heritability and environment to the variance in the symptoms and incidence of behavioral disorder diagnoses (Plomin et al., 2001). This core principle is evident in the assessment of typical behavioral characteristics, such as affiliative social behavior. Studies of twins highlight the remarkable variability in specific traits that make up affiliative social behavior (Ebstein et al., 2010), with some elements exhibiting high (~0.7) heritability (prosocial behavior; social responsiveness) and others low (~0.3) heritability (empathy; secure attachment). In animal studies, heritability of the behaviors that make up affiliative social behavior exhibits very similar genetic contributions (Knoll et al., 2018).

These studies also showed that environmental context plays a particularly important role in modifying behavior—even in those with moderate to high heritability. As Bush and Boyce (2016) note, the accumulating biological data from studies of humans and animals have changed the concept from the long-standing diathesis stress model of sensitivity to environment to one that focuses on determining factors that confer individual differences that affect susceptibility and resilience. Stress reactivity, which had been presumed to influence behavioral outcomes in a single direction—negatively—is an important individual difference that can influence responses to different environmental contexts in either a positive or negative direction (Bush and Boyce, 2014; Ellis et al., 2011; Obradović et al., 2010). Again, context appears to be a major moderator of biological predispositions, and an ongoing topic of study is why some children adhere to healthy developmental trajectories despite profoundly adverse circumstances while others do not (Cicchetti, 2013; Masten, 2014; NASEM, 2015; Rutter, 2012; Shonkoff, 2016).

The importance of individual differences in development points out lessons for practice and policies in efforts to prevent developmental problems and promote positive trajectories (Shonkoff, 2017). A key fact is that universal interventions will be more or less effective depending on the individual(s) being targeted. Thus, well-designed interventions are those that are sufficiently flexible to take individual differences and heterogeneity into account. The challenge continues to be predicting what specific changes are most likely to produce the best outcomes. For example, the New Hope Project, a welfare reform demonstration based in Milwaukee, Wisconsin, was designed to raise families out of poverty, using a work-support intervention that was tailored to the specific needs of each family (Huston et al., 2011). The intervention had multiple components that families would choose from over 3 years, and it was expected that the combination of benefits and services would increase parents' employment, income, and use of child care and health insurance. In a report to summarize effects over 8 years (i.e., 5 years after the intervention ended), researchers concluded that work supports can positively impact low-income parents and children, even though the economic effects of employment and income were not sustained beyond the 3 years of the intervention. Importantly, positive effects for children appeared during the intervention period and extended to the 8-year follow-up.[8]

Another example is *Filming Interactions to Nurture Development*, a 10-week video-feedback program to promote acquisition of developmentally supportive parenting skills (Fisher et al., 2016; Nese et al., 2016). This behavioral training program is tailored to address individual differences in the types of challenging parenting styles via weekly structured coaching sessions, and findings suggest that it is effective for improving caregiver skills (Fisher et al., 2016).

In some cases, individuals have different responses to social or environmental stimuli as the result of age of exposure. Specific time points in development represent "sensitive periods" when risk or protective factors have a maximal influence on cognitive capacities, biology, emotions, and behavior (Ben-Shlomo and Kuh, 2002; Hertzman and Boyce, 2010; Knudsen, 2004; Zeanah et al., 2011). The strongest evidence for the heightened importance of specific periods comes from experiments using laboratory animals (Hertzman and Boyce, 2010) because it is challenging to isolate sensitive periods within observational studies in humans (given that risk factors are often continuous and may in turn elicit subsequent risks). As noted in detail above, the prenatal, postnatal, and early childhood phases are recognized as having sensitive periods that result in brain and behavioral changes. Research is beginning to elucidate how risk factors at different time points may have varying impacts. Although it is generally accepted that developmental timing can influence the effect of a social or environmental risk factor on child health, the majority of studies do not consider how risk or protective factors vary by age.

---

[8] Although the positive effect of this personalized intervention on children's academic performance and test scores at the 2- and 5-year follow-ups faded, at the 8-year follow-up, children in families assigned to the intervention condition were more likely to be engaged in school and to show positive social behaviors relative to those in families assigned to the control condition, and they were less likely to have to repeat a grade, to be placed in special education, to receive poor grades, or to have cynical attitudes about work (Miller et al., 2008).

CONCLUSION

With advances in science emerging from different disciplines, now more than ever, there is a major need to facilitate new public–private–non-profit sector relations to build substantial opportunities for the fields of neuroscience, behavioral sciences, and psychology to collaborate. Therefore, the committee recommends:

Recommendation 2-1: The National Institutes of Health and other relevant research entities should support the development of public–private partnerships or other innovative collaborations to

- **Build multidisciplinary teams, including but not limited to researchers in neuroscience, endocrinology, immunology, physiology, metabolism, behavior, psychology, and primary care, to identify the most relevant factors in a child's complex environment that promote resilience and outcomes related to physical and mental health.**
- **Conduct research that measures the impact of chronic stress on all relevant organ systems and determines the specific molecular and biological pathways of interaction during the pre- and postnatal periods, which are directly relevant to potential interventions to address health disparities.**

This will require recruiting diverse populations, with explicit attention to addressing racial/ethnic and socioeconomic inequities in developmental outcomes. Research with these populations will require researchers and practitioners that are knowledgeable of theoretical models, measures, and the realities of these families and communities as co-investigators. For all studies that typically use expensive biological assessments (e.g., biomarkers as mediators, moderators, or outcomes) for use in interventions, researchers need to strongly consider the ability to apply measures within the context of scaled, community-based interventions to have the broadest possible impact on outcomes for children and their caregivers. For example, there is a major gap in research support for projects that combine modern, noninvasive technologies to measure key domains of brain, behavioral, and psychological development with clinical interventions that promote best outcomes for children and their caregivers.

In summary, research advances in neuroscience, immunology, endocrinology, behavior, and psychology in the past two decades provide a new depth of understanding regarding the impact of adverse experiences on developmental processes throughout the life course. Because of these advances, the fields of developmental neuroscience, behavior, and psychology are recognizing the trajectories of development in the context of racial, ethnic, and socioeconomic health disparities. Deciphering the mechanisms through which adversity disrupts foundational developmental processes of the whole child, and the long-term impact on health, wellness, personal and community relationships, and life-span productivity across the life course, is being achieved through multidisciplinary, longitudinally designed research that has incorporated principles of human development, including individual differences and differential sensitivity to context. With this foundation, the chapters that follow provide advances in the research that address the role of macro- and micro-level variables in influencing development and outcomes.

REFERENCES

Acevedo-Garcia, D., N. McArdle, E. F. Hardy, U. I. Crisan, B. Romano, D. Norris, M. Baek, and J. Reece. 2014. The Child Opportunity Index: Improving collaboration between community development and public health. *Health Affairs* 33(11):1948–1957.

Acevedo-Garcia, D., N. McArdle, E. Hardy, K.-N. Dillman, J. Reece, U. I. Crisan, D. Norris, and T. L. Osypuk. 2016. Neighborhood opportunity and location affordability for low-income renter families. *Housing Policy Debate* 26(4–5):607–645.

Akins, M. R., and T. Biederer. 2006. Cell-cell interactions in synaptogenesis. *Current Opinion in Neurobiology* 16(1):83–89.

Almas, A. N., L. J. Papp, M. R. Woodbury, C. A. Nelson, C. H. Zeanah, and N. A. Fox. 2018. The impact of caregiving disruptions of previously institutionalized children on multiple outcomes in late childhood. *Child Development.* doi: 10.1111/cdev.13169. [Epub ahead of print.]

Amrit, C., T. Paauw, R. Aly, and M. Lavric. 2017. Identifying child abuse through text mining and machine learning. *Expert Systems with Applications* 88:402–418.

Bae, B. I., D. Jayaraman, and C. A. Walsh. 2015. Genetic changes shaping the human brain. *Developmental Cell* 32(4):423–434.

Bagot, K. S., S. A. Matthews, M. Mason, L. M. Squeglia, J. Fowler, K. Gray, M. Herting, A. May, I. Colrain, J. Godino, S. Tapert, S. Brown, and K. Patrick. 2018. Current, future and potential use of mobile and wearable technologies and social media data in the ABCD Study to increase understanding of contributors to child health. *Developmental Cognitive Neuroscience* 32:121–129.

Bale, T. L. 2015. Epigenetic and transgenerational reprogramming of brain development. *Nature Reviews Neuroscience* 16(6):332–344.

Bartz, J. A., J. Zaki, N. Bolger, and K. N. Ochsner. 2011. Social effects of oxytocin in humans: Context and person matter. *Trends in Cognitive Sciences* 15(7):301–309.

Bastek, J. A., L. M. Gómez, and M. A. Elovitz. 2011. The role of inflammation and infection in preterm birth. *Clinics in Perinatology* 38(3):385–406.

Bath, K. G., G. Manzano-Nieves, and H. Goodwill. 2016. Early life stress accelerates behavioral and neural maturation of the hippocampus in male mice. *Hormones and Behavior* 82:64–71.

Beck, A. F., B. Huang, P. H. Ryan, M. T. Sandel, C. Chen, and R. S. Kahn. 2016. Areas with high rates of police-reported violent crime have higher rates of childhood asthma morbidity. *The Journal of Pediatrics* 173:175–182.

Beck, A. F., B. Huang, K. Wheeler, N. R. Lawson, R. S. Kahn, and C. L. Riley. 2017a. The Child Opportunity Index and disparities in pediatric asthma hospitalizations across one Ohio metropolitan area, 2011–2013. *The Journal of Pediatrics* 190:200–206.

Beck, A. F., M. T. Sandel, P. H. Ryan, and R. S. Kahn. 2017b. Mapping neighborhood health geomarkers to clinical care decisions to promote equity in child health. *Health Affairs* 36(6):999–1005.

Belfield, C. R., M. Nores, S. Barnett, and L. Schweinhart. 2006. The High/Scope Perry Preschool Program cost–benefit analysis using data from the age-40 followup. *Journal of Human Resources* 41(1):162–190.

Ben-Shlomo, Y., and D. Kuh. 2002. A life course approach to chronic disease epidemiology: Conceptual models, empirical challenges and interdisciplinary perspectives. *International Journal of Epidemiology* 31(2):285–293.

Ben-Shlomo, Y., G. Mishra, and D. Kuh. 2014. Life course epidemiology. In *Handbook of epidemiology*, edited by W. Ahrens and I. Pigeot. New York: Springer. Pp. 1521–1549.

Berbari, E. J., E. A. Bock, A. C. Chazaro, X. Sun, and L. Sornmo. 2005. High-resolution analysis of ambulatory electrocardiograms to detect possible mechanisms of premature ventricular beats. *IEEE Transactions on Biomedical Engineering* 52(4):593–598.

Bercury, K. K., and W. B. Macklin. 2015. Dynamics and mechanisms of CNS myelination. *Developmental Cell* 32(4):447–458.

Black, P. H. 2003. The inflammatory response is an integral part of the stress response: Implications for atherosclerosis, insulin resistance, type II diabetes and metabolic syndrome X. *Brain, Behavior, and Immunity* 17(5):350–364.

Bleil, M. E., C. Booth-LaForce, and A. D. Benner. 2017. Race disparities in pubertal timing: Implications for cardiovascular disease risk among African American women. *Population Research and Policy Review* 36(5):717–738.

Bleil, M. E., P. English, J. Valle, N. F. Woods, K. D. Crowder, S. E. Gregorich, and M. I. Cedars. 2018. Is in utero exposure to maternal socioeconomic disadvantage related to offspring ovarian reserve in adulthood? *Women's Midlife Health* 4(1):5.

Bonnin, A., and P. Levitt. 2011. Fetal, maternal, and placental sources of serotonin and new implications for developmental programming of the brain. *Neuroscience* 197:1–7.

Bonnin, A., N. Goeden, K. Chen, M. L. Wilson, J. King, J. C. Shih, R. D. Blakely, E. S. Deneris, and P. Levitt. 2011. A transient placental source of serotonin for the fetal forebrain. *Nature* 472(7343):347–350.

Bourgeois, J. P. 1997. Synaptogenesis, heterochrony and epigenesis in the mammalian neocortex. *Acta Paediatrica* 422:27–33.

Boyce, W. 2019. *The orchid and the dandelion: Why some children struggle and how all can thrive.* New York: Knopf.

Boyce, W. T., and M. S. Kobor. 2015. Development and the epigenome: The "synapse" of gene–environment interplay. *Developmental Science* 18(1):1–23.

Brikell, I., H. Larsson, Y. Lu, E. Pettersson, Q. Chen, R. Kuja-Halkola, R. Karlsson, B. B. Lahey, P. Lichtenstein, and J. Martin. 2018. The contribution of common genetic risk variants for ADHD to a general factor of childhood psychopathology. *Molecular Psychiatry* 1.

Brito, N. H., and K. G. Noble. 2014. Socioeconomic status and structural brain development. *Frontiers in Neuroscience* 8:276.

Bronfenbrenner, U. 1979. Contexts of child rearing: Problems and prospects. *American Psychologist* 34(10):844–850.

Bronfenbrenner, U., and G. W. Evans. 2000. Developmental science in the 21st century: Emerging questions, theoretical models, research designs and empirical findings. *Social Development* 9(1):115–125.

Bucci, M., S. S. Marques, D. Oh, and N. B. Harris. 2016. Toxic stress in children and adolescents. *Advances in Pediatrics* 63(1):403–428.

Burton, T., and N. B. Metcalfe. 2014. Can environmental conditions experienced in early life influence future generations? *Proceedings of the Royal Society B: Biological Sciences* 281(1785).

Bush, N. R., and T. Boyce. 2014. The contributions of early experience to biological development and sensitivity to context. In *Handbook of developmental psychopathology*, edited by M. Lewis and K. Rudolph. New York: Springer. Pp. 287–309.

Bush, N. R., and T. Boyce. 2016. Differential sensitivity to context: Implications for developmental psychopathology. In *Developmental psychopathology*, Vol. 2, edited by D. Cicchetti. Hoboken, NJ: John Wiley & Sons, Inc. Pp. 107–137.

Buss, C., S. Entringer, N. K. Moog, P. Toepfer, D. A. Fair, H. N. Simhan, C. M. Heim, and P. D. Wadhwa. 2017. Intergenerational transmission of maternal childhood maltreatment exposure: Implications for fetal brain development. *Journal of the American Academy of Child and Adolescent Psychiatry* 56(5):373–382.

Buttke, D. E., K. Sircar, and C. Martin. 2012. Exposures to endocrine-disrupting chemicals and age of menarche in adolescent girls in NHANES. *Environmental Health Perspectives* 120(11):1613–1618.

Bystron, I., C. Blakemore, and P. Rakic. 2008. Development of the human cerebral cortex: Boulder committee revisited. *Nature Reviews Neuroscience* 9:110.

Cameron, J. L., K. L. Eagleson, N. A. Fox, T. K. Hensch, and P. Levitt. 2017. Social origins of developmental risk for mental and physical illness. *Journal of Neuroscience* 37(45):10783–10791.

Cameron, O. G. 2009. Visceral brain–body information transfer. *Neuroimage* 47(3):787–794.

Campbell, F., G. Conti, J. J. Heckman, S. H. Moon, R. Pinto, E. Pungello, and Y. Pan. 2014. Early childhood investments substantially boost adult health. *Science* 343(6178):1478–1485.

Cance, J. D., S. T. Ennett, A. A. Morgan-Lopez, V. A. Foshee, and A. E. Talley. 2013. Perceived pubertal timing and recent substance use among adolescents: A longitudinal perspective. *Addiction* 108(10):1845–1854.

Canoy, D., V. Beral, A. Balkwill, F. L. Wright, M. E. Kroll, G. K. Reeves, J. Green, and B. J. Cairns. 2015. Age at menarche and risks of coronary heart and other vascular diseases in a large UK cohort. *Circulation* 131(3):237–244.

Carlyle, B. C., R. R. Kitchen, J. E. Kanyo, E. Z. Voss, M. Pletikos, A. M. M. Sousa, T. T. Lam, M. B. Gerstein, N. Sestan, and A. C. Nairn. 2017. A multiregional proteomic survey of the postnatal human brain. *Nature Neuroscience* 20(12):1787–1795.

Casillas, K. L., A. Fauchier, B. T. Derkash, and E. F. Garrido. 2016. Implementation of evidence-based home visiting programs aimed at reducing child maltreatment: A meta-analytic review. *Child Abuse & Neglect* 53:64–80.

Causadias, J. M., and A. J. Umaña-Taylor. 2018. Reframing marginalization and youth development: Introduction to the special issue. *American Psychologist* 73(6):707–712.

Center on the Developing Child at Harvard University. 2005. *Excessive stress disrupts the architecture of the developing brain.* Cambridge, MA: Harvard University. Pp. 1–9.

Center on the Developing Child at Harvard University. 2014. *A decade of science informing policy: The story of the National Scientific Council on the Developing Child.* Cambridge, MA: Harvard University.

Center on the Developing Child at Harvard University. n.d-a. *Brain architecture.* https://developingchild.harvard.edu/science/key-concepts/brain-architecture (accessed June 17, 2019).

Center on the Developing Child at Harvard University. n.d.-b. *Five numbers to remember about early childhood development.* https://pdg.grads360.org/services/PDCService.svc/GetPDCDocumentFile?fileId=16462 (accessed June 17, 2019).

Center on the Developing Child at Harvard University. n.d.-c. *What is early childhood development? A guide to the science.* https://developingchild.harvard.edu/guide/what-is-early-childhood-development-a-guide-to-the-science (accessed April 17, 2019).

Chan, J. C., B. M. Nugent, and T. L. Bale. 2018. Parental advisory: Maternal and paternal stress can impact offspring neurodevelopment. *Biological Psychiatry* 83(10):886–894.

Chen, M., and K. L. Chan. 2016. Effects of parenting programs on child maltreatment prevention: A meta-analysis. *Trauma, Violence, & Abuse* 17(1):88–104.

Chen, Y., and T. Z. Baram. 2016. Toward understanding how early-life stress reprograms cognitive and emotional brain networks. *Neuropsychopharmacology* 41(1):197–206.

Chetty, R., N. Hendren, and L. F. Katz. 2016. The effects of exposure to better neighborhoods on children: New evidence from the Moving to Opportunity experiment. *The American Economic Review* 106(4):855–902.

Cheung, K. L., and R. A. Lafayette. 2013. Renal physiology of pregnancy. *Advances in Chronic Kidney Disease* 20(3):209–214.

Christian, H., S. R. Zubrick, S. Foster, B. Giles-Corti, F. Bull, L. Wood, M. Knuiman, S. Brinkman, S. Houghton, and B. Boruff. 2015. The influence of the neighborhood physical environment on early child health and development: A review and call for research. *Health & Place* 33:25–36.

Chrousos, G. P. 2009. Stress and disorders of the stress system. *Nature Reviews Endocrinology* 5(7):374.

Cicchetti, D. 1996. Child maltreatment: Implications for developmental theory and research. *Human Development* 39(1):18–39.

Cicchetti, D. 2013. Annual research review: Resilient functioning in maltreated children—past, present, and future perspectives. *Journal of Child Psychology and Psychiatry* 54(4):402–422.

Cicchetti, D. 2015a. Neural plasticity, sensitive periods, and psychopathology. *Development and Psychopathology* 27(2):319–320.

Cicchetti, D. 2015b. Preventive intervention efficacy, development, and neural plasticity. *Journal of the American Academy of Child & Adolescent Psychiatry* 54(2):83–85.

Cicchetti, D., and J. A. Blender. 2006. A multiple-levels-of-analysis perspective on resilience: Implications for the developing brain, neural plasticity, and preventive interventions. *Annals of the New York Academy of Sciences* 1094:248–258.

Cicchetti, D., and W. J. Curtis. 2006. The developing brain and neural plasticity: Implications for normality, psychopathology, and resilience. In *Developmental psychopathology: Developmental neuroscience*, 2nd ed. Vol. 2, edited by D. J. Cohen. New York: Wiley. Pp. 1–64.

Cicchetti, D., and E. D. Handley. 2017. Methylation of the glucocorticoid receptor gene, nuclear receptor subfamily 3, group c, member 1 (NR3C1), in maltreated and nonmaltreated children: Associations with behavioral undercontrol, emotional lability/negativity, and externalizing and internalizing symptoms. *Development and Psychopathology* 29(5):1795–1806.

Clauss, J. A., S. N. Avery, and J. U. Blackford. 2015. The nature of individual differences in inhibited temperament and risk for psychiatric disease: A review and meta-analysis. *Progress in Neurobiology* 127–128:23–45.

Cohen, S., D. Janicki-Deverts, and G. E. Miller. 2007. Psychological stress and disease. *JAMA* 298(14):1685–1687.

Coll, C. G., and L. A. Szalacha. 2004. The multiple contexts of middle childhood. *Future of Children* 14(2):81–97.

Collins, F. S. 2004. What we do and don't know about "race," "ethnicity," genetics and health at the dawn of the genome era. *Nature Genetics* 36(Suppl 11):S13–S15.

Conture, E. G., E. M. Kelly, and T. A. Walden. 2013. Temperament, speech and language: An overview. *Journal of Communication Disorders* 46(2):125–142.

Corso, P. S., S. N. Visser, J. B. Ingels, and R. Perou. 2015. Cost-effectiveness of Legacy for Children for reducing behavioral problems and risk for ADHD among children living in poverty. *Journal of Child and Adolescent Behaviour* 3(5):240.

Costantine, M. M. 2014. Physiologic and pharmacokinetic changes in pregnancy. *Frontiers in Pharmacology* 5:65.

Council on Community Pediatrics. 2016. Poverty and child health in the United States. *Pediatrics* 137(4):e20160339.

Criado-Marrero, M., T. Rein, E. B. Binder, J. T. Porter, J. Koren, 3rd, and L. J. Blair. 2018. HSP90 and FKBP51: Complex regulators of psychiatric diseases. *Philosophical Transactions of the Royal Society B: Biological Sciences* 373(1738).

Cuffe, J. S., L. O'Sullivan, D. G. Simmons, S. T. Anderson, and K. M. Moritz. 2012. Maternal corticosterone exposure in the mouse has sex-specific effects on placental growth and MRNA expression. *Endocrinology* 153(11):5500–5511.

Cunningham, M. 2019. Introduction to myths and realities associated with research and theorizing for human development. *Research in Human Development* 16(1):1–4.

Danese, A., and J. R. Baldwin. 2017. Hidden wounds? Inflammatory links between childhood trauma and psychopathology. *Annual Review of Psychology* 68:517–544.

Danese, A., and B. S. McEwen. 2012. Adverse childhood experiences, allostasis, allostatic load, and age-related disease. *Physiology & Behavior* 106(1):29–39.

Danese, A., T. E. Moffitt, H. Harrington, B. J. Milne, G. Polanczyk, C. M. Pariante, R. Poulton, and A. Caspi. 2009. Adverse childhood experiences and adult risk factors for age-related disease: Depression, inflammation, and clustering of metabolic risk markers. *Archives of Pediatrics and Adolescent Medicine* 163(12):1135–1143.

Dantzer, R., J. C. O'Connor, G. G. Freund, R. W. Johnson, and K. W. Kelley. 2008. From inflammation to sickness and depression: When the immune system subjugates the brain. *Nature Reviews Neuroscience* 9(1):46–56.

Day, F. R., C. E. Elks, A. Murray, K. K. Ong, and J. R. Perry. 2015. Puberty timing associated with diabetes, cardiovascular disease and also diverse health outcomes in men and women: The UK Biobank Study. *Scientific Reports* 5:11208.

De Dreu, C. K., and M. E. Kret. 2016. Oxytocin conditions intergroup relations through upregulated in-group empathy, cooperation, conformity, and defense. *Biological Psychiatry* 79(3):165–173.

Dedovic, K., A. Duchesne, J. Andrews, V. Engert, and J. C. Pruessner. 2009. The brain and the stress axis: The neural correlates of cortisol regulation in response to stress. *Neuroimage* 47(3):864–871.

Detillion, C. E., T. K. S. Craft, E. R. Glasper, B. J. Prendergast, and A. C. DeVries. 2004. Social facilitation of wound healing. *Psychoneuroendocrinology* 29(8):1004–1011.

Diamond, A. 2013. Executive functions. *Annual Review of Psychology* 64(1):135–168.

Dinan, T. G., and J. F. Cryan. 2012. Regulation of the stress response by the gut microbiota: Implications for psychoneuroendocrinology. *Psychoneuroendocrinology* 37(9):1369–1378.

DiPietro, J. A., K. A. Costigan, and K. M. Voegtline. 2015. Studies in fetal behavior: Revisited, renewed, and reimagined. *Monographs of the Society for Research in Child Development* 80(3):vii, 1–94.

Doan, R. N., T. Shin, and C. A. Walsh. 2018. Evolutionary changes in transcriptional regulation: Insights into human behavior and neurological conditions. *Annual Review of Neuroscience* 41:185–206.

Donaldson, Z. R., and L. J. Young. 2008. Oxytocin, vasopressin, and the neurogenetics of sociality. *Science* 322(5903):900–904.

Donkin, I., S. Versteyhe, L. R. Ingerslev, K. Qian, M. Mechta, L. Nordkap, B. Mortensen, E. V. Appel, N. Jorgensen, V. B. Kristiansen, T. Hansen, C. T. Workman, J. R. Zierath, and R. Barres. 2016. Obesity and bariatric surgery drive epigenetic variation of spermatozoa in humans. *Cell Metabolism* 23(2):369–378.

Durbin, C. E., and B. M. Hicks. 2014. Personality and psychopathology: A stagnant field in need of development. *European Journal of Personality* 28(4):362–386.

Ebstein, R. P., S. Israel, S. H. Chew, S. Zhong, and A. Knafo. 2010. Genetics of human social behavior. *Neuron* 65(6):831–844.

Eisner, V., M. Picard, and G. Hajnoczky. 2018. Mitochondrial dynamics in adaptive and maladaptive cellular stress responses. *Nature Cell Biology* 20(7):755–765.

Elks, C. E., K. K. Ong, R. A. Scott, Y. T. Van Der Schouw, J. S. Brand, P. A. Wark, P. Amiano, B. Balkau, A. Barricarte, and H. Boeing. 2013. Age at menarche and type 2 diabetes risk: The Epic-Interact study. *Diabetes Care* 36(11):3526–3534.

Ellis, B. J., and M. D. Giudice. 2019. Developmental adaptation to stress: An evolutionary perspective. *Annual Review of Psychology* 70(1):111–139.

Ellis, B. J., W. T. Boyce, J. Belsky, M. J. Bakermans-Kranenburg, and M. H. van Ijzendoorn. 2011. Differential susceptibility to the environment: An evolutionary–neurodevelopmental theory. *Development and Psychopathology* 23(1):7–28.

Enoch, M. A., A. A. Rosser, Z. Zhou, D. C. Mash, Q. Yuan, and D. Goldman. 2014. Expression of glutamatergic genes in healthy humans across 16 brain regions; altered expression in the hippocampus after chronic exposure to alcohol or cocaine. *Genes, Brain and Behavior* 13(8):758–768.

Entringer, S. 2013. Impact of stress and stress physiology during pregnancy on child metabolic function and obesity risk. *Current Opinion in Clinical Nutrition and Metabolic Care* 16(3):320–327.

Entringer, S., C. Buss, and P. D. Wadhwa. 2010. Prenatal stress and developmental programming of human health and disease risk: Concepts and integration of empirical findings. *Current Opinion in Endocrinology Diabetes and Obesity* 17(6):507–516.

Entringer, S., E. S. Epel, J. Lin, C. Buss, B. Shahbaba, E. H. Blackburn, H. N. Simhan, and P. D. Wadhwa. 2013. Maternal psychosocial stress during pregnancy is associated with newborn leukocyte telomere length. *American Journal of Obstetrics and Gynecology* 208(2):134.e131–134.e137.

Entringer, S., C. Buss, and P. D. Wadhwa. 2015. Prenatal stress, development, health and disease risk: A psychobiological perspective—2015 Curt Richter Award paper. *Psychoneuroendocrinology* 62:366–375.

Evans, G. W. 2004. The environment of childhood poverty. *American Psychologist* 59:77–92.

Evans, G. W., N. M. Wells, and M. Schamberg. 2010. The role of the environment in socioeconomic status and obesity. In *Obesity prevention: The role of society and brain on individual behavior*, edited by L. Dube, A. Bechara, A. Dagher, D. Drewnowski, J. LeBel, P. James, R. Y. Yada, and M. C. Laflamme-Sanders. New York: Academic Press. Pp. 713–726.

Favuzzi, E., and B. Rico. 2018. Molecular diversity underlying cortical excitatory and inhibitory synapse development. *Current Opinion in Neurobiology* 53:8–15.

Feldman, R., and M. J. Bakermans-Kranenburg. 2017. Oxytocin: A parenting hormone. *Current Opinion in Psychology* 15:13–18.

Feldman, R., Z. Rosenthal, and A. I. Eidelman. 2014. Maternal-preterm skin-to-skin contact enhances child physiologic organization and cognitive control across the first 10 years of life. *Biological Psychiatry* 75(1):56–64.

Ferguson, K. T., R. C. Cassells, J. W. MacAllister, and G. W. Evans. 2013. The physical environment and child development: An international review. *International Journal of Psychology* 48(4):437–468.

Fisher, C. B., S. A. Wallace, and R. E. Fenton. 2000. Discrimination distress during adolescence. *Journal of Youth and Adolescence* 29(6):679–695.

Fisher, P. A., T. I. Frenkel, L. K. Noll, M. Berry, and M. Yockelson. 2016. Promoting healthy child development via a two-generation translational neuroscience framework: The Filming Interactions to Nurture Development video coaching program. *Child Development Perspectives* 10(4):251–256.

Flavell, J. H. 1963. *The developmental psychology of Jean Piaget*. Princeton, NJ: D. Van Nostrand.

Forsythe, P., J. Bienenstock, and W. A. Kunze. 2014. Vagal pathways for microbiome-brain-gut axis communication. In *Microbial endocrinology: The microbiota-gut-brain axis in health and disease*. Switzerland: Springer Nature. Pp. 115–133.

Foster, M. W., and R. R. Sharp. 2004. Beyond race: Towards a whole-genome perspective on human populations and genetic variation. *Nature Reviews Genetics* 5(10):790–796.

Franklin, T. B., H. Russig, I. C. Weiss, J. Gräff, N. Linder, A. Michalon, S. Vizi, and I. M. Mansuy. 2010. Epigenetic transmission of the impact of early stress across generations. *Biological Psychiatry* 68(5):408–415.

Frazier, T. W., E. W. Klingemier, S. Parikh, L. Speer, M. S. Strauss, C. Eng, A. Y. Hardan, and E. A. Youngstrom. 2018. Development and validation of objective and quantitative eye tracking-based measures of autism risk and symptom levels. *Journal of the American Academy of Child and Adolescent Psychiatry* 57(11):858–866.

Gabrieli, J. D. E., and S. A. Bunge. 2017. Does poverty shape the brain? *Scientific American*, https://www.scientificamerican.com/article/does-poverty-shape-the-brain (accessed April 17, 2019).

García Coll, C. T. 1990. Developmental outcome of minority infants: A process-oriented look into our beginnings. *Child Development* 61(2):270–289.

García Coll, C., G. Lamberty, R. Jenkins, H. P. McAdoo, K. Crnic, B. H. Wasik, and H. Vazquez Garcia. 1996. An integrative model for the study of developmental competencies in minority children. *Child Development* 67(5):1891–1914.

Garcia-Vargas, L., S. S. Addison, R. Nistala, D. Kurukulasuriya, and J. R. Sowers. 2012. Gestational diabetes and the offspring: Implications in the development of the cardiorenal metabolic syndrome in offspring. *Cardiorenal Medicine* 2(2):134–142.

Garner, A. S., J. P. Shonkoff, B. S. Siegel, M. I. Dobbins, M. F. Earls, L. McGuinn, J. Pascoe, D. L. Wood, Committee on Psychosocial Aspects of Child and Family Health, Committee on Early Childhood, Adoption, and Dependent Care, and Section on Developmental and Behavioral Pediatrics. 2012. Early childhood adversity, toxic stress, and the role of the pediatrician: Translating developmental science into lifelong health. *Pediatrics* 129(1):e224–e231.

Gascon, M., M. Vrijheid, and M. J. Nieuwenhuijsen. 2016. The built environment and child health: An overview of current evidence. *Current Environmental Health Reports* 3(3):250–257.

Geschwind, D. H., and P. Rakic. 2013. Cortical evolution: Judge the brain by its cover. *Neuron* 80(3):633–647.

Gillingham, P. 2016. Predictive risk modelling to prevent child maltreatment and other adverse outcomes for service users: Inside the "black box" of machine learning. *The British Journal of Social Work* 46(4):1044–1058.

Gilman, S. E., M. Hornig, A. Ghassabian, J. Hahn, S. Cherkerzian, P. S. Albert, S. L. Buka, and J. M. Goldstein. 2017. Socioeconomic disadvantage, gestational immune activity, and neurodevelopment in early childhood. *Proceedings of the National Academy of Sciences of the United States of America* 114(26):6728–6733.

Gluckman, P. D., M. A. Hanson, and A. S. Beedle. 2007. Early life events and their consequences for later disease: A life history and evolutionary perspective. *American Journal of Human Biology* 19(1):1–19.

Gobrogge, K., and Z. Wang. 2015. Neuropeptidergic regulation of pair-bonding and stress buffering: Lessons from voles. *Hormones and Behavior* 76:91–105.

Goeden, N., J. Velasquez, K. A. Arnold, Y. Chan, B. T. Lund, G. M. Anderson, and A. Bonnin. 2016. Maternal inflammation disrupts fetal neurodevelopment via increased placental output of serotonin to the fetal brain. *Journal of Neuroscience* 36(22):6041–6049.

Gogtay, N., J. N. Giedd, L. Lusk, K. M. Hayashi, D. Greenstein, A. C. Vaituzis, T. F. Nugent, D. H. Herman, L. S. Clasen, A. W. Toga, J. L. Rapoport, and P. M. Thompson. 2004. Dynamic mapping of human cortical development during childhood through early adulthood. *Proceedings of the National Academy of Sciences of the United States of America* 101(21):8174–8179.

Goldberg, A. D., C. D. Allis, and E. Bernstein. 2007. Epigenetics: A landscape takes shape. *Cell* 128(4):635–638.

Goldman-Mellor, S., C. Margerison–Zilko, K. Allen, and M. Cerda. 2016. Perceived and objectively-measured neighborhood violence and adolescent psychological distress. *Journal of Urban Health* 93(5):758–769.

Goll, M. G., and T. H. Bestor. 2005. Eukaryotic cytosine methyltransferases. *Annual Review of Biochemistry* 74:481–514.

Golub, M. S., G. W. Collman, P. M. Foster, C. A. Kimmel, E. Rajpert-De Meyts, E. O. Reiter, R. M. Sharpe, N. E. Skakkebaek, and J. Toppari. 2008. Public health implications of altered puberty timing. *Pediatrics* 121(Suppl 3):S218–S230.

Gonzalez, T. L., T. Sun, A. F. Koeppel, B. Lee, E. T. Wang, C. R. Farber, S. S. Rich, L. W. Sundheimer, R. A. Buttle, Y.-D. I. Chen, J. I. Rotter, S. D. Turner, J. Williams, M. O. Goodarzi, and M. D. Pisarska. 2018. Sex differences in the late first trimester human placenta transcriptome. *Biology of Sex Differences* 9(1):4.

Goodman, R. N., J. C. Rietschel, L.-C. Lo, M. E. Costanzo, and B. D. Hatfield. 2013. Stress, emotion regulation and cognitive performance: The predictive contributions of trait and state relative frontal EEG alpha asymmetry. *International Journal of Psychophysiology* 87(2):115–123.

Gorski Findling, M. T., J. A. Wolfson, E. B. Rimm, and S. N. Bleich. 2018. Differences in the neighborhood retail food environment and obesity among us children and adolescents by SNAP participation. *Obesity* 26(6):1063–1071.

Gramlich, E. M. 1986. Evaluation of education projects: The case of the Perry Preschool Program. *Economics of Education Review* 5(1):17–24.

Greenough, W. T., J. E. Black, and C. S. Wallace. 1987. Experience and brain development. *Child Development* 58(3):539–559.

Grindal, T., J. B. Bowne, H. Yoshikawa, H. S. Schindler, G. J. Duncan, K. Magnuson, and J. P. Shonkoff. 2016. The added impact of parenting education in early childhood education programs: A meta-analysis. *Children and Youth Services Review* 70:238–249.

Gunnar, M. R., and P. A. Fisher. 2006. Bringing basic research on early experience and stress neurobiology to bear on preventive interventions for neglected and maltreated children. *Development and Psychopathology* 18(3):651–677.

Gunnar, M. R., and C. E. Hostinar. 2015. The social buffering of the hypothalamic–pituitary–adrenocortical axis in humans: Developmental and experiential determinants. *Social Neuroscience* 10(5):479–488.

Hair, N. L., J. L. Hanson, B. L. Wolfe, and S. D. Pollak. 2015. Association of child poverty, brain development, and academic achievement. *JAMA Pediatrics* 169(9):822–829.

Halfon, N., K. Larson, M. Lu, E. Tullis, and S. Russ. 2014. Lifecourse health development: Past, present and future. *Maternal and Child Health Journal* 18(2):344–365.

Hammock, E. A., M. M. Lim, H. P. Nair, and L. J. Young. 2005. Association of vasopressin 1a receptor levels with a regulatory microsatellite and behavior. *Genes, Brain, and Behavior* 4(5):289–301.

Hanson, J. L., N. Hair, D. G. Shen, F. Shi, J. H. Gilmore, B. L. Wolfe, and S. D. Pollak. 2013. Family poverty affects the rate of human infant brain growth. *PLoS ONE* 8(12):e80954.

Hansson, G. K., and A. Hermansson. 2011. The immune system in atherosclerosis. *Nature Immunology* 12(3):204–212.

Hantsoo, L., S. Kornfield, M. C. Anguera, and C. N. Epperson. 2019. Inflammation: A proposed intermediary between maternal stress and offspring neuropsychiatric risk. *Biological Psychiatry* 85(2):97–106.

Harding, A. 2006. Fernando Martinez: Seeking to solve the puzzle of asthma. *The Lancet* 368(9537):725.

Heard-Garris, N. J., M. Cale, L. Camaj, M. C. Hamati, and T. P. Dominguez. 2018. Transmitting trauma: A systematic review of vicarious racism and child health. *Social Science & Medicine* 199:230–240.

Heim, C., and E. B. Binder. 2012. Current research trends in early life stress and depression: Review of human studies on sensitive periods, gene-environment interactions, and epigenetics. *Experimental Neurology* 233(1):102–111.

Heinrichs, M., T. Baumgartner, C. Kirschbaum, and U. Ehlert. 2003. Social support and oxytocin interact to suppress cortisol and subjective responses to psychosocial stress. *Biological Psychiatry* 54(12):1389–1398.

Hennessy, M. B., S. Kaiser, and N. Sachser. 2009. Social buffering of the stress response: Diversity, mechanisms, and functions. *Frontiers in Neuroendocrinology* 30(4):470–482.

Hensch, T. K. 2016a. Critical ingredients for brain development. *Scientific American*, https://www.scientificamerican.com/article/critical-ingredients-for-brain-development (accessed April 17, 2019).

Hensch, T. K. 2016b. The power of the infant brain. *Scientific American* 314(2):64–69.

Hensch, T. K., and P. M. Bilimoria. 2012. Re-opening windows: Manipulating critical periods for brain development. *Cerebrum* 11.

Herman-Giddens, M. E., E. J. Slora, R. C. Wasserman, C. J. Bourdony, M. V. Bhapkar, G. G. Koch, and C. M. Hasemeier. 1997. Secondary sexual characteristics and menses in young girls seen in office practice: A study from the pediatric research in office settings network. *Pediatrics* 99(4):505–512.

Herman-Giddens, M. E., J. Steffes, D. Harris, E. Slora, M. Hussey, S. A. Dowshen, R. Wasserman, J. R. Serwint, L. Smitherman, and E. O. Reiter. 2012. Secondary sexual characteristics in boys: Data from the pediatric research in office settings network. *Pediatrics* 130(5):e1058–e1068.

Hertzman, C., and T. Boyce. 2010. How experience gets under the skin to create gradients in developmental health. *Annual Review of Public Health* 31:329–347.

Heun-Johnson, H., and P. Levitt. 2018. Differential impact of MET receptor gene interaction with early-life stress on neuronal morphology and behavior in mice. *Neurobiology of Stress* 8:10–20.

Hiatt, R. A., S. L. Stewart, K. S. Hoeft, L. H. Kushi, G. C. Windham, F. M. Biro, S. M. Pinney, M. S. Wolff, S. L. Teitelbaum, and D. Braithwaite. 2017. Childhood socioeconomic position and pubertal onset in a cohort of multiethnic girls: Implications for breast cancer. *Cancer Epidemiology and Prevention Biomarkers* 26(12):1714–1721.

Hoffman, M. C. 2016. Stress, the placenta, and fetal programming of behavior: Genes' first encounter with the environment. *American Journal of Psychiatry* 173(7):655–657.

Hofmeyr, F., C. A. Groenewald, D. G. Nel, M. M. Myers, W. P. Fifer, C. Signore, G. D. Hankins, and H. J. Odendaal. 2014. Fetal heart rate patterns at 20 to 24 weeks gestation as recorded by fetal electrocardiography. *Journal of Maternal-Fetal and Neonatal Medicine* 27(7):714–718.

Hosseini, M., H. Soltanian-Zadeh, K. Elisevich, and D. Pompili. 2016. Cloud-based deep learning of big EEG data for epileptic seizure prediction. Paper read at 2016 IEEE Global Conference on Signal and Information Processing (GlobalSIP), December 7–9, 2016.

Hostinar, C. E., R. M. Sullivan, and M. R. Gunnar. 2014. Psychobiological mechanisms underlying the social buffering of the hypothalamic-pituitary-adrenocortical axis: A review of animal models and human studies across development. *Psychological Bulletin* 140(1):256–282.

Howerton, C. L., and T. L. Bale. 2012. Prenatal programing: At the intersection of maternal stress and immune activation. *Hormones and Behavior* 62(3):237–242.

Huston, A. C., A. E. Gupta, J. T. Walker, C. J. Dowsett, S. R. Epps, A. E. Imes, and V. C. McLoyd. 2011. The long-term effects on children and adolescents of a policy providing work supports for low-income parents. *Journal of Policy Analysis and Management* 30(4):729–754.

Iacono, W. G., S. M. Malone, and M. McGue. 2008. Behavioral disinhibition and the development of early-onset addiction: Common and specific influences. *Annual Review of Clinical Psychology* 4:325–348.

Insel, T. R. 2010. The challenge of translation in social neuroscience: A review of oxytocin, vasopressin, and affiliative behavior. *Neuron* 65(6):768–779.

IOM aqnd NRC (Institute of Medicine and National Research Council). 2015. *Transforming the workforce for children birth through age 8: A unifying foundation.* Washington, DC: The National Academies Press.

Israel, S., O. Weisel, R. P. Ebstein, and G. Bornstein. 2012. Oxytocin, but not vasopressin, increases both parochial and universal altruism. *Psychoneuroendocrinology* 37(8):1341–1344.

Jayaraman, D., B. I. Bae, and C. A. Walsh. 2018. The genetics of primary microcephaly. *Annual Review of Genomics and Human Genetics* 19:177–200.

Johnson, S. B., J. L. Riis, and K. G. Noble. 2016. State of the art review: Poverty and the developing brain. *Pediatrics* 137(4):e20153075.

Jones, C. E., R. A. Opel, M. E. Kaiser, A. Q. Chau, J. R. Quintana, M. A. Nipper, D. A. Finn, E. A. D. Hammock, and M. M. Lim. 2019. Early-life sleep disruption increases parvalbumin in primary somatosensory cortex and impairs social bonding in prairie voles. *Science Advances* 5(1):1–11.

Jones, S. 2019. Encyclopedia of cells in early pregnancy. *Nature Biotechnology* 37:26.

Juonala, M., J. S. Viikari, T. Ronnemaa, L. Taittonen, J. Marniemi, and O. T. Raitakari. 2006. Childhood C-reactive protein in predicting CRP and carotid intima-media thickness in adulthood: The Cardiovascular Risk in Young Finns Study. *Arteriosclerosis, Thrombosis, and Vascular Biology* 26(8):1883–1888.

Kalish, J. M., C. Jiang, and M. S. Bartolomei. 2014. Epigenetics and imprinting in human disease. *The International Journal of Developmental Biology* 58(2–4):291–298.

Kaminski, J. W., R. Perou, S. N. Visser, K. G. Scott, L. Beckwith, J. Howard, D. C. Smith, and M. L. Danielson. 2013. Behavioral and socioemotional outcomes through age 5 years of the Legacy for Children public health approach to improving developmental outcomes among children born into poverty. *American Journal of Public Health* 103(6):1058–1066.

Kast, R. J., and P. Levitt. 2019. Precision in the development of neocortical architecture: From progenitors to cortical networks. *Progress in Neurobiology* 175:77–95.

Katz, L. C., and C. J. Shatz. 1996. Synaptic activity and the construction of cortical circuits. *Science* 274(5290):1133–1138.

Kelly, Y., A. Zilanawala, A. Sacker, R. Hiatt, and R. Viner. 2017. Early puberty in 11-year-old girls: Millennium cohort study findings. *Archives of Disease in Childhood* 102(3):232–237.

Keshavan, M., J. Giedd, J. Lau, D. A. Lewis, and T. Paus. 2014. Changes in the adolescent brain and the pathophysiology of psychotic disorders. *The Lancet Psychiatry* 1(7):549–558.

Khan, N. A., and C. H. Hillman. 2014. The relation of childhood physical activity and aerobic fitness to brain function and cognition: A review. *Pediatric Exercise Science* 26(2):138–146.

Kikusui, T., J. T. Winslow, and Y. Mori. 2006. Social buffering: Relief from stress and anxiety. *Philosophical Transactions of the Royal Society B: Biological Sciences* 361(1476):2215–2228.

Kim, S., and L. Strathearn. 2017. Trauma, mothering, and intergenerational transmission: A synthesis of behavioral and oxytocin research. *The Psychoanalytic Study of the Child* 70(1):200–223.

King, L. B., H. Walum, K. Inoue, N. W. Eyrich, and L. J. Young. 2016. Variation in the oxytocin receptor gene predicts brain region-specific expression and social attachment. *Biological Psychiatry* 80(2):160–169.

Knoll, A. T., K. Jiang, and P. Levitt. 2018. Quantitative trait locus mapping and analysis of heritable variation in affiliative social behavior and co-occurring traits. *Genes, Brain, and Behavior* 17(5):e12431.

Knudsen, E. I. 2004. Sensitive periods in the development of the brain and behavior. *Journal of Cognitive Neuroscience* 16(8):1412–1425.

Kolodkin, A. L., and M. Tessier-Lavigne. 2011. Mechanisms and molecules of neuronal wiring: A primer. *Cold Spring Harbor Perspectives in Biology* 3(6).

Koss, K. J., and M. R. Gunnar. 2018. Annual research review: Early adversity, the hypothalamic–pituitary–adrenocortical axis, and child psychopathology. *Journal of Child Psychology and Psychiatry* 59(4):327–346.

Kostović, I., N. Jovanov-Milošević, M. Radoš, G. Sedmak, V. Benjak, M. Kostović-Srzentić, L. Vasung, M. Ćuljat, M. Radoš, P. Hüppi, and M. Judaš. 2014. Perinatal and early postnatal reorganization of the subplate and related cellular compartments in the human cerebral wall as revealed by histological and MRI approaches. *Brain Structure and Function* 219(1):231–253.

Krieger, N. 2012. Methods for the scientific study of discrimination and health: An ecosocial approach. *American Journal of Public Health* 102(5):936–944.

Krieger, N., D. Carney, K. Lancaster, P. D. Waterman, A. Kosheleva, and M. Banaji. 2010. Combining explicit and implicit measures of racial discrimination in health research. *American Journal of Public Health* 100(8):1485–1492.

Krishnan, M. L., Z. Wang, P. Aljabar, G. Ball, G. Mirza, A. Saxena, S. J. Counsell, J. V. Hajnal, G. Montana, and A. D. Edwards. 2017. Machine learning shows association between genetic variability in PPARG and cerebral connectivity in preterm infants. *Proceedings of the National Academy of Sciences of the United States of America* 114(52):13744–13749.

Krsnik, Ž., V. Majić, L. Vasung, H. Huang, and I. Kostović. 2017. Growth of thalamocortical fibers to the somatosensory cortex in the human fetal brain. *Frontiers in Neuroscience* 11:233.

Kubo, A., J. Deardorff, C. A. Laurent, A. Ferrara, L. C. Greenspan, C. P. Quesenberry, and L. H. Kushi. 2018. Associations between maternal obesity and pregnancy hyperglycemia and timing of puberty onset in adolescent girls: A population-based study. *American Journal of Epidemiology* 187(7):1362–1369.

Kudielka, B. M., and C. Kirschbaum. 2005. Sex differences in HPA axis responses to stress: A review. *Biological Psychology* 69(1):113–132.

Kuh, D., Y. Ben-Shlomo, J. Lynch, J. Hallqvist, and C. Power. 2003. Life course epidemiology. *Journal of Epidemiology and Community Health* 57(10):778–783.

Kumsta, R. 2019. The role of epigenetics for understanding mental health difficulties and its implications for psychotherapy research. *Psychology and Psychotherapy: Theory, Research and Practice* 92(2):190–207.

Leighton, A. H., and C. Lohmann. 2016. The wiring of developing sensory circuits—from patterned spontaneous activity to synaptic plasticity mechanisms. *Frontiers in Neural Circuits* 10:71.

Lerner, R. M., S. J. Schwartz, and E. Phelps. 2009. Problematics of time and timing in the Longitudinal Study of Human Development: Theoretical and methodological issues. *Human Development* 52(1):44–68.

Levitt, P., and K. L. Eagleson. 2018. The ingredients of healthy brain and child development. *Washington University Journal of Law and Policy* 57.

Li, M., G. Santpere, Y. Imamura Kawasawa, O. V. Evgrafov, F. O. Gulden, S. Pochareddy, S. M. Sunkin, Z. Li, Y. Shin, Y. Zhu, A. M. M. Sousa, D. M. Werling, R. R. Kitchen, H. J. Kang, M. Pletikos, J. Choi, S. Muchnik, X. Xu, D. Wang, B. Lorente-Galdos, S. Liu, P. Giusti-Rodriguez, H. Won, C. A. de Leeuw, A. F. Pardinas, M. Hu, F. Jin, Y. Li, M. J. Owen, M. C. O'Donovan, J. T. R. Walters, D. Posthuma, M. A. Reimers, P. Levitt, D. R. Weinberger, T. M. Hyde, J. E. Kleinman, D. H. Geschwind, M. J. Hawrylycz, M. W. State, S. J. Sanders, P. F. Sullivan, M. B. Gerstein, E. S. Lein, J. A. Knowles, and N. Sestan. 2018. Integrative functional genomic analysis of human brain development and neuropsychiatric risks. *Science* 362(6420).

Libby, P., P. M. Ridker, and A. Maseri. 2002. Inflammation and atherosclerosis. *Circulation* 105(9):1135–1143.

Loria, A. S., D. H. Ho, and J. S. Pollock. 2014. A mechanistic look at the effects of adversity early in life on cardiovascular disease risk during adulthood. *Acta Physiologica* 210(2):277–287.

Luby, J. L., D. M. Barch, A. Belden, M. S. Gaffrey, R. Tillman, C. Babb, T. Nishino, H. Suzuki, and K. N. Botteron. 2012. Maternal support in early childhood predicts larger hippocampal volumes at school age. *Proceedings of the National Academy of Sciences of the United States of America* 109(8):2854–2859.

Ludwig, J., L. Sanbonmatsu, L. Gennetian, E. Adam, G. J. Duncan, L. F. Katz, R. C. Kessler, J. R. Kling, S. T. Lindau, R. C. Whitaker, and T. W. McDade. 2011. Neighborhoods, obesity, and diabetes—a randomized social experiment. *New England Journal of Medicine* 365(16):1509–1519.

Luthar, S. S., and N. Eisenberg. 2017. Resilient adaptation among at-risk children: Harnessing science toward maximizing salutary environments. *Child Development* 88(2):337–349.

Luthar, S. S., N. E. Suchman, and M. Altomare. 2007. Relational psychotherapy mothers' group: A randomized clinical trial for substance abusing mothers. *Development and Psychopathology* 19(1):243–261.

Luthar, S., E. J. Crossman, and P. J. Small. 2015. Resilience and adversity. In *Handbook of child psychology and developmental science*, 7th ed. Vol. 3, edited by R. M. Lerner and M. E. Lamb. New York: Wiley. Pp. 247–286.

Luthar, S. S., A. Curlee, S. J. Tye, J. C. Engelman, and C. M. Stonnington. 2017. Fostering resilience among mothers under stress: "Authentic connections groups" for medical professionals. *Women's Health Issues* 27(3):382–390.

Lynch, S. V., and O. Pedersen. 2016. The human intestinal microbiome in health and disease. *New England Journal of Medicine* 375(24):2369–2379.

Mantella, R. C., R. R. Vollmer, L. Rinaman, X. Li, and J. A. Amico. 2004. Enhanced corticosterone concentrations and attenuated FOS expression in the medial amygdala of female oxytocin knockout mice exposed to psychogenic stress. *American Journal of Physiology: Regulatory, Integrative and Comparative Physiology* 287(6):1494–1504.

Masten, A. S. 2014. Global perspectives on resilience in children and youth. *Child Development* 85(1):6–20.

Masten, A. S. 2018. Resilience theory and research on children and families: Past, present, and promise. *Journal of Family Theory & Review* 10(1):12–31.

Matthews, S. G., and D. I. Phillips. 2012. Transgenerational inheritance of stress pathology. *Experimental Neurology* 233(1):95–101.

McCarty, C. A., R. L. Chisholm, C. G. Chute, I. J. Kullo, G. P. Jarvik, E. B. Larson, R. Li, D. R. Masys, M. D. Ritchie, D. M. Roden, J. P. Struewing, and W. A. Wolf. 2011. The eMERGE network: A consortium of biorepositories linked to electronic medical records data for conducting genomic studies. *BMC Medical Genomics* 4:13.

McCoy, D. C., C. C. Raver, and P. Sharkey. 2015. Children's cognitive performance and selective attention following recent community violence. *Journal of Health and Social Behavior* 56(1):19–36.

McCracken, D. S., D. A. Allen, and A. J. Gow. 2016. Associations between urban greenspace and health-related quality of life in children. *Preventive Medicine Reports* 3:211–221.

McEwen, B. S. 1998. Stress, adaptation, and disease: Allostasis and allostatic load. *Annals of the New York Academy of Sciences* 840(1):33–44.

McEwen, B. S. 2017. Allostasis and the epigenetics of brain and body health over the life course: The brain on stress. *JAMA Psychiatry* 74(6):551–552.

McEwen, B. S., and L. Getz. 2013. Lifetime experiences, the brain and personalized medicine: An integrative perspective. *Metabolism* 62(Suppl 1):S20–S26.

McEwen, C. A., and B. S. McEwen. 2017. Social structure, adversity, toxic stress, and inter-generational poverty: An early childhood model. *Annual Review of Sociology* 43(1):445–472.

McEwen, B. S., and J. H. Morrison. 2013. The brain on stress: Vulnerability and plasticity of the prefrontal cortex over the life course. *Neuron* 79(1):16–29.

McEwen, B. S., N. P. Bowles, J. D. Gray, M. N. Hill, R. G. Hunter, I. N. Karatsoreos, and C. Nasca. 2015. Mechanisms of stress in the brain. *Nature Neuroscience* 18(10):1353–1363.

McGee, A. W., Y. Yang, Q. S. Fischer, N. W. Daw, and S. M. Strittmatter. 2005. Experience-driven plasticity of visual cortex limited by myelin and NOGO receptor. *Science* 309(5744):2222–2226.

McGregor, T. L., S. L. Van Driest, K. B. Brothers, E. A. Bowton, L. J. Muglia, and D. M. Roden. 2013. Inclusion of pediatric samples in an opt-out biorepository linking DNA to de-identified medical records: Pediatric BioVU. *Clinical Pharmacology & Therapeutics* 93(2):204–211.

McKay, R. 2011. Developmental biology: Remarkable role for the placenta. *Nature* 472(7343):298–299.

McLanahan, S., I. Garfinkel, N. Reichman, J. Teitler, M. Carlson, and C. N. Audigier. 2003. The Fragile Families and Child Wellbeing Study: Baseline national report. Princeton, NJ: Center for Research on Child Wellbeing, Princeton University.

McLaughlin, K. A., M. A. Sheridan, and C. A. Nelson. 2017. Neglect as a violation of species-expectant experience: Neurodevelopmental consequences. *Biological Psychiatry* 82(7):462–471.

McLoyd, V. C. 1990. The impact of economic hardship on black families and children: Psychological distress, parenting, and socioemotional development. *Child Development* 61:311–346.

Meaney, M. J. 2001. Maternal care, gene expression, and the transmission of individual differences in stress reactivity across generations. *Annual Review of Neuroscience* 24(1):1161–1192.

Meaney, M. J., and A. C. Ferguson-Smith. 2010. Epigenetic regulation of the neural transcriptome: The meaning of the marks. *Nature Neuroscience* 13(11):1313–1318.

Medland, S. E., N. Jahanshad, B. M. Neale, and P. M. Thompson. 2014. Whole-genome analyses of whole-brain data: Working within an expanded search space. *Nature Neuroscience* 17(6):791–800.

Mendle, J., R. M. Ryan, and K. M. McKone. 2016. Early childhood maltreatment and pubertal development: Replication in a population-based sample. *Journal of Research on Adolescence* 26(3):595–602.

Miguel, P. M., L. O. Pereira, P. P. Silveira, and M. J. Meaney. 2019. Early environmental influences on the development of children's brain structure and function. *Developmental Medicine & Child Neurology*. doi: 10.1111/dmcn.14182. [Epub ahead of print.]

Miller, C., A. C. Huston, G. J. Duncan, V. C. McLoyd, and T. S. Weisner. 2008. New hope for the working poor: Effects after eight years for families and children. New York: MDRC.

Miller, D. J., T. Duka, C. D. Stimpson, S. J. Schapiro, W. B. Baze, M. J. McArthur, A. J. Fobbs, A. M. M. Sousa, N. Šestan, D. E. Wildman, L. Lipovich, C. W. Kuzawa, P. R. Hof, and C. C. Sherwood. 2012. Prolonged myelination in human neocortical evolution. *Proceedings of the National Academy of Sciences of the United States of America* 109(41):16480–16485.

Miller, E. M. 2017. Beyond passive immunity: Breastfeeding, milk and collaborative mother-infant immune systems. In *Breastfeeding*, edited by C. Tomori, A. E. L. Palmquist, and E. A. Quinn. Abindgon, UK: Routledge. Pp. 50–63.

Miller, G. E., E. Chen, and K. J. Parker. 2011. Psychological stress in childhood and susceptibility to the chronic diseases of aging: Moving toward a model of behavioral and biological mechanisms. *Psychological Bulletin* 137(6):959–997.

Morishita, H., J. H. Cabungcal, Y. Chen, K. Q. Do, and T. K. Hensch. 2015. Prolonged period of cortical plasticity upon redox dysregulation in fast-spiking interneurons. *Biological Psychiatry* 78(6):396–402.

Morrison, K. E., C. N. Epperson, M. D. Sammel, G. Ewing, J. S. Podcasy, L. Hantsoo, D. R. Kim, and T. L. Bale. 2017. Preadolescent adversity programs a disrupted maternal stress reactivity in humans and mice. *Biological Psychiatry* 81(8):693–701.

NASEM (National Academies of Sciences, Engineering, and Medicine). 2019. *The promise of adolescence: Realizing opportunity for all youth.* Washington, DC: The National Academies Press.

National Scientific Council on the Developing Child. 2010. *Early experiences can alter gene expression and affect long-term development. Working paper no. 10.* Cambridge, MA: Center on the Developing Child at Harvard University.

National Scientific Council on the Developing Child. 2014. *Excessive stress disrupts the architecture of the brain. Working paper no. 3.* Cambridge, MA: Center on the Developing Child at Harvard University.

Negi, S. K., and C. Guda. 2017. Global gene expression profiling of healthy human brain and its application in studying neurological disorders. *Scientific Reports* 7(1):897.

Nelson, C. A., 3rd, C. H. Zeanah, N. A. Fox, P. J. Marshall, A. T. Smyke, and D. Guthrie. 2007. Cognitive recovery in socially deprived young children: The Bucharest Early Intervention project. *Science* 318(5858):1937–1940.

Nelson, C. A., N. A. Fox, and C. Zeanah. 2014. *Romania's abandoned children. Deprivation, brain development, and the struggle for recovery.* Cambridge, MA: Harvard University Press.

Nese, R. N. T., C. M. Anderson, T. Ruppert, and P. A. Fisher. 2016. Effects of a video feedback parent training program during child welfare visitation. *Children and Youth Services Review* 71:266–276.

Noll, J. G., P. K. Trickett, J. D. Long, S. Negriff, E. J. Susman, I. Shalev, J. C. Li, and F. W. Putnam. 2017. Childhood sexual abuse and early timing of puberty. *Journal of Adolescent Health* 60(1):65–71.

Non, A. L., M. Rewak, I. Kawachi, S. E. Gilman, E. B. Loucks, A. A. Appleton, J. C. Roman, S. L. Buka, and L. D. Kubzansky. 2014. Childhood social disadvantage, cardiometabolic risk, and chronic disease in adulthood. *American Journal of Epidemiology* 180(3):263–271.

NRC and IOM. 2000. *From neurons to neighborhoods: The science of early childhood development.* Washington, DC: National Academy Press.

Nugent, B. M., and T. L. Bale. 2015. The omniscient placenta: Metabolic and epigenetic regulation of fetal programming. *Frontiers in Neuroendocrinology* 39:28–37.

Numan, M., and L. J. Young. 2016. Neural mechanisms of mother-infant bonding and pair bonding: Similarities, differences, and broader implications. *Hormones and Behavior* 77:98–112.

Nusslock, R., and G. E. Miller. 2016. Early-life adversity and physical and emotional health across the lifespan: A neuroimmune network hypothesis. *Biological Psychiatry* 80(1):23–32.

Obradović, J., N. R. Bush, J. Stamperdahl, N. E. Adler, and W. T. Boyce. 2010. Biological sensitivity to context: The interactive effects of stress reactivity and family adversity on socioemotional behavior and school readiness. *Child Development* 81(1):270–289.

O'Connor, T. G., J. A. Moynihan, and M. T. Caserta. 2014. Annual research review: The neuro-inflammation hypothesis for stress and psychopathology in children—developmental psychoneuroimmunology. *Journal of Child Psychology and Psychiatry* 55(6):615–631.

O'Donnell, K. J., A. Bugge Jensen, L. Freeman, N. Khalife, T. G. O'Connor, and V. Glover. 2012. Maternal prenatal anxiety and downregulation of placental 11beta-HSD2. *Psychoneuroendocrinology* 37(6):818–826.

O'Driscoll, A., J. Daugelaite, and R. D. Sleator. 2013. "Big data," Hadoop and cloud computing in genomics. *Journal of Biomedical Informatics* 46(5):774–781.

Ogbu, J. U. 1981. Racism and health I: Pathways and scientific evidence. *Child Development* 52(2):413–429.

Pachter, L. M., and C. G. Coll. 2009. Racism and child health: A review of the literature and future directions. *Journal of Developmental and Behavioral Pediatrics* 30(3):255–263.

Pachter, L. M., L. A. Szalacha, B. A. Bernstein, and C. G. Coll. 2010. Perceptions of Racism in Children and Youth (PRACY): Properties of a self-report instrument for research on children's health and development. *Ethnicity & Health* 15(1):33–46.

Padgett, D. A., and R. Glaser. 2003. How stress influences the immune response. *Trends in Immunology* 24(8):444–448.

Pager, D., and H. Shepherd. 2008. The sociology of discrimination: Racial discrimination in employment, housing, credit, and consumer markets. *Annual Review of Sociology* 34:181–209.

Painter, R. C., S. R. de Rooij, P. M. Bossuyt, D. I. Phillips, C. Osmond, D. J. Barker, O. P. Bleker, and T. J. Roseboom. 2006. Blood pressure response to psychological stressors in adults after prenatal exposure to the Dutch famine. *Journal of Hypertension* 24(9):1771–1778.

Paquette, A. G., H. M. Brockway, N. D. Price, and L. J. Muglia. 2017. Comparative transcriptomic analysis of human placentae at term and preterm delivery. *Biology of Reproduction* 98(1):89–101.

Paradies, Y., J. Ben, N. Denson, A. Elias, N. Priest, A. Pieterse, A. Gupta, M. Kelaher, and G. Gee. 2015. Racism as a determinant of health: A systematic review and meta-analysis. *PLoS ONE* 10(9):e0138511.

Pearson, T. A., G. A. Mensah, R. W. Alexander, J. L. Anderson, R. O. Cannon, M. Criqui, Y. Y. Fadl, S. P. Fortmann, Y. Hong, G. L. Myers, N. Rifai, S. C. Smith, K. Taubert, R. P. Tracy, and F. Vinicor. 2003. Markers of inflammation and cardiovascular disease application to clinical and public health practice—a statement for healthcare professionals from the Centers for Disease Control and Prevention and the American Heart Association. *Circulation* 107(3):499–511.

Peña, C. J., H. G. Kronman, D. M. Walker, H. M. Cates, R. C. Bagot, I. Purushothaman, O. Issler, Y.-H. E. Loh, T. Leong, D. D. Kiraly, E. Goodman, R. L. Neve, L. Shen, and E. J. Nestler. 2017. Early life stress confers lifelong stress susceptibility in mice via ventral tegmental area OTX2. *Science* 356:1185–1188.

Picard, M., and B. S. McEwen. 2018. Psychological stress and mitochondria: A conceptual framework. *Psychosomatic Medicine* 80(2):126–140.

Plomin, R., K. Asbury, and J. Dunn. 2001. Why are children in the same family so different? Nonshared environment a decade later. *The Canadian Journal of Psychiatry* 46(3):225–233.

Plotsky, P. M., and M. J. Meaney. 1993. Early, postnatal experience alters hypothalamic corticotropin-releasing factor (CRF) MRNA, median eminence CRF content and stress-induced release in adult rats. *Brain Research: Molecular Brain Research* 18(3):195–200.

Plotsky, P., K. Thrivikraman, C. Nemeroff, C. Caldji, S. Sharma, and M. Meaney. 2005. Long-term consequences of neonatal rearing on central corticotropin–releasing factor systems in adult male rat offspring. *Neuropsycho-pharmacology* 30(12):2192–2204.

Pollak, S. D., D. Cicchetti, R. Klorman, and J. T. Brumaghim. 1997. Cognitive brain event-related potentials and emotion processing in maltreated children. *Child Development* 68(5):773–787.

Poulton, R., T. E. Moffitt, and P. A. Silva. 2015. The Dunedin Multidisciplinary Health and Development Study: Overview of the first 40 years, with an eye to the future. *Social Psychiatry and Psychiatric Epidemiology* 50(5):679–693.

Priest, N., Y. Paradies, M. Stevens, and R. Bailie. 2012. Exploring relationships between racism, housing and child illness in remote indigenous communities. *Journal of Epidemiology and Community Health* 66(5):440–447.

Priest, N., Y. Paradies, B. Trenerry, M. Truong, S. Karlsen, and Y. Kelly. 2013. A systematic review of studies examining the relationship between reported racism and health and wellbeing for children and young people. *Social Science & Medicine* 95:115–127.

Quirin, M., J. Kuhl, and R. Düsing. 2011. Oxytocin buffers cortisol responses to stress in individuals with impaired emotion regulation abilities. *Psychoneuroendocrinology* 36(6):898–904.

Reagan, P. B., P. J. Salsberry, M. Z. Fang, W. P. Gardner, and K. Pajer. 2012. African-American/white differences in the age of menarche: Accounting for the difference. *Social Science & Medicine (1982)* 75(7):1263–1270.

Roberts, A. L., S. Galea, S. B. Austin, H. L. Corliss, M. A. Williams, and K. C. Koenen. 2014. Women's experience of abuse in childhood and their children's smoking and overweight. *American Journal of Preventive Medicine* 46(3):249–258.

Roden, D. M., J. M. Pulley, M. A. Basford, G. R. Bernard, E. W. Clayton, J. R. Balser, and D. R. Masys. 2008. Development of a large-scale de-identified DNA biobank to enable personalized medicine. *Clinical Pharmacology & Therapeutics* 84(3):362–369.

Rodgers, A. B., C. P. Morgan, N. A. Leu, and T. L. Bale. 2015. Transgenerational epigenetic programming via sperm microRNA recapitulates effects of paternal stress. *Proceedings of the National Academy of Sciences of the United States of America* 112(44):13699–13704.

Rodrigues, S. M., L. R. Saslow, N. Garcia, O. P. John, and D. Keltner. 2009. Oxytocin receptor genetic variation relates to empathy and stress reactivity in humans. *Proceedings of the National Academy of Sciences of the United States of America* 106(50):21437–21441.

Ross, H. E., and L. J. Young. 2009. Oxytocin and the neural mechanisms regulating social cognition and affiliative behavior. *Frontiers in Neuroendocrinology* 30(4):534–547.

Ross, H. E., C. D. Cole, Y. Smith, I. D. Neumann, R. Landgraf, A. Z. Murphy, and L. J. Young. 2009a. Characterization of the oxytocin system regulating affiliative behavior in female prairie voles. *Neuroscience* 162(4):892–903.

Ross, H. E., S. M. Freeman, L. L. Spiegel, X. Ren, E. F. Terwilliger, and L. J. Young. 2009b. Variation in oxytocin receptor density in the nucleus accumbens has differential effects on affiliative behaviors in monogamous and polygamous voles. *Journal of Neuroscience* 29(5):1312–1318.

Rowold, E. D., L. Schulze, S. Van der Auwera, and H. J. Grabe. 2017. Paternal transmission of early life traumatization through epigenetics: Do fathers play a role? *Medical Hypotheses* 109:59–64.

Rubenstein, J., and P. Rakic. 2013. *Patterning and cell type specification in the developing CNS and PNS*, Vol. 1, *Comprehensive developmental neuroscience*. Amsterdam, the Netherlands: Academic Press.

Rudolph, M. D., A. M. Graham, E. Feczko, O. Miranda-Dominguez, J. M. Rasmussen, R. Nardos, S. Entringer, P. D. Wadhwa, C. Buss, and D. A. Fair. 2018. Maternal IL-6 during pregnancy can be estimated from newborn brain connectivity and predicts future working memory in offspring. *Nature Neuroscience* 21(5):765–772.

Rundle, A. G., M. D. Bader, C. A. Richards, K. M. Neckerman, and J. O. Teitler. 2011. Using Google Street View to audit neighborhood environments. *American Journal of Preventive Medicine* 40(1):94–100.

Rutter, M. 2012. Resilience as a dynamic concept. *Development and Psychopathology* 24(2):335–344.

Rzotkiewicz, A., A. L. Pearson, B. V. Dougherty, A. Shortridge, and N. Wilson. 2018. Systematic review of the use of Google Street View in health research: Major themes, strengths, weaknesses and possibilities for future research. *Health & Place* 52:240–246.

Sallis, J. F., T. L. Conway, K. L. Cain, J. A. Carlson, L. D. Frank, J. Kerr, K. Glanz, J. E. Chapman, and B. E. Saelens. 2018. Neighborhood built environment and socioeconomic status in relation to physical activity, sedentary behavior, and weight status of adolescents. *Preventive Medicine* 110:47–54.

Sampson, J., J. D. Morenoff, and F. Earls. 1999. Beyond social capital: Spatial dynamics of collective efficacy for children. *American Sociological Review* 64:633–660.

Sampson, R. J., and S. W. Raudenbush. 1997. Neighborhoods and violent crime: A multilevel study of collective efficacy. *Science* 277(5328):918.

Sampson, R. J., and S. W. Raudenbush. 1999. Systematic social observation of public spaces: A new look at disorder in urban neighborhoods. *American Journal of Sociology* 105(3):603–651.

Santavirta, T., N. Santavirta, and S. E. Gilman. 2018. Association of the World War II Finnish evacuation of children with psychiatric hospitalization in the next generation. *JAMA Psychiatry* 75(1):21–27.

Schindler, H. S., J. Kholoptseva, S. S. Oh, H. Yoshikawa, G. J. Duncan, K. A. Magnuson, and J. P. Shonkoff. 2015. Maximizing the potential of early childhood education to prevent externalizing behavior problems: A meta-analysis. *Journal of School Psychology* 53(3):243–263.

Schwartz, I. M., P. York, E. Nowakowski-Sims, and A. Ramos-Hernandez. 2017. Predictive and prescriptive analytics, machine learning and child welfare risk assessment: The Broward County experience. *Children and Youth Services Review* 81:309–320.

Schweinhart, L. J., J. R. Berrueta-Clement, W. S. Barnett, A. S. Epstein, and D. P. Weikart. 1985. Effects of the Perry Preschool Program on youths through age 19: A summary. *Topics in Early Childhood Special Education* 5(2):26–35.

Shalev, I., and J. Belsky. 2016. Early-life stress and reproductive cost: A two-hit developmental model of accelerated aging? *Medical Hypotheses* 90:41–47.

Sharma, D., S. Shastri, and P. Sharma. 2016. Intrauterine growth restriction: Antenatal and postnatal aspects. Clinical medicine insights. *Pediatrics* 10:67–83.

Shonkoff, J. P. 2010. Building a new biodevelopmental framework to guide the future of early childhood policy. *Child Development* 81(1):357–367.

Shonkoff, J. P. 2016. Capitalizing on advances in science to reduce the health consequences of early childhood adversity. *JAMA Pediatrics* 170(10):1003–1007.

Shonkoff, J. P. 2017. Rethinking the definition of evidence-based interventions to promote early childhood development. *Pediatrics* 140(6):e20173136.

Shonkoff, J. P., and S. N. Bales. 2011. Science does not speak for itself: Translating child development research for the public and its policymakers. *Child Development* 82(1):17–32.

Shonkoff, J. P., and A. S. Garner. 2012. The lifelong effects of early childhood adversity and toxic stress. *Pediatrics* 129(1):e232–e246.

Shonkoff, J. P., and P. Levitt. 2010. Neuroscience and the future of early childhood policy: Moving from why to what and how. *Neuron* 67(5):689–691.

Shonkoff, J. P., W. T. Boyce, and B. S. McEwen. 2009. Neuroscience, molecular biology, and the childhood roots of health disparities: Building a new framework for health promotion and disease prevention. *JAMA* 301(21):2252–2259.

Silbereis, J. C., S. Pochareddy, Y. Zhu, M. Li, and N. Sestan. 2016. The cellular and molecular landscapes of the developing human central nervous system. *Neuron* 89(2):248–268.

Simon, A. K., G. A. Hollander, and A. McMichael. 2015. Evolution of the immune system in humans from infancy to old age. *Proceedings of the Royal Society B: Biological Sciences* 282(1821):1–9.

Slopen, N., K. C. Koenen, and L. D. Kubzansky. 2012. Childhood adversity and immune and inflammatory biomarkers associated with cardiovascular risk in youth: A systematic review. *Brain, Behavior, and Immunity* 26.

Slopen, N., K. A. McLaughlin, and J. P. Shonkoff. 2014. Interventions to improve cortisol regulation in children: A systematic review. *Pediatrics* 133(2):312–326.

Slopen, N., G. Strizich, S. Hua, L. C. Gallo, D. H. Chae, N. Priest, M. J. Gurka, S. I. Bangdiwala, J. I. Bravin, E. C. Chambers, M. L. Daviglus, M. M. Llabre, M. R. Carnethon, and C. R. Isasi. 2019. Maternal experiences of ethnic discrimination and child cardiometabolic outcomes in the study of Latino (SOL) youth. *Annals of Epidemiology* 34:52–57.

Snowdon, C. T., B. A. Pieper, C. Y. Boe, K. A. Cronin, A. V. Kurian, and T. E. Ziegler. 2010. Variation in oxytocin is related to variation in affiliative behavior in monogamous, pairbonded tamarins. *Hormones and Behavior* 58(4):614–618.

Social Programs That Work. 2017. *Social programs that work review: Evidence summary for the Perry Preschool Project.* https://evidencebasedprograms.org/document/perry-preschool-project-evidence-summary (accessed March 29, 2019).

Spencer, M. B., and C. Markstrom-Adams. 1990. Identity processes among racial and ethnic minority children in America. *Child Development* 61(2):290–310.

Sroufe, L. A. 2005. Attachment and development: A prospective, longitudinal study from birth to adulthood. *Attachment & Human Development* 7(4):349–367.

Stein, G. L., R. G. Gonzales, C. G. Coll, and J. I. Prandoni. 2016. Latinos in rural, new immigrant destinations: A modification of the integrative model of child development. In *Rural ethnic minority youth and families in the United States: Theory, research, and applications. Advancing responsible adolescent development*, edited by R. J. R. Levesque. Cham, Switzerland: Springer International Publishing. Pp. 37–56.

Stiles, J. 2008. The fundamentals of brain development: Integrating nature and nurture. Cambridge, MA: Harvard University Press.

Strohsnitter, W. C., E. E. Hatch, M. Hyer, R. Troisi, R. H. Kaufman, S. J. Robboy, J. R. Palmer, L. Titus-Ernstoff, D. Anderson, and R. N. Hoover. 2008. The association between in utero cigarette smoke exposure and age at menopause. *American Journal of Epidemiology* 167(6):727–733.

Sudhof, T. C. 2018. Towards an understanding of synapse formation. *Neuron* 100(2):276–293.

Sudhof, T. C., and R. C. Malenka. 2008. Understanding synapses: Past, present, and future. *Neuron* 60(3):469–476.

Sun, Y., F. K. Mensah, P. Azzopardi, G. C. Patton, and M. Wake. 2017. Childhood social disadvantage and pubertal timing: A national birth cohort from Australia. *Pediatrics* 139(6):e20164099.

Tang, Y., J. R. Nyengaard, D. M. De Groot, and H. J. Gundersen. 2001. Total regional and global number of synapses in the human brain neocortex. *Synapse* 41(3):258–273.

Taylor, S. E., B. M. Way, and T. E. Seeman. 2011. Early adversity and adult health outcomes. *Development and Psychopathology* 23(3):939–954.

Teicher, M. H., J. A. Samson, C. M. Anderson, and K. Ohashi. 2016. The effects of childhood maltreatment on brain structure, function and connectivity. *Nature Reviews Neuroscience* 17(10):652.

Thompson, B. L., P. Levitt, and G. D. Stanwood. 2009. Prenatal exposure to drugs: Effects on brain development and implications for policy and education. *Nature Reviews Neuroscience* 10(4):303–312.

Thompson, R. A. 2014. Stress and child development. *The Future of Children* 24(1):41–59.

Thompson, R. A. 2016. What more has been learned? The science of early childhood development 15 years after Neurons to Neighborhoods. *Zero to Three* 36(3):18–24.

Tom, S. E., R. Cooper, D. Kuh, J. M. Guralnik, R. Hardy, and C. Power. 2010. Fetal environment and early age at natural menopause in a British birth cohort study. *Human Reproduction* 25(3):791–798.

Tourangeau, K., C. Nord, T. Lê, A. G. Sorongon, and M. Najarian. 2009. Early Childhood Longitudinal Study, kindergarten class of 1998–99 (ECLS-K): Combined user's manual for the ECLS-K eighth-grade and K–8 full sample data files and electronic codebooks. NCES 2009-004. National Center for Education Statistics.

Tran, A. G. T. T. 2014. Family contexts: Parental experiences of discrimination and child mental health. *American Journal of Community Psychology* 53(1–2):37–46.

Tseng, P. H., I. G. Cameron, G. Pari, J. N. Reynolds, D. P. Munoz, and L. Itti. 2013. High-throughput classification of clinical populations from natural viewing eye movements. *Journal of Neurology* 260(1):275–284.

Turner, A. M., and W. T. Greenough. 1985. Differential rearing effects on rat visual cortex synapses. I. Synaptic and neuronal density and synapses per neuron. *Brain Research* 329(1–2):195–203.

Vaiserman, A. M. 2015. Epigenetic programming by early-life stress: Evidence from human populations. *Developmental Dynamics* 244(3):254–265.

Van Essen, D. C., S. M. Smith, D. M. Barch, T. E. Behrens, E. Yacoub, and K. Ugurbil. 2013. The WU-minn Human Connectome Project: An overview. *Neuroimage* 80:62–79.

Velez-Agosto, N. M., J. G. Soto-Crespo, M. Vizcarrondo-Oppenheimer, S. Vega-Molina, and C. García Coll. 2017. Bronfenbrenner's bioecological theory revision: Moving culture from the macro into the micro. *Perspectives on Psychological Science* 12(5):900–910.

Vied, C. M., F. Freudenberg, Y. Wang, A. A. Raposo, D. Feng, and R. S. Nowakowski. 2014. A multi-resource data integration approach: Identification of candidate genes regulating cell proliferation during neocortical development. *Frontiers in Neuroscience* 8:257.

Waddington, C. H. 1942. The epigenotype. *Endeavor* 1:18–20.

Waddington, C. H. 1957. *The strategy of the genes; a discussion of some aspects of theoretical biology.* London, UK: Allen & Unwin.

Wade, M., N. A. Fox, C. H. Zeanah, and C. A. Nelson. 2018. Effect of foster care intervention on trajectories of general and specific psychopathology among children with histories of institutional rearing: A randomized clinical trial. *JAMA Psychiatry* 75(11):1137–1145.

Wadhwa, P. D., S. Entringer, C. Buss, and M. C. Lu. 2011. The contribution of maternal stress to preterm birth: Issues and considerations. *Clinics in Perinatology* 38(3):351–384.

Wang, H., S. L. Lin, G. M. Leung, and C. M. Schooling. 2016. Age at onset of puberty and adolescent depression: "Children of 1997" birth cohort. *Pediatrics* 137(6):e20153231.

Wang, Y., and S. Zhao. 2010. Vascular biology of the placenta. *Colloquium Series on Integrated Systems Physiology: From Molecule to Function* 2(1):1–98.

Weber-Stadlbauer, U. 2017. Epigenetic and transgenerational mechanisms in infection-mediated neurodevelopmental disorders. *Translational Psychiatry* 7(5):e1113.

Wee, C. Y., T. A. Tuan, B. F. Broekman, M. Y. Ong, Y. S. Chong, K. Kwek, L. P. Shek, S. M. Saw, P. D. Gluckman, M. V. Fortier, M. J. Meaney, and A. Qiu. 2017. Neonatal neural networks predict children behavioral profiles later in life. *Human Brain Mapping* 38(3):1362–1373.

Welberg, L. A., K. V. Thrivikraman, and P. M. Plotsky. 2005. Chronic maternal stress inhibits the capacity to up-regulate placental 11beta-hydroxysteroid dehydrogenase type 2 activity. *Journal of Endocrinology* 186(3):R7–R12.

Welch, M. G. 2016. Calming cycle theory: The role of visceral/autonomic learning in early mother and infant/child behaviour and development. *Acta Paediatrica* 105(11):1266–1274.

Welch, M. G., M. M. Myers, P. G. Grieve, J. R. Isler, W. P. Fifer, R. Sahni, M. A. Hofer, J. Austin, R. J. Ludwig, and R. I. Stark. 2014. Electroencephalographic activity of preterm infants is increased by family nurture intervention: A randomized controlled trial in the NICU. *Clinical Neurophysiology* 125(4):675–684.

Welch, M. G., M. R. Firestein, J. Austin, A. A. Hane, R. I. Stark, M. A. Hofer, M. Garland, S. B. Glickstein, S. A. Brunelli, R. J. Ludwig, and M. M. Myers. 2015. Family nurture intervention in the neonatal intensive care unit improves social-relatedness, attention, and neurodevelopment of preterm infants at 18 months in a randomized controlled trial. *Journal of Child Psychology and Psychiatry* 56(11):1202–1211.

Williams, D. R., and S. A. Mohammed. 2009. Discrimination and racial disparities in health: Evidence and needed research. *Journal of Behavioral Medicine* 32(1):20–47.

Williams, D. R., and S. A. Mohammed. 2013. Racism and health I: Pathways and scientific evidence. *American Behavioral Scientist* 57(8).

Williams, D. R., Y. Yan, J. S. Jackson, and N. B. Anderson. 1997. Racial differences in physical and mental health: Socio-economic status, stress and discrimination. *Journal of Health Psychology* 2(3):335–351.

Williams, D. R., J. A. Lawrence, and B. A. Davis. 2019. Racism and health: Evidence and needed research. *Annual Review of Public Health* 40(1):105–125.

Woo Baidal, J. A., L. M. Locks, E. R. Cheng, T. L. Blake-Lamb, M. E. Perkins, and E. M. Taveras. 2016. Risk factors for childhood obesity in the first 1,000 days: A systematic review. *American Journal of Preventive Medicine* 50(6):761–779.

Yarde, F., F. Broekmans, K. Van der Pal-de Bruin, Y. Schönbeck, E. Te Velde, A. Stein, and L. Lumey. 2013. Prenatal famine, birthweight, reproductive performance and age at meno-pause: The Dutch Hunger Winter Families Study. *Human Reproduction* 28(12):3328–3336.

Yehuda, R., and L. M. Bierer. 2007. Transgenerational transmission of cortisol and PTSD risk. In *Stress hormones and post traumatic stress disorder: Basic studies and clinical perspectives*, Vol. 167, edited by E. R. DeKloet and E. Vermetten. Amsterdam, the Netherlands: Elsevier Science. Pp. 121–135.

Yehuda, R., S. M. Engel, S. R. Brand, J. Seckl, S. M. Marcus, and G. S. Berkowitz. 2005. Trans-generational effects of posttraumatic stress disorder in babies of mothers exposed to the World Trade Center attacks during pregnancy. *The Journal of Clinical Endocrinology & Metabolism* 90(7):4115–4118.

Yehuda, R., N. P. Daskalakis, A. Lehrner, F. Desarnaud, H. N. Bader, I. Makotkine, J. D. Flory, L. M. Bierer, and M. J. Meaney. 2014. Influences of maternal and paternal PTSD on epi-genetic regulation of the glucocorticoid receptor gene in Holocaust survivor offspring. *American Journal of Psychiatry* 171(8):872–880.

Yeung, M. S., S. Zdunek, O. Bergmann, S. Bernard, M. Salehpour, K. Alkass, S. Perl, J. Tisdale, G. Possnert, L. Brundin, H. Druid, and J. Frisen. 2014. Dynamics of oligodendrocyte generation and myelination in the human brain. *Cell* 159(4):766–774.

Yudell, M., D. Roberts, R. DeSalle, and S. Tishkoff. 2016. Taking race out of human genetics. *Science* 351(6273):564–565.

Zeanah, C. H., C. A. Nelson, N. A. Fox, A. T. Smyke, P. Marshall, S. W. Parker, and S. Koga. 2003. Designing research to study the effects of institutionalization on brain and behavioral development: The Bucharest Early Intervention Project. *Development and Psychopathology* 15(4):885–907.

Zeanah, C. H., M. R. Gunnar, R. B. McCall, J. M. Kreppner, and N. A. Fox. 2011. VI. Sensitive periods. *Monographs of the Society for Research in Child Development* 76(4):147–162.

Zhang, C., A. Paolozza, P. H. Tseng, J. N. Reynolds, D. P. Munoz, and L. Itti. 2019. Detec-tion of children/youth with fetal alcohol spectrum disorder through eye movement, psychometric, and neuroimaging data. *Frontiers in Neurology* 10:80.

Zhao, L., X. Zheng, J. Liu, R. Zheng, R. Yang, Y. Wang, and L. Sun. 2019. The placental transcriptome of the first-trimester placenta is affected by in vitro fertilization and embryo transfer. *Reproductive Biology and Endocrinology* 17(1):50.

3

Development Happens in Contexts: Overview of Early Life Critical Influences

INTRODUCTION

To ensure healthy and optimal development for all children, there is a need to understand how the context that a child grows in and the cumulative risk associated with that specific context shape the odds for thriving. Sir Michael Rutter, the first professor of child psychiatry in the United Kingdom, is credited as one of the first to bring the concept of cumulative risk to the study of child development. In his now classic work studying 10-year-old children, he documented that children who had two or more risk factors had a four-fold risk for having a psychiatric disorder (Rutter, 1979). Approximately a decade later, Sameroff and colleagues extended this work to young children's social and emotional competences (Sameroff et al., 1987a) and cognitive outcomes (Sameroff et al., 1987b). Since these studies, and the subsequent publication of *From Neurons to Neighborhoods* (NRC and IOM, 2000), there has been a rapid increase of cross-disciplinary research using an accumulation of risk models to assess early childhood social risk factors in relation to outcomes across the life course. Understanding the origins and mechanisms of the contextual factors and cumulative risk that produce inequities for children and families is a prerequisite to advance health equity.

While Chapter 2 discusses the mechanisms of healthy development within the growing child, this chapter provides an overview of the key early life protective and risk factors associated with development, as indicated in the committee's Statement of Task. This chapter discusses how each of these factors and conditions shapes health and safety, mental

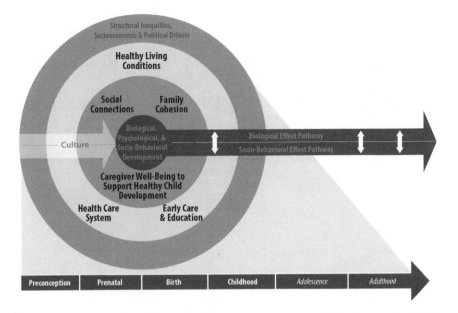

FIGURE 3-1 Mapping Chapter 3 early life protective and risk factors for child development to conceptual model and solution-driven chapters.
NOTES: The domains of focus in this chapter are reflected in the second and third rings in the model. These elements are bolded for emphasis.

and emotional well-being, and cognitive health during the prenatal and early childhood phases by mapping each factor to both the conceptual model and the forthcoming solution-driven Chapters 4–8 (see Figure 3-1 and Table 3-1 for how the content in this chapter maps to the conceptual model and the following chapters, and Box 3-1 for a high-level chapter overview). The committee identified domains by which to group these critical influences, with a focus on factors that shape inequities at the

TABLE 3-1 Mapping Chapter 3 Content to Chapters 4–7

Critical Influences in Prenatal and/or Early Childhood Stages Discussed in This Chapter	Corresponding "Action" Chapter
Family cohesion and social connections	Chapter 4
Health care	Chapter 5
Economic security	Chapter 6
Neighborhood conditions (e.g., concentrated disadvantage, physical and social environments, violence and crime, housing, environmental exposures)	Chapter 6
Early care and education	Chapter 7

BOX 3-1
Chapter in Brief

This chapter provides an overview of the key external influences that affect brain development in early life to either promote or hinder a child's opportunity to achieve optimal health and well-being. The chapter summarizes the evidence for the way multiple domains (family cohesion and healthy social connections; health care; healthy living conditions including economic security, and nutrition and food security; neighborhood conditions, housing, and environmental safety; early care and education) converge to create an accumulation of risk. This composite risk is heavily influenced by racism and discrimination and affects outcomes across a child's entire life course. A review of the epidemiology of risk and protective factors, prenatal and childhood outcomes, and evidence-based mechanisms (when known) are included.

Key findings on early life critical influences:

• There are specific risk and protective factors that affect health and development at multiple levels (e.g., individual, family, neighborhood, and systems/ policies).
• Racism and discrimination are crosscutting factors that perpetuate structural inequities and thwart healthy development for specific groups of children.
• Exposure to multiple risk factors discussed in this chapter can lead to an accumulation of risk over the life course and ultimately result in poor health outcomes in adulthood. Conversely, exposure to positive exposures and buffering experiences can promote health and resilience for children and adults.

child, family, community, and population levels. These domains include family cohesion and healthy social connections (see Chapter 4); health care (see Chapter 5); healthy living conditions (i.e., economic security, nutrition and food security, housing, and environmental safety) (see Chapter 6); and early care and education (ECE) (see Chapter 7).

Committee's Approach to Early Life Critical Influences

While there are many critical factors that shape development, the committee limited the scope of this chapter to include those with strong evidence for shaping affecting outcomes from the prenatal through early childhood periods. Where possible, the committee relied on high-quality systematic reviews and meta-analyses to provide a brief overview. To the extent possible, this chapter includes data and outcomes specific to the prenatal through early childhood periods; however, when those data are not available, data for caregivers and families are presented. The committee takes a life course approach in this report (see Figure 1-1), so, as such, it is important to note that many of the influences discussed in this chapter manifest in adolescent and adult outcomes. In each domain, critical factors are addressed in terms of definition, overall prevalence and disparities, and prenatal, birth, and early childhood outcomes, including information on potential mechanisms when the evidence points to these.

Crosscutting Elements: Discrimination and Racism

Across all of the critical factors in this chapter, there are two crosscutting elements that the committee has identified as being pervasive and rooted in health inequities—discrimination and racism—that can be thought of as the mechanisms by which structural inequities operate. (See Box 3-2 for a description of the root causes of health inequities and key definitions from a related report.) The crosscutting elements operate at multiple levels (i.e., intrapersonal, interpersonal, institutional, structural) and shape the experiences of children and families across the domains discussed in the rest of this chapter (and this report). While race is considered a social rather than biological construct (i.e., created from prevailing social perceptions, historical policies, and practices), the consequences of racism and the experiences of racial and ethnic minorities have psychological, biological, and social consequences (NASEM, 2017a). For example, historical policies and practices, such as residential segregation, redlining of districts, and discriminatory banking practices, are structural

---

BOX 3-2
Key Terms and Concepts from
Communities in Action: Pathways to Health Equity

The 2017 report *Communities in Action: Pathways to Health Equity* examined the root causes of health inequities in the United States. The authoring committee identified two clusters of root causes:

1. The intrapersonal, interpersonal, institutional, and systemic mechanisms that organize the distribution of power and resources differentially across lines of race, gender, class, sexual orientation, gender expression, and other dimensions of individual and group identity and
2. The unequal allocation of power and resources—including goods, services, and societal attention—which manifests in unequal social, economic, and environmental conditions.

This report defines structural inequities as the systemic disadvantage of one social group compared to other groups with whom it coexists, encompassing policy, law, governance, and culture.

SOURCE: NASEM, 2017a.

forms of racism that have long-lasting ramifications for the health of communities of color (NASEM, 2017a). This type of structural racism unfolds across many of the domains discussed in this chapter, including housing, economic stability, physical environment, and community violence. Furthermore, structural racism has been linked to historical trauma, which manifests from past treatment of specific racial or ethnic groups (NASEM, 2017a). This type of trauma is an important yet often "invisible" context that sets the stage for risk and resilience. Another example of a crosscutting element that is salient for this chapter is immigration-related experiences and challenges. For immigrant children or children of immigrants, there are unique barriers to achieving optimal health that play out at multiple levels and have serious implications for food security, housing stability, safety, and access to quality health care services. These important crosscutting elements will be highlighted throughout the chapter as they relate to the various factors that influence early development. The chapter will also discuss specific subgroups with unique needs or circumstances as they relate to these crosscutting elements, where appropriate.

FAMILY COHESION AND SOCIAL CONNECTIONS

Relationships in early childhood form the foundation for how children interact with their environment and other individuals across the life-span. This section discusses key influences that exist within the most proximal microsystem for children, consisting of family and peers. The following discussions include the scientific findings on experiences or factors that either enhance or undermine family cohesion and healthy social connections. Chapter 4 describes the interventions and mechanisms needed to support the family and promote healthy relationships. See Figure 3-2 for a visual of how this section ties to the report conceptual model.

Parental Factors

Parental well-being is a critical determinant of child health and developmental outcomes; therefore, what happens to the parent before, during, and after pregnancy has serious implications for the child. Parental mental health is inextricably linked to child well-being and there is consistent evidence that maternal depression compromises healthy child development (Center on the Developing Child at Harvard University, 2009; Goodman and Garber, 2017). Estimates show that 10–20 percent of mothers have lifetime prevalence of depression and the rates are much higher for mothers in low-income households. Because of the socioeconomic disparities in maternal depression and the implications for children's development, maternal depression has been thought of as a contributing factor to the cycle of intergenerational poverty (Reeves and Krause, 2019).

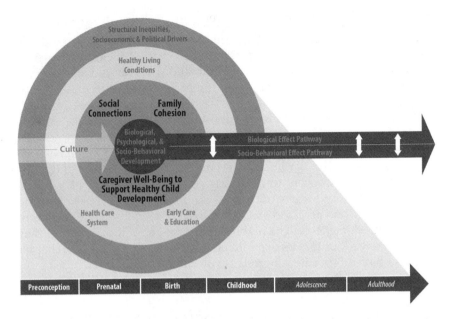

FIGURE 3-2 Leveraging early opportunities to achieve health equity across the life course: A conceptual framework.
NOTES: The elements of focus in this section are reflected in the second innermost ring in the model: caregiver well-being and support, family cohesion, and social connections. These elements are bolded for emphasis.

For children, the consequences of maternal depression include neuro-developmental and other biological disruptions and psychological and behavioral difficulties. Postpartum maternal depression specifically has been linked to the neurobiological pathways that shape emotional regulation, cognitive and executive function, and physiological stress response systems—all of which are critical functions and systems for ensuring optimal development (Drury et al., 2016). The Center on the Developing Child at Harvard University (2009) published a paper on the effects of maternal depression that indicated the following:

- Chronic depression can manifest in two types of problematic parenting patterns that disrupt the "serve and return"[1] interaction that is essential for healthy brain development: hostile or intrusive, and disengaged or withdrawn.

---

[1] "Serve and return" interactions occur when young children innately reach out for connection by babbling, using facial expressions, and gestures (i.e., serve), and adults respond with similar vocalization or gestures (i.e., return) (National Scientific Council on the Developing Child, 2004).

- Children who experience maternal depression early in life may have lasting effects on their brain architecture and persistent disruptions of their stress response systems.
- Maternal depression may begin to affect brain development in the fetus before birth.

While evidence exists that maternal depression is significantly related to children's behavioral and emotional functioning, more research is needed to better understand moderating effects for various subgroups of children (Goodman et al., 2011). In addition to maternal depression, paternal depression has also been shown to negatively affect parenting behaviors and child developmental outcomes (Gutierrez-Galve et al., 2015; Ramchandani et al., 2011; Wilson and Durbin, 2010). Sweeney and MacBeth (2016) identify the following mediators of the effect of paternal depression on children: paternal negative expressiveness, hostility, and involvement and marital conflict. There are other aspects of parental well-being for which evidence exists of an association with child health and well-being (e.g., parental alcohol or substance abuse or incarceration) (Conners et al., 2004; Lieb et al., 2002; Luthar et al., 2007; Nichols and Loper, 2012; VanDeMark et al., 2005). Additional select parent-specific factors that have been shown to be associated with child health and well-being outcomes include incarceration (see Chapter 4), interaction with the welfare system (see Chapter 4), adverse childhood experiences (ACEs) (see the Adverse Childhood Experiences section at the end of this chapter), and intimate partner violence (IPV).

IPV has adverse effects on pregnancy and birth outcomes (Boy and Salihu, 2004; Iliopoulou et al., 2012). A systematic review found that pregnant women who have experienced IPV are more likely to suffer from maternal mortality and have children who suffer from low birth weight (LBW) and infant mortality when compared to women who have not experienced IPV (Boy and Salihu, 2004). Research also suggests that children can suffer from harmful consequences associated with exposure to IPV, even if they have not directly observed the violence (Wathen and Macmillan, 2013). These consequences include social, emotional, and behavioral problems, such as mood and anxiety disorders, posttraumatic stress disorders, substance abuse, and school-related problems in childhood and adolescence. Rates of comorbidity between exposure to IPV and child maltreatment are high—some data show that 60–75 percent of families that have experiences of IPV also include children exposed to maltreatment (Osofsky, 2003).

Child Maltreatment

In the absence of safe and nurturing relationships, children are vulnerable to the effects of maltreatment, or child abuse and neglect.

BOX 3-3
Defining Common Types of Child Maltreatment

- *Physical abuse* is the intentional use of physical force that can result in physical harm. Examples include hitting, kicking, shaking, burning, or other shows of force against a child.
- *Sexual abuse* involves pressuring or forcing a child to engage in sexual acts. It includes behaviors such as fondling, penetration, and exposing a child to other sexual activities.
- *Emotional abuse* refers to behaviors that harm a child's self-worth or emotional well-being. Examples include name-calling, shaming, rejection, withholding love, and threatening.
- *Neglect* is the failure to meet a child's basic physical and emotional needs. These needs include housing, food, clothing, education, and access to medical care.

SOURCE: Excerpted from CDC, 2019.

The Child Abuse Prevention and Treatment Act defines child abuse and neglect as

> any recent act or set of acts or failure to act on the part of a parent or caretaker, which results in death, serious physical or emotional harm, sexual abuse or exploitation, or an act or failure to act, which presents an imminent risk of serious harm.[2]

Generally, child abuse and neglect are grouped into four types: neglect and physical, sexual, and emotional abuse. See Box 3-3 for descriptions of the four types of maltreatment. Despite this definition, there remain challenges related to varying state legal definitions, data collection, and calculating accurate incidence and prevalence rates in population-based studies (IOM and NRC, 2014). Therefore, the magnitude of child abuse and neglect is more than likely underestimated in the United States (Fortson et al., 2016). Not only is child maltreatment detrimental to children's health and well-being, it is also costly for the United States. Data from 2008 indicate that the total lifetime economic cost associated with child abuse and neglect amounted to approximately $124 billion (Fang et al., 2012).

Trends and Disparities

Despite the well-known consequences, child maltreatment is still too common today. At least one in seven children have experienced child abuse

---

[2] 42 U.S.C. § 5101 note.

or neglect in the past year, which is likely an underestimate (Finkelhor et al., 2015). State-level data on reports of child abuse and neglect show a 2.7 percent increase in the national rate of victims of child maltreatment from 2013 to 2017 (HHS, 2019).

Disparities in child maltreatment exist across groups by race and ethnicity, age, and socioeconomic status (SES). According to 2017 data from the National Child Abuse and Neglect Data System, rates of child abuse or neglect were reported to be highest for American Indian/Alaska Native (AI/AN) children (14.3 per 1,000 children). Following those are rates for African American (13.9 per 1,000), multiracial (11.3 per 1,000), Pacific Islander (8.7 per 1,000), white (8.1 per 1,000), Hispanic (8.0 per 1,000), and Asian (1.6 per 1,000) children. Likewise, the rate of fatalities due to maltreatment for African American children (4.86 per 100,000 children) is 2.6 times greater than that of white children and 3.1 times higher than that of Hispanic children (HHS, 2019).

Young children are the most vulnerable to child maltreatment (HHS, 2019), and more than one-fourth (28.5 percent) of child maltreatment victims are younger than 3 years. Overall, children under the age of 1 year are most likely to die from child abuse or neglect (see Figure 3-3). Very young children with disabilities have increased risk of child maltreatment when compared to children without disabilities—and rates of disability are higher among low-income populations that experience higher rates of pre-term birth (Hibbard et al., 2007; NASEM, 2015a). Children living in poverty are disproportionately exposed to child abuse and neglect and experience five times the risk of child abuse or neglect as children from higher SES

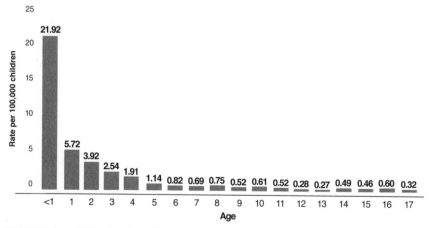

FIGURE 3-3 Child fatalities due to maltreatment by age, 2017.
NOTE: Based on data from 44 states.
SOURCE: HHS, 2019.

households (Sedlak et al., 2010).[3] It is important to note that disparities in child maltreatment have been attributed to other social, environmental, or economic factors, pointing to the need for a multilevel approach to preventing maltreatment (Fortson et al., 2016; Gilbert et al., 2009).

Outcomes Related to Child Maltreatment

Child maltreatment has a pervasive and harmful influence on many aspects of development and children who are exposed to a certain type of maltreatment are frequently exposed to others (Gilbert et al., 2009). Exposure to child abuse and neglect has serious ramifications for a child's biological, behavioral, cognitive, and emotional development (Cicchetti and Handley, 2017). The relationship between child abuse and neglect and physiological, psychological, and behavioral outcomes has been well documented throughout the child development literature, and a comprehensive review was published in the 2014 Institute of Medicine (IOM) and National Research Council (NRC) report *New Directions in Child Abuse and Neglect Research*. Therefore, the literature review is not repeated here; key findings related to the effects of maltreatment from the 2014 IOM and NRC report are provided in Box 3-4. See Chapter 2 for more on biological mechanisms of development that can be hindered or enhanced through early experiences.

Peer Social Connections

For children, an important source of social connections is the peer group that they interact with. After experiences with primary caregivers and family members, peers are the most proximal interpersonal relationships for young children. Through peer relationships and interactions, young children learn and reinforce notions of reciprocal interactions. For example, young children learn how to share, take turns, and give and receive from interactions with other young children. From these experiences, they can also learn to interpret and take into account the needs and desires of others and to manage their own impulses (National Scientific Council on the Developing Child, 2004). From early on, peer interactions can have positive and/or negative effects on children's mental, behavioral, and emotional health. (See Box 3-5 for findings and conclusions from a report on preventing bullying.)

---

[3] In the *Fourth National Incidence Study of Child Abuse and Neglect (NIS-4): Report to Congress,* a low-socioeconomic status household was defined as having a household income below $15,000 per year; parent education level less than high school; or any member of the household receiving poverty program benefits (e.g., Temporary Assistance for Needy Families, food stamps, public housing, energy assistance, or subsidized school meals) (Sedlak et al., 2010).

BOX 3-4
Key Findings from the 2014 IOM and NRC Report
New Directions in Child Abuse and Neglect Research

- Across human and nonhuman primate studies, perturbations to the hypothalamic-pituitary-adrenal axis system often are seen to be associated with child abuse and neglect. The findings are complex, moderated by a number of factors, and seen at some ages and not others.
- Abused and neglected children show behavioral and emotional difficulties that are consistent with effects on the amygdala, such as internalizing problems, heightened anxiety and emotional reactivity, and deficits in emotional processing.
- Despite mixed evidence regarding structural changes in the prefrontal cortex, a number of studies suggest that abuse and neglect are associated with functional changes in the prefrontal cortex and associated brain regions, often affecting inhibitory control.
- Abuse and neglect have profound effects on selected aspects of children's cognitive development. Although many attempts have been made to disentangle the effects of abuse and neglect, the balance of findings suggests that severe neglect may interfere with the development of executive functioning, and both neglect and abuse increase the risk for attention regulation problems and attention-deficit/hyperactivity disorder, lower IQ, and poorer school performance.
- Children who experience abuse or neglect have been found to be at higher risk for the development of externalizing behavior problems, including oppositional defiant disorder, conduct disorder, and aggressive behaviors. Abused and neglected children also have been found to be at increased risk for internalizing problems, particularly depression, in childhood, adolescence, and adulthood.
- A number of studies have found elevated rates of posttraumatic stress disorder (PTSD) among individuals with a history of abuse and neglect. PTSD has been associated with physical, cognitive, psychological, social, and behavioral problems among youth who were abused or neglected in childhood.
- Experiences of child abuse and neglect have effects on many health outcomes, including risks for long-term chronic and debilitating diseases and, in extreme cases, stunted growth.
- Experiences of abuse and neglect in childhood have a large effect on delinquency, violence, and suicide attempts in adolescence and adulthood.
- Adolescents and adults with a history of child abuse and neglect have higher rates of alcohol abuse and alcoholism than those without a history of abuse and neglect, although this relationship has been found most frequently in women.
- Not all children who experience abuse or neglect show problematic outcomes. Factors that influence resilience among abused and neglected children have been identified at the level of the individual child, the family, and the child's broader social context. These factors, along with risks and stressors at each level, interact with one another to predict resilient outcomes.
- The timing, chronicity, and severity of child abuse and neglect, as well as the context in which they occur, have been shown to impact the associated outcomes.

SOURCE: IOM and NRC, 2014.

BOX 3-5
The Effects of Bullying in Early Childhood

The 2016 report *Preventing Bullying Through Science, Policy, and Practice* makes the case that bullying is not a normal aspect of childhood, as it is commonly thought to be. Bullying—unwanted aggressive behavior repeated (or likely to be repeated) by another youth or group of youths that involves a power imbalance—can be thought of as a public health issue. In fact, the report draws the following findings and conclusions about the serious development effects and implications of being the victim or perpetrator of bullying behavior at a young age:

- Although the effects of being bullied on the brain are not yet fully understood, there are changes in the stress response systems and in the brain that are associated with increased risk for mental health problems, cognitive function, self-regulation, and other physical health problems.
- The long-term consequences of being bullied extend into adulthood, and the effects can be more severe than other forms of being maltreated as a child.
- Bullying has significant short- and long-term internalizing and externalizing psychological consequences for the children who are involved in bullying behavior.
- Existing evidence suggests that both social-cognitive and emotion regulation processes may mediate the relation between being bullied and adverse mental health outcomes.
- Although genes appear to modulate humans' response to being either a target or a perpetrator of bullying behavior, it is still unclear what aspects of these experiences are interacting with genes and which genes are implicated to produce the variability in outcomes. Examining the role of genes in bullying in the context of the environment is essential to providing meaningful information on the genetic component of individual differences in outcomes from being a target or a perpetrator of bullying behavior.

See Chapter 7 in this report on Promoting Health Equity Through Early Care and Education for more on the role of educators in preventing bullying.

SOURCE: NASEM, 2016b.

Safe, Stable, Nurturing Relationships and Environments

While child abuse and neglect increase the risk for a host of mental and physical ailments, lifelong mental and/or physical anguish is not a foregone conclusion. There is clear scientific evidence that the presence of safe, stable, and nurturing relationships is critical to healthy development and can buffer the mechanisms of adversity and support positive trajectories (Bornstein and Leventhal, 2015; Bronfenbrenner and Morris, 2006; CDC, 2014; Luthar, 2006; Masten, 2014; National Scientific Council on the Developing Child, 2004). (For information on mechanisms of buffering the stress response, see Chapter 2.) Safe, stable, and nurturing relationships are also important for preventing maltreatment, as they have been identified as a moderator of intergenerational child maltreatment. A meta-analysis found that adult relationships and parent–child relationships had a protective effect against intergenerational child maltreatment when they were safe, stable, and nurturing (Schofield et al., 2013). A stable relationship with caring adults is also important in child care settings, which can affect social competence, behavioral issues, and thinking and reasoning skills. In a 2004 summary of key scientific findings on relationships, the National Scientific Council on the Developing Child identified nurturing and stable relationships with caring adults as a cornerstone of healthy development. The Council identified "serve and return" as a key mechanism of healthy interactions between parents and babies, by which the brain architecture is strengthened. This is also important in child care settings, which can affect social competence, behavioral issues, and thinking and reasoning skills. Finally, the Council concluded based on the science that secure and stable relationships can protect children from illness, chronic stress, exposure to toxicants, and preventable injuries.

HEALTH CARE

In addition to the social determinants of health (SDOH) described throughout this report, health care itself plays a major role in child development through the life course. From preconception through early childhood, there are several aspects of health care that are critically important from an equity perspective: access to quality care, coverage, provider bias (or lack thereof), and provider cultural/linguistic competency. The following section provides an introduction to these issues along the continuum of preconception, prenatal, and pediatric health care; Chapter 5 provides a more in-depth look into opportunities to enhance these systems. See Figure 3-4 for a visual of how this section ties to the report conceptual model.

Preconception Care

The number of studies devoted to understanding preconception health and the interventions intended to improve health among women who may become pregnant have increased in recent years, but there is still a general paucity of data. According to a 2016 review of this research, results are mixed, and the studies themselves are generally of moderate to poor quality (Hussein et al., 2016). While preconception care may increase women's knowledge about certain health conditions and pregnancy (Callec et al., 2014; Chuang et al., 2010), it is not clear if this translates to healthier outcomes for infants and children. Across eight randomized

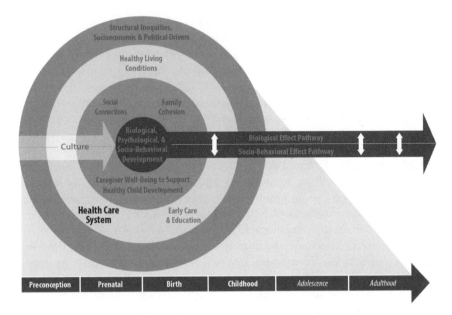

FIGURE 3-4 Leveraging early opportunities to achieve health equity across the life course: A conceptual framework.
NOTES: The element of focus in this section is reflected in the second outermost ring in the model: the health care system. This element is bolded for emphasis.

controlled trials (RCTs) of preconception health care interventions, there was little evidence that interventions reduced adverse pregnancy outcomes (Hussein et al., 2016). This was true even though the interventions appeared to increase maternal knowledge and locus of control and reduce risky behaviors (Hussein et al., 2016).

It is also true that only a small minority of women receive preconception care, making it difficult to draw broad generalizations about its effectiveness (Hemsing et al., 2017). This is likely because access to preconception care is not widespread (Hemsing et al., 2017), and a recent review outlined several reasons why (Goossens, 2018). First, a lack of reimbursement mechanisms for administering preconception care reduces providers' incentive to deliver it. Lack of reimbursement, payment mechanisms, or insurance are also reasons that preventive services and health promotion services are not delivered more generally (Goossens, 2018). Limited time and heavy workloads were a second reason that health care providers do not engage in preconception care with widespread frequency. A third reason was simply a lack of knowledge on the part of clients themselves (i.e., they were not aware of preconception care or did not seek it out) (Goossens, 2018). A fourth reason was that providers themselves did not think it was their duty to provide preconception care; primary care providers, for instance, were likely to think it was the role of the obstetrician, and vice versa (Goossens, 2018). A final reason could be that, given the lack of strong evidence for improving birth outcomes (Hussein et al., 2016), women simply choose not to engage in preconception care because they do not think it will be effective.

Preconception care as currently conceptualized—typically a single medical visit initiated when one wants to become pregnant—is likely insufficient to address the accumulated life and medical risks up to that point for both parents. Thus, a broader, multisector view of preconception care seen through an SDOH lens is likely necessary to achieve the significant impact that would be expected when one mitigates potential risks prior to achieving pregnancy.

Prenatal Care

Delivered early and often, prenatal care increases the chances of delivering a healthy baby (Kilpatrick et al., 2017). Conversely, women who do not receive prenatal care are three to four times as likely to die from pregnancy-related issues compared to women who do receive such care (Bingham et al., 2011). There are well-documented negative effects on babies as well (Cox et al., 2011). Women who do not receive prenatal care are more likely to deliver babies that are underweight, preterm, and are more likely to die in infancy from respiratory problems, sudden infant death syndrome, and gastrointestinal issues; however, these outcomes are not solely due to lack of prenatal care (Association of Maternal & Child Health Programs, 2016).

In contrast to preconception care, prenatal care is one of the most common types of health care in the United States. In 2016, 77 percent of pregnant women initiated prenatal care in the first trimester of pregnancy (Osterman and Martin, 2018). Despite advances in prenatal care, there are significant disparities in coverage and access. Women who are young, are not white, have low educational attainment, or lack private insurance are more likely to have late or inadequate prenatal care (Osterman and Martin, 2018), and issues related to insurance coverage and access persist into postnatal life for the baby.

Pediatric Care

In general, the preponderance of evidence suggests that higher rates of health insurance have led to higher rates of pediatric health care access and better health outcomes for children (Leininger and Levy, 2015). Still, disparities in health care access remain, especially among those who do not have health insurance or have intermittent coverage (Leininger and Levy, 2015). While the number of children who are uninsured is low

(~5 percent of children 0–18 years old), this varies from 1 to 11 percent based on state of residence (Kaiser Family Foundation, 2017). Immigrant children, including those who are undocumented, are less likely to be insured than children of the same age with U.S. citizenship (Leininger and Levy, 2015). Some studies suggest that intermittent losses of coverage—which is more common among families with income near the Medicaid eligibility line—decreases children's use of care (Leininger and Levy, 2015). For instance, one study found that even small gaps in insurance coverage decrease a visit to any doctor or a well-child visit by 4 and 9 percent, respectively (Leininger, 2009). Importantly, minority children are disproportionately likely to be from low-income families, particularly African American, AI/AN, and Hispanic children (Jiang et al., 2016). As a consequence of periodic bouts of being uninsured due to poverty (Leininger and Levy, 2015), these groups are less likely to receive routine pediatric care or treatment for medical conditions (Hodgkinson et al., 2017). These disparities in use are reflected in reported health statistics from parents: ethnic minority children are at least four times as likely to be described as in "fair or poor health" by their parents compared to white children. Similarly, children living in poverty are less likely to be described as in "excellent or very good health" by their parents (71 percent) compared to those not living in poverty (87 percent) (Kuo et al., 2012).

Barriers to Accessing Quality Health Care

There are a number of plausible reasons for the existing disparities in access to care, including lack of time and flexibility to seek services, long wait times, or the requirement of multiple appointments (Hodgkinson et al., 2017), and the decline of prenatal care in rural settings (Hung et al., 2017). These factors may make prioritizing pediatric care or treatment untenable for those living in poverty or enduring stress (Hodgkinson et al., 2017; Santiago et al., 2013).

It is important to note that, just as with other aspects of health care, bias and unequal treatment may play a role in women's preventative services and prenatal care (IOM, 2002). Stereotyping and bias on the part of health care providers may increase disparities in preconception care, as has been suggested of prenatal care (Kogan et al., 1994). In particular, messaging that places all of the responsibility for the fetus' health on mothers may serve to exacerbate stigmas among those already facing significant societal disparities (Greaves et al., 2014; Sue, 2019).

Stigma, bias, or lack of training on the part of health care professionals may also exacerbate pediatric health care disparities (Sue, 2019). Some studies have shown that providers for lower-income families admit to these challenges, including a lack of understanding and training about the effects of poverty on children, confrontation of their own personal prejudice and biases, stigma that comes with working with low-income families and children, and difficulty applying typical diagnostic frameworks to children from low-income families (Smith et al., 2011, 2013).

As outlined in the 2016 National Academies report *Parenting Matters: Supporting Parents of Children Ages 0–8*, medical providers (and service providers more generally) are met with increasing pressure to provide care in a culturally and linguistically sensitive way. Because of rapid changes in demographics, medical providers may face difficulty in adapting to language barriers or cultural norms, which may in turn reduce the willingness of ethnic minorities and families in poverty to access the health care system (NASEM, 2016a). Medical providers require the knowledge and tools to provide appropriate care to diverse populations in order to address the aforementioned health care disparities. Chapter 5 provides a more in-depth look into opportunities to enhance systems along the continuum of preconception, prenatal, and pediatric health care.

HEALTHY LIVING CONDITIONS

In the report's conceptual model, the committee identifies healthy living conditions as an important domain for study and intervention (see Figure 3-5 for a visual of how this section ties to the conceptual model). For the purposes of this report, healthy living conditions are the social, economic, cultural, and environmental factors that shape the odds for optimal child health and development. Specifically, these include economic security, nutrition and food security, neighborhood conditions, housing, and environmental exposures. These living conditions interact with multiple levels of the conceptual model. For example, adequate nutrition and food security encompass individual behaviors, such as breastfeeding, but they can also be shaped by the larger policy context, such as government programs (e.g., the Supplemental Nutrition Assistance Program [SNAP] and the Special Supplemental Nutrition Program for Women, Infants, and Children [WIC]). The following sections delve into the evidence on how healthy living conditions are critical for early development. Chapter 6 follows this thread and discusses the evidence for interventions (i.e., programs, policies, and systems) that show the most promise for promoting equitable healthy living conditions for all children.

ECONOMIC SECURITY

Household Socioeconomic Status

Household SES, a construct often measured using income, occupation, and education, is an important social determinant of child health and well-being. For children, SES not only reflects household income but is

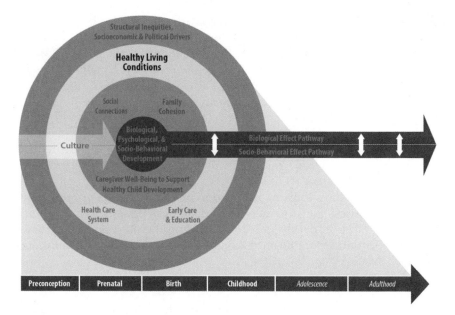

FIGURE 3-5 Leveraging early opportunities to achieve health equity across the life course: A conceptual framework.

NOTES: The element of focus in this section is reflected in the second outermost ring in the model: healthy living conditions (i.e., economic security, nutrition and food security, housing, and environmental safety). This element is bolded for emphasis.

also indicative of their neighborhood and housing conditions, food security, parental well-being and educational attainment, exposure to violence and other stressors, quality of ECE, and more. This section specifically explores how household SES as it relates to income, poverty, wealth, class, and education affects early developmental outcomes.

Poverty can be defined broadly as the lack of financial resources or material possessions to meet basic needs, such as shelter, food, and clothing. Poverty, income, and wealth are considered to be determinants of health, and there is a robust literature base that ties income and wealth to key health indicators, such as life expectancy, risk of chronic disease, and health-promoting behaviors (e.g., physical activity, healthy eating) (Chetty et al., 2016; NASEM, 2017a; Woolf et al., 2015). Poverty is a multidimensional construct that has many implications for the living conditions and environment that shape health and development.

For children, living in poverty is associated with negative health and developmental outcomes. The existing research suggests at least two pathways by which living in poverty can influence child outcomes (Evans, 2004). The first is through access to material resources and services (e.g., safe housing, nutrition, exercise, health care) (Braveman et al., 2018;

Johnson et al., 2016; Woolf et al., 2015). The second is through psychosocial stress (e.g., parental job strain, exposure to violence, housing instability, food insecurity) (Braveman et al., 2018; Johnson et al., 2016; Lefmann and Combs-Orme, 2014). The convergence of these factors shapes early living conditions, which can lead to cumulative risk exposure for those living in poverty. Therefore, income and poverty can be conceptualized as upstream determinants of many of the social, economic, and environmental factors discussed in this chapter.

Trends and Disparities

While children under the age of 18 represent 23 percent of the nation's population, they make up 32 percent of people living in poverty (Koball and Jiang, 2018a). In 2016, 44 percent of young children (i.e., under the age of 9) lived in low-income households (i.e., below 200 percent of the federal poverty threshold). In addition, approximately one in five young children lived in poor households (i.e., below 100 percent of the federal poverty threshold) (Koball and Jiang, 2018b). It is important to note that child poverty, and poverty in general, can be measured in a variety of ways, which has implications for how trends are measured. For example, consumption-based measures of poverty—as opposed to those based on income alone—reflect permanent income and government benefits, and some argue that these are more likely to capture the effects of saving, ownership of goods (e.g., property), and access to credit (Meyer and Sullivan, 2009).

Socioeconomic disparities exist across race, ethnicity, age group, and geographic region. For example, black, AI/AN, and Hispanic children disproportionately live in low-income and poor households; they are also most likely to live in deep poverty (below 50 percent of the federal poverty threshold). In terms of upward economic mobility, there are differences among racial groups as well. In particular, research suggests that black and AI/AN children have the lowest rates of upward mobility, even when controlling for parental income (Chetty et al., 2018). When looking across age groups, younger children (up to 11 years old) are more likely to live in low-income or poor households. However, when stratified by racial or ethnic group, there are stark differences in the proportions (see Table 3-2).

Effects of Income and Poverty

Pregnancy and birth outcomes Blumenshine et al. (2010) conducted a systematic review examining the association between socioeconomic disadvantage and adverse birth outcomes (e.g., outcomes related to birth weight, gestational age, or growth restriction). The authors determined that 91 studies found significant associations between at least one measure of socioeconomic disadvantage and one adverse birth outcome.

TABLE 3-2 Percentage of Children (ages 0–11 years) Living in High Poverty Areas from 2013 to 2017, by Race and Ethnicity

Race or Ethnicity	Percentage of Children (0–11 years) Living in Low-Income or Poor Households
American Indian/Alaska Native	28%
Asian and Pacific Islander	6%
Black or African American	28%
Hispanic or Latino	19%
Multiracial	10%
Non-Hispanic White	4%

NOTES: High poverty areas are defined as census tracts with poverty rates of 30 percent or more. These data are sourced from the Population Reference Bureau analysis of data from the 2013–2017 American Community Survey 5-year data.
SOURCE: Kids Count Data Center, 2019.

While differences in birth outcomes based on individual-level socioeconomic factors were almost always observed among non-Hispanic white women, the results were less consistent for African American and Hispanic women. For example, no studies included in this review found birth outcomes to be associated with individual-level socioeconomic factors among foreign-born Hispanic women. However, other studies show associations between neighborhood-level poverty and pregnancy and birth outcomes across racial and ethnic groups. The authors postulate that the cumulative effects of neighborhood conditions (e.g., poor housing, crime, pollution, stress), which are more common for communities of color, may have stronger health impacts than those associated with individual-level income or educational attainment, pointing to the need for community-level interventions (see the section Concentrated Disadvantage for more discussion of these studies at the neighborhood level).

Childhood outcomes Living in poverty during early childhood can have long-lasting implications for health and well-being. Family income has been found to be associated with risk of child maltreatment, where families with limited economic resources are at a higher risk (Berger et al., 2017; Cancian, 2010). Other research points to allostatic load as an important proximal outcome of living in an environment in the context of poverty. Blair et al. (2011) found that two aspects of the poverty environment were related to salivary cortisol (a measure of the stress response) in infancy: adult exits from the home and perceived economic insufficiency. In terms of neurodevelopmental and cognitive outcomes, the existing literature suggests that poverty affects the developing brain. This includes the structure and function of areas that regulate memory, emotion,

---

BOX 3-6
Conclusions from *A Roadmap to Reducing Child Poverty:*
The Consequences of Child Poverty

The 2019 report *A Roadmap to Reducing Child Poverty* presents the current evidence on the health and well-being consequences of growing up in childhood poverty. Based on this evidence the authoring committee reached the following conclusions:

- The weight of the causal evidence indicates that income poverty itself causes negative child outcomes, especially when it begins in early childhood and/or persists throughout a large share of a child's life.
- Poverty alleviation can promote children's development, both because of the goods and services that parents can buy for their children and because it may promote a more responsive, less stressful environment in which more positive parent–child interactions can take place.

See Chapter 6 in this report for a summary of the antipoverty packages evaluated in this report for their potential to reduce child poverty by half in 10 years.

SOURCE: NASEM, 2019.

---

cognitive functioning, and language and literacy (Johnson et al., 2016). There is also research that demonstrates the impact of family income on academic achievement, whereby a $1,000 increase in annual income could increase achievement by 5–6 percent of a standard deviation (Duncan et al., 2011; Wolf et al., 2017). Box 3-6 enumerates a few conclusions on the consequences of poverty from the 2019 National Academies report *A Roadmap to Reducing Child Poverty.*

Implications of the Wealth Gap

Income is often the target of many policies and interventions and is important for short-term outcomes, but a focus on the more encompassing construct of wealth is important for a health equity agenda because it has long-term and intergenerational implications. That is, income is necessary for building wealth, and wealth could buffer families from periods of income instability and low income.

> Wealth, or economic assets accumulated over time, is calculated by subtracting outstanding debts and liabilities from the cash value of currently owned assets—such as houses, land, cars, savings accounts, pension plans, stocks and other financial investments, and businesses. Wealth measured at a single time period may provide a more complete picture than income of a person's economic resources. (NASEM, 2017a, p. 127)

U.S. Census data show that the median household wealth in 2013 was $1,700 for black families, $2,000 for Latinos, and an astonishing $116,800 for whites. The median household wealth in 1983 was $6,800 for black families, $4,000 for Latinos, and $102,200 for whites (Asante-Muhammad et al., 2017). Using data from the Panel Study of Income Dynamics, Williams (2004) found that level of income was not as good of an indicator for black children's outcomes as it was for white children. Rather, having assets such as stocks or an IRA mattered more for black than for white children. Though focused on older individuals, Zhan and Sherraden (2010) found that household income was more associated with white children's college attendance and graduation, whereas wealth seemed to be more salient for black and Latino college students. This is also consistent with findings from Williams Shanks (2007) that family income is associated with white children's test scores but not those of black children. Kaushal and Nepomnyaschy (2009) find that although wealth, along with family sociodemographics and parental resources, accounts for the disparities in the black-white and Hispanic-white gap in children's participation in gifted programs, extracurricular activities, and grade retention, black children continued to face high risk of expulsion or suspension from school relative to white children regardless of wealth status. Furthermore, inter-generational transmission of wealth may not be as common, especially for black families (Chetty et al., 2018). While Latino families are moving up in their incomes across generation, black families have substantially lower rates of upward mobility and higher rates of downward mobility (Chetty et al., 2018). That is, black children from higher-income households are likely to become poor as adults compared to their white peers. This indicates that the pathway to wealth accumulation and maintenance differs across racial groups, which has implications for policies that are developed and implemented, especially if they do not address the continued loss of wealth for minority families and communities.

Parental Educational Attainment

Evidence shows that higher levels of caregiver/parental educational attainment are associated with positive child educational outcomes (e.g., school readiness, educational achievement), physical health outcomes (e.g., rates of LBW), and health behaviors (e.g., rates of smoking and binge drinking) (Child Trends, 2015). Research indicates that caregiver/parental educational attainment may also serve as a protective factor for outcomes in childhood, adolescence, and adulthood (Dubow et al., 2009).

Higher levels of maternal educational attainment, in particular, have been linked with improved health and well-being for children (Cutler and Lleras-Muney, 2006). Conversely, low levels of maternal educational attainment have been found to be significantly associated with negative

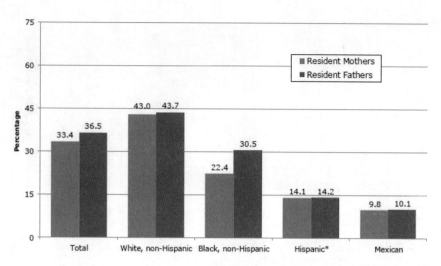

FIGURE 3-6 Percentage of school-age children whose parents have at least a bachelor's degree, by child's race and Hispanic origin and parent's gender, 2015. NOTES: * Hispanic includes Mexican. Data are sourced from Child Trends analysis of Current Population Survey, March Supplement.
SOURCE: Child Trends, 2015.

infant and child outcomes. Infants whose mothers have not completed high school have been found to have twice the risk of dying before their first birthday compared to those of mothers who have completed college (Egerter et al., 2011b; Mathews and MacDorman, 2007).

Since 1974, the percentage of parents (with children ages 6–18) with less than a high school diploma has decreased, while the percent of those with a bachelor's degree or higher has increased (Child Trends, 2015). However, disparities by race and ethnicity have persisted, particularly for African American and Hispanic mothers and fathers (see Figure 3-6).

Education is often touted as the gateway to prosperity or ensuring stability for families and children. However, accumulating evidence shows that there are racial differences in the impact of college attainment on income and wealth. Asante-Muhammad and colleagues of Prosperity Now show that

> [w]hite families whose head of household holds a high school diploma have nearly enough wealth ($64,200) to be considered middle class [see Figure 3-7]. A typical black or Latino family whose head of household has a college degree, however, owns just $37,600 and $32,600, respectively, in wealth. In fact, only black and Latino households at the median with an advanced degree have enough wealth to fit into [their] middle-class definition. By contrast, all white households except those who fail to attain a high school diploma could be considered middle class. (Asante-Muhammad et al., 2017, p. 10)

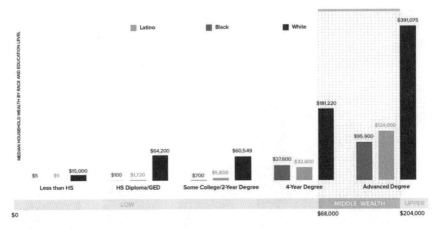

FIGURE 3-7 Having a college education is not enough to guarantee middle-class wealth for many black and Latino families.
NOTES: Wealth figures depicted above exclude durable goods. Data are sourced from the U.S. Census Bureau Survey of Income and Program Participation, 2014.
SOURCE: Asante-Muhammad et al., 2017.

Black and Latino families with college degrees have less than half of the wealth of white families with a high school diploma. This differential impact of higher education is also seen with unemployment rates: black individuals with college degrees have a 19, 65, 31, and 31 percent greater chance of unemployment than Latinos, Hispanics, whites, and Asian Americans, respectively (Andolfatto, 2017). This is particularly concerning when many blacks and Latinos are less likely to have higher education degrees compared to their white peers. Thus, while educational attainment is associated with better child outcomes, more research is needed to better uncover how racial disparities in education coupled with availability of wealth may be associated with the racial disparities in health and education.

NUTRITION AND FOOD SECURITY

Although access to adequate and nutritious foods affects development across the life course, it is particularly important for the preconception, prenatal, and early childhood periods. Furthermore, the period from conception to 2 years of age (about the first 1,000 days) is especially critical, as the brain undergoes significant developmental changes during this period that may not be possible later in life (Schwarzenberg and Georgieff, 2018). In addition to macronutrients (protein, fat, and glucose), certain micronutrients (zinc, copper, iodine, iron, and selenium) and vitamins and cofactors (vitamin B_6, vitamin B_{12}, vitamin A, vitamin K, folate, and choline) are particularly important for healthy early brain development (American Pregnancy Association, 2017; Cusick and Georgieff, 2016; Georgieff et al., 2015; IOM, 1990; March of Dimes, 2018; Schwarzenberg and Georgieff, 2018). Malnutrition can take the form of undernutrition (inadequate intake of macro- and/or micronutrients) and/or overweight/ obesity (excessive intake of calories but not necessarily adequate intake of macro- and micronutrients). Inadequate intake of macro- and micro-nutrients during critical or sensitive periods of development can result in negative developmental effects across the life course, with long-term effects being more likely the earlier such nutrient deficiencies occur (Georgieff et al., 2015; Schwarzenberg and Georgieff, 2018).

Access to healthy and nutritious foods for pregnant mothers is impor-tant to ensure healthy birth and developmental outcomes for their infants (Borge et al., 2017; Ramakrishnan et al., 2012; Thorne-Lyman and Fawzi, 2012; Veena et al., 2016; Yakoob and Lo, 2017; Zerfu and Ayele, 2013). In an overview of systematic reviews of international interventions to improve nutrition during pregnancy, infants of pregnant women who were provided oral supplements of vitamin A, low-dose calcium, zinc, and multiple micronutrients as well as nutrition education and preven-tive antimalarials were found to have a lower risk of LBW (da Silva Lopes et al., 2017).

Maternal nutrition during pregnancy can also affect overweight and obesity in children (Lau, 2014; Leonard et al., 2017). Tabacchi et al. (2007) describe that "the prenatal interactions between genetics and environ-ment play an important role in determining the postnatal phenotype related to obesity" (see Chapter 2 for more detailed information on fetal programming and the interplay of genetics and environment). Evidence also suggests a correlation between maternal obesity and poor infant and birth outcomes (e.g., higher risk of preterm birth, being large for gesta-tional age, fetal defects, perinatal death) (Aviram et al., 2011; Marchi et al., 2015), poor health outcomes in infancy and early childhood, including childhood obesity (Beckhaus et al., 2015; Mameli et al., 2016; Marques et al., 2013; Monasta et al., 2010; Nyaradi et al., 2013; Van Lieshout et al., 2011; Woo Baidal et al., 2016), and negative implications for dis-ease and other poor health outcomes in adulthood (Langley-Evans, 2015; Poston et al., 2011).

Despite clear evidence linking maternal and infant nutrition with positive health and development outcomes, many communities, par-ticularly low-income communities and communities of color, do not have access to affordable, high-quality, nutritious food (Harrington et al., 2009). The lack of access in these communities is compounded by greater exposure to unhealthy foods and beverages, including targeted

---

BOX 3-7
Statistics on Child Food Insecurity

In 2016:

- 13 million (one in six) children were food insecure.
- Fifty states and Washington, DC, were home to food-insecure children. The number of food-insecure children living in Los Angeles and New York City was 800,000.
- The rate of food insecurity among households with children was 16.5 percent.
- The rate of food insecurity among households with children headed by a single woman was 31.6 percent, compared to 22.2 percent among households with children.
- In households headed by non-Hispanic blacks and Hispanics, the rate of food insecurity was 22.5 and 18.5 percent, respectively.
- 85 percent of counties with high child food insecurity were rural.
- In households with income less than 185 percent of the poverty threshold, the rate of food insecurity was 31.6 percent.

SOURCES: Coleman-Jensen et al., 2017; Medlin and McDonald, 2018.

---

advertising for such products (NASEM, 2017b). To achieve health equity for all children, it is critically important for all families to have access to healthy and nutritious foods. (For a discussion of the policies and programs in the United States that aim to decrease food insecurity and improve nutrition and healthy eating in the prenatal and early childhood periods, e.g., Temporary Assistance for Needy Families, SNAP, and WIC, see Chapter 6.) See Box 3-7 for statistics on food insecurity during childhood.

Breastfeeding

Exclusive breastfeeding[4] offers complete nutrition for infants during the first 6 months of life. Because of this, the World Health Organization (WHO) and the American Academy of Pediatrics (AAP) recommend that infants receive only breast milk during this time to achieve optimal growth, development, and health. After that, WHO and AAP recommend continued breastfeeding combined with complementary foods up until at least 1 year of age.

---

[4] Exclusive breastfeeding is defined by WHO as not giving the infant any other food or drink, including water, except needed vitamins and medications (WHO, n.d.-b). WHO recommends that infants start receiving complementary foods at 6 months of age, in addition to breast milk (WHO, n.d.-a).

Breastfeeding provides important health benefits for mothers and children, but it is important to note methodological difficulties in studying the health impact of breastfeeding. RCTs comparing breastfeeding to formula would be unethical, and observational study designs limit causal inferences. However, this is an area that has been studied for many decades, and there are several areas where the science has converged on the understanding of how breastfeeding promotes healthy outcomes for children and breastfeeding mothers.

There is evidence that exclusively breastfed infants have lower rates of infant mortality, otitis media, and gastrointestinal infections (Bowatte et al., 2015; Kramer and Kakuma, 2012; Sankar et al., 2015). The impact of breastfeeding on the child's health seems to endure, because breastfeeding (and longer breastfeeding duration) is protective against overweight and obesity in children, although reviews and meta-analyses describe such correlations as small (but consistent) and difficult to prove, with research needed to further elucidate the relationship (Arenz et al., 2004; Beyerlein and von Kries, 2011; Dewey, 2003; Harder et al., 2005; Horta et al., 2015; Lodge et al., 2015; Ryan, 2007; Wang et al., 2017). A growing body of research demonstrates important psychological effects of breastfeeding on children, including an impact on brain, cognitive, and socio-emotional development (Krol and Grossmann, 2018).

Breastfeeding may also be protective for mothers, with lower rates of breast and ovarian carcinoma, type 2 diabetes, and postpartum depression (Chowdhury et al., 2015; Dias and Figueiredo, 2015; Hahn-Holbrook et al., 2013; Ip et al., 2007). However, a study by Borra et al. (2015) showed that there is an increased risk of postpartum depression when women who had planned to breastfeed had not gone on to breastfeed, and it concluded that breastfeeding intentions during pregnancy and mothers' mental health during pregnancy both mediated the effect of breastfeeding on maternal depression. This aspect points to the need to provide not only "expert breastfeeding support to women who want to breastfeed but also . . . compassionate support for women who had intended to breastfeed, but who find themselves unable to."

Breastfeeding Disparities

In the United States, breastfeeding rates as a whole have been increasing (CDC, 2018a). According to the Centers for Disease Control and Prevention (CDC), of infants born in 2015 in the United States, 83.2 percent started to breastfeed, more than half (57.6 percent) were breastfeeding at 6 months, and 35.9 percent were breastfeeding at 12 months. However, there are disparities in breastfeeding rates along a number of demographics.

Breastfeeding rates are lowest among African American mothers and mothers living in rural areas. From 2011 to 2015, the percentage of women who initiated breastfeeding was 64.3 percent for African Americans, 81.5 percent for whites, and 81.9 percent for Hispanics (Anstey et al., 2017). Rates of breastfeeding are also lower in mothers who are young, have lower educational attainment, and have lower incomes (ASTHO, 2017). Roughly 80 percent of higher-income women were still breastfeeding at 1 year compared to 20 percent of lower-income women (ASTHO, 2017).

A multitude of factors impact a woman's decision to start and continue breastfeeding. Social factors, such as unsupportive cultural and social norms, concerns about milk supply, poor family and social support, and unsupportive work and child care arrangements, can make it difficult for many mothers to meet their breastfeeding goals (HHS, 2011). Black women disproportionally experience some of these barriers, such as returning to work soon after a child is born, lack of breastfeeding information from providers, and lack of access to professional breastfeeding support (Johnson et al., 2015). Black mothers also might not have consistent access to evidence-based supportive practices. A study by Chapman and Pérez-Escamilla (2012) on hospital support for breastfeeding indicated that facilities in areas with higher proportions of black residents were less likely to fulfill supportive breastfeeding practices than those located in areas with lower percentages of black residents. Health care provider practices may also account for reduced rates of breastfeeding among black mothers, particularly with respect to breastfeeding encouragement and information (Jones et al., 2015). For mothers in rural communities, factors such as poverty and inadequate access to needed maternity and health services may serve as obstacles to breastfeeding (CDC, n.d.-b). Supportive programs and policies for mothers who plan to breastfeed are needed; see Chapter 6 for a discussion of some of these interventions (e.g., paid parental leave) (Pac et al., 2019).

NEIGHBORHOOD AND COMMUNITY CONDITIONS

A community is the place where a child lives, learns, and plays. By this notion, communities serve as the bedrock of health where experiences and behaviors are shaped by the conditions in which a child lives (NASEM, 2017a). The conditions that make up a community or neighborhood are critical for supporting healthy behaviors and providing safe environments for children. This section of the chapter explores the community conditions that can either promote or hinder optimal development during the prenatal through early childhood periods. These include factors that are deeply rooted in historical policies and structural inequities (as was introduced in the beginning of the chapter) and protective factors that can prevent or mitigate the manifestation of negative developmental outcomes among children. The following sections discuss disparities and scientific evidence related to developmental outcomes, including mechanisms across a number of neighborhood-level factors: concentrated disadvantage, physical environment, social environment, and exposure to violence. These factors are all interrelated, and despite the serious effects that some can have on early development, it is important to note that they are not immutable circumstances or effects (NASEM, 2017a).

Concentrated Disadvantage

Trends and Disparities

Beyond poverty at the household level, which was discussed in the previous section, nationally, 12 percent of children live in neighborhoods with concentrated poverty (i.e., Census tracts with poverty rates of 30 percent or more) (Kids Count Data Center, 2019). Concentrated disadvantage and neighborhood-level deprivation are important factors to examine because of the cumulative risk that is associated with these neighborhood conditions. Data from the Early Childhood Longitudinal Study indicate that the proportion of kindergarten children living in moderate and high-poverty neighborhoods increased from 1998 to 2010, which has important implications for school readiness (Wolf et al., 2017).

Neighborhood Disadvantage and Prenatal Through Childhood Outcomes

Individual-, household-, and neighborhood-level economic deprivation shows a graded relationship to health outcomes (Pickett and Pearl, 2001). The Whitehall (Kumari et al., 2004) and GLOBE (Global Leadership and Organizational Behaviour Effectiveness) studies (van Lenthe et al., 2004) both offer strong evidence that individual and neighborhood-level economic conditions each contribute to health outcomes. Twin studies offer other compelling evidence; one such study of 3,738 same-sex twin pairs found that neighborhood deprivation had a significant within-pair association with depression after adjusting for individual socioeconomic indicators and other factors (Cohen-Cline et al., 2018). There is a strong body of associational evidence linking neighborhood economic environments to depression (Paczkowski and Galea, 2010) and other chronic diseases (Pickett and Pearl, 2001). Box 3-8 describes asthma disparities as an example of a health outcome in the context of neighborhood disadvantage.

Neighborhood-level economic deprivation has also been widely associated with pregnancy and birth outcomes, including reduced use of prenatal care (Schempf et al., 2009) and an increased risk of a range of adverse birth outcomes (Messer et al., 2006; O'Campo et al., 2008; Zeka et al., 2008). Studies have linked neighborhood-level economic deprivation

---

BOX 3-8
Concentrated Poverty Case Study: Asthma

Childhood asthma disparities by neighborhoods are one example of the importance of neighborhood conditions. There are significant disparities in the rates of asthma between African American and white children. In 2016, the prevalence of asthma was 15.7 percent in African American children under 18 years old and 7.1 percent in white children (CDC, 2018b); the prevalence among African American children has remained about double that of white children since 2007 (Akinbami et al., 2009, 2014). Some evidence shows that this disparity in asthma prevalence may in fact stem from neighborhood conditions. For example, a study of children living in New Jersey between 2006 and 2010 found that in zip codes in which the highest fraction of the sample was African American, higher rates of asthma among low birth weight children were present regardless of race. As the authors state, "this distinction is important because unlike race, it is possible to change neighborhoods either by finding and remediating the hazards that are causing higher asthma prevalence or by helping vulnerable children to move" (Alexander and Currie, 2017). Furthermore, it is difficult to parse the effects of specific neighborhood factors (e.g., poor housing quality or exposure to environmental pollutants) in studies that examine zip codes or Census tracts because harmful neighborhood conditions or factors tend to cluster in the same areas.

---

indicators with birth weight (Buka et al., 2003; Morenoff, 2003; Pearl et al., 2001; Rich-Edwards et al., 2003; Subramanian et al., 2006), preterm birth (Ahern et al., 2003; Kaufman et al., 2003; O'Campo et al., 2008), and gestational age and fetal growth (Farley et al., 2006). However, this is not to suggest that neighborhood economic deprivation is the cause of poor health—Jokela's (2014, 2015) analyses of data from the British Household Panel Survey suggest that the observed associations may in fact reflect more fundamental social inequalities that shape health and hinder some people's ability to move to less deprived neighborhoods. Research has consistently shown an association between neighborhood deprivation and health, but a firm causal connection has not been established.

While there is evidence connecting neighborhood-level poverty and birth outcomes, the mechanism of this link remains unclear; one theory is allostatic load due to stress (Lefmann and Combs-Orme, 2014; Wallace et al., 2013). Wallace and colleagues (2013) found that while African American mothers who resided in poor neighborhoods had higher allostatic load than white mothers, allostatic load was not associated with preterm birth or LBW after accounting for race, neighborhood SES, maternal education, maternal age at time of birth, and smoking during pregnancy, among other things. This lack of link between allostatic load and pregnancy was also found in another study (Morrison et al., 2013). Nevertheless, African American women living in low-poverty neighborhoods were more than five times as likely to have an LBW infant and to have given birth preterm than white women in low-poverty neighborhoods. This racial disparity link between neighborhood disadvantage and LBW and preterm birth was also found in a systematic review and meta-analysis of population-based studies (Ncube et al., 2016). Margerison-Zilko and colleagues (2015) stress that it is not just about living in a poor neighborhood that is related to preterm birth but the length of time spent in a low-resourced, high-poverty neighborhood. In their systemic review and meta-analysis examining the link between residential segregation and adverse birth outcomes, Mehra et al. (2017) found that black mothers living in segregated neighborhoods have the highest risk of LBW and multiple adverse birth outcomes.

Physical Environment

A number of studies have assessed how various physical characteristics of neighborhoods—the "built environment"—may shape health or birth outcomes, either through direct exposure or by limiting access to or the effectiveness of traditional health care strategies. Green infrastructure, such as vegetation or tree canopy, has been associated with reduced depression rates (Cohen-Cline et al., 2018; Fan et al., 2011), which may in turn impact birth outcomes (Accortt et al., 2015). The presence of active living attributes, such as walkability, mixed land use, and active transit options, has been associated with increased physical activity and reduced obesity in general (Feng et al., 2010; Saelens et al., 2003a,b). However, the evidence is unclear on whether this ultimately affects birth outcomes: the one study assessing built environments in terms of adverse birth outcomes did not yield clear evidence of impact (Vinikoor-Imler et al., 2011). It is possible that the condition of early built environments could be associated with "sleeper effects," whereby outcomes are observed later in life.

The importance of food security and nutrition has long been identified as a key determinant of prenatal and postnatal health outcomes. However, the *food environment* people live in—the accessibility of healthy food options in their neighborhoods—is an additional contextual factor that may shape their prenatal outcomes by facilitating or limiting their ability to follow prenatal nutritional advice. A few studies have found positive effects of healthy food environments on reducing obesity (Auchincloss et al., 2013), hypertension (Kaiser et al., 2016), and type 2 diabetes (Christine et al., 2015). However, a number of other studies of the food environment's impact on health outcomes have reported null results, leading to an overall mixed body of evidence (Cobb et al., 2015), and few such studies have moved beyond overall health outcomes to assess specific adverse birth outcomes. Two studies have found associational evidence that women living in neighborhoods with a high concentration of convenience stores versus healthier food sources (Ma et al., 2016) or in areas lacking proximity to supermarkets (Lane et al., 2008) had increased risk of some adverse birth outcomes. However, other studies have not found evidence that neighborhood food environments significantly impacted birth outcomes (Farley et al., 2006). Overall, the evidence in this area remains preliminary and somewhat mixed.

Social Neighborhood Environment

The social environment people live in can be as important as their physical environment. Social support has been hypothesized to benefit birth outcomes both by moderating or buffering the stress of pregnancy (or of other contextual challenges to a healthy pregnancy) and by exerting a direct positive influence on the health of a prospective mother (Cohen and Wills, 1985). Social isolation has been associated with whether women receive adequate prenatal care (Heaman et al., 2018) and with late antenatal presentation (i.e., delayed access to antenatal care) and poor fetal outcomes (Kapaya et al., 2015), while better social support has been associated with higher birth weight and Apgar scores at birth (Collins et al., 1993), reduced risk of maternal depression (Uebelacker et al., 2013), and improved fetal growth (Hoffman and Hatch, 1996). However, studies of interventions aimed at improving social support for pregnant women have not been uniformly shown to be effective (Lu et al., 2005), and the mechanisms by which social support may impact birth outcomes remains somewhat unclear.

Social support can refer to personal networks but also to neighborhood environmental context. These "neighborhood cohesion" measures have been associated with physical and mental health and well-being outcomes in some studies (Bures, 2003; Fone et al., 2007; Hutchinson et al., 2009), perhaps acting to help protect individuals from the harmful or stressful effects of neighborhood deprivation (Robinette et al., 2013). They have also been specifically associated with improved birth weight outcomes in several studies (Buka et al., 2003; Morenoff, 2003).

Exposure to Violence

Childhood exposure to violence can take on many forms, including primary exposure or direct victimization (e.g., maltreatment or abuse by an adult caregiver or bullying by peers) and secondary exposure (e.g., witnessing IPV between parents or community violence) (Gilbert et al., 2009). Regardless of the mechanism, the body of evidence on early exposure to violence shows that this is harmful to children's health and well-being (Egerter et al., 2011a; Moffitt and Tank, 2013; Shonkoff et al., 2012). Data also show that specific subgroups are at higher risk of being exposed to violence based on certain demographics, such as race and ethnicity, gender, SES, and parental education level. Research also indicates that children who are exposed to one incident of violent victimization are likely to be exposed to violence again, including other forms (Finkelhor et al., 2007, 2009, 2015).

Trends and Disparities

Data from the National Survey of Children's Exposure to Violence (2013–2014) including a nationally representative sample of children (n = 4,000; 0–17 years old) showed that 37.3 percent had experienced any physical assault in the past year, 51.4 percent had experienced physical assault in their lifetime, and 24.5 and 38.3 percent witnessed violence in the past year and in their lifetime, respectively (Finkelhor et al., 2015). For women, disparities in violence have been documented. For example, for 2003–2014, non-Hispanic black and AI/AN women experienced the highest homicide rates nationally, at 4.4 and 4.3 per 100,000, respectively (Petrosky et al., 2017). Furthermore, more than half of all female homicides (55.3 percent) were related to IPV, which is considered an ACE for children who are exposed to it. (See the section at the end of this chapter on Accumulation of Risk for more on ACEs.)

Neighborhood Violence and Child Well-Being

Research has linked neighborhood violence with negative health and well-being outcomes across the continuum of early development. For example, there is evidence to suggest that high rates of youth violence (e.g., assault, kidnapping, homicide, robbery, larceny, destruction of property) measured at the Census tract level are associated with elevated odds of preterm birth (Masho et al., 2017). The presence of community violence has also been shown to have a direct negative relationship with children's self-regulatory behavior and cognitive performance indicators (Sharkey, 2010; Sharkey et al., 2012). A systematic review of studies examined exposure to community violence and health outcomes in youth (0–18 years old) (Wright et al., 2017). Across the 28 studies included, the most consistent finding was that early exposure to community violence was associated with elevated blood pressure, asthma, and sleep disturbance, which the authors note can contribute to other health-related problems when it persists over an extended period. Among the studies in this review, one found that the level of collective efficacy[5] in a community moderated the effect of exposure to community violence on increased asthma risk, particularly among African Americans (Sternthal et al., 2010). In addition, social support has been identified as a critical buffer for children against the negative effects of violence (Margolin and Gordis, 2004).

More recent studies have begun to examine the underlying pathways through which violence specifically influences health outcomes (Finegood et al., 2017; Theall et al., 2017). For example, a 2012–2013 study of African American children in New Orleans found that reports of domestic violence and rates of violent crime within a 500-meter radius of a child's home were associated with decreases in mean telomere length and the likelihood of reducing cortisol levels after a stress reactivity test (Theall et al., 2017). Some research suggests that underlying disadvantage (e.g., poverty, high unemployment, lower levels of educational attainment) associated with neighborhood violence partially explains the relationship between exposure to violence and negative cognitive and behavioral outcomes (Aizer, 2008). Egerter et al. (2011a) postulate that social and economic disadvantage increases the likelihood of exposure to violence, which can diminish levels of trust, social cohesion, and perceptions of safety in a community.

Limitations of the Evidence on Neighborhood Effects

Despite these associations, the relationship between neighborhood characteristics and health outcomes is complex, making causal connections difficult to establish in this literature. Associations may vary based on individual-level characteristics, such as age or sex (Meijer et al., 2013), and may be quite sensitive to the inclusion of other covariates in the models (Auchincloss et al., 2013; Blair et al., 2014; Paczkowski and Galea, 2010). As stated previously, it is also difficult to separate out the effects of factors that tend to cluster together (i.e., concentrated disadvantage) or are systematically present for specific populations, such as poor housing quality, poverty, and exposure to environmental toxicants. Results also vary widely depending on how a specific health domain is measured or how a neighborhood is defined (Paczkowski and Galea, 2010), and many studies capture only limited domains of neighborhood characteristics, leaving unanswered the question of which characteristics are most

---

[5] Collective efficacy can be defined as the level of trust among residents and their perceived willingness to engage in collective action (Sternthal et al., 2010).

important or how those characteristics interplay with one another to shape outcomes. Last, few studies establish a causal connection between these endogenous neighborhood characteristics and health (Dohrenwend et al., 1992; Jokela, 2014; Ritsher et al., 2001).

HOUSING

Housing affordability, stability, and quality are well studied and documented SDOH across the life-span. This is also true, of course, during the prenatal and early childhood years. Quality, stability, affordability, and loss of housing in the prenatal and childhood periods can have significant effects on health, cognition, and neurodevelopment. As described previously, residential segregation has had persistent effects on communities, including limiting the availability of safe and affordable housing for some. In this section, housing instability, quality of housing, and affordability will be addressed in turn.

Housing Instability

According to a 2017 report from the U.S. Department of Housing and Urban Development, there were more than 550,000 individuals considered to be homeless on any given night in the United States in that year. More than 1.4 million people were homeless in sheltered locations (e.g., emergency shelter, transitional housing, safe haven) at some point in 2017 (Henry et al., 2017). Moreover, the risk of homelessness is high for many individuals: according to recent studies, nearly 3 million individuals renting are at risk of eviction, which indicates high rates of potential instability (Sandel and Desmond, 2017). The data indicate a vast imbalance in equitable access to stable housing, such that those experiencing homelessness are disproportionately likely to be black. Only 13 percent of the general population is black, compared to more than 40 percent of the homeless population (Olivet et al., 2018).

While housing instability and homelessness are notoriously difficult to measure accurately, families with children are estimated to make up 33 percent of homeless populations (Henry et al., 2017). A 2008 cross-sectional study of 12,746 children from low-income families suggests that nearly 30 percent of children from these households are in households with housing instability (Ma et al., 2008). This includes frequent moves, difficulty paying bills or rent, spending a large proportion of income on rent, being evicted, or living in overcrowded conditions.

Housing instability—either chronic or intermittent homelessness— has well-documented negative health effects on developing children. A 2014 study of nearly 10,000 women found that mothers who were homeless while pregnant were more likely to deliver LBW children compared to those who were homeless after delivery (Cutts et al., 2015). Following birth, housing instability is associated with a wide range of cognitive, emotional, and behavioral outcomes. In a nationally representative, longitudinal study of children 2–21 years old, Coley and colleagues (2013) found that residential instability was associated with negative internalizing and externalizing behaviors—particularly for children with multiple housing moves. It was hypothesized that the negative effects of housing instability are due to changes in social structures, schooling, and the emotional health of the family (Coley et al., 2013). In a 2008 study, housing instability was associated with delays in seeking medical care or medications and increased emergency department (ED) visits among children from low-income families (Ma et al., 2008).

More broadly, it has been shown that homeless children—or children with frequent moves—are at increased risk for conduct problems at school, social difficulties, and low academic achievement (Buckner, 2008; Miller, 2011; NRC and IOM, 2010). These effects appear to be independent of low-income status; data on academic achievement and improvement on standardized tests suggest that students with frequent moves perform consistently worse in reading and math compared to other low-income students without frequent moves or housing instability (Masten et al., 2014; Obradović et al., 2009). Overall, the picture of housing instability is one of pervasive and sometimes long-term outcomes on children's health and well-being.

Housing Affordability

Housing is widely considered "affordable" if less than 30 percent of pretax income is required to own or rent (Schwartz and Wilson, n.d.; The Pew Charitable Trusts, 2018). By this definition, approximately 31.8 million U.S. households are living in housing that is unaffordable (Joint Center for Housing Studies of Harvard University, 2018). This population is generally low income. In 2015, 84 percent of renters in the lowest quintile of income were living in unaffordable housing; 70 percent of this group spent more than 50 percent of their income on housing costs (Fenelon et al., 2018). In 2016, 47 percent of all renters, and more than three-quarters of families earning between $15,000 and $30,000, had unaffordable housing (Joint Center for Housing Studies of Harvard University, 2017).

According to the most recent data available, racial/ethnic minorities and single-parent families disproportionately experience high housing cost burden, with 55 and 54 percent of black and Hispanic renters in unaffordable housing, respectively, compared to 43 percent of white renters. Furthermore, 63 percent of single-parent renters are in unaffordable homes, compared to 39 percent for married or partnered parents, and finding affordable housing in large metropolitan areas is particularly challenging (Joint Center for Housing Studies of Harvard University, 2017). Across the United States, there are only 37 available and affordable rentals for every 100 low-income households that require housing (National Low Income Housing Coalition, 2018).

There is mixed evidence for housing affordability on health and well-being outcomes among children. A 2010 critical review of housing characteristics and child development found that affordability was not well studied and was only marginally associated with children's health (Leventhal and Newman, 2010). These findings suggest that affordability, per se, is not the primary concern; rather, the amount invested in a child's health and enrichment may be a more robust predictor of developmental trajectories (Newman and Holupka, 2016). This includes spending in other domains that are important for optimal child development (Newman and Holupka, 2016), such as quality child care (Campbell et al., 2014), schools, and neighborhoods (Beyers et al., 2003; Knopf et al., 2016; Theall et al., 2017; Xue et al., 2005). Research suggests that a high housing cost burden is associated with lower spending on child enrichment (Newman and Holupka, 2016) and elevated maternal stress (Warren and Font, 2015), but its impact on maternal depression or anxiety is unclear (Harkness and Newman, 2005; Newman and Holupka, 2014). Families in unaffordable housing are more likely to miss rent payments (Warren, 2018) and therefore may be forced to move (Crowley, 2003; Desmond and Shollenberger, 2015). At the same time, research also suggests that by allocating a higher fraction of household income to housing, families may gain access to higher-quality homes (Kull and Coley, 2014), neighborhoods (Acevedo-Garcia et al., 2016b), and/or schools, and these contextual advantages of high housing costs may outweigh any negatives (Kull and Coley, 2014).

While high housing costs can be problematic, very low housing costs for low-income families may also present risks for healthy child development because they can be indicative of substandard or poor-quality housing conditions (Newman and Holupka, 2014, 2016). Accordingly, for low-income families, high or low housing cost burden could be harmful (Newman, 2008). Although prior research suggests risk associated with high and low housing cost burden (Newman and Holupka, 2014, 2016), we focus our discussion on high housing cost burden because this is the main problem for low-income families.

Economic and developmental theories used in child research (Becker and Tomes, 1986; Garner and Shonkoff, 2012; Shonkoff et al., 2012) and the scientific literature on the influence of poverty and child development (Brooks-Gunn and Duncan, 1997; Duncan, 2012; Duncan et al., 1994) suggest that understanding the role of housing affordability for child development requires considering (a) the multiple and interacting contexts in which children develop into adults (Bronfenbrenner, 1979; Bronfenbrenner and Evans, 2000; Bronfenbrenner and Morris, 2007), such as the home, school, and neighborhood; (b) the developmental timing and duration of unaffordable housing across childhood (Ben-Schlomo and Kuh, 2002; Ben-Schlomo et al., 2014; Brooks-Gunn and Duncan, 1997; Coley et al., 2013; Harkness and Newman, 2005; Hicks et al., 2018; Slopen et al., 2010); and (c) unequal health or educational benefits associated with a given level of parental income or education across racial/ethnic groups (Acevedo-Garcia et al., 2005; Assari, 2018; Assari et al., 2018; Chen et al., 2006; Shervin, 2018; Williams et al., 2010). For example, research suggests that youth are particularly influenced by socioeconomic variables during early childhood (Duncan et al., 1998; Ziol-Guest et al., 2009). Other research suggests that black and Hispanic children may be disproportionately harmed by unaffordable housing because investments in housing costs may have smaller returns for minority families (i.e., these investments may have diminished returns to school and neighborhood quality for minority children, relative to those for white children) (Assari, 2018; Shervin, 2018; Williams et al., 2010).

Housing Quality and Crowding

Families living in poverty are less likely to be able to afford high-quality housing, a factor clearly associated with child health (Rauh et al., 2008; Sandel et al., 2004). Although causal relationships are not always clear because most research is observational (Leventhal and Newman, 2010), many studies have explored the connection between child health and conditions in old and inadequately maintained residences, such as dampness, disrepair, poor ventilation, and lead paint. For instance, a study of low-income families waiting for housing vouchers found that poor-quality housing was associated with parents rating their child's health as "fair" or "poor" (Sharfstein et al., 2001). Overall, poor housing quality is consistently associated with "worse emotional and behavioral functioning and lower cognitive skills" (Coley et al., 2013). In addition, another common feature of low-income housing is overcrowding, which has been demonstrated to negatively impact children's well-being (Solari and Mare, 2012). The three subsections below focus on the relationship between child health and (1) exposure to allergens that cause asthma, (2) exposure to lead, and (3) overcrowding.

Allergens and Asthma

According to the National Health Interview Survey, more than 6 million (8.4 percent) of U.S. children under the age of 18 had asthma in 2017 (Black and Benson, 2018). While the management of childhood asthma improved from 2001 to 2016, its prevalence remained relatively consistent (Zahran et al., 2018). This warrants an increased focus on the root causes and triggers, and especially on the housing conditions of children who are disparately impacted.

Poor housing conditions can lead to increased risk of asthma. Several studies have found connections between asthma and exposure to allergens, such as cockroaches (Rauh et al., 2008; Wu and Takaro, 2007). Other research has found a causal association between dust mite exposure and asthma (IOM, 2000). Dampness and mold are also associated with asthma and other respiratory conditions (Rauh et al., 2008; Wu and Takaro, 2007). One study found that density in housing code violations was associated with a greater likelihood of a revisit to an ED or a hospital readmission (Beck et al., 2014). Another study found that children living in improved public housing were less likely to experience repeat ED and urgent care visits for conditions unrelated to an initial visit (Kersten et al., 2014). Some researchers have estimated that eliminating specific asthma triggers in older children could reduce asthma prevalence by more than 40 percent (Lanphear et al., 2001). Previous IOM studies have explored these connections in detail (IOM, 2000, 2004).

Exposure to Lead

While there is no known safe amount of lead exposure, in 2012, CDC established a reference level of 5 micrograms per deciliter to identify children who have been exposed (Wheeler and Brown, 2013). The percentage of children estimated to have blood lead levels (BLLs) greater than this amount has decreased significantly over the past decades, from an estimated 8.6 percent for 1999–2002 to 2.6 percent for 2007–2010 (Wheeler and Brown, 2013). These reductions are attributed to the phased elimination of lead from gasoline from the mid-1970s to the mid-1980s (President's Task Force on Environmental Health Risks and Safety Risks to Children, 2018) and from paint in 1978 (Markowitz and Rosner, 2014). Lead paint was banned in 1978, but older homes, primarily in the Northeastern and Midwestern parts of the country, have a higher prevalence of lead paint (Rauh et al., 2008). When these homes are poorly maintained, this paint can chip or peel, and a child may ingest it or breathe in dust, resulting in elevated BLLs (Muller et al., 2018). In addition, lead remains in the soil in areas that were in close proximity to certain manufacturing sites (Muller et al., 2018).

Despite some improvements over time, current estimates suggest that more than 500,000 children ages 1–5 have BLLs over the reference level. Young black children are more than twice as likely (5.6 percent) than white children (2.4 percent) to have a BLL greater than 5 micrograms (Wheeler and Brown, 2013). Children who are living in poverty or who have Medicaid coverage are up to eight times more likely to have elevated BLLs (Wheeler and Brown, 2013).

Young children are particularly susceptible to absorption of lead (Lidsky and Schneider, 2003). Reviews of multiple studies have associated exposure to lead—even in low amounts—with IQ, test scores, impulsivity, and attention-deficit/hyperactivity disorder (Leventhal and Newman, 2010; Muller et al., 2018; Rauh et al., 2008). Some studies have linked perinatal or childhood lead exposure to adolescent body mass index (BMI), impulsivity, anxiety, and depression (Kim and Williams, 2017; Winter and Sampson, 2017).

Overcrowding

The U.S. Census collects information on the number of occupants per unit and defines crowding at more than one occupant per room within a single unit. By this metric, 4.3 percent of houses in the United States are overcrowded (U.S. Census Bureau, 2015). Units are most likely to be overcrowded in regions with disproportionately high rental prices. According to the U.S. Census from 2000, for instance, Los Angeles had more than four times the number of crowded units per capita compared to the United States as a whole (Solari and Mare, 2012).

Research has shown that living in a crowded home may have several detrimental effects on child development, although the overall picture is decidedly mixed. Solari and Mare (2012) found that living in a crowded home negatively impacts children's academic achievement, externalizing behaviors, and physical health, even when controlling for several dimensions of SES. While this research is cross-sectional, making causal interpretations difficult, it does suggest several mechanisms by which crowding could impact child development. One hypothesis is that living in a crowded home reduces time spent studying and reading for school, thereby decreasing comprehension and test scores. Another is that overcrowding may disrupt a child's sleep, leading to mood changes and difficulty concentrating on academics. A final hypothesis is that overcrowding increases the chances that children will become sick, preventing them from attending school or concentrating while there. All of this, coupled with a lack of privacy, could impact a child's sociability and increase stress and behavioral problems. Each of these hypotheses need to be studied in more detail.

Other studies have shown mixed results. A 2010 study found that crowding during infancy was linked to negative cognitive and social skills, mediated primarily by mothers being less responsive to children in crowded homes (Evans et al., 2010). On the other hand, in 2012, Martin and colleagues found that overcrowding at age 2 was not a significant predictor of age 5 vocabulary, attention, or control of effortful behavior when accounting for other measures of household chaos (e.g., noise, family instability, lack of routine, and television watching) (Martin et al., 2012). This particular factor of housing requires more research, particularly because children growing up in crowded homes are more likely than their peers to end up in similar situations as adults (Leventhal and Newman, 2010), thereby "contributing to the intergenerational transmission of social inequality" (Solari and Mare, 2012, p. 3).

ENVIRONMENTAL EXPOSURES

While environmental exposures to toxicants and limited access to green spaces and healthy living areas have been found to be associated with poor health outcomes at multiple stages throughout the life course, the preconception, prenatal, neonatal, and early childhood periods represent several key developmental phases when humans may be particularly vulnerable to toxic environmental exposures. To best protect women, men, and children, it is important to understand how these substances can affect health and the methods to limit toxic exposures at these critical phases in development.

Environmental Toxicants

There are thousands of potential environmental toxicants that may be transmitted through the air we breathe, the water we use, and the soil and consumer products with which we, our food, and our water come into contact (Giudice et al., 2017). Many of these substances occur naturally in the environment (e.g., arsenic, radon, etc.), and many more are released through human-based processes (e.g., heavy metals, chemicals from plastic production and degradation, and particulates), such as through manufacturing by-products, fossil fuel use, mining, and disposal of waste (Di Renzo et al., 2015).

Several of these compounds are associated with poor preconception and prenatal outcomes. In particular, lead, methyl mercury, polybrominated biphenyls, polychlorinated biphenyls, and the pesticide chlorpyrifos have been shown to result in developmental neurotoxicity, leading experts in fetal development, obstetrics and gynecology, and fertility to conclude that there is no "safe" exposure. Furthermore, endocrine disrupters, such as the pesticides and herbicides atrazine, glyphosate, and chlorpyrifos, are associated with cancer and neurodevelopmental disorders (Diamanti-Kandarakis et al., 2009; Gore et al., 2015). Animal models align with these human studies; endocrine disruptors in animal studies indicate that in-utero exposure leads to obesity (Manikkam et al., 2013), abnormal sexual anatomy and sexual performance (Vandenbergh, 2004), and abnormal neuronal migration (Nakamura et al., 2012), similar to that seen in children with autism. Moreover, chemicals in personal products, such as phthalates, bisphenol A (BPA), and fluoroacetic acid, are related to reproductive outcomes (Giudice et al., 2017). However, hundreds of these chemicals remain untested, and researchers estimate that the markedly rapid increase in noncommunicable diseases, particularly those related to endocrine disruption, exceeds the expected natural occurrence of change due to evolution alone. Researchers conclude that these chemicals, on their own or in combination, are likely the drivers of this change (Di Renzo et al., 2015).

In addition, several substances are associated with poor early childhood development outcomes and long-term health problems. For example, particulate matter, ozone, and carbon monoxide are associated with poor child health outcomes (Giudice et al., 2017), including impaired lung function and neurodevelopment, as well as exacerbation of existing issues, such as asthma (Webb et al., 2016). Lead, mercury, and arsenic are associated with cognitive disorders and kidney disease among children (Weidemann et al., 2016). Certain groups in the United States are more likely than others to come into contact with these environmental toxicants or to be unable to access healthy living areas and green space. In particular, certain racial and ethnic groups and families and children living in poverty are disproportionally more likely to experience exposures and see poor health outcomes related to contact with environmental toxicants (ACOG Committee Opinion, 2013; Oberg et al., 2016). For example, a Chicago longitudinal study documented marked, persistent disparities in elevated BLLs of African American children compared to white children (Sampson and Winter, 2016). African American women exposed to higher levels of $PM_{2.5}$ were more likely to report higher depression severity during pregnancy and postpartum (Sheffield et al., 2018). In addition, African Americans and other people of color experienced higher $PM_{2.5}$ exposure compared to whites, as did those living in poverty (Mikati et al., 2018).

Specifically, the research literature has documented strong evidence of adverse pregnancy outcomes, such as increased risk of preterm delivery, related to exposure to certain metals, including lead, which may be transmitted to the fetus through maternal BLLs (Taylor et al., 2015). This study also documented an increased risk of reduced birth weight, smaller head circumference, and reduced crown to heel infant length related to exposure to lead from maternal BLLs. Similarly, higher maternal blood cadmium levels are associated with reduced birth weight, smaller head circumference, and reduced crown to heel length (Taylor et al., 2016), particularly for female infants. Mercury has long been shown to have negative effects on the developing fetus. One study demonstrated that levels greater than or equal to 10 parts per million of mercury can be harmful to fetal development, causing brain pathologies that result in Minamata disease, microencephaly, seizures, intellectual disability, and stillbirth, as evidenced by methylmercury poisoning in Japan and Iraq from industrial waste and the use of an imported grain treated with a fungicide containing methylmercury (Cox et al., 1989; Kalter, 2003).

Higher exposure to phthalates, chemicals added to plastics to increase flexibility and make other physical changes for use in consumer products, is associated with an increased risk of preterm delivery and spontaneous preterm delivery (Ferguson et al., 2014). In a Swedish case-control study, higher levels of butyl benzyl phthalate (BBzP), bis(2-ethylhexyl) phthalate (DEHP), and polyvinyl chloride were more likely to be found in children with a diagnosis of rhinitis and eczema; asthma; and asthma, rhinitis, and eczema, respectively (Bornehag et al., 2004). A Bulgarian case-control study found evidence of a higher risk of asthma among cases with high levels of DEHP (Kolarik et al., 2008). The presence of urinary concentrations of phthalate metabolites, particularly diethyl phthalate and BBzP, was associated with 6.6 and 8.7 percent increases, respectively, of fractional nitric oxide, a biomarker of airway inflammation. The BBzP association with fractional nitric oxide levels was particularly strong for children who wheeze (Just et al., 2012).

Phenols, particularly BPA, have been found to be associated with endocrine and neurodevelopmental problems. Prenatal BPA exposure among boys is significantly associated with a risk of decreased anogenital distance, a marker of testosterone production (Miao et al., 2011). The odds of preterm birth among infants with mothers who had higher plasma BPA levels was between 4.12 and 4.78 times higher than those without high BPA levels (Behnia et al., 2016). Each 10-fold increase in maternal urinary BPA level is associated with an increased risk of anxious and depressed behavior and poorer emotional control among 3-year-old girls (Braun et al., 2017). There is evidence that exposure to composite fillings that leach BPA can have detrimental effects on early neurodevelopment, including a heightened risk of internalizing, problem, and delinquent behaviors in children, along with increased risk of anxiety, depression, social stress, and problems with interpersonal relationships (Bellinger et al., 2008). Heightened risk of asthma is associated with prenatal exposure to BPA, depending on the phase of fetal development in which the exposure took place (Spanier et al., 2012). Prenatal exposure among male infants is associated with a higher risk of high BMI, increased waist circumference, higher fat mass, and overweight/obesity (Gascon et al., 2015; Midoro-Horiuti et al., 2010; Spanier et al., 2012). Higher maternal blood BPA levels are associated with lower thyroid-stimulating hormone levels in male infants, suggesting poorer thyroid function (Chevrier et al., 2013; Harley et al., 2013). Higher maternal blood levels of 2,4-DCP (dichlorophenols), 2,5-DCP, and triclosan (phenols other than BPA) are associated with lower weight among male infants. A higher maternal blood level of bisphenol-S is associated with lower weight among female infants (Ferguson et al., 2018). In the same study, Ferguson et al. (2018) also demonstrated that higher maternal blood levels of parabens and benxophenone-3 are associated with lower weight among male infants.

Among young children, postnatal exposure to BPA is associated with a heightened risk of asthma, depending on the phase of child development in which the exposure took place (Donohue et al., 2013). In studies of African American, Dominican American, and Chinese children, high BPA levels were associated with a higher risk of obesity (Donohue et al., 2013; Wang et al., 2012). Increased urinary BPA levels among children is also associated with an increased risk of albuminuria, which is an indicator of future health problems, including type 2 diabetes and cardiovascular disease (Trasande et al., 2013).

Limited and Developing Evidence

A number of studies have established a relationship between poor health or birth outcomes and living in places with close proximity to potential pollution challenges. Air quality through the gestational period has been associated with increased risk of LBW, preterm birth, and infant death (Padula et al., 2012). Exposure to metals such as cadmium and arsenic has been shown to increase incidence of LBW and preterm birth (Ahmad et al., 2001; Hopenhayn et al., 2003), as have other measures of poor water quality (ChangeLab Solutions, 2017). Maternal residences near power plants have been associated with high risk for preterm birth and LBW (Ha et al., 2015; Tsai et al., 2004), while women living in neighborhoods with high exposure to natural gas wells were 1.4 times more likely to have preterm birth outcomes (Casey et al., 2016). Living in areas with high traffic density, or near high-traffic roadways, has also been associated with increased risk of preterm births in a number of studies (Currie and Walker, 2011; Fleisch et al., 2017; Harris et al., 2016; Miranda et al., 2013; Woodward et al., 2015), as has living near landfill sites (Elliott et al., 2001) or being exposed to pesticides (Wolff et al., 2007).

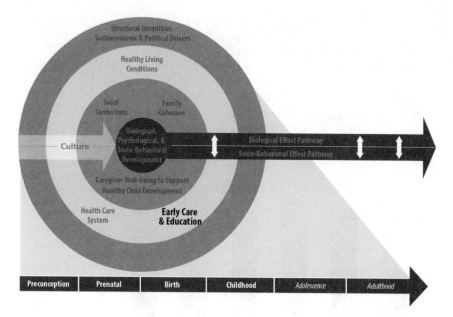

FIGURE 3-8 Leveraging early opportunities to achieve health equity across the life course: A conceptual framework.
NOTES: The element of focus in this section is reflected in the second outermost ring in the model: healthy living conditions (i.e., economic security, nutrition and food security, housing, and environmental safety). This element is bolded for emphasis.

EARLY CARE AND EDUCATION

ECE[6] has significant effects on children's academic readiness and cognitive and socio-emotional development. ECE also impacts children's physical, emotional, and mental health and well-being, and access to high-quality ECE creates many pathways through which greater health equity can be achieved (Hahn et al., 2016). The following section describes disparities in access to ECE, including specific programs such as Head Start/ Early Head Start and state-funded preschool programs. See Chapter 7 for a more detailed discussion of the link between ECE interventions and outcomes related to children's health, development, and well-being as well as recommendations to advance health equity through ECE. See Figure 3-8 for a visual of how this section ties to the report conceptual model.

_____

[6] Early care and education can be defined as nonparental care that occurs outside the child's home. ECE services may be delivered in center-, school-, or home-based settings (NASEM, 2018).

Access to Early Care and Education

Currently, about 60 percent of all children age 5 or younger who are not in kindergarten are enrolled in at least one nonparental care arrangement. The most common *primary* arrangement of early child care for all children was center-based care (29 percent), followed by home-based relative care (19 percent), home-based nonrelative care (10 percent), and multiple arrangements (2 percent) (de Brey et al., 2019). These percentages varied by race and ethnicity—see Figure 3-9 for the percentages of

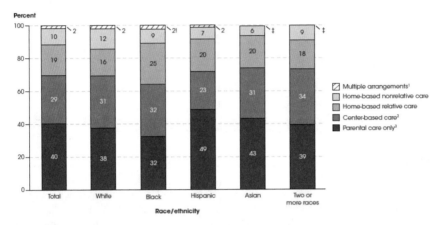

FIGURE 3-9 Percentage distribution of children under 6 years old who are not enrolled in kindergarten, by race/ethnicity of child and type of primary care arrangement, 2016.

[!] Interpret data with caution. The coefficient of variation (CV) for this estimate is between 30 and 50 percent.

[‡] Reporting standards not met. The CV for this estimate is 50 percent or greater.

[1] Children who spent an equal number of hours per week in multiple nonparental care arrangements.

[2] Center-based arrangements include day care centers, Head Start programs, preschools, pre-kindergartens, and other early childhood programs.

[3] Children who had no regularly scheduled nonparental care arrangement and mainly received care only from their parents.

NOTES: A child's primary arrangement is the regular nonparental care arrangement or early childhood education program in which the child spent the most time per week. Data for Pacific Islanders and American Indians/Alaska Natives not shown because reporting standards were not met. Race categories exclude persons of Hispanic ethnicity. Although rounded numbers are displayed, the figures are based on unrounded estimates. Detail may not sum to totals because of rounding. Data are sourced from the U.S. Department of Education, National Center for Education Statistics, Early Childhood Program Participation Survey of the National Household Education Surveys Program (ECPP-NHES:2016). See *Digest of Education Statistics 2017*, Table 202.30.

SOURCE: de Brey et al., 2019.

white, black, Hispanic, Asian, and two or more race children by type of early child care. In the United States, children under 2 years spend several more hours in informal care when compared to children in other Organisation for Economic Co-operation and Development countries (25 hours per week compared to 3.5 hours per week) (Mathur, 2016).

Enrollment in ECE (including home-based care by a relative or a nonrelative and center/school-based arrangements) is associated with the following:

- Age: Preschool-aged children from 3 to 5 years old are more likely to participate than younger children.
- Race: White and black children are more likely to participate in one of these arrangements (62 and 68 percent of all young children, respectively) than Hispanic and Asian children (51 and 57 percent, respectively). However, white and Asian children are more likely to be placed in center/school-based programs (61 and 63 percent, respectively) than black and Hispanic children (57 and 52 percent, respectively).
- Home language: Children from homes where no parents or guardians speak English are less likely to participate in any ECE.
- Parental education: The lower the level of education of the parents, the less likely their children are to participate in ECE.
- Income: The lower the level of income of the parents, the less likely their children are to participate in ECE (see Figure 3-10).

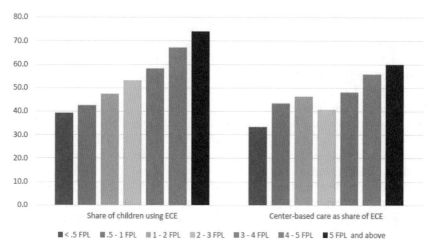

FIGURE 3-10 Patterns of ECE use by income category, all children age 0–5 years (not in kindergarten).
NOTE: ECE = early care and education; FPL = federal poverty level.
SOURCE: NASEM, 2018.

Fifty-four percent of poor children do not participate in any non-parental care arrangements, compared to 31 percent of nonpoor children (de Brey et al., 2019). While about three-quarters of 4-year-olds from the highest income quintile attend preschool, only half of those from the lowest-income quintile do (Cascio and Schanzenbach, 2016). However, the relationship is not completely linear. Children from households with an income from $50,001 to $75,000 are less likely to participate in center/school-based programs than those from the poorest ($20,000 or less) or highest ($100,001 or more) income groups. That said, poor children are much less likely than their nonpoor peers to be enrolled in center-based care or home-based nonrelative care as their *primary* form of ECE, defined as the arrangement where the child spends most of his or her time per week (Corcoran et al., 2019).

It is important to note that access to ECE does not guarantee access to quality care, especially for children from poor households and black and Hispanic children, who are more likely to be in lower-quality care than white and Asian children (Barnett et al., 2013; Valentino, 2018). Quality of access is also not available for AI/AN children.

The federal government subsidizes the cost of child care and provides early education programs for some low-income families through the Child Care & Development Block Grant (CCDBG) and Head Start,[7] which may explain the greater access to ECE among low-income families compared to those who earn slightly more. CCDBG provides child care subsidies to low-income families whose parents are working, going to school, or in a job training program. Children up to 13 years of age can be served in centers or family child care settings. (Two-thirds of children served are younger than six [Office of Child Care, n.d.].) These funds are also used to improve the quality of care, coordinate resources, conduct research and evaluation, and provide technical assistance to grantees. There have been limited studies linking child care subsidies and child health and well-being, with mixed findings. In their econometric analyses drawing on the Early Childhood Longitudinal Study, Herbst and Tekin (2010) found that subsidy use was associated with poor outcomes (i.e., reading, math, externalizing problems, approaches to learning, and interpersonal skills) for children compared to peers in the year prior to kindergarten entry. This was also found by Hawkinson et al. (2013) for math outcomes using the same dataset. The authors hypothesize that these

---

[7] Head Start is a program of the U.S. Department of Health and Human Services that provides comprehensive early childhood education, health, nutrition, and parent involvement services to low-income children and their families. See the following section and Box 7-3 for more information on Head Start.

negative findings linking subsidy use and poor child outcomes may be due to the quality of care that children with subsidies are likely to receive and the lack of availability of high-quality child care meeting the needs of low-resource families. In contrast, Krafft et al. (2017), using a fixed effects approach that sought to adjust for selection bias, found that children receiving a child care subsidy experienced higher-quality care as reported by parents but there were no differences in the stability of arrangements or having multiple arrangements. The differences in these findings may be due to data used, methodology, analytical procedures, and how quality was defined and measured. However, these studies underscore the importance of ensuring that children from low-income families are able to access high-quality programs that meet their unique cognitive, emotional, social, and health needs.

Head Start is a federally funded preschool program for 3- and 4-year-olds from low-income households, created as part of President Lyndon Johnson's War on Poverty. In addition to focusing on children's learning and development, it also provides a range of services that address the holistic needs of children and families, such as health, nutrition, and parent education. Early Head Start was created in 1995 to focus on pregnant women and younger children from birth to age 3 (Office of Head Start, 2018a). Families receive services in homes, centers, or sometimes both settings (Office of Head Start, 2018b).

As of 2012, only about 15 percent of eligible families received CCDBG subsidies (Walker and Matthews, 2017), and Head Start serves less than half of all eligible 3- and 4-year-olds due to insufficient funding (Barnett and Friedman-Krauss, 2016). Early Head Start reaches about 5 percent of all eligible children (Schmit and Walker, 2016). Children from ages 2 to 4 and those living in deep poverty receive the highest rates of CCDBG subsidies (Chien, 2017). See Figure 3-11 for the percentage of children eligible for federal subsidies who receive such subsidies, by age and household income in 2013.

In terms of race and ethnicity, Latino, Asian, and AI/AN children tend to be underrepresented among eligible CCDBG recipients and Head Start children. In fiscal year 2016, 15 percent of eligible black children had access to CCDBG, but only 3 percent of eligible Asian children, 6 percent of eligible Hispanic children, and 7 percent of eligible AI/AN children were served (Ullrich et al., 2019).[8] As for Head Start, Asian and Latino children are somewhat underrepresented at 36 and 38 percent of eligible children served, respectively, while 54 percent of eligible African American children are enrolled in the program (Schmit and Walker, 2016). It is important to note that these patterns differ markedly across states.

---

[8] These data reflect federal eligibility parameters for CCDBG (Ullrich et al., 2019).

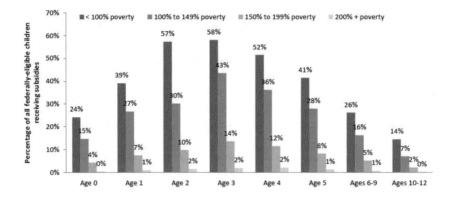

FIGURE 3-11 Percentage of federally eligible children receiving subsidies by age and income.
NOTES: Poverty figures are based on 2013 poverty thresholds published by the U.S. Census Bureau. For families with one adult and two children, 150 percent of poverty is $28,154 ($2,346 monthly).
SOURCE: Chien, 2017.

Pre-K programs are funded and regulated by the state. Currently, 43 states and Washington, DC, provide pre-K programs to 4-year-olds, with many also extending the program to 3-year-olds. Policies governing these programs are highly variable across states. Generally, unlike child care programs, state pre-K does not have any work or education requirements for the parents. Programs also tend to be more focused on early learning and school readiness and less on other needs of children and families, although there are exceptions.

Access data for state pre-K programs are less available, since eligibility levels and data collection vary by state. Nationwide, 5 percent of 3-year-olds and 33 percent of 4-year-olds are served in a state-funded pre-K program. More than half of all programs target low-income children, with eligibility criteria ranging from 100 to 300 percent of the federal poverty line. About half of the programs also take other risk factors or family backgrounds into consideration, including disabilities, abuse and neglect, homelessness, linguistic background, military duty, LBW, substance abuse, and teen parent status (Friedman-Krauss et al., 2018). Enrollment varies greatly by state. For 4-year-olds, 12 states[9] enrolled less than 10 percent, 10 states enrolled more than 50 percent, and 5 states enrolled more than 70 percent. Only Washington, DC, and Vermont

_____
[9] Alaska, Arizona, Delaware, Hawaii, Indiana, Massachusetts, Minnesota, Mississippi, Missouri, Nevada, Rhode Island, and Washington.

enrolled more than 50 percent of 3-year-olds. Seven states[10] continued to lack state-funded preschool programs. Washington, DC, enrolled the highest percentages of 3- and 4-year-olds (66 and 88 percent, respectively) (Friedman-Krauss et al., 2018).

Head Start and state pre-K programs tend to have higher quality standards in terms of teacher qualifications and supports, learning standards for children, curriculum, group size, and adult–child ratios than child care programs outside those systems. To the extent that higher-quality programs are more likely to promote children's health and well-being, it is important for these programs to serve those with experiences of concentrated disadvantage, ACEs, and chronic stress. As mentioned earlier, while Head Start targets poor children, it currently serves only about half of all eligible children, and access by different racial groups is uneven.

Access to Special Education Services

About 2.9 percent of children from birth through age 2 are served under Part C (the Program for Infants and Toddlers with Disabilities) of the Individuals with Disabilities Education Act (IDEA), and most were served at home in 2014 (Davis, 2016). Native Hawaiian or Other Pacific Islander and white infants and toddlers had risk ratios of 1.4 and 1.2, respectively, indicating that those in each of these racial/ethnic groups were slightly more likely than those in all other racial/ethnic groups combined to be served under Part C. In 2014, 6.1 percent of children ages 3 through 5 were served under Part B (Assistance for Education of All Children with Disabilities) of IDEA. In 2014, AI/AN, Native Hawaiian or Other Pacific Islander, and white children ages 3–5 had risk ratios above 1 (1.4, 1.5, and 1.2, respectively), indicating they were more likely to be served under Part B than were children ages 3 through 5 in all other racial/ethnic groups combined. In 2014, 8.7 percent of individuals ages 6 through 21 were served under Part B, with the most in specific learning disabilities. AI/AN, black or African American, and Native Hawaiian or Other Pacific Islander children ages 6–21 had risk ratios above 1 (1.7, 1.4, and 1.6, respectively), indicating that they were more likely to be served under Part B than children in all other racial/ethnic groups combined.

Unfortunately, access to early intervention and special education services is variable due to the wide discrepancy in eligibility criteria (Twardzik et al., 2017). Using data from the 2007 National Survey of Children's Health, Bethell and colleagues (2011) found that 19.5 percent of children received a parent-completed developmental screening. This varied across states and demographics. Screening was highest for

---

[10] Idaho, Montana, New Hampshire, North Dakota, South Dakota, Utah, and Wyoming.

children who were young, black, and publicly insured and lowest for children who were uninsured and had gaps in insurance coverage. They also found a significant gap between the developmental screening that is recommended by the American Academic of Pediatrics and what is reported nationally.

Public Education

Educational attainment is correlated with health outcomes (NASEM, 2017a). Studies indicate that individuals with more education are more likely to have economic stability and better health outcomes (Heckman et al., 2018). Yet, disparities exist among income and racial groups in terms of both education inputs and outcomes. For example, recent data indicate increasing school segregation, with a growing trend of more schools that are high poverty and high minority, from 10 percent of schools in 2000 to 17 percent in 2013 (Chang, 2018). Other research examining longitudinal data established an association between court-ordered desegregation of schools (from 1954 to 1990) and subsequent adult outcomes for African Americans (e.g., educational attainment, adult earnings, probability of incarceration) through 2013 (Johnson, 2011). However, some contend that it is not segregation that is increasing but rather the number of non-minority students in public schools. Regardless, research also indicates that school districts serving the largest populations of minority (e.g., black, Latino, or AI/AN) students receive approximately $1,800, or 13 percent, less per student in state and local funding than those serving the fewest students of color. The United States spends approximately 7 percent—or $1,000—less per pupil on students in the highest poverty districts than those educated in the wealthiest (Morgan and Amerikaner, 2018). Another estimate suggests a funding gap of $23 billion between school districts serving predominantly nonwhite students and those with mostly white students, despite serving the same number of children (EdBuild, 2019).

Funding inequities between rich and poor or majority-white and majority-minority schools are likely one factor contributing to the achievement gaps. Numerous studies have shown a relationship between school socioeconomic and racial/ethnic composition and student achievement outcomes (Kainz and Pan, 2014; Ready and Silander, 2011). Specifically, schools with large proportions of poor, African American, and Hispanic students have been shown to have lower rates of learning growth compared to schools serving larger proportions of white and high-income students. There are conflicting patterns of evidence regarding unique and overlapping effects of racial/ethnic and poverty concentrations on children's academic achievement. However, recent analyses of test data from the national public K–12 system have indicated that concentrations of poverty are the proximal explanation for observed negative associations between racial concentration and student achievement (Reardon, 2016). That is, racial segregation has a negative effect on education performance precisely because racial segregation is an indicator of students' exposure to poverty concentration and isolation and limited access to needed supports.

For example, data from the U.S. Department of Education's National Center for Education Statistics show that graduation rates collected from 2010–2011 to 2015–2016 increased from 79 to 84 percent (National Center for Education Statistics, n.d.). That is, more than four out of five students who were first-time 9th-graders in 2012–2013 had completed high school by 2015–2016 (within 4 years). There are some racial differences, with Asian/Pacific Islanders and white students graduating at higher rates, 91 and 88 percent, respectively, compared to Hispanic (79 percent), black (76 percent), and AI/AN (72 percent) students.

Similarly, the dropout rate has declined from 15 percent in 1970 to 6 percent in 2016. The youth dropout rate in 1972 was 12 percent for whites, 21 percent for blacks, and 34 percent for Hispanics. In 2016, the youth dropout rate for blacks was 6 percent (close to the national average) and 9 percent for Hispanics, compared to 5 percent for whites and 3 percent for Asians (Child Trends DataBank, 2018). It is important to note that these estimates do not include those who were institutionalized, which is particularly pronounced for black and Hispanic male youth. There is a link between non-graduation and incarcerations (Kearney et al., 2014; Skiba et al., 2014).

There are many factors that lead to educational attainment or lack of education (i.e., dropout). However, one predictor of high school graduation or dropout is reading proficiency at the end of 3rd grade. In a study of nearly 4,000 students born between 1979 and 1989, Hernandez (2012) found that those who did not read proficiently by 3rd grade were four times more likely to leave school without a diploma than proficient readers, with the rates increasing for those who could not master basic reading skills. According to the National Assessment of Education Progress, in 2017, while 47 percent of white and 59 percent of Asian 4th graders were proficient in reading, only 20 percent of African American and AI/AN students and 23 percent of Hispanic students achieved at that level (The Nation's Report Card, 2017). (A similar gap exists between low-income and nonpoor students.) Furthermore, the relationship between reading proficiency and dropout was particularly pronounced for students from poor households. Hernandez found that 31 percent of African American students and 33 percent of Hispanic students from poor households who were not proficient in 3rd grade reading did not graduate, compared to 22 percent for white children from poor households. The racial and education gaps disappear when students are proficient in 3rd-grade reading and not living in poverty. However, the confound between poverty and race and ethnicity often makes it difficult to isolate the unique effects of each characteristic.

REVISITING CROSSCUTTING ELEMENTS

Racism and Discrimination

The 2017 report *Communities in Action: Pathways to Health Equity* describes racism as "an umbrella concept that encompasses specific mechanisms that operate at the intrapersonal, interpersonal, institutional, and systemic levels of a socioecological framework" (NASEM, 2017a, pp. 104–105) (see Figure 3-12 for examples of how racism plays out at these levels). The report makes the distinction that racism is "not an

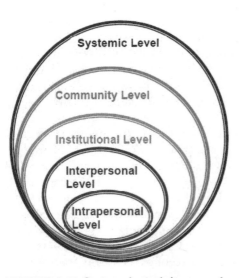

Systemic Level
- Immigration policies
- Incarceration policies
- Civil rights
- Predatory banking

Community Level
- Differential resource allocation
- Racially or class segregated schools

Institutional Level
- Hiring and promotion practices
- Under- or over-valuation of contributions

Interpersonal Level
- Overt discrimination
- Implicit bias

Intrapersonal Level
- Internalized racism
- Stereotype threat
- Embodying inequities

FIGURE 3-12 Socioecological framework with examples of racism constructs by level.
NOTES: The mechanisms by which the social determinants of health operate differ with respect to the level. For the intrapersonal level, these mechanisms are individual knowledge, attitudes/beliefs, and skills. At the interpersonal level, they are families, friends, and social networks. At the institutional level, they are organizations and social institutions. At the community level, they are relationships among organizations. At the systemic level, the mechanisms are national, state, and local policies, laws, and regulations.
SOURCE: Adapted from NASEM, 2017a.

attribute of minority groups; rather it is an aspect of the social context and is linked with differential power relations among racial and ethnic groups" (NASEM, 2017a, p. 105; see also Guess, 2006). Camara Jones's (2000) theoretic framework for racism uses an allegory of a garden to illustrate the relationships between these multiple levels and to provide a framework to guide interventions that would address these mechanisms of racism. It is also important to note that discrimination can affect a variety of racial and ethnic minority groups. For example, Asian Americans are often ascribed the stereotype of "model minority"; however, they can experience discrimination and its effects, as well as social or economic conditions that affect health (Chou and Feagin, 2015).

Reported racism[11] has been documented as a determinant of poor health outcomes across the life-span, particularly for mental health (e.g., depression, anxiety, psychological stress), with weaker evidence for physical health (Paradies et al., 2015). Bailey et al. (2017) highlight structural racism as an important but understudied driver of inequities, defining structural racism as "the totality of ways in which societies foster racial discrimination, via mutually reinforcing inequitable systems (e.g., in housing, education, employment, earnings, benefits, credit, media, health care, criminal justice, etc.) that in turn reinforce discriminatory beliefs, values, and distribution of resources, reflected in history, culture, and interconnected institutions" (p. 1454). For more information on racism and discrimination as root causes of inequities, see Chapter 3 of *Communities in Action: Pathways to Health Equity* (NASEM, 2017a).

Childhood exposure to racism is mostly documented as experiences of discrimination. For example, the National Survey of Children's Health includes an item that asks parents if their child has ever been treated or judged unfairly because of their race or ethnic group. Data from 2016–2017 indicate that the overall prevalence of exposure to discrimination is low, at 3.7 percent nationwide. However, when these data are examined by subgroups, there are disparities. For instance, black and other, non-Hispanic children were most likely to be treated or judged unfairly due to their race or ethnicity. (See Table 3-3 for a breakdown by race and ethnicity.)

---

[11] This meta-analysis defined reported racism as self-reported racism experienced directly in interpersonal contact; racism directed toward a group (e.g., based on ethnicity/race/nationality) of which the person is a member; vicarious experiences of racism (e.g., witnessing racism experienced by family members or friends); proxy reports of racism (e.g., a child's experiences of racism as reported by their parent); and internalized racism (i.e., the incorporation of racist attitudes and/or beliefs within an individual's worldview) (Paradies et al., 2015).

TABLE 3-3 Childhood Experiences of Discrimination by Race and Ethnicity

Race or Ethnicity	Percent of Children Who Have Ever Been Treated or Judged Unfairly Because of Their Race or Ethnic Group
Black, non-Hispanic	10.4
Hispanic	4.2
Other, non-Hispanic	7.4
White, non-Hispanic	1.0

SOURCE: National Survey of Children's Health, 2016–2017, from the Data Resource Center for Child and Adolescent Health, 2019.

There is an existing literature stream that draws connections between racism and early development and well-being outcomes. Specifically, negative prenatal and birth outcomes have been shown to be associated with discrimination or unfair treatment. An integrative review of 15 studies assessing adverse birth outcomes and discrimination found significant relationships between racial discrimination and LBW, preterm birth, and small size for gestational age (Alhusen et al., 2016). Studies in this review that examined mediating variables that are proximally related to birth outcomes (e.g., prenatal care, employment opportunities, neighborhood characteristics, or inflammatory markers) also found a significant association between these specific variables and racial discrimination. Another review found similar outcomes when investigating the relationship between racial discrimination and black-white disparities in birth outcomes, showing a consistent positive relationship between discrimination and preterm birth and LBW or very LBW (Giurgescu et al., 2011). The review findings also suggest that parental lifetime and childhood experiences of discrimination could have a stronger association with birth weight than experiences of discrimination reported during pregnancy.

For childhood outcomes, the available evidence suggests that discrimination affects children through two pathways: (1) direct transmission to the child and (2) discrimination that affects the parent directly (sometimes called "vicarious racism"). A systematic review examining mostly cross-sectional studies synthesized the study findings related to racial discrimination and child health and well-being outcomes (Priest et al., 2013). Associations were most salient among mental health outcomes (e.g., depression and anxiety). The authors reported statistically significant associations between discrimination and 76 percent of the mental health outcomes studied. The findings also showed a consistent relationship between discrimination and reduced positive mental health outcomes, such as self-esteem, self-worth, and psychological adaption and adjustment. The authors reported weaker results for child physical health outcomes, but they also note that this likely reflects the extended period of time that it takes for physical health outcomes to manifest. With respect to vicarious racism effects, there is some evidence to suggest that there is a link between secondhand exposure to racism and socio-emotional (e.g., externalizing behavior) and mental health (e.g., depression) outcomes among children (Heard-Garris et al., 2018). Acevedo-Garcia et al. (2013) identify three directions for research on interpersonal and institutional discrimination and child health:

1. Incorporating a life course perspective into studies of discrimination and children's health,
2. Linking residential segregation with geography of opportunity[12] conceptual frameworks and measure, and
3. Considering residential segregation along with segregation in other contexts that influence children's health.

American Indian/Alaska Native Children and Children of Immigrant Background: A Closer Look

This section describes two populations of children and families for whom the crosscutting elements in this chapter are particularly salient: AI/AN children and children of an immigrant background. While there are many subgroups that have unique needs and historical contexts related to health equity, these are two that the committee has identified as important to highlight here because of the lack of attention given to these groups, often due to data collection or sampling issues (ASPE, 2007; NASEM, 2017a; National Congress of American Indians, n.d.). For these subgroups, racism and discrimination operate at multiple levels, including interpersonal, everyday experiences of discrimination and policies that obstruct access to health-promoting goods and services or induce historical trauma that can affect multiple generations. Their experiences across the domains discussed in this chapter (e.g., family cohesion, access to health care, neighborhood conditions) are amplified when examined with the additional lens of structural inequities.

---

[12] One tool for measuring opportunity by units of geography is the Child Opportunity Index, a data resource that compiles neighborhood-level indicators related to educational, health and environmental, and social and economic opportunity (Acevedo-Garcia et al., 2016a).

American Indians and Alaska Natives

Health outcomes across AI/AN populations AI/AN populations experience stark disparities across a number of health indicators. Researchers hypothesize that a combination of factors may be related to these disparities, including the SDOH (i.e., poverty, unemployment, and education) (Elder et al., 2016), the effect of high rates of obesity and inactivity, alcohol and tobacco use, and a lack of access to health care (Bhaskar and O'Hara, 2017; Cobb et al., 2014; Rutman et al., 2016), particularly care that is culturally congruent (Lewis and Myhra, 2018; Rentner et al., 2012). This stems in large part from the population's unique history in relation to U.S. policies, historical trauma, and the consequences for the health and well-being of generations (for more information on the historical and legal context of AI/ANs, see Appendix A in NASEM, 2017a). Moreover, health disparities and inequities vary by region, with some tribes experiencing high levels and intensity of alcohol use (Fortin et al., 2016), poor birth outcomes (Coughlin et al., 2013; Hwang et al., 2013; Kim et al., 2014), and poorer reproductive health (Rutman et al., 2012). AI/AN communities also experience higher levels of racial misclassification, which reduce the reliability of existing health data for these populations (Jim et al., 2014). In addition, certain SDOH, such as violence against AI/AN women, is not consistently tracked across jurisdictions, making the justification for systemic changes challenging. For example, in some counties in the United States, AI/AN women are 10 times more likely to be murdered as compared to the national average, are 3 times as likely to be raped in their lifetimes compared to any other racial or ethnic group, and the perpetrator of rape against AI/AN women is more likely to be white compared to other racial and ethnic groups. More research is needed to fully explicate the potential health impacts for AI/AN women living with the disproportionate level of violence specific to their race and gender in these contexts (Bachman et al., 2008).

Birth and postpartum outcomes While the research on AI/AN populations remains limited, major disparities have been documented, particularly concerning birth outcomes. The mortality rate for AI/AN infants aged 0 to 1 year of age is 1.61 times higher than that of white children, with sudden infant death syndrome, unintentional injuries, and influenza/pneumonia being the top three causes of death (Wong et al., 2014). Concomitantly, AI/AN women experience some of the highest rates of diabetes and hypertension in the nation, as well as preeclampsia-eclampsia (Zamora-Kapoor et al., 2016), which are related to poor birth outcomes (Anderson et al., 2016; Dorfman et al., 2015). In a comparison between AI/AN, black, and Hispanic women, significantly lower rates of fetal and first-day mortality were found among black and Hispanic women for

2005–2008 as compared to 1995–1998 rates. However, among AI/AN, the rates did not decline significantly for AI/AN women.

Studies have found that preterm birth rates among AI/AN women (13.0 percent) are significantly higher as compared to the rate for all women in the United States (11.4 percent). Stress before and during pregnancy constitutes one of the biggest contributors to preterm birth. Research has demonstrated that AI/AN women experience the highest number of major stressors in the 12 months before becoming pregnant and in the 12 months before giving birth. Interpersonal violence rates, including rates of childhood physical abuse, rape, and multiple victimizations, are highest among AI/AN women. Access to prenatal care is limited for AI/AN women, with twice the rate of AI/AN women accessing prenatal care late or receiving no prenatal care compared with other women (Raglan et al., 2016). In a study of nearly 300 AI/AN women, about 30 percent reported depressive symptoms 13–24 months postpartum. Nearly 70 percent of the sample reported financial events, 60 percent reported emotional events, 46 percent reported partner-related events, 38 percent reported traumatic events, and 19 percent reported IPV. Having had at least one partner-related or traumatic stressful life event or at least one traumatic stressful life event was significantly related to depression symptoms (Ness et al., 2017).

Adverse childhood experiences In data from the 2011–2012 National Survey of Children's Health, AI/AN children were more likely to report eight of nine ACEs, including income deprivation, witnessing or experiencing violent victimization, racial/ethnic discrimination, household substance abuse, domestic violence, parental incarceration, divorce, and death of a parent. AI/AN children were also more likely to report more than one ACE compared to non-Hispanic white children. After adjusting for sociodemographic factors, the difference between AI/AN and white children was no longer significant, which suggests that the heightened risk for AI/AN children was explained by family and neighborhood factors. For AI/AN children reporting with one or more ACE, parents reported an increasing prevalence of behavioral issues, including arguing, lack of emotional control, and school problems, and more provider-diagnosed behavioral disorders, such as depression, anxiety, and attention-deficit/hyperactivity disorder (Kenney and Singh, 2016).

Health system challenges Studies of health systems issues within AI/AN communities remain limited. The Indian Health Service provides national access to care statistics, but updated reports are lacking, and few focus specifically on the needs of early childhood. In one study of 59 emergency medical service agencies, or ambulance services, 46,761 annual emergency responses were reported, with 9,981 annual inter-facility transports. Pediatric emergency responses represented 15 percent (n = 7,190) of the total emergency responses, with an annual average of 180 pediatric responses per agency. Nine agencies (15 percent) reported that their agency did not have a medical director. Agencies with a medical director were more likely to report availability of pediatric medical direction than agencies without one. About 80 percent of agencies reported that their emergency medical services (EMS) providers needed pediatric continuing education for certification and recertification. About one-quarter of agencies reported that all of their EMS providers received pediatric continuation education training, while six agencies reported that no providers had received pediatric training. About half of agencies reported having a mass casualties plan, and of these, 15 had participated in a pediatric-focused mass casualties drill within 2 years of the survey. About 30 percent of all agencies had responded to a mass casualty incident involving a large number of pediatric patients that overwhelmed their service. Of these, about half of the agencies reported that they did not have enough pediatric equipment available when they responded to the incident at that time (Genovesi et al., 2014).

Resilience Few studies examine factors contributing to resilience among AI/AN people; however, one review found that, across eight relevant research studies examining resilience among AI/ANs, resilience was an ongoing, dynamic process that responds to a changing environment, is evident within the life course, and can be accessed through culture. Cultural values, beliefs, and practices were identified as essential resources for AI/AN resilience along the life course and across generations. Three studies found culture could be best accessed through the use of narratives, lived experiences, and traditional stories (Ore et al., 2016).

Children of Immigrant Backgrounds

Children of immigrant backgrounds are one of the largest growing population segments among the U.S. population of 0- to 10-year-olds. Nearly 90 percent of children in immigrant families are U.S. citizens, and about one-quarter of them have an unauthorized immigrant parent (Koball et al., 2015). Thus, many children who live in immigrant families—irrespective of their own citizenship status—are greatly impacted by not only the household context but also the larger policy context for immigrant families (Filindra et al., 2011; Koball et al., 2015; Yoshikawa, 2011). In addition, research suggests that the United States will increasingly need to depend on immigrants and their children to maintain its workforce (Singer, 2012). To that end, supporting children of immigrant background and their families is essential to ensure not only individual healthy developmental trajectories, but also the future of the country. Much of the following discussion applies to documented immigrants, unless otherwise specified.

Many children of immigrant background face unique stressors that influence their development. For example, many parents who are first-generation immigrants have fled extreme poverty, political persecution, sexual violence, and other sources of oppression, which are traumatic experiences with long-term consequences (Petrosky et al., 2017). In addition, many have experienced discrimination in housing and employment, as well as overt expressions of racism in their daily lives. These traumatic experiences can have implications for their parenting.

Residential segregation, among other factors, is one contributing factor as to why immigrants tend to end up living in concentrated poverty, which might lead to unhealthy levels of stress during pregnancy and in the infant's first years of life (NASEM, 2015b). Living in poverty in addition to an undocumented status may result in inadequate supports for caregiving: lack of high-quality day care, preschool, and elementary/middle school; and lack of access to adequate housing and health care (Yoshikawa and Kalil, 2011). There is growing evidence that documents the harm to children of parents with unauthorized status in terms of economic and socio-emotional hardship. For example, children fearing the deportation of a parent may show psychological distress by experiencing problems eating or sleeping, increases in headaches and stomachaches, anger or detachment, and depression and anxiety (Artiga and Ubri, 2017; Rojas-Flores et al., 2017).

The current policies toward immigrants in the United States have become another source of the toxic stress response for these families and their children. In particular, the dramatic recent increases in deportation of U.S. immigrants and the detention of parents at the borders seeking asylum have resulted in the separation of thousands of children from their parents (HHS Office of Inspector General, 2019). Research conducted since the 1950s shows that the scientific evidence is clear: separating children from families has long-term damaging health consequences for the children (Acker et al., 2019). These traumatic experiences can have cascading effects in multiple areas, even after reunification. Furthermore, recent immigration policies have had a documented effect on parents' willingness to enroll their children of immigrant background in public programs, including those in ECE settings (Cervantes et al., 2018). This could have serious implications because it increases the environmental barriers for these families; they refrain from using programs that could ameliorate or prevent educational and health problems (Koball et al., 2015; Yoshikawa, 2011). These barriers could be exacerbated as the increasing efforts to limit access to government services, such as education and health care, take effect at the federal or state levels.

However, research conducted both in the United States and internationally shows that if the right conditions are attainable and present, children of immigrant background can not only thrive, but also excel (García Coll et al., 2012; Motti-Stefanidi and García Coll, 2018). Many countries have policies that support children of immigrant backgrounds at the state and national levels (Bachega, 2018; Line and Poon, 2013; OECD, 2018; Shinkman, 2018). Domestic and international studies show that policies providing support for immigrant families facilitate increases in positive outcomes, such as high school graduation rates. A U.S. national study showed that state family-supportive policies, such as allowing immigrant families to obtain driver's licenses and health care benefits, among others, lead to higher high school graduation rates (Filindra et al., 2011). An international study showed that immigrant-supportive public policies at the country level also contribute to more optimal health outcomes in children of immigrants (Marks et al., 2018).

At the community and neighborhood levels, research shows that school programs that support dual-language learners facilitate positive developmental trajectories for children of immigrant background (NASEM, 2017b). In addition, interventions with a two-generation preventive focus also provide promising models and strategies to further support the healthy development of children of immigrant background (Valdez et al., 2013; Williamson et al., 2014).

ACCUMULATION OF RISK

This chapter has provided an overview of how family cohesion and social connections (see Chapter 4), health care (see Chapter 5), early living conditions (i.e., economic security, nutrition and food security, housing, and environmental exposures) (see Chapter 6), ECE (see Chapter 7), and racism converge through an accumulation of risk factors that influence a child's entire life course. Extensive evidence shows that exposure to multiple social risk factors or continuous exposure to a single risk factor is more harmful to children than one-time exposure to a single risk, across a broad range of outcomes (Evans et al., 2013; Sameroff, 1998). It is most common for researchers to calculate composite scores to represent the accumulation of risk factors by summing dichotomous indicators for each risk factor, although other, more complex methods exist (Evans et al., 2013). Across studies, there is variation in what is included within cumulative risk scores; in some studies, researchers focus on information about the family and residential context, whereas other studies may include information about the residential neighborhood context and/or school experiences.

Cumulative risk scores offer an easily interpreted measure and are strong predictors of child health (Evans et al., 2013). Notably, however, studies using cumulative risk scores typically do not consider the sequential timing or intensity of risk factors and are limited by the assumption that each type of risk is equally weighted and additive (i.e., not considering synergistic or interactive effects between risk and/or protective factors) (Dohrenwend, 2006; Evans et al., 2013). Longitudinal birth cohort studies with frequent assessments, such as the Dunedin Multidisciplinary Health and Development Study (Poulton et al., 2015) or the Avon Longitudinal Study of Parents and Children (Boyd et al., 2012; Fraser et al., 2012), provide an opportunity to investigate the chronicity of multiple risk factors over time (Danese et al., 2009; Dunn et al., 2018). The next section of this chapter explores the Adverse Childhood Experiences (ACEs) Study as an example of a composite approach to investigate the relationship between cumulative risk through childhood experiences and outcomes in adulthood (Felitti et al., 1998).

Adverse Childhood Experiences

As elaborated in Chapter 2, prenatal and early life environments have a profound role in shaping life course health, and even the health of the next generation, through a complex interplay of contextual and biological factors, including individual genetic characteristics, gene–environment interactions, family supports or stressors, environmental factors, and developmental experiences. This chapter looks more closely at the social and environmental contexts in which the aforementioned biological processes unfold and which structures promote the accumulation of risk or resilience. Perhaps the most well-known study of accumulated risk is the ACEs Study conducted by CDC and Kaiser Permanente and published by Felitti et al. in 1998 (see Box 3-9).

Since the publication of the ACEs Study, subsequent research has demonstrated that the health impacts of ACEs are evident as early as infancy, and even in the prenatal and preconception periods. Parental ACEs are associated with increased risk of negative preconception and prenatal outcomes, including menstrual irregularity, reduced odds of conception, chronic health complications, preeclampsia, psychological risk (prenatal and postpartum depression), social risk (age at first pregnancy, education level, income, relational resilience, perceived stress, IPV, partner's drug abuse, maternal hostile behavior in infancy), behavioral risk (alcohol use, drug use, smoking), and negative pregnancy outcomes (miscarriage, premature delivery, reduced birth weight, shorter gestational age) (Ångerud

---

BOX 3-9
Adverse Childhood Experiences Study

The phrase "adverse childhood experiences" was coined in 1998 following the publication of the Adverse Childhood Experiences (ACEs) Study, a large epidemiological study conducted by the Centers for Disease Control and Prevention and Kaiser Permanente, and refers specifically to the 10 categories of adverse events evaluated in the study, which include

1. Emotional abuse (recurrent),
2. Physical abuse (recurrent),
3. Sexual abuse (contact),
4. Physical neglect,
5. Emotional neglect,
6. Substance abuse in the household (e.g., living with an alcoholic or a person with a substance abuse problem),
7. Mental illness in the household (e.g., living with someone who suffers from depression or mental illness or had attempted suicide),
8. Mother treated violently,
9. Divorce or parental separation, and
10. Criminal behavior in household (e.g., a household member going to prison).

The ACEs Study's findings were substantial and important, revealing that ACEs are common within the population (two-thirds of study participants had experienced at least one ACE and 12.6 percent had experienced four or more) and are associated with a broad array of long-term negative health outcomes in a dose–response relationship. Numerous epidemiological studies have supported these findings and demonstrated that those with an ACE Score of 4 or more are at dramatically increased odds for many of the leading causes of death in the United States (see Table 3-4).

SOURCES: CDC, n.d.-a; Felitti et al., 1998.

---

et al., 2018; Brunton, 2013; Christiaens et al., 2015; Leeners et al., 2014; Li et al., 2018; Liu et al., 2018; Olsen, 2018; Racine et al., 2018; Smith et al., 2016).

Outcomes related to prenatal and early childhood exposure to ACEs in children include altered neurodevelopment, neurocognitive function, cerebral processing, functional and structural brain connectivity involving the amygdala and (pre)frontal cortex, hypothalamic-pituitary-adrenal axis, and autonomous nervous system (Brunton, 2013; McGowan and Matthews, 2018; Provençal and Binder, 2015; van den Bergh et al., 2018). Infants and children exposed to ACEs demonstrate increased risk of sleep disturbance, failure to thrive, growth and developmental delays, viral and bacterial infection, atopic disease (including asthma, allergies,

TABLE 3-4 Leading Causes of Death in 2015 and Their Relationship with the Experience of Four or More ACES

Leading Causes of Death in the United States, 2015	Odds Ratio Associated with ≥4 ACEs[a]
1 Heart disease	2.1
2 Cancer	2.3
3 Chronic lower respiratory disease	3.0
4 Accidents	—
5 Stroke	2.4
6 Alzheimer's disease	11.2
7 Diabetes	1.5
8 Influenza and pneumonia	—
9 Kidney disease	—
10 Suicide	30.1

[a] Hughes et al., 2017, for all odds ratios except for stroke and Alzheimer's disease; Felitti et al., 1998, for stroke; Center for Youth Wellness, 2014, for Alzheimer's disease. SOURCE: CDC, 2017.

and eczema), overweight and obesity, and learning and behavioral difficulties (Björkenstam et al., 2015; Burke et al., 2011; Giordano et al., 2014; Kerker et al., 2015; Matheson et al., 2016; Oh et al., 2017; Rhodes et al., 2012; Ryan et al., 2016; Shen et al., 2016; Thompson et al., 2017). Studies have also shown that ACEs are associated with increased risk-taking behaviors in adolescents, including early sexual initiation, teen pregnancy, teen paternity, substance use, and victimization (Hughes et al., 2017; Shin et al., 2009; Thompson et al., 2017).

Evidence points to several mechanisms by which ACEs and other early life stressors affect preconception, prenatal, and postnatal health:

1. Neuro-endocrine-immune dysregulation, metabolic regulation, and gene expression (as discussed in Chapter 2);
2. Increased risk of health problems that may affect pregnancy outcomes, including obesity, diabetes, and autoimmune disease;
3. Increased risk of parental mental health disorders;
4. Increased risk behaviors, such as smoking, and substance use and risk exposures, such as victimization;
5. Changes in epigenetic regulation that may be passed down via maternal or paternal germ lines; and
6. Difficulty with emotional regulation.

Beginning in 2009, many states began to systematically collect population-based representative data on ACEs, beginning with adults via the Behavioral Risk Factor Surveillance System (BRFSS). In 2011–2012, a modified ACE inventory was introduced into the National Survey of Children's Health. These surveillance activities provide scientists and policy makers with information on the prevalence of ACEs and data to study associations with health outcomes. According to the most recent published CDC data reporting from the BRFSS, in 23 states, 62 percent of American adults have experienced at least one of the eight ACEs, and 15 percent have experienced four or more (Merrick et al., 2018). In 2012, the Institute for Safe Families formed the ACE Task Force to assess the prevalence of ACEs in Philadelphia in order to broaden the concept of ACEs to reflect the experiences of children of color in urban communities (Public Health Management Corporation, 2013).[13]

While the term refers specifically to the 10 categories identified in the ACEs Study, it is recognized that other forms of early life adversity, such as economic hardship, food and housing insecurity, unsafe toxic environments, and discrimination, are also critical in shaping health and developmental outcomes. Cumulative exposure to negative experiences increases the risk of negative outcomes, but the converse is also true—supportive, nurturing, and buffering experiences also add up in a manner that is protective of health and neurodevelopmental outcomes. Thus, family, social, neighborhood, and structural environmental factors play an important role in shaping life course health and the health of future generations.

CONCLUSION

This chapter provides an overview of the risk and protective factors relevant to each level of the committee's conceptual model (see Figure 1-9). These factors are interrelated and complex, but they also demonstrate critical areas where there are opportunities for change and the science may be applied to inform interventions for children and families. In the chapters that follow, the committee takes the vast science base described in Chapters 2 and 3 and applies it to the necessary actions to advance child and family health outcomes and health equity across the domains discussed in this chapter (see Table 3-1 at the beginning of this chapter).

---

[13] The original ACEs study sample was composed of primarily white, middle-class, and educated individuals (Felitti et al., 1998).

REFERENCES

Accortt, E. E., A. C. Cheadle, and C. Dunkel Schetter. 2015. Prenatal depression and adverse birth outcomes: An updated systematic review. *Maternal and Child Health Journal* 19(6):1306–1337.

Acevedo-Garcia, D., M. J. Soobader, and L. F. Berkman. 2005. The differential effect of foreign-born status on low birth weight by race/ethnicity and education. *Pediatrics* 115(1):e20–e30.

Acevedo-Garcia, D., L. E. Rosenfeld, E. Hardy, N. McArdle, and T. L. Osypuk. 2013. Future directions in research on institutional and interpersonal discrimination and children's health. *American Journal of Public Health* 103(10):1754–1763.

Acevedo-Garcia, D., E. F. Hardy, N. McArdle, U. I. Crisan, B. Romano, D. Norris, M. Baek, and J. Reece. 2016a. *The Child Opportunity Index: Measuring and mapping neighborhood-based opportunities for children.* Waltham, MA, and Columbus, OH: diversitydatakids. org and Kirwan Institute for the Study of Race and Ethnicity.

Acevedo-Garcia, D., N. McArdle, E. Hardy, K.-N. Dillman, J. Reece, U. I. Crisan, D. Norris, and T. L. Osypuk. 2016b. Neighborhood opportunity and location affordability for low-income renter families. *Housing Policy Debate* 26(4–5):607–645.

Acker, J., P. Braveman, E. Arkin, L. Leviton, J. Parsons, and G. Hobor. 2019. *Mass incarceration threatens health equity in America.* Princeton, NJ: Robert Wood Johnson Foundation.

ACOG (American College of Obstetricians and Gynecologists) Committee Opinion No. 575. 2013. Exposure to toxic environmental agents. *Fertility and Sterility* 122(4):931–935.

Ahern, J., K. E. Pickett, S. Selvin, and B. Abrams. 2003. Preterm birth among African American and white women: A multilevel analysis of socioeconomic characteristics and cigarette smoking. *Journal of Epidemiology and Community Health* 57(8):606–611.

Ahmad, S. A., M. H. Sayed, S. Barua, M. H. Khan, M. H. Faruquee, A. Jalil, S. A. Hadi, and H. K. Talukder. 2001. Arsenic in drinking water and pregnancy outcomes. *Environmental Health Perspectives* 109(6):629–631.

Aizer, A. 2008. *Neighborhood violence and urban youth: NBER working paper no. 13773.* https://www.nber.org/papers/w13773 (accessed April 18, 2019).

Akinbami, L. J., J. E. Moorman, P. L. Garbe, and E. J. Sondik. 2009. Status of childhood asthma in the United States, 1980–2007. *Pediatrics* 123:S131–S145.

Akinbami, L. J., J. E. Moorman, A. E. Simon, and K. C. Schoendorf. 2014. Trends in racial disparities for asthma outcomes among children 0 to 17 years, 2001–2010. *Journal of Allergy and Clinical Immunology* 134(3):547–553.

Alexander, D., and J. Currie. 2017. Is it who you are or where you live? Residential segregation and racial gaps in childhood asthma. *Journal of Health Economics* 55:186–200.

Alhusen, J. L., K. M. Bower, E. Epstein, and P. Sharps. 2016. Racial discrimination and adverse birth outcomes: An integrative review. *Journal of Midwifery & Women's Health* 61(6):707–720.

American Pregnancy Association. 2017. *Nutrients & vitamins for pregnancy.* https://americanpregnancy.org/pregnancy-health/nutrients-vitamins-pregnancy (accessed April 22, 2019).

Anderson, K., P. Spicer, and M. Peercy. 2016. Obesity, diabetes, and birth outcomes among American Indians and Alaska Natives. *Maternal and Child Health Journal* 20(12):2548–2556.

Andolfatto, D. 2017. *Why do unemployment rates vary by race and ethnicity?* https://www.stlouisfed.org/on-the-economy/2017/february/why-unemployment-rates-vary-races-ethnicity (accessed April 18, 2019).

Ångerud, K., E. M. Annerbäck, T. Tydén, S. Boddeti, and P. Kristiansson. 2018. Adverse childhood experiences and depressive symptomatology among pregnant women. *Acta Obstetricia et Gynecologica Scandinavica* 97(6):701–708.

Anstey, E. H., J. Chen, L. D. Elam-Evans, and C. G. Perrine. 2017. Racial and geographic differences in breastfeeding—United States, 2011–2015. *Morbidity Mortality Weekly Report* 66:723–727.

Arenz, S., R. Ruckerl, B. Koletzko, and R. von Kries. 2004. Breast-feeding and childhood obesity—a systematic review. *International Journal of Obesity and Related Metabolic Disorders* 28(10):1247–1256.

Artiga, S., and P. Ubri. 2017. *Living in an immigrant family in America: How fear and toxic stress are affecting daily life, well-being, and health.* Menlo Park, CA: Kaiser Family Foundation.

Asante-Muhammad, D., C. Collins, J. Hoxie, and E. Nieves. 2017. *The road to zero wealth: How the racial wealth divide is hollowing out America's middle class.* Washington, DC: Prosperity Now and Institute for Policy Studies.

ASPE (Assistant Secretary for Planning and Evaluation). 2007. *Gaps and strategies for improving American Indian/Alaska Native/Native American data.* Washington, DC: Office of the Assistant Secretary for Planning and Evaluation.

Assari, S. 2018. Diminished economic return of socioeconomic status for black families. *Social Sciences* 7(5):74.

Assari, S., A. Thomas, C. H. Caldwell, and R. B. Mincy. 2018. Blacks diminished health return of family structure and socioeconomic status; 15 years of follow-up of a national urban sample of youth. *Journal of Urban Health* 95:21–35.

Association of Maternal & Child Health Programs. 2016. *Opportunities to optimize access to prenatal care through health transformation.* Washington, DC: Association of Maternal & Child Health Programs.

ASTHO (Association of State and Territorial Health Officials). 2017. *Enhancing health equity in breastfeeding opportunities and outcomes. Issue brief.* Arlington, VA: Association of State and Territorial Health Officials.

Auchincloss, A. H., M. S. Mujahid, M. Shen, E. D. Michos, M. C. Whitt-Glover, and A. V. Diez Roux. 2013. Neighborhood health-promoting resources and obesity risk (the Multi-ethnic Study of Atherosclerosis). *Obesity* 21(3):621–628.

Aviram, A., M. Hod, and Y. Yogev. 2011. Maternal obesity: Implications for pregnancy outcome and long-term risks—a link to maternal nutrition. *International Journal of Gynecology & Obstetrics* 115:S6–S10.

Bachega, H. 2018. Separation of migrant families: What other countries do. *BBC News,* https://www.bbc.com/news/world-us-canada-44374756 (accessed April 23, 2019).

Bachman, R., H. Zaykowski, R. Kallmyer, M. Poteyeva, and C. Lanier. 2008. *Violence against American Indian and Alaska Native women and the criminal justice response: What is known.* Washington, DC: U.S. Department of Justice, Office of Justice Programs, National Institute of Justice.

Bailey, Z. D., N. Krieger, M. Agenor, J. Graves, N. Linos, and M. T. Bassett. 2017. Structural racism and health inequities in the USA: Evidence and interventions. *The Lancet* 389(10077):1453–1463.

Barnett, S., M. Carolan, and D. Johns. 2013. *Equity and excellence: African-American children's access to quality preschool.* New Brunswick, NJ: Center on Enhancing Early Learning Outcomes.

Barnett, W. S., and A. H. Friedman-Krauss. 2016. *State(s) of Head Start.* New Brunswick, NJ: National Institute for Early Education Research.

Beck, A. F., B. Huang, R. Chundur, and R. S. Kahn. 2014. Housing code violation density associated with emergency department and hospital use by children with asthma. *Health Affairs* 33(11):1993–2002.

Becker, G. S., and N. Tomes. 1986. Human capital and the rise and fall of families. *Journal of Labor Economics* 4:S1–S39.

Beckhaus, A. A., L. Garcia-Marcos, E. Forno, R. M. Pacheco-Gonzalez, J. C. Celedón, and J. A. Castro-Rodriguez. 2015. Maternal nutrition during pregnancy and risk of asthma, wheeze, and atopic diseases during childhood: A systematic review and meta-analysis. *Allergy* 70(12):1588–1604.

Behnia, F., M. Peltier, D. Getahun, C. Watson, G. Saade, and R. Menon. 2016. High bisphenol A (BPA) concentration in the maternal, but not fetal, compartment increases the risk of spontaneous preterm delivery. *Journal of Maternal-Fetal and Neonatal Medicine* 29(22):3583–3589.

Bellinger, D. C., F. Trachtenberg, A. Zhang, M. Tavares, D. Daniel, and S. McKinlay. 2008. Dental amalgam and psychosocial status: The New England Children's Amalgam Trial. *Journal of Dental Research* 87(5):470–474.

Ben-Schlomo, Y., and D. Kuh. 2002. A life course approach to chronic disease epidemiology: Conceptual models, empirical challenges and interdisciplinary perspectives. *International Journal of Epidemiology* 31(2):285–293.

Ben-Schlomo, Y., G. Mishra, and D. Kuh. 2014. Life course epidemiology, 1521–1549. In *Handbook of epidemiology*, edited by W. Ahrens and I. Pigeot. New York: Springer.

Berger, L. M., S. A. Font, K. S. Slack, and J. Waldfogel. 2017. Income and child maltreatment in unmarried families: Evidence from the Earned Income Tax Credit. *Review of Economics of the Household* 15(4):1345–1372.

Bethell, C., C. Reuland, E. Schor, M. Abrahms, and N. Halfon. 2011. Rates of parent-centered developmental screening: Disparities and links to services access. *Pediatrics* 128(1):146–155.

Beyerlein, A., and R. von Kries. 2011. Breastfeeding and body composition in children: Will there ever be conclusive empirical evidence for a protective effect against overweight? *American Journal of Clinical Nutrition* 94(6 Suppl):1772s–1775s.

Beyers, J. M., J. E. Bates, G. S. Pettit, and K. A. Dodge. 2003. Neighborhood structure, parenting processes, and the development of youths' externalizing behaviors: A multilevel analysis. *American Journal of Community Psychology* 31(1–2):35–53.

Bhaskar, R., and B. O'Hara. 2017. Indian health service coverage among American Indians and Alaska Natives in federal tribal areas. *Journal of Health Care for the Poor and Underserved* 28(4):1361.

Bingham, D., N. Strauss, and F. Coeytaux. 2011. Maternal mortality in the United States: A human rights failure. *Contraception* 83(3):189–193.

Björkenstam, E., B. Burström, L. Brännström, B. Vinnerljung, C. Björkenstam, and A. R. Pebley. 2015. Cumulative exposure to childhood stressors and subsequent psychological distress. An analysis of US panel data. *Social Science & Medicine* 142:109–117.

Black, L. I., and V. Benson. 2018. *Tables of summary health statistics for U.S. children: 2017 National Health Interview Survey.* https://www.cdc.gov/nchs/nhis/SHS/tables.htm (accessed May 21, 2019).

Blair, A., N. A. Ross, G. Gariepy, and N. Schmitz. 2014. How do neighborhoods affect depression outcomes? A realist review and a call for the examination of causal pathways. *Social Psychiatry and Psychiatric Epidemiology* 49(6):873–887.

Blair, C., C. C. Raver, D. Granger, R. Mills-Koonce, and L. Hibel. 2011. Allostasis and allostatic load in the context of poverty in early childhood. *Development and Psychopathology* 23(3):845–857.

Blumenshine, P., S. Egerter, C. J. Barclay, C. Cubbin, and P. A. Braveman. 2010. Socioeconomic disparities in adverse birth outcomes: A systematic review. *American Journal of Preventive Medicine* 39(3):263–272.

Borge, T. C., H. Aase, A. L. Brantsaeter, and G. Biele. 2017. The importance of maternal diet quality during pregnancy on cognitive and behavioural outcomes in children: A systematic review and meta-analysis. *BMJ Open* 7(9):e016777.

Bornehag, C. G., J. Sundell, C. J. Weschler, T. Sigsgaard, B. Lundgren, M. Hasselgren, and L. Hägerhed-Engman. 2004. The association between asthma and allergic symptoms in children and phthalates in house dust: A nested case-control study. *Environmental Health Perspectives* 112(14):1393–1397.

Bornstein, M. H., and T. Leventhal. 2015. Children in bioecological landscapes of development. In *Handbook of child psychology and developmental science*, 7th ed. Vol. 4, *Ecological settings and processes*, edited by R. M. Lerner. Hoboken, NJ: Wiley. Pp. 1–5.

Borra, C., M. Iacovou, and A. Sevilla. 2015. New evidence on breastfeeding and postpartum depression: The importance of understanding women's intentions. *Maternal and Child Health Journal* 19(4):897–907.

Bowatte, G., R. Tham, K. J. Allen, D. J. Tan, M. X. Z. Lau, X. Dai, and C. J. Lodge. 2015. Breastfeeding and childhood acute otitis media: A systematic review and meta-analysis. *Acta Paediatrica* 104(S467):85–95.

Boy, A., and H. M. Salihu. 2004. Intimate partner violence and birth outcomes: A systematic review. *International Journal of Fertility and Women's Medicine* 49(4):159–164.

Boyd, A., J. Golding, J. Macleod, D. A. Lawlor, A. Fraser, J. Henderson, L. Molloy, A. Ness, S. Ring, and G. Davey Smith. 2012. Cohort profile: The "children of the 90s"—the index offspring of the Avon Longitudinal Study of Parents and Children. *International Journal of Epidemiology* 42(1):11–127.

Braun, J. M., G. Muckle, T. Arbuckle, M. F. Bouchard, W. D. Fraser, E. Ouellet, J. R. Seguin, Y. Oulhote, G. M. Webster, and B. P. Lanphear. 2017. Associations of prenatal urinary bisphenol a concentrations with child behaviors and cognitive abilities. *Environmental Health Perspectives* 125(6):067008.

Braveman, P., J. Acker, E. Arkin, J. Bussel, K. Wehr, and D. Proctor. 2018. *Early childhood is critical to health equity*. Princeton, NJ: Robert Wood Johnson Foundation.

Bronfenbrenner, U. 1979. Contexts of child rearing: Problems and prospects. *American Psychologist* 34(10):844–850.

Bronfenbrenner, U., and G. W. Evans. 2000. Developmental science in the 21st century: Emerging questions, theoretical models, research designs and empirical findings. *Social Development* 9(1):115–125.

Bronfenbrenner, U., and P. A. Morris. 2006. The bioecological model of human development. In *Handbook of child psychology and developmental science*, 7th ed. Vol. 1, *Theory and method*, edited by R. M. Lerner. New York: Wiley. Pp. 793–828.

Bronfenbrenner, U., and P. A. Morris. 2007. *The bioecological model of human development. Handbook of child psychology*. Hoboken, NJ: John Wiley & Sons, Inc.

Brooks-Gunn, J., and G. J. Duncan. 1997. The effects of poverty on children. *The Future of Children* 7(2):55–71.

Brunton, P. J. 2013. Effects of maternal exposure to social stress during pregnancy: Consequences for mother and offspring. *Reproduction* 146(5):R175–R189.

Buckner, J. 2008. Understanding the impact of homelessness on children: Challenges and future research directions. *American Behavioral Scientist* 51(6):721–736.

Buka, S. L., R. T. Brennan, J. W. Rich-Edwards, S. W. Raudenbush, and F. Earls. 2003. Neighborhood support and the birth weight of urban infants. *American Journal of Epidemiology* 157(1):1–8.

Bures, R. M. 2003. Childhood residential stability and health at midlife. *American Journal of Public Health* 93(7):1144–1148.

Burke, N. J., J. L. Hellman, B. G. Scott, C. F. Weems, and V. G. Carrion. 2011. The impact of adverse childhood experiences on an urban pediatric population. *Child Abuse & Neglect* 35(6):408–413.

Callec, R., E. Perdriolle-Galet, G.-A. Sery, and O. Morel. 2014. Type 2 diabetes in pregnancy: Rates of fetal malformations and level of preconception care. *Journal of Obstetrics and Gynaecology* 34(7):648–649.

Campbell, F., G. Conti, J. J. Heckman, S. H. Moon, R. Pinto, E. Pungello, and Y. Pan. 2014. Early childhood investments substantially boost adult health. *Science* 343(6178):1478–1485.

Cancian, M. 2010. *The effect of family income on risk of child maltreatment*. Madison, WI: Institute for Research on Poverty.

Cascio, E. U., and D. W. Schanzenbach. 2016. *Expanding preschool access for disadvanaged children*. Washington, DC: The Brookings Institution.

Casey, J. A., D. A. Savitz, S. G. Rasmussen, E. L. Ogburn, J. Pollak, D. G. Mercer, and B. S. Schwartz. 2016. Unconventional natural gas development and birth outcomes in Pennsylvania, USA. *Epidemiology* 27(2):163–172.

CDC (Centers for Disease Control and Prevention). 2014. *Essentials for childhood: Steps to create safe, stable, and nurturing relationships and environments*. Atlanta, GA: Centers for Disease Control and Prevention.

CDC. 2017. *Leading causes of death*. https://www.cdc.gov/nchs/fastats/leading-causes-of-death.htm (accessed April 23, 2019).

CDC. 2018a. *Breastfeeding report card, United States, 2018*. https://www.cdc.gov/breastfeeding/data/reportcard.htm (accessed April 18, 2019).

CDC. 2018b. *Table 4-1 Current Asthma Prevalence Percents by Age, United States: National Health Interview Survey, 2016*. https://www.cdc.gov/asthma/nhis/2016/table4-1.htm (accessed July 15, 2019).

CDC. 2019. *Preventing child abuse & neglect*. https://www.cdc.gov/violenceprevention/pdf/CAN-factsheet.pdf (accessed April 22, 2019).

CDC. n.d.-a. *About the CDC-Kaiser ACE study*. https://www.cdc.gov/violenceprevention/acestudy/about.html (accessed July 18, 2018).

CDC. n.d.-b. *Breastfeeding practices and policies*. https://www.cdc.gov/nccdphp/dnpao/state-local-programs/health-equity-guide/pdf/health-equity-guide/Health-Equity-Guide-sect-3-5.pdf (accessed July 13, 2019).

Center for Youth Wellness. 2014. *Data report: A hidden crisis. Findings on adverse childhood experiences in California*. https://centerforyouthwellness.org/wp-content/themes/cyw/build/img/building-a-movement/hidden-crisis.pdf (accessed July 15, 2019).

Center on the Developing Child at Harvard University. 2009. *Maternal depression can undermine the development of young children: Working paper no. 8*. Cambridge, MA: Harvard University.

Cervantes, W., R. Ullrich, and H. Matthews. 2018. *Our children's fear: Immigration policy's effects on young children*. Washington, DC: Center for Law and Social Policy.

Chang, A. 2018. The data proves that school segregation is getting worse. *Vox*, https://www.vox.com/2018/3/5/17080218/school-segregation-getting-worse-data (accessed April 22, 2019).

ChangeLab Solutions. 2017. *Closing the water quality gap: Using policy to improve drinking water in federally-unregulated water systems*. Oakland, CA: ChangeLab Solutions.

Chapman, D. J., and R. Pérez-Escamilla. 2012. Breastfeeding among minority women: Moving from risk factors to interventions. *Advances in Nutrition* 3:95–104.

Chen, E., A. D. Martin, and K. A. Matthews. 2006. Understanding health disparities: The role of race and socioeconomic status in children's health. *American Journal of Public Health* 96(4):702–708.

Chetty, R., M. Stepner, S. Abraham, S. Lin, B. Scuderi, N. Turner, A. Bergeron, and D. Cutler. 2016. The association between income and life expectancy in the United States, 2001–2014. *JAMA* 315(16):1750–1766.

Chetty, R., N. Hendren, M. R. Jones, and S. R. Porter. 2018. *Race and economic opportunity in the United States: An intergenerational perspective*. NBER working paper no. 24441. National Bureau of Economic Research.

Chevrier, J., R. B. Gunier, A. Bradman, N. T. Holland, A. M. Calafat, B. Eskenazi, and K. G. Harley. 2013. Maternal urinary bisphenol A during pregnancy and maternal and neonatal thyroid function in the Chamacos Study. *Environmental Health Perspectives* 121(1):138–144.

Chien, N. 2017. *Factsheet: Estimates of child care eligibility & receipt for fiscal year 2013.* Washington, DC: U.S. Department of Health and Human Services, Office of the Assistant Secretary for Planning and Evaluation.

Child Trends. 2015. *Parental education. Indicators of child and youth well-being.* Bethesda, MD: Child Trends.

Child Trends DataBank. 2018. *High school dropout rates.* https://www.childtrends.org/indicators/high-school-dropout-rates (accessed April 22, 2019).

Chou, R. S., and J. R. Feagin. 2015. *The myth of the model minority: Asian Americans facing racism.* Boulder, CO: Paradigm Publishers.

Chowdhury, R., B. Sinha, M. J. Sankar, S. Taneja, N. Bhandari, N. Rollins, R. Bahl, and J. Martines. 2015. Breastfeeding and maternal health outcomes: A systematic review and meta-analysis. *Acta Paediatrica* 104(467):96–113.

Christiaens, I., K. Hegadoren, and D. M. Olson. 2015. Adverse childhood experiences are associated with spontaneous preterm birth: A case-control study. *BMC Medicine* 13:124.

Christine, P. J., A. H. Auchincloss, A. G. Bertoni, M. R. Carnethon, B. N. Sanchez, K. Moore, S. D. Adar, T. B. Horwich, K. E. Watson, and A. V. Diez Roux. 2015. Longitudinal associations between neighborhood physical and social environments and incident type 2 diabetes mellitus: The Multi-Ethnic Study of Atherosclerosis (MESA). *JAMA Internal Medicine* 175(8):1311–1320.

Chuang, C. H., D. L. Velott, and C. S. Weisman. 2010. Exploring knowledge and attitudes related to pregnancy and preconception health in women with chronic medical conditions. *Maternal and Child Health Journal* 14(5):713–719.

Cicchetti, D., and E. D. Handley. 2017. Methylation of the glucocorticoid receptor gene, nuclear receptor subfamily 3, group c, member 1 (NR3C1), in maltreated and non-maltreated children: Associations with behavioral undercontrol, emotional lability/negativity, and externalizing and internalizing symptoms. *Development and Psychopathology* 29(5):1795–1806.

Cobb, L. K., L. J. Appel, M. Franco, J. C. Jones-Smith, A. Nur, and C. A. Anderson. 2015. The relationship of the local food environment with obesity: A systematic review of methods, study quality, and results. *Obesity* 23(7):1331–1344.

Cobb, N., D. Espey, and J. King. 2014. Health behaviors and risk factors among American Indians and Alaska Natives, 2000–2010. *American Journal of Public Health* 104(S3):S481–S489.

Cohen, S., and T. A. Wills. 1985. Stress, social support, and the buffering hypothesis. *Psychological Bulletin* 98(2):310–357.

Cohen-Cline, H., S. A. A. Beresford, W. E. Barrington, R. L. Matsueda, J. Wakefield, and G. E. Duncan. 2018. Associations between neighbourhood characteristics and depression: A twin study. *Journal of Epidemiology and Community Health* 72(3):202–207.

Coleman-Jensen, A., M. P. Rabbitt, C. A. Gregory, and A. Singh. 2017. *Household food security in the United States in 2016, ERR-237.* Washington, DC: U.S. Department of Agriculture, Economic Research Service.

Coley, R. L., T. Leventhal, A. D. Lynch, and M. Kull. 2013. Relations between housing characteristics and the well-being of low-income children and adolescents. *Developmental Psychology* 49(9):1775–1789.

Collins, N. L., C. Dunkel-Schetter, M. Lobel, and S. C. Scrimshaw. 1993. Social support in pregnancy: Psychosocial correlates of birth outcomes and postpartum depression. *Journal of Personality and Social Psychology* 65(6):1243–1258.

Conners, N. A., R. H. Bradley, L. W. Mansell, J. Y. Liu, T. J. Roberts, K. Burgdorf, and J. M. Herrell. 2004. Children of mothers with serious substance abuse problems: An accumulation of risks. *American Journal of Drug and Alcohol Abuse* 30(1):85–100.

Corcoran, L., K. Steinley, and S. Grady. 2019. *Early childhood program participation, results from the national household education surveys program of 2016.* Washington, DC: U.S. Department of Education, National Center for Education Statistics, Institute of Education Sciences.

Coughlin, R., E. Kushman, G. Copeland, and M. Wilson. 2013. Pregnancy and birth outcome improvements for American Indians in the healthy start project of the inter-tribal council of Michigan, 1998–2008. *Maternal and Child Health Journal* 17(6):1005–1015.

Cox, C., T. W. Clarkson, D. O. Marsh, L. Amin-Zaki, S. Tikriti, and G. G. Myers. 1989. Dose-response analysis of infants prenatally exposed to methyl mercury: An application of a single compartment model to single-strand hair analysis. *Environmental Research* 49(2):318–332.

Cox, R. G., L. Zhang, M. E. Zotti, and J. Graham. 2011. Prenatal care utilization in Mississippi: Racial disparities and implications for unfavorable birth outcomes. *Maternal and Child Health Journal* 15(7):931–942.

Crowley, S. 2003. The affordable housing crisis: Residential mobility of poor families and school mobility of poor children. *Journal of Negro Education* 72(1):22–38.

Currie, J., and R. Walker. 2011. Traffic congestion and infant health: Evidence from E-ZPass *American Economic Journal: Applied Economics* 3(1):65–90.

Cusick, S. E., and M. K. Georgieff. 2016. The role of nutrition in brain development: The golden opportunity of the "first 1000 days." *The Journal of Pediatrics* 175:16–21.

Cutler, D. M., and A. Lleras-Muney. 2006. *Education and health: Evaluating theories and evidence. National Bureau of Economic Research Working Paper no. 12352.* https://www.nber.org/papers/w12352 (accessed February 10, 2019).

Cutts, D. B., S. Coleman, M. M. Black, M. M. Chilton, J. T. Cook, S. E. de Cuba, T. C. Heeren, A. Meyers, M. Sandel, P. H. Casey, and D. A. Frank. 2015. Homelessness during pregnancy: A unique, time-dependent risk factor of birth outcomes. *Maternal and Child Health Journal* 19(6):1276–1283.

da Silva Lopes, K., E. Ota, P. Shakya, A. Dagvadorj, O. O. Balogun, J. P. Pena-Rosas, L. M. De-Regil, and R. Mori. 2017. Effects of nutrition interventions during pregnancy on low birth weight: An overview of systematic reviews. *BMJ Global Health* 2(3):e000389.

Danese, A., T. E. Moffitt, H. Harrington, B. J. Milne, G. Polanczyk, and C. M. Pariante. 2009. Adverse childhood experiences and adult risk factors for age-related disease: Depression, inflammation, and clustering of metabolic risk markers. *Archives of Pediatric & Adolescent Medicine* 163(12):1135–1143.

Data Resource Center for Child and Adolescent Health. 2019. *Explore the data > NSCH interactive data query (2016–present) > data search results.* https://www.childhealthdata.org/browse/survey/results?q=5554&r=1&g=652 (accessed April 5, 2019).

Davis, R. 2016. *38th annual report to Congress on the implementation of the Individuals with Disabilities Education Act, 2016.* Washington, DC: U.S. Department of Education.

de Brey, C., L. Musu, J. McFarland, S. Wilkinson-Flicker, M. Diliberti, A. Zhang, C. Branstetter, and X. Wang. 2019. *Status and trends in the education of racial and ethnic groups 2018. NCES 2019-038.* Washington, DC: U.S. Department of Education, National Center for Education Statistics.

Desmond, M., and T. Shollenberger. 2015. Forced displacement from rental housing: Prevalence and neighborhood consequences. *Demography* 52(5):1751–1772.

Dewey, K. G. 2003. Is breastfeeding protective against child obesity? *Journal of Human Lactation* 19(1):9–18.

Di Renzo, G. C., J. A. Conry, J. Blake, M. S. Defrancesco, N. Denicola, J. N. Martin, K. A. McCue, D. Richmond, A. Shah, P. Sutton, T. J. Woodruff, S. Z. Van Der Poel, and L. C. Giudice. 2015. International Federation of Gynecology and Obstetrics opinion on reproductive health impacts of exposure to toxic environmental chemicals. *International Journal of Gynecology & Obstetrics* 131(3):219–225.

Diamanti-Kandarakis, E., J.-P. Bourguignon, L. C. Giudice, R. Hauser, G. S. Prins, A. M. Soto, R. T. Zoeller, and A. C. Gore. 2009. Endocrine-disrupting chemicals: An Endocrine Society scientific statement. *Endocrine Reviews* 30(4):293.

Dias, C. C., and B. Figueiredo. 2015. Breastfeeding and depression: A systematic review of the literature. *Journal of Affective Disorders* 171:142–154.

Dohrenwend, B. P. 2006. Inventorying stressful life events as risk factors for psychopathology: Toward resolution of the problem of intracategory variability. *Psychological Bulletin* 132(3):477–495.

Dohrenwend, B. P., I. Levav, P. E. Shrout, S. Schwartz, G. Naveh, B. G. Link, A. E. Skodol, and A. Stueve. 1992. Socioeconomic status and psychiatric disorders: The causation-selection issue. *Science* 255(5047):946–952.

Donohue, K. M., R. L. Miller, M. S. Perzanowski, A. C. Just, L. A. Hoepner, S. Arunajadai, S. Canfield, D. Resnick, A. M. Calafat, F. P. Perera, and R. M. Whyatt. 2013. Prenatal and postnatal bisphenol A exposure and asthma development among inner-city children. *Journal of Allergy and Clinical Immunology* 131(3):736–742.

Dorfman, H., M. Srinath, K. Rockhill, and C. Hogue. 2015. The association between diabetes mellitus among American Indian/Alaska Native populations with preterm birth in eight US states from 2004–2011. *Maternal and Child Health Journal* 19(11):2419–2428.

Drury, S. S., L. Scaramella, and C. H. Zeanah. 2016. The neurobiological impact of postpartum maternal depression: Prevention and intervention approaches. *Child and Adolescent Psychiatric Clinics of North America* 25(2):179–200.

Dubow, E. F., P. Boxer, and L. R. Huesmann. 2009. Long-term effects of parents' education on children's educational and occupational success: Mediation by family interactions, child aggression, and teenage aspirations. *Merrill-Palmer Quarterly* 55(3):224–249.

Duncan, G. J. 2012. Give us this day our daily breadth. *Child Development* 83(1):6–15.

Duncan, G. J., J. Brooks-Gunn, and P. K. Klebanov. 1994. Economic deprivation and early childhood development. *Child Development* 65(2 Spec No):296–318.

Duncan, G. J., W. J. Yeung, J. Brooks-Gunn, and J. R. Smith. 1998. How much does childhood poverty affect the life chances of children? *American Sociological Review* 63(3):406–423.

Duncan, G. J., P. A. Morris, and C. Rodrigues. 2011. Does money really matter? Estimating impacts of family income on young children's achievement with data from random-assignment experiments. *Developmental Psychology* 47(5):1263–1279.

Dunn, E. C., T. W. Soare, M. R. Raffeld, D. S. Busso, K. M. Crawford, K. A. Davis, V. A. Fisher, N. Slopen, A. D. Smith, and H. Tiemeier. 2018. What life course theoretical models best explain the relationship between exposure to childhood adversity and psychopathology symptoms: Recency, accumulation, or sensitive periods? *Psychological Medicine* 48(15):2562–2572.

EdBuild. 2019. *Nonwhite school districts get $23 billion less than white districts despite serving the same number of students.* https://edbuild.org/content/23-billion/full-report.pdf (accessed July 14, 2019).

Egerter, S., C. Barclay, R. Grossman-Kahn, and P. A. Braveman. 2011a. *Violence, social disadvantage and health.* Princeton, NJ: Robert Wood Johnson Foundation.

Egerter, S., P. Braveman, T. Sadegh-Nobari, R. Grossman-Kahn, and M. Dekker. 2011b. *Education and health.* Princeton, NJ: Robert Wood Johnson Foundation.

Elder, T. E., J. H. Goddeeris, and S. J. Haider. 2016. Racial and ethnic infant mortality gaps and the role of socio-economic status. *Labour Economics* 43:42–54.

Elliott, P., D. Briggs, S. Morris, C. de Hoogh, C. Hurt, T. K. Jensen, I. Maitland, S. Richardson, J. Wakefield, and L. Jarup. 2001. Risk of adverse birth outcomes in populations living near landfill sites. *BMJ* 323(7309):363–368.

Evans, G. W. 2004. The environment of childhood poverty. *American Psychologist* 59(2):77–92.

Evans, G. W., H. N. Ricciuti, S. Hope, I. Schoon, R. H. Bradley, R. F. Corwyn, and C. Hazan. 2010. Crowding and cognitive development: The mediating role of maternal responsiveness among 36-month-old children. *Environment and Behavior* 42(1):135–148.

Evans, G. W., D. Li, and S. Sepanski Whipple. 2013. Cumulative risk and child development. *Psychological Bulletin* 139(6):1342–1396.

Fan, Y., K. V. Das, and Q. Chen. 2011. Neighborhood green, social support, physical activity, and stress: Assessing the cumulative impact. *Health and Place* 17(6):1202–1211.

Fang, X., D. S. Brown, C. S. Florence, and J. A. Mercy. 2012. The economic burden of child maltreatment in the United States and implications for prevention. *Child Abuse & Neglect* 36(2):156–165.

Farley, T. A., K. Mason, J. Rice, J. D. Habel, R. Scribner, and D. A. Cohen. 2006. The relationship between the neighbourhood environment and adverse birth outcomes. *Paediatric and Perinatal Epidemiology* 20(3):188–200.

Felitti, V. J., R. F. Anda, D. Nordenberg, D. F. Williamson, A. M. Spitz, V. Edwards, M. P. Koss, and J. S. Marks. 1998. Relationship of childhood abuse and household dysfunction to many of the leading causes of death in adults: The Adverse Childhood Experiences (ACE) Study. *American Journal of Preventive Medicine* 14(4):245–258.

Fenelon, A., N. Slopen, M. Boudreaux, and S. J. Newman. 2018. The impact of housing assistance on the mental health of children in the United States. *Journal of Health and Social Behavior* 59(3):447–463.

Feng, J., T. A. Glass, F. C. Curriero, W. F. Stewart, and B. S. Schwartz. 2010. The built environment and obesity: A systematic review of the epidemiologic evidence. *Health and Place* 16(2):175–190.

Ferguson, K. K., T. F. McElrath, and J. D. Meeker. 2014. Environmental phthalate exposure and preterm birth. *JAMA Pediatrics* 168(1):61–67.

Ferguson, K. K., J. D. Meeker, D. E. Cantonwine, B. Mukherjee, G. G. Pace, D. Weller, and T. F. McElrath. 2018. Environmental phenol associations with ultrasound and delivery measures of fetal growth. *Environment International* 112:243–250.

Filindra, A., D. Blanding, and C. García Coll. 2011. The power of context: State-level policies and politics and the educational performance of the children of immigrants in the United States. *Harvard Educational Review* 81(3):407–438.

Finegood, E. D., J. R. D. Rarick, and C. Blair. 2017. Exploring longitudinal associations between neighborhood disadvantage and cortisol levels in early childhood. *Development and Psychopathology* 29(5):1649–1662.

Finkelhor, D., R. K. Ormrod, and H. A. Turner. 2007. Re-victimization patterns in a national longitudinal sample of children and youth. *Child Abuse & Neglect* 31:479–502.

Finkelhor, D., R. K. Ormrod, and H. A. Turner. 2009. Lifetime assessment of poly-victimization in a national sample of children and youth. *Child Abuse & Neglect* 33:403–411.

Finkelhor, D., H. A. Turner, A. Shattuck, and S. L. Hamby. 2015. Prevalence of childhood exposure to violence, crime, and abuse: Results from the national survey of children's exposure to violence. *JAMA Pediatrics* 169(8):746–754.

Fleisch, A. F., H. Luttmann-Gibson, W. Perng, S. L. Rifas-Shiman, B. A. Coull, I. Kloog, P. Koutrakis, J. D. Schwartz, A. Zanobetti, C. S. Mantzoros, M. W. Gillman, D. R. Gold, and E. Oken. 2017. Prenatal and early life exposure to traffic pollution and cardiometabolic health in childhood. *Pediatric Obesity* 12(1):48–57.

Fone, D., F. Dunstan, K. Lloyd, G. Williams, J. Watkins, and S. Palmer. 2007. Does social cohesion modify the association between area income deprivation and mental health? A multilevel analysis. *International Journal of Epidemiology* 36(2):338–345.

Fortin, M., G. Muckle, E. Anassour-Laouan-Sidi, S. W. Jacobson, J. L. Jacobson, and R. E. Belanger. 2016. Trajectories of alcohol use and binge drinking among pregnant Inuit women. *Alcohol and Alcoholism* 51(3):339–346.

Fortson, B. L., J. Klevens, M. T. Merrick, L. K. Gilbert, and S. P. Alexander. 2016. *Preventing child abuse and neglect: A technical package for policy, norm, and programmatic activities.* Atlanta, GA: National Center for Injury Prevention and Control, Centers for Disease Control and Prevention.

Fraser, A., C. Macdonald-Wallis, K. Tilling, A. Boyd, J. Golding, G. Davey Smith, J. Henderson, J. Macleod, L. Molloy, A. Ness, S. Ring, S. M. Nelson, and D. A. Lawlor. 2012. Cohort profile: The Avon Longitudinal Study of Parents and Children: ALSPAC mothers cohort. *International Journal of Epidemiology* 42(1):97–110.

Friedman-Krauss, A. H., W. S. Barnett, G. G. Weisenfeld, R. Kasmin, N. DiCrecchio, and M. Horowitz. 2018. *The state of preschool 2017. State preschool yearbook.* New Brunswick, NJ: National Institute for Early Education Research.

García Coll, C., F. Patton, A. K. Marks, R. Dimitrova, H. Yang, G. Suarez-Aviles, and A. Batchelor. 2012. Understanding the immigrant paradox in youth: Developmental and contextual considerations. In *Realizing the potential of immigrant youth*, edited by A. S. Masten, K. Liebkind, and D. J. Hernandez. New York: Cambridge University Press.

Garner, A. S., and J. P. Shonkoff. 2012. Early childhood adversity, toxic stress, and the role of the pediatrician: Translating developmental science into lifelong health. *Pediatrics* 129(1):e224–e231.

Gascon, M., D. Valvi, J. Forns, M. Casas, D. Martinez, J. Julvez, N. Monfort, R. Ventura, J. Sunyer, and M. Vrijheid. 2015. Prenatal exposure to phthalates and neuropsychological development during childhood. *International Journal of Hygiene and Environmental Health* 218(6):550–558.

Genovesi, A. L., B. Hastings, E. Edgerton, and L. Olson. 2014. Pediatric emergency care capabilities of Indian health service emergency medical service agencies serving American Indians/Alaska Natives in rural and frontier. *Rural and Remote Health* 14(2):2688.

Georgieff, M. K., K. E. Brunette, and P. V. Tran. 2015. Early life nutrition and neural plasticity. *Development and Psychopathology* 27(2):411–423.

Gilbert, R., A. Kemp, J. Thoburn, P. Sidelbotham, L. Radford, and D. Glaser. 2009. Recognising and responding to child maltreatment. *The Lancet* 373:167–180.

Giordano, G. N., H. Ohlsson, K. S. Kendler, K. Sundquist, and J. Sundquist. 2014. Unexpected adverse childhood experiences and subsequent drug use disorder: A Swedish population study (1995–2011). *Addiction* 109(7):1119–1127.

Giudice, L., T. Woodruff, and J. Conry. 2017. Reproductive and developmental environmental health. *Obstetrics, Gynaecology & Reproductive Medicine* 27(3):99–101.

Giurgescu, C., B. L. McFarlin, J. Lomax, C. Craddock, and A. Albrecht. 2011. Racial discrimination and the black-white gap in adverse birth outcomes: A review. *Journal of Midwifery & Women's Health* 56(4):362–370.

Goodman, S. H., and J. Garber. 2017. Evidence-based interventions for depressed mothers and their young children. *Child Development* 88(2):368–377.

Goodman, S. H., M. H. Rouse, A. M. Connell, M. R. Broth, C. M. Hall, and D. Heyward. 2011. Maternal depression and child psychopathology: A meta-analytic review. *Clinical Child and Family Psychology Review* 14(1):1–27.

Goossens, J. 2018. Barriers and facilitators to the provision of preconception care by healthcare providers: A systematic review. *International Journal of Nursing Studies* 87C:113–130.

Gore, A., V. A. Chappell, S. Fenton, J. Flaws, A. Nadal, G. Prins, J. Toppari, and R. Zoeller. 2015. Executive summary to EDC-2: The Endocrine Society's second scientific statement on endocrine-disrupting chemicals. *Endocrine Reviews* 36(6):593–602.

Greaves, L., A. P. Pederson, and N. Poole. 2014. *Making it better: Gender-transformative health promotion.* Toronto, Ontario: Canadian Scholars' Press.

Guess, T. J. 2006. The social construction of whiteness: Racism by intent, racism by consequence. *Critical Sociology* 32(4):649–673.

Gutierrez-Galve, L., A. Stein, L. Hanington, J. Heron, and P. Ramchandani. 2015. Paternal depression in the postnatal period and child development: Mediators and moderators. *Pediatrics* 135(2):e339–e347.

Ha, S., H. Hu, J. Roth, H. Kan, and X. Xu. 2015. Associations between residential proximity to power plants and adverse birth outcomes. *American Journal of Epidemiology* 182(3):215–224.

Hahn, R. A., W. S. Barnett, J. A. Knopf, B. I. Truman, R. L. Johnson, J. E. Fielding, C. Muntaner, C. P. Jones, M. T. Fullilove, and P. C. Hunt. 2016. Early childhood education to promote health equity: A community guide systematic review. *Journal of Public Health Management and Practice* 22(5):e1–e8.

Hahn-Holbrook, J., M. G. Haselton, C. Dunkel Schetter, and L. M. Glynn. 2013. Does breastfeeding offer protection against maternal depressive symptomatology?: A prospective study from pregnancy to 2 years after birth. *Archives of Women's Mental Health* 16(5):411–422.

Harder, T., R. Bergmann, G. Kallischnigg, and A. Plagemann. 2005. Duration of breastfeeding and risk of overweight: A meta-analysis. *American Journal of Epidemiology* 162(5):397–403.

Harkness, J., and S. J. Newman. 2005. Housing affordability and children's well-being: Evidence from the national survey of America's families. *Housing Policy Debate* 16(2):223–255.

Harley, K. G., R. B. Gunier, K. Kogut, C. Johnson, A. Bradman, A. M. Calafat, and B. Eskenazi. 2013. Prenatal and early childhood bisphenol A concentrations and behavior in school-aged children. *Environmental Research* 126:43–50.

Harrington, J., J. Lutomski, M. Molcho, and I. J. Perry. 2009. Food poverty and dietary quality: Is there a relationship? *Journal of Epidemiology and Community Health* 63(Suppl 2):16.

Harris, M. H., D. R. Gold, S. L. Rifas-Shiman, S. J. Melly, A. Zanobetti, B. A. Coull, J. D. Schwartz, A. Gryparis, I. Kloog, P. Koutrakis, D. C. Bellinger, M. B. Belfort, T. F. Webster, R. F. White, S. K. Sagiv, and E. Oken. 2016. Prenatal and childhood traffic-related air pollution exposure and childhood executive function and behavior. *Neurotoxicology & Teratology* 57:60–70.

Hawkinson, L. E., A. S. Griffen, N. Dong, and R. A. Maynard. 2013. The relationship between child care subsidies and children's cognitive development. *Early Childhood Research Quarterly* 28(2):388–404.

Heaman, M. I., P. J. Martens, M. D. Brownell, M. J. Chartier, K. R. Thiessen, S. A. Derksen, and M. E. Helewa. 2018. Inequities in utilization of prenatal care: A population-based study in the Canadian province of Manitoba. *BMC Pregnancy Childbirth* 18(1):430.

Heard-Garris, N. J., M. Cale, L. Camaj, M. C. Hamati, and T. P. Dominguez. 2018. Transmitting trauma: A systematic review of vicarious racism and child health. *Social Science & Medicine* 199:230–240.

Heckman, J. J., J. E. Humphries, and G. Veramendi. 2018. Returns to education: The causal effects of education on earnings, health, and smoking. *Journal of Political Economy* 126(Suppl 1):S197–S246.

Hemsing, N., L. Greaves, and N. Poole. 2017. Preconception health care interventions: A scoping review. *Sexual and Reproductive Healthcare* 14:24–32.

Henry, M., R. Watt, L. Rosenthal, and A. Shivji. 2017. *The 2017 Annual Homeless Assessment Report (AHAR) to Congress.* Washington, DC: U.S. Department of Housing and Urban Development.

Herbst, C. M., and E. Tekin. 2010. Child care subsidies and child development. *Economics of Education Review* 29(4):618–638.

Hernandez, D. J. 2012. *Double jeopardy: How third-grade reading skills and poverty influence high school graduation.* Baltimore, MD: The Annie E. Casey Foundation.

HHS (U.S. Department of Health and Human Services). 2011. *The Surgeon General's call to action to support breastfeeding.* Rockville, MD: Office of the Surgeon General, Centers for Disease Control and Prevention, Office on Women's Health.

HHS. 2019. *Child maltreatment 2017.* Washington, DC: U.S. Department of Health and Human Services, Administration for Children and Families, Administration on Children, Youth and Families, Children's Bureau.

HHS Office of Inspector General. 2019. *Separated children placed in office of refugee resettlement care.* Washington, DC: U.S. Department of Health and Human Services.

Hibbard, R. A., L. W. Desch, and the Committee on Child Abuse and Neglect, and Council on Children with Disabilities. 2007. Maltreatment of children with disabilities. *Pediatrics* 119(5):1018–1025.

Hicks, A. L., M. S. Handcock, N. Sastry, and A. R. Pebley. 2018. Sequential neighborhood effects: The effect of long-term exposure to concentrated disadvantage on children's reading and math test scores. *Demography* 55(1):1–31.

Hodgkinson, S., L. Godoy, L. S. Beers, and A. Lewin. 2017. Improving mental health access for low-income children and families in the primary care setting. *Pediatrics* 139(1):e20151175.

Hoffman, S., and M. C. Hatch. 1996. Stress, social support and pregnancy outcome: A reassessment based on recent research. *Paediatric and Perinatal Epidemiology* 10(4):380–405.

Hopenhayn, C., C. Ferreccio, S. R. Browning, B. Huang, C. Peralta, H. Gibb, and I. Hertz-Picciotto. 2003. Arsenic exposure from drinking water and birth weight. *Epidemiology* 14(5):593–602.

Horta, B. L., C. Loret de Mola, and C. G. Victora. 2015. Long-term consequences of breast-feeding on cholesterol, obesity, systolic blood pressure and type 2 diabetes: A systematic review and meta-analysis. *Acta Paediatrica* 104(467):30–37.

Hughes, K., M. A. Bellis, K. A. Hardcastle, D. Sethi, A. Butchart, C. Mikton, L. Jones, and M. P. Dunne. 2017. The effect of multiple adverse childhood experiences on health: A systematic review and meta-analysis. *Lancet Public Health* 2(8):e356–e366.

Hung, P., K. B. Kozhimannil, M. Casey, and C. Henning-Smith. 2017. *State variability in access to hospital-based obstetric services in rural U.S. counties.* Minneapolis, MN: University of Minnesota Rural Health Research Center.

Hussein, N., J. Kai, and N. Qureshi. 2016. The effects of preconception interventions on improving reproductive health and pregnancy outcomes in primary care: A systematic review. *European Journal of General Practice* 22(1):42–52.

Hutchinson, R. N., M. A. Putt, L. T. Dean, J. A. Long, C. A. Montagnet, and K. Armstrong. 2009. Neighborhood racial composition, social capital and black all-cause mortality in Philadelphia. *Social Science & Medicine* 68(10):1859–1865.

Hwang, M., A. Shrestha, S. Yazzie, and M. Jackson. 2013. Preterm birth among American Indian/Alaskan Natives in Washington and Montana: Comparison with non-Hispanic whites. *Maternal and Child Health Journal* 17(10):1908–1912.

Iliopoulou, I. M. S. M., P. Kanavidis, I. Matsoukis, and E. Petridou. 2012. Pregnancy outcomes linked to intimate partner violence: A systematic review. *Injury Prevention* 18(Suppl 1):A184.

IOM (Institute of Medicine). 1990. *Nutrition during pregnancy. Part I: Weight gain, part II: Nutrient supplements.* Washington, DC: National Academy Press.

IOM. 2000. *Clearing the air: Asthma and indoor air exposures.* Washington, DC: National Academy Press.

IOM. 2002. *Unequal treatment: Confronting racial and ethnic disparities in health care.* Washington, DC: The National Academies Press.

IOM. 2004. *Damp indoor spaces and health.* Washington, DC: The National Academies Press.

IOM and NRC (National Research Council). 2014. *New directions in child abuse and neglect research.* Washington, DC: The National Academies Press.

Ip, S., M. Chung, G. Raman, P. Chew, N. Magula, D. DeVine, T. Trikalinos, and J. Lau. 2007. Breastfeeding and maternal and infant health outcomes in developed countries. *Evidence Report/Technology Assessment* 153:1–186.

Jiang, Y., M. Ekono, and C. Skinner. 2016. *Basic facts about low-income children: Children under 18 years*. New York: National Center for Children in Poverty, Mailman School of Public Health, Columbia University.

Jim, M., E. Arias, D. Seneca, M. Hoopes, C. Jim, N. Johnson, and C. Wiggins. 2014. Racial misclassification of American Indians and Alaska Natives by Indian Health Service contract health service delivery area. *American Journal of Public Health* 104(Suppl 3):S295–S302.

Johnson, A., R. Kirk, K. L. Rosenblum, and M. Muzik. 2015. Enhancing breastfeeding rates among African American women: A systematic review of current psychosocial interventions. *Breastfeeding Medicine: The Official Journal of the Academy of Breastfeeding Medicine* 10:45–62.

Johnson, R. C. 2011. *Long-run impacts of school desegregation & school quality*. Cambridge, MA: National Bureau of Economic Research.

Johnson, S. B., J. L. Riis, and K. G. Noble. 2016. State of the art review: Poverty and the developing brain. *Pediatrics* 137(4):e20153075.

Joint Center for Housing Studies of Harvard University. 2017. *America's rental housing 2017*. Cambridge, MA: Harvard University.

Joint Center for Housing Studies of Harvard University. 2018. The state of the nation's housing 2018. Cambridge, MA: Harvard University.

Jokela, M. 2014. Are neighborhood health associations causal? A 10-year prospective cohort study with repeated measurements. *American Journal of Epidemiology* 180(8):776–784.

Jokela, M. 2015. Does neighbourhood deprivation cause poor health? Within-individual analysis of movers in a prospective cohort study. *Journal of Epidemiology and Community Health* 69(9):899–904.

Jones, C. P. 2000. Levels of racism: A theoretic framework and a gardener's tale. *American Journal of Public Health* 90(8):1212–1215.

Jones, K. M., M. L. Power, J. T. Queenan, and J. Schulkin. 2015. Racial and ethnic disparities in breastfeeding. *Breastfeeding Medicine: The Official Journal of the Academy of Breastfeeding Medicine* 10(4):186–196.

Just, A. C., R. M. Whyatt, R. L. Miller, A. G. Rundle, Q. Chen, A. M. Calafat, A. Divjan, M. J. Rosa, H. Zhang, F. P. Perera, I. F. Goldstein, and M. S. Perzanowski. 2012. Children's urinary phthalate metabolites and fractional exhaled nitric oxide in an urban cohort. *American Journal of Respiratory and Critical Care Medicine* 186(9):830–837.

Kainz, K., and Y. Pan. 2014. Segregated school effects on first grade reading gains: Using propensity score matching to disentangle effects for African-American, Latino, and European-American students. *EARCHI Early Childhood Research Quarterly* 29(4):531–537.

Kaiser, P., A. V. Diez Roux, M. Mujahid, M. Carnethon, A. Bertoni, S. D. Adar, S. Shea, R. McClelland, and L. Lisabeth. 2016. Neighborhood environments and incident hypertension in the Multi-ethnic Study of Atherosclerosis. *American Journal of Epidemiology* 183(11):988–997.

Kaiser Family Foundation. 2017. *Health insurance coverage of children 0–18*. https://www.kff.org/other/state-indicator/children-0-18/?currentTimeframe=0&sortModel=%7B%22colId%22:%22Uninsured%22,%22sort%22:%22desc%22%7D (accessed April 12, 2019).

Kalter, H. 2003. Teratology in the 20th century: Environmental causes of congenital malformations in humans and how they were established. *Neurotoxicology and Teratology* 25(2):131–282.

Kapaya, H., E. Mercer, F. Boffey, G. Jones, C. Mitchell, and D. Anumba. 2015. Deprivation and poor psychosocial support are key determinants of late antenatal presentation and poor fetal outcomes—a combined retrospective and prospective study. *BMC Pregnancy Childbirth* 15:309.

Kaufman, J. S., N. Dole, D. A. Savitz, and A. H. Herring. 2003. Modeling community-level effects on preterm birth. *Annals of Epidemiology* 13(5):377–384.

Kaushal, N., and L. Nepomnyaschy. 2009. Wealth, race/ethnicity, and children's educational outcomes. *Children and Youth Services Review* 31(9):963–971.

Kearney, M. S., B. H. Harris, E. Jácome, and L. Parker. 2014. *Ten economic facts about crime and incarceration in the United States.* Washington, DC: The Hamilton Project.

Kenney, M. K., and G. K. Singh. 2016. Adverse childhood experiences among American Indian/Alaska Native children: The 2011–2012 national survey of children's health. *Scientifica* 2016:7424239.

Kerker, B. D., J. Zhang, E. Nadeem, R. E. Stein, M. S. Hurlburt, A. Heneghan, and S. McCue Horwitz. 2015. Adverse childhood experiences and mental health, chronic medical conditions, and development in young children. *Academic Pediatrics* 15:510–517.

Kersten, E. E., K. Z. LeWinn, L. Gottlieb, D. P. Jutte, and N. E. Adler. 2014. San Francisco children living in redeveloped public housing used acute services less than children in older public housing. *Health Affairs* 33(12):2230–2237.

Kids Count Data Center. 2019. *Children living in high poverty areas by race and ethnicity in the United States.* https://datacenter.kidscount.org/data/tables/7753-children-living-in-areas-of-concentrated-poverty-by-race-and-ethnicity (accessed July 15, 2019).

Kilpatrick, S. J., L.-A. Papile, and G. A. Macones. 2017. *Guidelines for perinatal care.* Washington, DC: American Academy of Pediatrics.

Kim, M. A., and K. A. Williams. 2017. Lead levels in landfill areas and childhood exposure: An integrative review. *Public Health Nursing* 34(1):87–97.

Kim, S., L. England, C. Shapiro-Mendoza, H. Wilson, J. Klejka, M. Tucker, C. Lewis, and J. Kendrick. 2014. Community and federal collaboration to assess pregnancy outcomes in Alaska Native women, 1997–2005. *Maternal and Child Health Journal* 18(3):634–639.

Knopf, J. A., R. K. Finnie, Y. Peng, R. A. Hahn, B. I. Truman, M. Vernon-Smiley, V. C. Johnson, R. L. Johnson, J. E. Fielding, C. Muntaner, P. C. Hunt, C. Phyllis Jones, M. T. Fullilove, and Community Preventive Services Task Force. 2016. School-based health centers to advance health equity: A community guide systematic review. *American Journal of Preventive Medicine* 51(1):114–126.

Koball, H., and Y. Jiang. 2018a. *Basic facts about low-income children. Children under 18 years, 2016.* New York: National Center for Children in Poverty, Columbia University Mailman School of Public Health.

Koball, H., and Y. Jiang. 2018b. *Basic facts about low-income children: Children under 9 years, 2016.* New York: National Center for Children in Poverty, Columbia University Mailman School of Public Health.

Koball, H., R. Capps, S. Hooker, K. Perreira, A. Campetella, J. M. Pedroza, W. Monson, and S. Huerta. 2015. *Health and social service needs of U.S. citizen children with detained or deported immigrant parents.* Washington, DC: Migration Policy Institute.

Kogan, M. D., M. Kotelchuck, G. R. Alexander, and W. E. Johnson. 1994. Racial disparities in reported prenatal care advice from health care providers. *American Journal of Public Health* 84(1):82–88.

Kolarik, B., K. Naydenov, M. Larsson, C. G. Bornehag, and J. Sundell. 2008. The association between phthalates in dust and allergic diseases among Bulgarian children. *Environmental Health Perspectives* 116(1):98–103.

Krafft, C., E. E. Davis, and K. Tout. 2017. Child care subsidies and the stability and quality of child care arrangements. *Early Childhood Research Quarterly* 39:14–34.

Kramer, M. S., and R. Kakuma. 2012. Optimal duration of exclusive breastfeeding. *Cochrane Database of Systematic Reviews* 8:CD003517.

Krol, K. M., and T. Grossmann. 2018. Psychological effects of breastfeeding on children and mothers. *Bundesgesundheitsblatt Gesundheitsforschung Gesundheitsschutz* 61(8):977–985.

Kull, M. A., and R. L. Coley. 2014. Housing costs and child functioning: Processes through investments and financial strains. *Children and Youth Services Review* 39:25–38.

Kumari, M., J. Head, and M. Marmot. 2004. Prospective study of social and other risk factors for incidence of type 2 diabetes in the Whitehall II Study. *Archives of Internal Medicine* 164(17):1873–1880.

Kuo, A. A., R. A. Etzel, L. A. Chilton, C. Watson, and P. A. Gorski. 2012. Primary care pediatrics and public health: Meeting the needs of today's children. *American Journal of Public Health* 102(12):e17–e23.

Lane, S. D., R. H. Keefe, R. Rubinstein, B. A. Levandowski, N. Webster, D. A. Cibula, A. K. Boahene, O. Dele-Michael, D. Carter, T. Jones, M. Wojtowycz, and J. Brill. 2008. Structural violence, urban retail food markets, and low birth weight. *Health and Place* 14(3):415–423.

Langley-Evans, S. C. 2015. Nutrition in early life and the programming of adult disease: A review. *Journal of Human Nutrition and Dietetics* 28(Suppl 1):1–14.

Lanphear, B. P., R. S. Kahn, O. Berger, P. Auinger, S. M. Bortnick, and R. W. Nahhas. 2001. Contribution of residential exposures to asthma in US children and adolescents. *Pediatrics* 107(6):e98.

Lau, E. Y., J. Liu, E. Archer, S. M. McDonald, and J. Liu. 2014. Maternal weight gain in pregnancy and risk of obesity among offspring: A systematic review. *Journal of Obesity* 2014(524939).

Leeners, B., W. Rath, E. Block, G. Gorres, and S. Tschudin. 2014. Risk factors for unfavorable pregnancy outcome in women with adverse childhood experiences. *Journal of Perinatal Medicine* 42(2):171–178.

Lefmann, T., and T. Combs-Orme. 2014. Prenatal stress, poverty, and child outcomes. *Child and Adolescent Social Work Journal* 31(6):577–590.

Leininger, L. J. 2009. Partial-year insurance coverage and the health care utilization of children. *Medical Care Research and Review* 66(1):49–67.

Leininger, L., and H. Levy. 2015. Child health and access to medical care. *The Future of Children* 25(1):65–90.

Leonard, S. A., K. M. Rasmussen, J. C. King, and B. Abrams. 2017. Trajectories of maternal weight from before pregnancy through postpartum and associations with childhood obesity. *American Journal of Clinical Nutrition* 106(5):1295–1301.

Leventhal, T., and S. Newman. 2010. Housing and child development. *Children and Youth Services Review* 32(9):1165–1174.

Lewis, M., and L. Myhra. 2018. Integrated care with indigenous populations: Considering the role of health care systems in health disparities. *Journal of Health Care for the Poor and Underserved* 29(3):1083–1107.

Li, Y., C. Margerison-Zilko, K. L. Strutz, and C. Holzman. 2018. Life course adversity and prior miscarriage in a pregnancy cohort. *Women's Health Issues* 28(3):232–238.

Lidsky, T. I., and J. S. Schneider. 2003. Lead neurotoxicity in children: Basic mechanisms and clinical correlates. *Brain* 126(1):5–19.

Lieb, R., K. R. Merikangas, M. Hofler, H. Pfister, B. Isensee, and H. U. Wittchen. 2002. Parental alcohol use disorders and alcohol use and disorders in offspring: A community study. *Psychological Medicine* 32(1):63–78.

Line, B., and L. Poon. 2013. How other countries handle immigration. *National Geographic*, https://news.nationalgeographic.com/news/2013/06/130630-immigration-reform-world-refugees-asylum-canada-japan-australia-sweden-denmark-united-kingdom-undocumented-immigrants (accessed April 23, 2019).

Liu, C., B. Vinnerljung, V. Östberg, K. Gauffin, S. Juarez, S. Cnattingius, and A. Hjern. 2018. Out-of-home care and subsequent preterm delivery: An intergenerational cohort study. *Pediatrics* 142(2):e20172729.

Lodge, C. J., D. J. Tan, M. X. Lau, X. Dai, R. Tham, A. J. Lowe, G. Bowatte, K. J. Allen, and S. C. Dharmage. 2015. Breastfeeding and asthma and allergies: A systematic review and meta-analysis. *Acta Paediatrica* 104(467):38–53.

Lu, Q., M. C. Lu, and C. D. Schetter. 2005. Learning from success and failure in psychosocial intervention: An evaluation of low birth weight prevention trials. *Journal of Health Psychology* 10(2):185–195.

Luthar, S. 2006. Resilience in development: A synthesis of research across five decades. In *Developmental psychopathology*, 3rd ed. Vol. 2, *Risk, disorder, and adaptation*, edited by D. Cicchetti and D. J. Cohen. New York: Wiley. Pp. 740–795.

Luthar, S. S., N. E. Suchman, and M. Altomare. 2007. Relational psychotherapy mothers' group: A randomized clinical trial for substance abusing mothers. *Development and Psychopathology* 19(1):243–261.

Ma, C. T., L. Gee, and M. B. Kushel. 2008. Associations between housing instability and food insecurity with health care access in low-income children. *Ambulatory Pediatrics* 8(1):50–57.

Ma, X., J. Liu, J. W. Hardin, G. Zhao, and A. D. Liese. 2016. Neighborhood food access and birth outcomes in South Carolina. *Maternal and Child Health Journal* 20(1):187–195.

Mameli, C., S. Mazzantini, and G. V. Zuccotti. 2016. Nutrition in the first 1000 days: The origin of childhood obesity. *International Journal of Environmental Research and Public Health* 13(9):838.

Manikkam, M., R. Tracey, C. Guerrero-Bosagna, and M. K. Skinner. 2013. Plastics derived endocrine disruptors (BPA, DEHP and DBP) induce epigenetic transgenerational inheritance of obesity, reproductive disease and sperm epimutations. *PLoS ONE* 8(1):e55387.

March of Dimes. 2018. *Vitamins and other nutrients during pregnancy.* https://www.marchofdimes.org/pregnancy/vitamins-and-other-nutrients-during-pregnancy.aspx (accessed April 22, 2019).

Marchi, J., M. Berg, A. Dencker, E. K. Olander, and C. Begley. 2015. Risks associated with obesity in pregnancy, for the mother and baby: A systematic review of reviews. *Obesity Reviews* 16(8):621–638.

Margerison-Zilko, C., C. Cubbin, J. Jun, K. Marchi, K. Fingar, and P. Braveman. 2015. Beyond the cross-sectional: Neighborhood poverty histories and preterm birth. *American Journal of Public Health* 105(6):1174–1180.

Margolin, G., and E. B. Gordis. 2004. Children's exposure to violence in the family and community. *Current Directions in Psychological Science* 13(4):152–155.

Markowitz, G., and D. Rosner. 2014. *Lead wars: The politics of science and the fate of America's children*, Vol. 24. Berkeley, CA: University of California Press.

Marks, A. K., J. L. McKenna, and C. García Coll. 2018. National immigration receiving contexts: A critical aspect of native-born, immigrant, and refugee youth well-being. *European Psychologist* 23(1):6–20.

Marques, A., T. O'Connor, C. Roth, E. Susser, and A.-L. Bjørke-Monsen. 2013. The influence of maternal prenatal and early childhood nutrition and maternal prenatal stress on offspring immune system development and neurodevelopmental disorders. *Frontiers in Neuroscience* 7:120.

Martin, A., R. A. Razza, and J. Brooks-Gunn. 2012. Specifying the links between household chaos and preschool children's development. *Early Child Development and Care* 182(10):1247–1263.

Masho, S. W., S. Cha, D. A. Chapman, and D. Chelmow. 2017. Understanding the role of violence as a social determinant of preterm birth. *American Journal of Obstetrics and Gynecology* 216(2):183.e1–183.e7.

Masten, A. S. 2014. *Ordinary magic: Resilience in development.* New York: Guilford Press.

Masten, A. S., J. J. Cutuli, J. E. Herbers, E. Hinz, J. Obradović, and A. J. Wenzel. 2014. Academic risk and resilience in the context of homelessness. *Child Development Perspectives* 8(4):201–206.

Matheson, S. L., M. Kariuki, M. J. Green, K. Dean, F. Harris, S. Tzoumakis, M. Tarren-Sweeney, S. Brinkman, M. Chilvers, T. Sprague, V. J. Carr, and K. R. Laurens. 2017. Effects of maltreatment and parental schizophrenia spectrum disorders on early childhood social-emotional functioning: A population record linkage study. *Epidemiology and Psychiatric Sciences* 26(6):612–623.

Mathews, T. J., and M. F. MacDorman. 2007. Infant mortality statistics from the 2004 period linked birth/infant death data set. *National Vital Statistics Reports* 55(14):1–32. Hyattsville, MD: National Center for Health Statistics.

Mathur, A. 2016. *Childcare costs: Yet another way we're failing the poor.* http://www.aei.org/publication/childcare-costs-yet-another-way-were-failing-the-poor (accessed July 14, 2019).

McGowan, P. O., and S. G. Matthews. 2018. Prenatal stress, glucocorticoids, and developmental programming of the stress response. *Endocrinology* 159(1):69–82.

Medlin, C., and E. McDonald. 2018. *Map the meal gap 2018. A report on county and congressional district food insecurity and county food cost in the United States in 2016.* Chicago, IL: Feeding American.

Mehra, R., L. M. Boyd, and J. R. Ickovics. 2017. Racial residential segregation and adverse birth outcomes: A systematic review and meta-analysis. *Social Science & Medicine* 191:237–250.

Meijer, M., K. Bloomfield, and G. Engholm. 2013. Neighbourhoods matter too: The association between neighbourhood socioeconomic position, population density and breast, prostate and lung cancer incidence in Denmark between 2004 and 2008. *Journal of Epidemiology and Community Health* 67(1):6–13.

Merrick, M. T., D. C. Ford, K. A. Ports, and A. S. Guinn. 2018. Prevalence of adverse childhood experiences from the 2011–2014 Behavioral Risk Factor Surveillance System in 23 states. *JAMA Pediatrics* 172(11):1038–1044.

Messer, L. C., J. S. Kaufman, N. Dole, A. Herring, and B. A. Laraia. 2006. Violent crime exposure classification and adverse birth outcomes: A geographically-defined cohort study. *International Journal of Health Geographics* 5:22.

Meyer, B. D., and J. X. Sullivan. 2009. *Five decades of consumption and income poverty.* Working paper 14827. Cambridge, MA: National Bureau of Economic Research.

Miao, M., W. Yuan, Y. He, Z. Zhou, J. Wang, E. Gao, G. Li, and D. K. Li. 2011. In utero exposure to bisphenol-A and anogenital distance of male offspring. *Birth Defects Research (Part A)* 91(10):867–872.

Midoro-Horiuti, T., R. Tiwari, C. S. Watson, and R. M. Goldblum. 2010. Maternal bisphenol A exposure promotes the development of experimental asthma in mouse pups. *Environmental Health Perspectives* 118(2):273–277.

Mikati, I., A. F. Benson, T. J. Luben, J. D. Sacks, and J. Richmond-Bryant. 2018. Disparities in distribution of particulate matter emission sources by race and poverty status. *American Journal of Public Health* 108(4):480–485.

Miller, P. 2011. A critical analysis of the research on student homelessness. *Review of Educational Research* 81(3):308–337.

Miranda, M. L., S. E. Edwards, H. H. Chang, and R. L. Auten. 2013. Proximity to roadways and pregnancy outcomes. *Journal of Exposure Science & Environmental Epidemiology* 23(1):32–38.

Moffitt, T. E., and K.-G. T. Tank. 2013. Childhood exposure to violence and lifelong health; clinical intervention science and stress-biology research join forces. *Developmental Psychopathology* 24:1619–1634.

Monasta, L., G. D. Batty, A. Cattaneo, V. Lutje, L. Ronfani, F. J. Van Lenthe, and J. Brug. 2010. Early-life determinants of overweight and obesity: A review of systematic reviews. *Obesity Reviews* 11(10):695–708.

Morenoff, J. D. 2003. Neighborhood mechanisms and the spatial dynamics of birth weight. *American Journal of Sociology* 108(5):976–1017.

Morgan, I., and A. Amerikaner. 2018. *An Analysis of School Funding Equity across the U.S. and within Each State.* Washington, DC: The Education Trust.

Morrison, S., E. D. Shenassa, P. Mendola, T. Wu, and K. Schoendorf. 2013. Allostatic load may not be associated with chronic stress in pregnant women, NHANES 1999–2006. *Annals of Epidemiology* 23(5):294–297.

Motti-Stefanidi, F., and C. García Coll. 2018. We have come a long way, baby: "Explaining positive adaptation of immigrant youth across cultures." *Journal of Adolescence* 62:218–221.

Muller, C., R. J. Sampson, and A. S. Winter. 2018. Environmental inequality: The social causes and consequences of lead exposure. *Annual Review of Sociology* 44:263–282.

Nakamura, K., K. Itoh, H. Dai, L. Han, X. Wang, S. Kato, T. Sugimoto, and S. Fushiki. 2012. Prenatal and lactational exposure to low-doses of bisphenol A alters adult mice behavior. *Brain and Development* 34(1):57–63.

NASEM (National Academies of Sciences, Engineering, and Medicine). 2015a. *Mental disorders and disabilities among low-income children.* Washington, DC: The National Academies Press.

NASEM. 2015b. *The integration of immigrants into American society.* Washington, DC: The National Academies Press.

NASEM. 2016a. *Parenting matters: Supporting parents of children ages 0–8.* Washington, DC: The National Academies Press.

NASEM. 2016b. *Preventing bullying through science, policy, and practice.* Washington, DC: The National Academies Press.

NASEM. 2017a. *Communities in action: Pathways to health equity.* Washington, DC: The National Academies Press.

NASEM. 2017b. *Promoting the educational success of children and youth learning English: Promising futures.* Washington, DC: The National Academies Press.

NASEM. 2018. *Transforming the financing of early care and education.* Washington, DC: The National Academies Press.

NASEM. 2019. *A roadmap to reducing child poverty.* Washington, DC: The National Academies Press.

National Center for Education Statistics. n.d. *Trends in high school dropout and completion rates in the United States.* https://nces.ed.gov/programs/dropout/ind_05.asp (accessed April 22, 2019).

National Congress of American Indians. n.d. *Data disaggregation. The asterisk nation.* http://www.ncai.org/policy-research-center/research-data/data (accessed April 23, 2019).

National Low Income Housing Coalition. 2018. *The gap: A shortage of affordable rental homes.* https://reports.nlihc.org/gap (accessed July 15, 2019).

National Scientific Council on the Developing Child. 2004. *Young children develop in an environment of relationships (working paper 1).* Cambridge, MA: Harvard University.

Ncube, C. N., D. A. Enquobahrie, S. M. Albert, A. L. Herrick, and J. G. Burke. 2016. Association of neighborhood context with offspring risk of preterm birth and low birthweight: A systematic review and meta-analysis of population-based studies. *Social Science & Medicine* 153:156–164.

Ness, M. N., K. D. Rosenberg, T. Abrahamson-Richards, A. P. Sandoval, T. M. Weiser, and V. Warren-Mears. 2017. Stressful life events and self-reported postpartum depressive symptoms 13–24 months after live birth among non-Hispanic American Indian/Alaska Native mothers in Oregon: Results from a population-based survey. *American Indian and Alaska Native Mental Health Research* 24(2):76–98.

Newman, S. J. 2008. Does housing matter for poor families? A critical summary of research and issues still to be resolved. *Journal of Policy Analysis and Management* 27(4):895–925.

Newman, S. J., and C. S. Holupka. 2014. Housing affordability and investments in children. *Journal of Housing Economics* 24:89–100.

Newman, S., and C. S. Holupka. 2016. Housing affordability and children's cognitive achievement. *Health Affairs* 35(11):2092–2099.

Nichols, E. B., and A. B. Loper. 2012. Incarceration in the household: Academic outcomes of adolescents with an incarcerated household member. *Journal of Youth and Adolescence* 41(11):1455–1471.

NRC and IOM. 2000. *From neurons to neighborhoods: The science of early childhood development.* Washington, DC: National Academy Press.

NRC and IOM. 2010. *Student mobility: Exploring the impacts of frequent moves on achievement: Summary of a workshop.* Washington, DC: The National Academies Press.

Nyaradi, A., J. Li, S. Hickling, J. Foster, and W. Oddy. 2013. The role of nutrition in children's neurocognitive development, from pregnancy through childhood. *Frontiers in Human Neuroscience* 7:97.

Oberg, C., S. Colianni, and L. King-Schultz. 2016. Child health disparities in the 21st century. *Current Problems in Pediatric and Adolescent Health Care* 46(9):291–312.

Obradović, J., J. D. Long, J. Cutuli, C.-K. Chan, E. Hinz, D. Heistad, and A. S. Masten. 2009. Academic achievement of homeless and highly mobile children in an urban school district: Longitudinal evidence on risk, growth, and resilience. *Development Psychopathology* 21(2):493–518.

O'Campo, P., J. G. Burke, J. Culhane, I. T. Elo, J. Eyster, C. Holzman, L. C. Messer, J. S. Kaufman, and B. A. Laraia. 2008. Neighborhood deprivation and preterm birth among non-Hispanic black and white women in eight geographic areas in the United States. *American Journal of Epidemiology* 167(2):155–163.

OECD (Organisation for Economic Co-operation and Development). 2018. Policies and practices to support the resilience of students with an immigrant background. In *The resilience of students with an immigrant background: Factors that shape well-being.* Paris, France: OECD Publishing.

Office of Child Care. n.d. *Quick fact.* https://www.acf.hhs.gov/occ/quick-fact (accessed April 22, 2019).

Office of Head Start. 2018a. *History of Head Start.* https://www.acf.hhs.gov/ohs/about/history-of-head-start (accessed April 22, 2019).

Office of Head Start. 2018b. *Head Start program facts. Fiscal year 2017.* https://eclkc.ohs.acf.hhs.gov/about-us/article/head-start-program-facts-fiscal-year-2017 (accessed April 22, 2019).

Oh, D. L., P. Jerman, S. Silverio Marques, K. Koita, S. K. Purewal Boparai, N. Burke Harris, and M. Bucci. 2018. Systematic review of pediatric health outcomes associated with childhood adversity. *BMC Pediatrics* 18(1):83.

Olivet, J., M. Dones, M. Richard, C. Wilkey, S. Yampolskaya, M. Beit-Arie, and L. Joseph. 2018. *Supporting partnerships for anti-racist communities: Phase one study findings.* Needham, MA: Center for Social Innovation.

Olsen, J. M. 2018. Integrative review of pregnancy health risks and outcomes associated with adverse childhood experiences. *Journal of Obstetric, Gynecologic, & Neonatal Nursing* 47(6):783–794.

Ore, C. E., N. Teufel-Shone, and T. M. Chico-Jarillo. 2016. American Indian and Alaska Native resilience along the life course and across generations: A literature review. *American Indian and Alaska Native Mental Health Research* 23(3):134–157.

Osofsky, J. D. 2003. Prevalence of children's exposure to domestic violence and child maltreatment: Implications for prevention and intervention. *Clinical Child and Family Psychology Review* 6(3):161–170.

Osterman, M. J. K., and J. A. Martin. 2018. Timing and adequacy of prenatal care in the United States, 2016. *National Vital Statistics Reports* 67(3):1–14.

Pac, J. E., A. P. Bartel, C. J. Ruhm, and J. Waldfogel. 2019. *Paid family leave and breastfeeding— evidence from California.* Cambridge, MA: National Bureau of Economic Research.

Paczkowski, M. M., and S. Galea. 2010. Sociodemographic characteristics of the neighborhood and depressive symptoms. *Current Opinion in Psychiatry* 23(4):337–341.

Padula, A. M., O. Humblet, K. Mortimer, F. Lurmann, and I. Tager. 2012. Exposure to air pollution during pregnancy and pulmonary function growth in the FACES LiTE Cohort. Meeting Abstracts. *American Journal of Respiratory and Critical Care Medicine. Conference: American Thoracic Society International Conference, ATS* 185(1):A1725.

Paradies, Y., J. Ben, N. Denson, A. Elias, N. Priest, A. Pieterse, A. Gupta, M. Kelaher, and G. Gee. 2015. Racism as a determinant of health: A systematic review and meta-analysis. *PLoS ONE* 10(9):e0138511.

Pearl, M., P. Braveman, and B. Abrams. 2001. The relationship of neighborhood socioeconomic characteristics to birthweight among 5 ethnic groups in California. *American Journal of Public Health* 91(11):1808–1814.

Petrosky, E., J. M. Blair, C. J. Betz, K. A. Fowler, S. P. D. Jack, and B. H. Lyons. 2017. Racial and ethnic differences in homicides of adult women and the role of intimate partner violence—United States, 2003–2014. *Morbidity and Mortality Weekly Report* 66(28):741–746.

Pickett, K. E., and M. Pearl. 2001. Multilevel analyses of neighbourhood socioeconomic context and health outcomes: A critical review. *Journal of Epidemiology and Community Health* 55(2):111–122.

Poston, L., L. F. Harthoorn, and E. M. Van Der Beek. 2011. Obesity in pregnancy: Implications for the mother and lifelong health of the child. A consensus statement. *Pediatric Research* 69(2):175–180.

Poulton, R., T. E. Moffitt, and P. A. Silva. 2015. The Dunedin Multidisciplinary Health and Development Study: Overview of the first 40 years, with an eye to the future. *Social Psychiatry and Psychiatric Epidemiology* 50(5):679–693.

President's Task Force on Environmental Health Risks and Safety Risks to Children. 2018. *Federal action plan to reduce childhood lead exposure.* Washington, DC: U.S. Environmental Protection Agency.

Priest, N., Y. Paradies, B. Trenerry, M. Truong, S. Karlsen, and Y. Kelly. 2013. A systematic review of studies examining the relationship between reported racism and health and wellbeing for children and young people. *Social Science & Medicine* 95:115–127.

Provençal, N., and E. B. Binder. 2015. The effects of early life stress on the epigenome: From the womb to adulthood and even before. *Experimental Neurology* 268:10–20.

Public Health Management Corporation. 2013. *Findings from the Philadelphia Urban ACE Survey.* Philadelphia, PA: The Research and Evaluation Group at Public Health Management Corporation.

Racine, N., A. Plamondon, S. Madigan, S. McDonald, and S. Tough. 2018. Maternal adverse childhood experiences and infant development. *Pediatrics* 141(4):e20172495.

Raglan, G., S. Lannon, K. Jones, and J. Schulkin. 2016. Racial and ethnic disparities in preterm birth among American Indian and Alaska Native women. *Maternal and Child Health Journal* 20(1):16–24.

Ramakrishnan, U., F. Grant, T. Goldenberg, A. Zongrone, and R. Martorell. 2012. Effect of women's nutrition before and during early pregnancy on maternal and infant outcomes: A systematic review. *Paediatric and Perinatal Epidemiology* 26(Suppl 1):285–301.

Ramchandani, P. G., L. Psychogiou, H. Vlachos, J. Iles, V. Sethna, E. Netsi, and A. Lodder. 2011. Paternal depression: An examination of its links with father, child and family functioning in the postnatal period. *Depression and Anxiety* 28(6):471–477.

Rauh, V. A., P. J. Landrigan, and L. Claudio. 2008. Housing and health. *Annals of the New York Academy of Sciences* 1136(1):276–288.

Ready, D., and M. Silander. 2011. School racial and ethnic composition and young children's cognitive development. In *Integrating schools in a changing society: New policies and legal options for a multiracial generation,* edited by E. Frankenberg and E. Debray-Pelot. Chapel Hill, NC: University of North Carolina. Pp. 91–113.

Reardon, S. F. 2016. *School district socioeconomic status, race, and academic achievement.* Stanford, CA: Stanford Center for Educational Policy Analysis.

Reeves, R. V., and E. Krause. 2019. *The effects of maternal depression on early childhood development and implications for economic mobility.* Washington, DC: The Brookings Institution.

Rentner, T. L., L. D. Dixon, and L. Lengel. 2012. Critiquing fetal alcohol syndrome health communication campaigns targeted to American Indians. *Journal of Health Communication* 17(1):6–21.

Rhodes, A. E., M. H. Boyle, J. Bethell, C. Wekerle, D. Goodman, L. Tonmyr, and I. Manion. 2012. Child maltreatment and onset of emergency department presentations for suicide-related behaviors. *Child Abuse and Neglect* 36:542–551.

Rich-Edwards, J. W., S. L. Buka, R. T. Brennan, and F. Earls. 2003. Diverging associations of maternal age with low birthweight for black and white mothers. *International Journal of Epidemiology* 32(1):83–90.

Ritsher, J. E., V. Warner, J. G. Johnson, and B. P. Dohrenwend. 2001. Inter-generational longitudinal study of social class and depression: A test of social causation and social selection models. *The British Journal of Psychiatry* 40:S84–S90.

Robinette, J. W., S. T. Charles, J. A. Mogle, and D. M. Almeida. 2013. Neighborhood cohesion and daily well-being: Results from a diary study. *Social Science & Medicine* 96:174–182.

Rojas-Flores, L., M. L. Clements, J. H. Koo, and J. London. 2017. Trauma and psychological distress in Latino citizen children following parental detention and deportation. *Psychological Trauma: Theory, Research, Practice, and Policy* 9(3):352–361.

Rutman, S., M. Taualii, D. Ned, and C. Tetrick. 2012. Reproductive health and sexual violence among urban American Indian and Alaska Native young women: Select findings from the National Survey of Family Growth (2002). *Maternal and Child Health Journal* 16(Suppl 2):347–352.

Rutman, S., L. Phillips, and A. Sparck. 2016. Health care access and use by urban American Indians and Alaska Natives: Findings from the national health interview survey (2006–09). *Journal of Health Care for the Poor and Underserved* 27(3):1521–1536.

Rutter, M. 1979. Protective factors in children's responses to stress and disadvantage. In *Primary prevention of psychopathology,* Vol. 3, edited by W. M. Kent and J. E. Rolf. Hanover, NH: University Press of New England. Pp. 49–74.

Ryan, A. S. 2007. Breastfeeding and the risk of childhood obesity. *Collegium Antropologicum* 31(1):19–28.

Ryan, J. P., B. E. Perron, and H. Huang. 2016. Child welfare and the transition to adulthood: Investigating placement status and subsequent arrests. *Journal of Youth and Adolescence* 45(1):172–182.

Saelens, B. E., J. F. Sallis, J. B. Black, and D. Chen. 2003a. Neighborhood-based differences in physical activity: An environment scale evaluation. *American Journal of Public Health* 93(9):1552–1558.

Saelens, B. E., J. F. Sallis, and L. D. Frank. 2003b. Environmental correlates of walking and cycling: Findings from the transportation, urban design, and planning literatures. *Annals of Behavioral Medicine* 25(2):80–91.

Sameroff, A. J. 1998. Environmental risk factors in infancy. *Pediatrics* 102(Suppl E1):1287–1292.

Sameroff, A., R. Seifer, M. Zax, and R. Barocas. 1987a. Early indicators of developmental risk: Rochester longitudinal study. *Schizophrenia Bulletin* 13(3):383–394.

Sameroff, A. J., R. Seifer, R. Barocas, M. Zax, and S. Greenspan. 1987b. Intelligence quotient scores of 4-year-old children: Social-environmental risk factors. *Pediatrics* 79(3):343–350.

Sampson, R. J., and A. S. Winter. 2016. The racial ecology of lead poisoning. *Du Bois Review* 13(2):261–283.

Sandel, M., and M. Desmond. 2017. Investing in housing for health improves both mission and margin. *JAMA* 318(23):2291–2292.

Sandel, M., K. Phelan, R. Wright, H. P. Hynes, and B. P. Lanphear. 2004. The effects of housing interventions on child health. *Pediatric Annals* 33(7):474–481.

Sankar, M. J. S., R. B. Chowdhury, R. N. Bhandari, S. Teneja, and J. Martines. 2015. Optimal breastfeeding practices and infant and child mortality: A systematic review and meta-analysis. *Acta Paediatrica* 104:3–13.

Santiago, C. D., S. Kaltman, and J. Miranda. 2013. Poverty and mental health: How do low-income adults and children fare in psychotherapy? *Journal of Clinical Psychology* 69(2):115–126.

Schempf, A., D. Strobino, and P. O'Campo. 2009. Neighborhood effects on birthweight: An exploration of psychosocial and behavioral pathways in Baltimore, 1995–1996. *Social Science & Medicine* 68(1):100–110.

Schmit, S., and C. Walker. 2016. *Disparate access. Head Start and CCDBG data by race and ethnicity.* Washington, DC: Center for Law and Social Policy.

Schofield, T. J., R. D. Lee, and M. T. Merrick. 2013. Safe, stable, nurturing relationships as a moderator of intergenerational continuity of child maltreatment: A meta-analysis. *Journal of Adolescent Health* 53:S32–S38.

Schwartz, M., and E. Wilson. n.d. *Who can afford to live in a home? A look at data from the 2006 American community survey.* https://www.census.gov/housing/census/publications/who-can-afford.pdf (accessed April 22, 2019).

Schwarzenberg, S. J., and M. K. Georgieff. 2018. Advocacy for improving nutrition in the first 1000 days to support childhood development and adult health. *Pediatrics* 141(2):e20173716.

Sedlak, A. J., J. Mettenburg, M. Basena, I. Petta, K. McPherson, A. Greene, and S. Li. 2010. *Fourth National Incidence Study of Child Abuse and Neglect (NIS-4): Report to Congress.* Washington, DC: U.S. Department of Health and Human Services, Administration for Children and Families.

Sharfstein, J., M. Sandel, R. Kahn, and H. Bauchner. 2001. Is child health at risk while families wait for housing vouchers? *American Journal of Public Health* 91(8):1191–1192.

Sharkey, P. 2010. The acute effect of local homicides on children's cognitive performance. *Proceedings of the National Academy of Sciences of the United States of America* 107(26):11733–11738.

Sharkey, P. T., N. Tirado-Strayer, A. V. Papachristos, and C. C. Raver. 2012. The effect of local violence on children's attention and impulse control. *American Journal of Public Health* 102(12):2287–2293.

Sheffield, P. E., R. A. Coulombe, R. Speranza, Y.-H. M. Chiu, H.-H. L. Hsu, P. C. Curtin, S. Renzetti, A. Pajak, B. Coull, J. Schwartz, I. Kloog, and R. J. Wright. 2018. Association between particulate air pollution exposure during pregnancy and postpartum maternal psychological functioning. *PLoS ONE* 13(4):e0195267.

Shen, H., C. Magnusson, D. Rai, M. Lundberg, F. Lê-Scherban, C. Dalman, and B. K. Lee. 2016. Associations of parental depression with child school performance at age 16 years in Sweden. *JAMA Psychiatry* 7:239–246.

Shervin, A. 2018. Health disparities due to diminished return among black Americans: Public policy solutions. *Social Issues and Policy Review* 12(1):112–145.

Shin, S. H., E. Edwards, T. Heeren, and M. Amodeo. 2009. Relationship between multiple forms of maltreatment by a parent or guardian and adolescent alcohol use. *The American Journal on Addictions* 18(3):226–234.

Shinkman, P. D. 2018. Comparing the policies and practices of detaining children. *U.S. News & World Report.* https://www.usnews.com/news/best-countries/articles/2018-06-25/how-other-countries-treatment-of-detained-migrant-children-compare-to-the-us (accessed April 23, 2019).

Shonkoff, J. P., A. S. Garner, Committee on Psychosocial Aspects of Child and Family Health, Committee on Early Childhood, Adoption, and Dependent Care, Section on Developmental and Behavioral Pediatrics. 2012. The lifelong effects of early childhood adversity and toxic stress. *Pediatrics* 129(1):e232–e246.

Singer, A. 2012. *Immigrant workers in the U.S. labor force.* Washington, DC: The Brookings Institution.

Skiba, R. J., M. I. Arredondo, and M. K. Rausch. 2014. *Discipline disparities: A research-to-practice collaborative.* Bloomington, IN: The Equity Project at Indiana University, Center for Evaluation and Education Policy.

Slopen, N., G. Fitzmaurice, D. R. Williams, and S. E. Gilman. 2010. Poverty, food insecurity, and the behavior for childhood internalizing and externalizing disorders. *Journal of the American Academy of Child and Adolescent Psychiatry* 49(5):444–452.

Smith, L., V. Li, S. Dykema, D. Hamlet, and A. Shellman. 2013. "Honoring somebody that society doesn't honor": Therapists working in the context of poverty. *Journal of Clinical Psychology* 69(2):138–151.

Smith, M. V., N. Gotman, and K. A. Yonkers. 2016. Early childhood adversity and pregnancy outcomes. *Maternal and Child Health Journal* 20(4):790–798.

Smith, S., S. Stagman, S. Blank, C. Ong, and K. McDow. 2011. *Building strong systems of support for young children's mental health: Key strategies for states and a planning tool.* New York: National Center for Children in Poverty, Mailman School of Public Health, Columbia University.

Solari, C. D., and R. D. Mare. 2012. Housing crowding effects on children's wellbeing. *Social Science Research* 41(2):464–476.

Spanier, A. J., R. S. Kahn, A. R. Kunselman, R. Hornung, Y. Xu, A. M. Calafat, and B. P. Lanphear. 2012. Prenatal exposure to bisphenol A and child wheeze from birth to 3 years of age. *Environmental Health Perspectives* 120(6):916–920.

Sternthal, M. J., H. J. Jun, F. Earls, and R. J. Wright. 2010. Community violence and urban childhood asthma: A multilevel analysis. *European Respiratory Journal* 36(6):1400–1409.

Subramanian, S. V., J. T. Chen, D. H. Rehkopf, P. D. Waterman, and N. Krieger. 2006. Comparing individual- and area-based socioeconomic measures for the surveillance of health disparities: A multilevel analysis of Massachusetts births, 1989–1991. *American Journal of Epidemiology* 164(9):823–834.

Sue, D. W. 2019. *Counseling the culturally diverse: Theory and practice,* 8th ed. Hoboken, NJ: John Wiley & Sons.

Sweeney, S., and A. MacBeth. 2016. The effects of paternal depression on child and adolescent outcomes: A systematic review. *Journal of Affective Disorders* 205:44–59.

Tabacchi, G., S. Giammanco, M. La Guardia, and M. Giammanco. 2007. A review of the literature and a new classification of the early determinants of childhood obesity: From pregnancy to the first years of life. *NTR Nutrition Research* 27(10):587–604.

Taylor, C. M., J. Golding, and A. M. Emond. 2015. Adverse effects of maternal lead levels on birth outcomes in the ALSPAC study: A prospective birth cohort study. *BJOG: An International Journal of Obstetrics and Gynaecology* 122(3):322–328.

Taylor, C. M., J. Golding, and A. M. Emond. 2016. Moderate prenatal cadmium exposure and adverse birth outcomes: A role for sex-specific differences? *Paediatric and Perinatal Epidemiology* 30(6):603–611.

The Nation's Report Card. 2017. *National achievement-level results.* https://www.nationsreportcard.gov/reading_2017/nation/achievement/?grade=4 (accessed April 22, 2019).

The Pew Charitable Trusts. 2018. *American families face a growing rent burden.* Washington, DC: The Pew Charitable Trusts.

Theall, K. P., E. A. Shirtcliff, A. R. Dismukes, M. Wallace, and S. S. Drury. 2017. Association between neighborhood violence and biological stress in children. *JAMA Pediatrics* 171(1):53–60.

Thompson, R., T. Lewis, E. C. Neilson, D. J. English, A. J. Litrownik, B. Margolis, and H. Dubowitz. 2017. Child maltreatment and risky sexual behavior. *Child Maltreatment* 22:69–78.

Thorne-Lyman, A. L., and W. W. Fawzi. 2012. Vitamin A and carotenoids during pregnancy and maternal, neonatal and infant health outcomes: A systematic review and meta-analysis. *Paediatric and Perinatal Epidemiology* 26(Suppl 1):36–54.

Trasande, L., T. M. Attina, and H. Trachtman. 2013. Bisphenol A exposure is associated with low-grade urinary albumin excretion in children of the United States. *Kidney International* 83(4):741–748.

Tsai, S. S., H. S. Yu, C. C. Chang, H. Y. Chuang, and C. Y. Yang. 2004. Increased risk of preterm delivery in women residing near thermal power plants in Taiwan. *Archives of Environmental Health* 59(9):478–483.

Twardzik, E., C. Cotto-Negron, and M. MacDonald. 2017. Factors related to early intervention Part C enrollment: A systematic review. *Disability and Health Journal* 10(4):467–474.

Uebelacker, L. A., C. B. Eaton, R. Weisberg, M. Sands, C. Williams, D. Calhoun, J. E. Manson, N. L. Denburg, and T. Taylor. 2013. Social support and physical activity as moderators of life stress in predicting baseline depression and change in depression over time in the Women's Health Initiative. *Social Psychiatry and Psychiatric Epidemiology* 48(12):1971–1982.

Ullrich, R., S. Schmitt, and R. Cosse. 2019. *Inequitable access to child care subsidies.* Washington, DC: Center for Law and Social Policy.

U.S. Census Bureau. 2015. *American Community Survey.* https://www.census.gov/topics/housing.html (accessed July 14, 2019).

Valdez, C. R., B. Padilla, S. M. Moore, and S. Magana. 2013. Feasibility, acceptability, and preliminary outcomes of the Fortalezas Familiares intervention for Latino families facing maternal depression. *Family Process* 52(3):394–410.

Valentino, R. 2018. Will public pre-K really close achievement gaps? Gaps in prekindergarten quality between students and across states. *American Educational Research Journal* 55(1):79–116.

van den Bergh, B. R. H., R. Dahnke, and M. Mennes. 2018. Prenatal stress and the developing brain: Risks for neurodevelopmental disorders. *Development and Psychopathology* 30(3):743–762.

van Lenthe, F. J., C. T. Schrijvers, M. Droomers, I. M. Joung, M. J. Louwman, and J. P. Mackenbach. 2004. Investigating explanations of socio-economic inequalities in health: The Dutch Globe Study. *European Journal of Public Health* 14(1):63–70.

Van Lieshout, R. J., V. H. Taylor, and M. H. Boyle. 2011. Pre-pregnancy and pregnancy obesity and neurodevelopmental outcomes in offspring: A systematic review. *Obesity Reviews* 12(5):e548–e559.

VanDeMark, N. R., L. A. Russell, M. O'Keefe, N. Finkelstein, C. D. Noether, and J. C. Gampel. 2005. Children of mothers with histories of substance abuse, mental illness, and trauma. *Journal of Community Psychology* 33(4):445–459.

Vandenbergh, J. G. 2004. Animal models and studies of in utero endocrine disruptor effects. *ILAR Journal* 45(4):438–442.

Veena, S. R., C. R. Gale, G. V. Krishnaveni, S. H. Kehoe, K. Srinivasan, and C. H. Fall. 2016. Association between maternal nutritional status in pregnancy and offspring cognitive function during childhood and adolescence; a systematic review. *BMC Pregnancy Childbirth* 16:220.

Vinikoor-Imler, L. C., L. C. Messer, K. R. Evenson, and B. A. Laraia. 2011. Neighborhood conditions are associated with maternal health behaviors and pregnancy outcomes. *Social Science & Medicine* 73(9):1302–1311.

Walker, C., and H. Matthews. 2017. *CCDBG participation drops to historic low.* Washington, DC: Center for Law and Social Policy.

Wallace, M., E. Harville, K. Theall, L. Webber, W. Chen, and G. Berenson. 2013. Neighborhood poverty, allostatic load, and birth outcomes in African American and white women: Findings from the Bogalusa Heart Study. *Health and Place* 24:260–266.

Wang, H. X., Y. Zhou, C. X. Tang, J. G. Wu, Y. Chen, and Q. W. Jiang. 2012. Association between bisphenol A exposure and body mass index in Chinese school children: A cross-sectional study. *Environmental Health* 11:79.

Wang, L., C. Collins, M. Ratliff, B. Xie, and Y. Wang. 2017. Breastfeeding reduces childhood obesity risks. *Childhood Obesity* 13(3):197–204.

Warren, E. J. 2018. Housing affordability and material hardship: Does affordability measurement matter? *Journal of Poverty* 22(3):228–247.

Warren, E. J., and S. A. Font. 2015. Housing insecurity, maternal stress, and child maltreatment: An application of the family stress model. *Social Service Review* 89(1):9–39.

Wathen, C. N., and H. L. Macmillan. 2013. Children's exposure to intimate partner violence: Impacts and interventions. *Paediatrics & Child Health* 18(8):419–422.

Webb, E., J. Hays, L. Dyrszka, B. Rodriguez, C. Cox, K. Huffling, and S. Bushkin-Bedient. 2016. Potential hazards of air pollutant emissions from unconventional oil and natural gas operations on the respiratory health of children and infants. *Reviews on Environmental Health* 31(2):225–243.

Weidemann, D., V. Weaver, and J. Fadrowski. 2016. Toxic environmental exposures and kidney health in children. *Pediatric Nephrology* 31(11):2043–2054.

Wheeler, W., and M. J. Brown. 2013. Blood lead levels in children aged 1–5 years—United States, 1999–2010. *Morbidity and Mortality Weekly Report* 62(13):245.

WHO (World Health Organization). n.d.-a. *Breastfeeding.* https://www.who.int/nutrition/topics/exclusive_breastfeeding/en (accessed April 22, 2019).

WHO. n.d.-b. *Exclusive breastfeeding for optimal growth, development and health of infants.* https://www.who.int/elena/titles/exclusive_breastfeeding/en (accessed April 19, 2019).

Williams, D. R., S. A. Mohammed, J. Leavell, and C. Collins. 2010. Race, socioeconomic status, and health: Complexities, ongoing challenges, and research opportunities. *Annals of the New York Academy of Sciences* 1186:69–101.

Williams, T. R. 2004. *The impacts of household wealth on child development* (CSD Working Paper No. 04-07). St. Louis, MO: Washington University, Center for Social Development.

Williams Shanks, T. R. 2007. The impacts of household wealth on child development. *Journal of Poverty* 11(2):93–116.

Williamson, A. A., L. Knox, N. G. Guerra, and K. R. Williams. 2014. A pilot randomized trial of community-based parent training for immigrant Latina mothers. *American Journal of Community Psychology* 53(1–2):47–59.

Wilson, S., and C. E. Durbin. 2010. Effects of paternal depression on fathers' parenting behaviors: A meta-analytic review. *Clinical Psychology Review* 30(2):167–180.

Winter, A. S., and R. J. Sampson. 2017. From lead exposure in early childhood to adolescent health: A Chicago birth cohort. *American Journal of Public Health* 107(9):1496–1501.

Wolf, S., K. A. Magnuson, and R. T. Kimbro. 2017. Family poverty and neighborhood poverty: Links with children's school readiness before and after the Great Recession. *Children and Youth Services Review* 79:368–384.

Wolff, M. S., S. Engel, G. Berkowitz, S. Teitelbaum, J. Siskind, D. B. Barr, and J. Wetmur. 2007. Prenatal pesticide and PCB exposures and birth outcomes. *Pediatric Research* 61(2):243–250.

Wong, C., F. Gachupin, R. Holman, M. Macdorman, J. Cheek, S. Holve, and R. Singleton. 2014. American Indian and Alaska Native infant and pediatric mortality, United States, 1999–2009. *American Journal of Public Health* 104(Suppl 3):S320–S328.

Woo Baidal, J. A., L. M. Locks, E. R. Cheng, T. L. Blake-Lamb, M. E. Perkins, and E. M. Taveras. 2016. Risk factors for childhood obesity in the first 1,000 days: A systematic review. *American Journal of Preventive Medicine* 50(6):761–779.

Woodward, N., C. E. Finch, and T. E. Morgan. 2015. Traffic-related air pollution and brain development. *Aims Environmental Science* 2(2):353–373.

Woolf, S. H., L. Aron, D. L, S. M. Simon, E. Zimmerman, and K. X. Luk. 2015. *How are income and wealth linked to health and longevity?* Washington, DC, and Richmond, VA: Urban Institute and Center on Society and Health.

Wright, A. W., M. Austin, C. Booth, and W. Kliewer. 2017. Systematic review: Exposure to community violence and physical health outcomes in youth. *Journal of Pediatric Psychology* 42(4):364–378.

Wu, F., and T. K. Takaro. 2007. Childhood asthma and environmental interventions. *Environmental Health Perspectives* 115(6):971–975.

Xue, Y., T. Leventhal, J. Brooks-Gunn, and F. J. Earls. 2005. Neighborhood residence and mental health problems of 5- to 11-year-olds. *Archives of General Psychiatry* 62(5):554–563.

Yakoob, M. Y., and C. W. Lo. 2017. Nutrition (micronutrients) in child growth and development: A systematic review on current evidence, recommendations and opportunities for further research. *Journal of Developmental and Behavioral Pediatrics* 38(8):665–679.

Yoshikawa, H. 2011. *Immigrants raising citizens: Undocumented parents and their children.* New York: Russell Sage Foundation.

Yoshikawa, H., and A. Kalil. 2011. The effects of parental undocumented status on the developmental contexts of young children in immigrant families. *Child Development Perspectives* 5(4):291–297.

Zahran, H. S., C. M. Bailey, S. A. Damon, P. L. Garbe, and P. N. Breysse. 2018. Vital signs: Asthma in children—United States, 2001–2016. *Morbidity and Mortality Weekly Report* 67(5):149.

Zamora-Kapoor, A., L. Nelson, D. Buchwald, L. Walker, and B. Mueller. 2016. Pre-eclampsia in American Indians/Alaska Natives and whites: The significance of body mass index. *Maternal and Child Health Journal* 20(11):2233–2238.

Zeka, A., S. J. Melly, and J. Schwartz. 2008. The effects of socioeconomic status and indices of physical environment on reduced birth weight and preterm births in eastern Massachusetts. *Environmental Health* 7:60.

Zerfu, T. A., and H. T. Ayele. 2013. Micronutrients and pregnancy; effect of supplementation on pregnancy and pregnancy outcomes: A systematic review. *Nutrition Journal* 12:20.

Zhan, M., and M. Sherraden. 2010. *Assets and liabilities, race/ethnicity, and children's college education: Working paper.* https://openscholarship.wustl.edu/csd_research/115 (accessed April 18, 2019).

Ziol-Guest, K. M., G. J. Duncan, and A. Kalil. 2009. Early childhood poverty and adult body mass index. *American Journal of Public Health* 99(3):527–532.

4

Fostering Caregiver Well-Being Toward Healthy Child Development

INTRODUCTION

The focus of this chapter is on how to best foster children's healthy psychosocial development, emotional adjustment, and physical health using what science has shown about risk and resilience among children and families in high-risk contexts. With the goal of systematically addressing inequities, the broad question to address is, "For those children who are at risk for negative outcomes, what can be done—guided by science-based evidence—to expediently and effectively move them toward positive developmental trajectories?" In other words, how can the playing field be leveled so that all children have the best possible opportunity to flourish and thrive in terms of their social-emotional, behavioral adjustment?

This chapter is structured in the following sections. At the outset is an overview of what developmental theory and research has demonstrated about "universals" in child development, beginning with a definition of core concepts in the phenomenon of resilience, followed by descriptions of risk and protective processes that are pervasive across diverse types of life adversities, with large and long-standing effects. Front and center among these universals are positive, supportive relationships and access to other basic and critical resources, such as good nutrition, health care, and early childhood education; these are all essential for developing children and for those charged with their care, and relevant theory and empirical evidence are provided on each. The primary focus is on fostering caregiver well-being and support, family cohesion, and social connections to promote healthy child development. This is reflected in the most proximal level to the individual child's development in the report conceptual model (see Figure 1-9). After discussions on these universals, the chapter continues with a consideration of some context-specific pathways to healthy child development: influences that are potent in and unique to particular subgroups of the population. As an example, issues of discrimination and segregation warrant attention for racial, ethnic, and sexual minorities. See Box 4-1 for an overview of this chapter.

The majority of this chapter is devoted to describing intervention programs that carry great promise in promoting positive outcomes among children in high-risk contexts. The focus is on interventions that are well grounded in developmental theory and research; have demonstrated significant improvements with replications; have moderate or substantial effect sizes with a meaningful impact for the population; and, importantly, can feasibly be taken to large scale. Methods used to deliver the interventions, to ensure fidelity (to intervention strategies), and to assess outcomes are described in detail to provide "blueprints" of science-based programs most likely to promote positive outcomes among young children and their caregivers who negotiate challenging life circumstances. For parameters and operational definitions used in this chapter, see Box 4-2.

Resilience

Under the definition of inequities (see Box 4-2) as *unequal likelihood of thriving or attaining positive adjustment outcomes* over time, the construct of resilience from developmental science is directly relevant to discussions here, as it implies correcting what otherwise might have been negative trajectories given major life stressors. Resilience can be defined as a dynamic process encompassing positive adaptation within the context of significant adversity (Cicchetti, 2010; Luthar et al., 2015; Masten, 2014). By this definition, there are two essential conditions that make up resilience: "a) exposure to significant threat, severe adversity, or trauma; and b) the achievement of positive adaptation despite major assaults on the developmental process" (Cicchetti, 2010, p. 145). With respect to a child's health, resilience is evident when physical, behavioral, and emotional well-being and development tip toward positive outcomes, even when a heavy accumulation of negative influences or risk factors exists.

Reviewing the body of accumulated scientific literature on resilience and socio-emotional functioning, Luthar et al. (2015) summarize the following core findings:

- Resilience happens across risk and age groups; there will be a subset of individuals who show some positive adaptation.
- Resilience relies fundamentally on relationships, and this is true for children and adults.

BOX 4-1
Chapter in Brief: Fostering Caregiver Well-Being

Maximizing the well-being of young children and their primary caregivers within the context of the family, and with a focus on optimizing development in circumstances that place them at risk, is of utmost importance. The committee identified nine principles of psychological and behavioral human development. For example, for all children, the single most important factor in promoting positive psychosocial, emotional, and behavioral well-being is having a strong, secure attachment to their primary caregivers; in most instances, this is their biological mother. This chapter also examines the evidence on interventions that support strong relationships and highlights promising examples.

Chapter conclusions in brief:

• The primary caretakers of children—usually the mothers—are critical to fostering child well-being, especially in high-risk circumstances. Ensuring the well-being of caretakers through ongoing support, extending beyond meeting basic needs, is necessary for child well-being.
• The most urgent parenting concern for families experiencing chronic stress and adversity is the potential for children's exposure to maltreatment.
• There is an urgent need to develop interventions well suited for fathers and other male caregivers; existing approaches that are developed for and tested with women cannot be assumed to generalize to other caregivers.
• Specific subgroups of children have unique needs and challenges when adjusting to adversity. Careful attention to potent subculture-specific processes should be considered when working with subgroups well known to face serious inequities in relation to mental health.
• A tiered approach is needed for families known to be at risk due to their life adversities, with appropriate investment of resources to expand delivery of promising cost-effective programs and assessments via scientifically sound measures of critical constructs.

Chapter recommendations in brief:

• Implement programs that ensure mothers and families have access to high-quality, cost-effective community programs, including interventions to foster strong attachments and group-based supports in communities.
• Strengthen and expand evidence-based home visiting programs.
• Support research on
  o the development of preventive interventions that target fathers and other male caregivers (with an emphasis on those that can be scaled up in the future); and
  o the development of culturally sensitive interventions that are tailored to meet the needs of subgroups of children known to be vulnerable.
• Routinely track levels of risk among mothers and children over time using periodic assessments.

BOX 4-2
Maximizing the Well-Being of Young Children and Their
Primary Caregivers: Parameters and Operational Definitions

As described in Chapter 1, "inequities" are operationally defined for the purpose of this report, in part, as the *unequal likelihood of thriving or attaining positive adjustment outcomes over time because of differences in opportunity leading to unfair and avoidable differences in health outcomes* (NASEM, 2017).

The focus in this chapter is on behavioral/psychological/socio-emotional outcomes, rather than physical health or education; there are obviously some common "protective processes" involved in affecting all of these outcomes, but there are unique important issues for health (such as immunizations, primary care, and access to safe housing) or education (such as early Head Start and high-quality child care for early education) that are addressed in the following chapters.

The focus of this chapter is on discussing how to best maximize well-being among young children and families that are vulnerable at the outset. These are individuals whose life circumstances have rendered them statistically more likely—compared to national normative samples—to be on negative adjustment trajectories from early in life onward. In the field of risk and resilience, any group demonstrated to be at significantly higher odds for negative outcomes is described as being "at risk." For the purpose of this report, the term "children in high-risk contexts" will be used, as it is the contexts in which children live, grow, and play that put them at risk.

The goal of this chapter is to describe how best to intervene to *optimize developmental trajectories across diverse groups of young children and their families in life circumstances that place them at risk for poor health outcomes.*

- Children's resilience is shaped by multiple transactional systems (i.e., proximal and distal processes and environments affect the child, and the developing child in turn affects each of these).
- Resilience is not fixed over time but is dynamic; periods of positive adaptation can be interrupted by times of struggles.

Resilience is not a unidimensional construct; among those at risk, successful adaptation in some areas (such as overt behaviors) can co-occur with difficulties in others (e.g., covert anxiety or depression). For information on physiological resilience and variability in susceptibility, see Chapter 2.

As noted above, there are important considerations for *the context within which a child exists* and how that environment affects resilience. As is true for all children—facing adversities or not—the developing child's lived experience is shaped by the family, caregivers, community, and systems that the child interacts with on a daily basis. Reis et al. (2000) identify four propositions to describe this phenomenon: (1) from conception forward, individuals exist within the context of their social relationships; (2) each relationship is nested in a social and physical environment system; (3) each relationship is embedded in larger societal and cultural systems; and (4) all of these systems are continuously changing and interacting with each other over time. For these reasons, taking a multilevel, transactional, and relationship-centered approach to understanding resilience and its determinants for children is important (Luthar et al., 2015; Reis et al., 2000).

Of particular salience and proximity are family-level influences of relationships on resilience in childhood, as will be described in detail within discussions that follow. While risk factors such as exposure to significant adversity often unfold within the context of the family, so too do the protective factors that have been shown to foster resilience, such as parental warmth, responsiveness, and sensitivity (Hamoudi et al., 2015). Therefore, the parent or primary caregiver is a major target for interventions to promote resilience in children.

Across socioeconomic strata and in most parts of the United States (and the world), the primary caregiver is generally the mother or a mother figure. It is certainly true that in general, it is better for children to have two parents in the home to share the responsibilities of child care and running the household. At the same time, even when there are two co-residing parents, one typically shoulders most of the child care, and this is generally the mother (e.g., see Ramey and Ramey, 2010). However, it should be clarified that in the discussions that follow, the term "mother" is used as a proxy for the primary caregiver who is a woman—whether that is the biological mother, grandmother, older sister, or other female relative. Considerations around men and fathers as primary caregivers are discussed separately later in this chapter, as the literature clearly indicates that there are distinct needs and issues that warrant specific, careful attention in interventions for men.

The critical importance of the parent–child relationship, specifically, is underscored in a 2017 special section published in *Child Development*, which highlights evidence-based interventions to maximize resilience in children and families. In their overview article, Luthar and Eisenberg (2017) outlined the key findings and recommendations that emerged from the collection of papers. Across these 11 papers, the single theme that most consistently recurred was the need to support the well-being of the primary caregiver—typically the mother. Contributing authors emphasized the importance of psychological and emotional support for mothers, particularly for single mothers (Taylor and Conger, 2017), those struggling with depression (Goodman and Garber, 2017), those at risk for maltreating their children (Valentino, 2017), and those living in poverty (Morris et al., 2017). A second important target for intervention identified from this set of articles was specific types of parenting behaviors that most urgently warranted attention among at-risk families. It was particularly important to minimize harsh, rejecting, or neglectful parenting behaviors (e.g., Goodman and Garber, 2017; Harold et al., 2017; Reynolds et al., 2017), because the ill effects of maltreatment on children can be profound, pervasive across areas of adjustment, and long-standing, especially when it starts early in development and is prolonged. A third target area identified as beneficial for interventions was self-regulation and coping skills among adults—parents and teachers—as well as children (e.g., Domitrovich et al., 2017; Modecki et al., 2017; Morris et al., 2017; Smith et al., 2017). Promoting self-regulation and coping for both the parent and child is essential because parents are likely to adjust their parenting behavior based on their children's behavior. Of course, for all parents living in challenging circumstances, there needs to be attention to not only their personal well-being and parenting but also the social and economic conditions that provoke the toxic stress response (discussed later in this chapter in the section on group difference).

HUMAN DEVELOPMENT IN THE CONTEXT OF RELATIONSHIPS

This chapter and the associated conclusions and recommendations are based on what is known from extant scientific literature about the major, critical building blocks to optimize the child's development from pregnancy through puberty (approximately 8–10 years of age). Sections that follow begin with a synthesis of this literature providing the basis for what are considered the universal principles of human child development, that is, principles that are largely generalizable to most children and families in the United States. Following this is a discussion of instances where children and families in discrete subcultural groups have important, unique needs, given the presence of potent risk or protective processes in their particular contexts. The remainder of this chapter is focused on a review of interventions that have been proven to be effective to promote relational supports and well-being of caregivers toward maximizing resilient adaptation.

Universals of Human Development

Universals: The Interplay of Biology and Environment in Human Development

As described in Chapter 2, during prenatal development, genetic and environmental factors work together to build organ systems that promote the ability of the individual and species to thrive and survive (Center on the Developing Child at Harvard University, 2010; National Scientific Council on the Developing Child, 2010). It is an evolutionary conserved

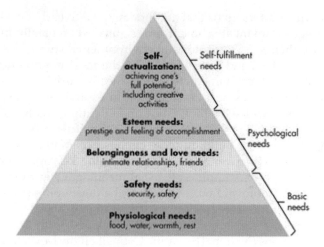

FIGURE 4-1 Maslow's hierarchy of needs.
NOTE: Concepts from Maslow, 1943.
SOURCE: McLeod, 2018.

core principle that prenatal through early childhood development is both experience dependent and experience expectant.[1] Thus, the adaptability of the organism to future challenges is influenced substantially by genetic and epigenetic factors that contribute to homeostatic boundaries within which the brain and other organ systems operate over the life course and the experiences that occur during development that the organism anticipates as the "future" contexts in which it will need to operate to survive and thrive. This core principle relates to both physical survival, which Maslow's (1943) hierarchy of needs indicates is the most basic need for all humans (children and their caregivers), and relationships that contribute to physical and behavioral well-being. See Figure 4-1 for Maslow's hierarchy pyramid.

All human circuits are built from the bottom up, with simple skills forming the foundation for the emergence of more complex skills (Center on the Developing Child at Harvard University, 2011). For sociability, the interaction between humans starts after birth, but the initial circuits

---

[1] "Experience dependent" describes the aspects of development that depend on the quality of the environmental input (e.g., while babies are born with a capacity for language development, their ability to communicate verbally will depend on their exposure to language during early development). "Experience expectant" describes the normal, generalized development when the environment provides infants with the needed input to develop neural connections that enable function in certain domains (such as vision and hearing). If input during these critical periods of development is not received, these functions will be lost permanently (Gallagher and Nelson, 2003).

needed to direct interactions that are fundamental to early development, such as caregiver–infant attachment, are established prenatally. Infants are ready to use their senses to attend to environmental stimuli—what they hear, see, smell, feel, and taste—to receive the most important information that supports their immediate internal needs, such as hunger, thirst, and arousal (Hammock and Levitt, 2006). In essence, early experiences drive a process in which the motivation and attention circuits focus more and more on those stimuli that are most meaningful—a process known as contingent learning. Building these circuits occurs in a social context with the primary caregiver and others, providing key opportunities for the infant to associate stimuli with social meaning. Over time, as social context becomes more and more complex, the developing child engages cognitive and emotional regulatory processes to infer social meaning and ultimately, social responsiveness to cues—back and forth or "serve and return" interactions (National Scientific Council on the Developing Child, 2004). These skills develop over an extended period, through adolescence (Casey et al., 2016; Dahl, 2004).

There are extended discussions pertaining to the importance of all children having their basic needs met and the existing problems that place children and families at risk, including those related to access to adequate housing, good nutrition, and health care (along with the associated barriers, ranging from parents' inability to take time off of work and lack of transportation to logistical problems deriving from the spread of critical services across physical locations and delivery systems). These issues are discussed extensively in Chapters 3 and 6.

Universals: Development in the Context of Proximal Family Relationships

The focus of this chapter is the next most basic need in Maslow's (1943) hierarchy: belongingness and love. To set the foundation for the committee's discussions on this topic, the following section outlines nine committee-generated, universal principles of human development that are derived from the scientific literature on child development in the context of relationships. To reiterate, these principles all pertain to the broad domain encompassing children's psychological and behavioral adjustment. See Box 4-3 for a list of the nine universal principles of human development.

The first principle, deriving from more than eight decades of research on resilience, is the following, mentioned earlier: *For all children, the single most important factor in promoting positive psychosocial, emotional, and behavioral well-being is having a strong, secure attachment to their primary caregivers; in most instances, this is their biological mother.* This conclusion makes good sense intuitively, as it is the primary caregiver who is the most constant and proximal person who has everyday contact with the young child

BOX 4-3
Nine Universal Principles of Psychological
and Behavioral Human Development

1. For all children, the single most important factor in promoting positive psychosocial, emotional, and behavioral well-being is having a strong, secure attachment to their primary caregivers; in most instances, this is their biological mother.
2. This strong attachment presupposes effective parenting behaviors in everyday life, and "effective parenting" changes in nature and complexity and with development over time.
3. Effective parenting presupposes the caregivers' own well-being.
4. It is critical to ensure that children's mothers have the necessary supports for maintaining good mental health and psychological well-being.
5. If there is any concern about a parent "faltering," the single most important dimension of parenting in which parents need to be helped is maltreatment (by parent figures or others).
6. The early childhood years are critical in shaping subsequent child development—but at the same time, there remains much room to change course and impact these trajectories in a positive fashion.
7. The ill effects of toxic early environments (e.g., unhealthy relationships) can manifest in physical health problems in childhood and throughout life.
8. The ill effects of early childhood adversities (e.g., abuse or neglect by caregivers) can become most visibly apparent later in life (i.e., there can be latent or "sleeper" effects that are seen at later points in development).
9. Biology is not "destiny;" rather, while indicating relative risk rates, it sets "confidence limits" within which environmental influence can lead to relatively positive versus negative adaptation.

and long-standing influence on the developing child from conception through late childhood. In most settings, this is typically the mother (relationships with fathers are also extremely important, and are discussed below). Even in families where they are employed outside the home, across socioeconomic contexts, it is typically mothers who have the earliest, most constant, and most prolonged everyday contact with the child. However, it should be noted that even when the primary caregiver is another adult, the universals that are described here would largely generalize to these other main caregivers (with a few exceptions that are discussed explicitly). See Box 4-4 for discussion of gender specificity.

Following this first universal—that a strong attachment to primary caregivers is critical for the child's well-being—the second major universal is that *this strong attachment presupposes effective parenting behaviors in everyday life, and "effective parenting" changes in nature and complexity and with development over time.* In infancy, parenting is extremely demanding

---

BOX 4-4
The Need for Gender Specificity in Referring to Parents

Developmental scientists have increasingly emphasized the need to avoid using gender-neutral terms in referring to parents in at-risk circumstances, and, instead, to describe patterns specific to fathers and mothers (see Cabrera et al., 2014; Luthar and Eisenberg, 2017; Phares et al., 2005; Rotheram-Borus et al., 2001; Yogman and Garfield, 2016). By far, most of the existing developmental studies on parenting have focused on mothers, as it is mothers who are typically primary caregivers of young children and who usually enroll and participate in intervention programs (Pruett et al., 2017). Yet, there are many instances where fathers are primarily responsible for raising their children, and their unique needs require attention: *It cannot be presumed that what helps fathers do well as parents is the same as what most benefits mothers* (Cabrera et al., 2014; Luthar and Eisenberg, 2017). To that end, differences between mothers and fathers render it critical to better understand the unique factors that shape fatherhood and child development to inform interventions. To illustrate, fathering is more affected by the quality of the marital relationship (levels of satisfaction and support) than is mothering (Lamb, 2004; Lewis and Lamb, 2003). Similarly, programs based in supportive, close relationships among women (service providers and community-based "mentor mothers") can effectively recruit mothers (Luthar, 2015; Valentino, 2017) but are unlikely to attract men as strongly. For fathers, recruitment efforts in community settings where they are commonly found, including soccer games, employment centers, and shopping malls, are more effective (Pruett et al., 2017).

---

on physical energy, and, of course, on sleep; at a psychological level, it calls for sensitivity to the child's needs and appropriate responsiveness (e.g., soothing/comforting when the child is in discomfort or pain). Often, parents are physically exhausted and not sure about how to soothe a baby who might cry inconsolably for hours. As children grow into the toddler years, in addition to providing love and comfort, effective parenting calls for constant vigilance and appropriate limit setting. During the toddler years, children are physically very mobile, oblivious to physical dangers (e.g., sharp objects or electrical outlets), increasingly and energetically willing to explore the world around them, rarely responsive to a simple "no" from adults, and prone to tantrums. The use of language as a mediator of appropriate parent–child interactions becomes increasingly complex and important. In early childhood through the onset of kindergarten and formal schooling, in addition to the primary caregiver providing love and comfort and appropriate, consistent limit setting at home, a new developmental task for the child—and thus for that caregiver—is adjustment to external influences. This subsumes the transition to child care and then to kindergarten with separation from the primary caregiver and learning to handle routines and a new set of socializing influences, including other adults plus children. During the elementary school years, failures and successes in various areas—academics, peer relations, sports, or other specialized arenas—need to be processed at the socio-emotional level. Peers and others adults can provide support to children and parents as they navigate increasingly diverse and demanding contexts.

The third universal is that *effective parenting presupposes the caregivers' own well-being*. Being able to deal with the various tasks and demands of parenting is difficult at the best of times, and this becomes particularly challenging in the presence of high levels of life stress. Chronic exposure to poverty or prolonged periods of limited resources, as well as life events involving high levels of trauma, can lead to maternal depression, anxiety, and other mental health problems, which in turn can greatly compromise the quality of parenting. There are multiple studies showing that when mothers struggle with mental illness, this can significantly affect all of their parenting behaviors (Knitzer, 2000; Luthar and Sexton, 2007; Rahman et al., 2013). In particular, maternal depression and high stress have been linked consistently with tendencies to neglectful or harsh parenting, increasing the likelihood of the child's exposure to adverse child experiences (ACEs) (Goodman and Garber, 2017; Plant et al., 2013; Toth et al., 2013; Valentino, 2017). Another important psychological element of effective parenting is parent agency or self-efficacy (i.e., the parent's perceived ability to influence the development of the child) (Jones and Prinz, 2005). The report *Parenting Matters: Supporting Parents of Children Ages 0–8* highlights parent self-efficacy as a contributing factor in shaping parenting competence and child self-regulation, social, and cognitive skills (NASEM, 2016). The report identifies one possible mechanism for this association as increased competence-promoting parenting practices (e.g., family routines or involvement with children in schools). As the current report's conceptual model in Chapter 1 suggests (see Figure 1-9), caregivers and families live in the context of their social circumstances and living conditions; therefore, they need support in coping with related stressors or eliminating such sources of stress, in addition to efficacy-promoting supports.

The first three universals have been long cited in the developmental literature; the next has been more recently emphasized explicitly: from as early in a child's life as possible, *it is critical to ensure that mothers have the necessary supports for maintaining good mental health and psychological well-being*. Resilience researchers have clearly articulated that in order to achieve positive mental health and functioning, the same principles that apply for children apply to their mothers. Just as children need ongoing unconditional love from their mothers, so do the mothers need ongoing love and support from other adults to function well across their life roles

(Luthar et al., 2015). In developmental science, for too many years, the tendency in studying families has been to discuss what parents should do and should not do, with little attention to what it is that allows parents themselves to function well and develop resilience at this daunting, decades-long task. In other words, what has been missing is mothers' well-being as the dependent variable.

In the past few years, this has changed (see Balaji et al., 2007; Jolly et al., 2014; Luthar and Ciciolla, 2015; Taylor and Conger, 2017). There is now much more explicit emphasis on the need to understand what helps mothers do well over time, especially in highly stressful life circumstances. With accumulating evidence from both basic research and intervention trials, the answer is clear: the single most important need is dependable supports in their role as parents—emotional/intangible and tangible—from a dependable, reliable network of others in their lives (for a review on this topic, see Luthar and Eisenberg, 2017). The nature of these supports, furthermore, is both perceived (e.g., the expectation that comfort will be available when distressed or help will be forthcoming if needed for parenting/running the household) and instrumental (e.g., actual receipt of help with child care or aspects of running the home; see Balaji et al., 2007; Goodman and Garber, 2017, for more information). See Box 4-5 for more on supporting caregivers.

BOX 4-5
Providing Supports for Caregivers

Recognizing the critical importance of supports for caregivers by no means implies parent blaming or minimizing parents' agency. Rather, it is intended to draw much needed attention to the great challenges of this life role and what even the most well-meaning caregiver needs, on an ongoing basis, to do this job well. As an analogy, consider the role of a surgeon. Ultimately, the physical manipulation of nerves, arteries, etc., is in his or her hands. Yet, it is common knowledge that for any surgery to go well, there needs to be high-level, ongoing supportive conditions—ranging from the assistants in the room to a sterile operating room and appropriate medications. It would be illogical to turn to any "surgeon-blaming" if a procedure failed in the absence of these various essential supports. In the same way, the first order of business in ensuring optimal child development is to ensure that all primary caregivers have the necessary supports on an ongoing basis if they are to sustain optimal parenting. Providing supports (e.g., in the form of services) does not assume any weakness on the part of the caregiver; instead, it promotes parents' agency to care for their children in the face of increasing demands as parents (e.g., work, child care) (Lino et al., 2017; NASEM, 2016; National Partnership for Women & Families, 2018).

A fifth universal, and also one more recently emphasized specifically in the literature, is that if there is *any concern about a parent "faltering," the single most important dimension of parenting in which parents need to be helped is maltreatment (by parent figures or others).*[2] In general, psychologists have shown that "bad is stronger than good" (Baumeister et al., 2001); that is, the ill effects of harsh behaviors are much stronger than the positive effects of praise (see also Fredrickson and Losada, 2005; Sparks and Baumeister, 2008). Additionally, the accumulated literature on resilience has shown that early and chronic maltreatment is the one category of adversity in which it is rare to find children who "do well" over time, showing little to no trouble across major adjustment domains; in fact, this has many serious long-term effects across salient aspects of child development (see Bolger and Patterson, 2003; Cicchetti, 2013).

Therefore, as a society, prevention of maltreatment needs to be a top priority in promoting the well-being of children in high-risk contexts. This again implies attentiveness when primary caregivers are stretched too thin, because they are at the most risk for maltreatment. As noted earlier, living with chronically high stress or mental illnesses, such as untreated depression, can lead the most well-meaning and loving parent to become angry and slip into neglectful or harsh parenting behaviors. If caregivers are believed to be at risk for abusing or neglecting their children—or of not being able to protect them from maltreatment by other adults—the situation needs to be treated as urgent and the appropriate help identified. Most importantly, the best help would be providing supports and/or mental treatment for the primary caregiver to address the root cause of maltreatment or neglect (Cicchetti, 2013; Cicchetti et al., 2006; Lieberman et al., 2005; Luthar et al., 2007; Toth et al., 2013). In the most extreme cases, continued high risk for maltreatment or actual maltreatment could entail removing the child from the home; however, there is evidence that suggests that this is not always the best course of action for the child (Toth et al., 2016).

Implicit within the above universals is that the well-being of the young child inherently involves the well-being of the primary caregiver; in fact, Seifer (2003) explicitly pointed out that it does not make sense to think about resilience of infants. Rather, we should consider the positive functioning of the mother–child dyad. Additionally, in many countries other than the United States, people think about the needs of the child through the needs of the caretaker: if the child is to be helped, that help is most effectively offered if it goes through the caretaker (e.g., see Hrdy, 1999).

---

[2] The Centers for Disease Control and Prevention (CDC) defines child maltreatment as any type of abuse (e.g., physical, sexual, or emotional) and neglect of a child under 18 years of age by a parent, caregiver, or another person in a custodial role (CDC, 2014).

In many cultural contexts, pregnancy, childbirth, and motherhood are embedded in a system of multiple generations of women who provide support and troubleshooting to the younger generations in all aspects of caretaking. Extended family systems and/or fictive kin are available and ready to help with any problem that arises; they affect the development and well-being of the child and also the mother (see Barlow and Chapin, 2010; Kopp, 2013).

To reiterate the caveat noted earlier—that in many instances, it may not be the mother but another family member (or caretaker) who serves as the primary caregiver—the principles described above are still the same; that is, whomever is charged with primary (or salient) responsibility of taking care of the young child needs to receive regular replenishment and support. Child care providers and educators also need ongoing support, including teachers from preschool onward through the K–12 system. These are all jobs that are among the lowest paid and with high levels of burnout and turnover, especially for early childhood educators. Once again, research has shown that these care and education professionals can serve critical protective functions, stepping in to provide the nurturance and support that complement or supplement what mothers, fathers, or other primary caregivers are able to offer. Yet, solutions rarely consider what it is that can and should be done to help replenish these professionals who are the primary adults during significant portions of children's daily lives. (For a more in-depth discussion of early care and education [ECE] professionals, see Chapter 7.)

Sixth, developmental research has clearly shown that *relationships in the early childhood years are critical in shaping subsequent child development— but at the same time, there remains much room to change course and impact these trajectories in a positive fashion*, with those starting out as negative changing to be more positive as well as the reverse. Without question, early attachments form the lens through which subsequent relationships are viewed (Lieberman et al., 2005; Sroufe et al., 2005; Yates et al., 2003; Zeanah and Zeanah, 1989), so that children with adverse early experiences are less likely to be open to or trusting of other nurturing people in their lives. Yet, there are certainly opportunities for reversals (e.g., at times of transition in life, including moves to new schools for children, and, later in life, marriage or employment changes). Many years ago, Rutter (1987) showed that women who were institutionalized as children were more likely to display positive parenting themselves if they married supportive spouses, and Sampson and Laub (2003) showed that for delinquent children followed over decades, both marriage and entry into the military conferred significant benefits to their well-being and adaptation. In short, even if subjected to early trauma, human beings are capable of recovering and healing.

The seventh universal principle is that *the ill effects of toxic early environments (e.g., unhealthy relationships) can manifest in physical health problems in childhood and throughout life.* Common health problems include asthma, headaches and backaches, and even elevated risk for heart disease and compromised immune functioning (e.g., Dong et al., 2004; Dube et al., 2009; Kalmakis and Chandler, 2015; Purewal et al., 2016; Wing et al., 2015). Therefore, once again, preventing exposure to such toxic experiences is of the essence, even if children appear to be adapting well behaviorally or psychologically to these adverse circumstances in their early years of childhood.

In a related vein is universal number eight: *The ill effects of early childhood adversities (e.g., abuse or neglect by caregivers) can become most visibly apparent later in life (i.e., there can be latent or "sleeper" effects that are seen at later points in development).* (See Chapter 2 for more information on sleeper effects.) For example, attachment insecurities developed in infancy could manifest in severe separation anxiety from the parent on starting kindergarten or significant difficulties in relating well with peers (Cicchetti and Toth, 2015, 2016). Other examples include behaviors that become relevant or salient closer to puberty or adolescence, such as delinquent behaviors or abuse of drugs and alcohol as a function of early relationship disturbances (Cicchetti and Toth, 2015, 2016). Perhaps the most obvious example is impaired parenting as adults; in general, there tends to be some intergenerational continuity of maltreatment (Adams et al., 2019; Cicchetti and Rizley, 1981; Kaufman and Ziegler, 1987; Pears and Capaldi, 2001; Rutter, 1987).

Universal nine—*biology is not "destiny;" rather, while indicating relative risk rates, it sets "confidence limits" within which environmental influence can lead to relatively positive versus negative adaptation.* Genetic factors, for example, can heighten children's vulnerability to disorders (physical and psychological) that afflict their parents. At the same time, intergenerational transmission of disorders is far from inevitable. As noted earlier, the notion of resilience encompasses the phenomenon wherein children who are at risk for psychopathology—or mothers who are at risk for negative parenting behaviors—can show healthy outcomes if they have the appropriate corrective or buffering influences in their lives. In other words, biological factors affect children's development, but they always operate in interaction with forces in the environment (Wise, 2009). The burgeoning field of epigenetics has shown that early life environments can lead to long-lasting changes in gene expression that "can leave indelible chemical marks on the brain and influence both physical and mental health later in life even when the initial trigger is long gone" (Murgatroyd and Spengler, 2011, p. 1; see also Dudley et al., 2011; Lerner and Overton, 2017; and Chapter 2 for more information).

To summarize, there are key take-home messages from the above discussion of universals to ensure positive psychological, behavioral, health, and social outcomes in early childhood. First, ensure the psychological well-being of the primary caregiver, as this will inevitably affect his or her parenting and the quality of attachment; this is best done by ensuring *ongoing* support for mothers in their everyday lives and communities (support during the child's early infancy will not protect the mother for the child's entire life). One population of particular importance for intervention is mothers under a high level of chronic stress and at risk for depression as this is strongly related to increased risk for neglect and maltreatment, which, of all parenting behaviors, are the ones that most urgently require prevention. Finally, in considering whether a child or parent has done well in spite of early adversities, it should be noted that ill effects of these adversities can become manifest later in life. At the same time, significant healing can happen, even well past childhood and adolescence, so that mothers who experience suboptimal care themselves as children can be effective caregivers if they receive appropriate support and help as they negotiate the challenges of motherhood.

Conclusion 4-1: The primary caretakers of children—usually the mothers—are critical to fostering the well-being of children, especially in high-risk circumstances. Ensuring the well-being of caretakers through ongoing support, extending beyond meeting basic needs, is necessary for child well-being.

Conclusion 4-2: The most urgent parenting concern for families experiencing chronic stress and adversity is the potential for children's exposure to maltreatment (by others within and outside of the family).

Fathers

For the most part, this chapter has focused on mothers (or mother figures) because across cultures and socioeconomic settings, they are typically the primary caregivers of young children (e.g., Hrdy, 2011; Luthar and Eisenberg, 2017); however, there are many instances where fathers are primarily responsible for raising children. This section reviews the importance of fathers for children's development. Following this, the extant evidence on interventions with fathers is reviewed and future needs are discussed.

While some research shows that fathers experience exclusion regarding parental involvement in child health and development (Plantin et al., 2011; Steen et al., 2012), there is empirical evidence that suggests they have an integral role in promoting the health and well-being of their children.

Some evidence points to a direct relationship between fathers and specific childhood outcomes. For example, research suggests that father education and supportiveness shapes language and cognitive development in children (Cabrera et al., 2007). Furthermore, varying levels of father involvement or connectedness with children are associated with differential self-regulation and aggression in children (Vogel et al., 2006). One study has even found that positive father–child relationships, as reported by fathers, are protective from pediatric injury (Schwebel and Brezausek, 2010). In terms of father well-being, paternal depression has been associated with increased odds of child neglect (Lee et al., 2012).

Other evidence suggests an indirect pathway by which fathers can influence their children's well-being—through their mothers. Bloch et al. (2010) found that poor-quality relationships between fathers and mothers are associated with depressive symptoms, stress, substance use, and smoking among low-income mothers. Other research indicates that father involvement has a positive association with a mother's health behaviors (e.g., seeking prenatal care in the first trimester, abstaining from drinking, drug use, and smoking) (Teitler, 2001). Finally, fathers can support maternal well-being and birth outcomes. For mothers, a supportive relationship with the father can have buffering effects on maternal depression and preterm birth (Giurgescu et al., 2018).

Involving Fathers in Preventive Interventions

As noted earlier in this chapter, developmental scientists have increasingly emphasized that it cannot be presumed that what helps fathers do well as parents is the same as what most benefits mothers (e.g., Grusec and Davidov, 2010). To illustrate, Lamb and his colleagues have shown that fathering can be more affected by the quality of the marital relationship (levels of satisfaction and support) than is mothering (see Lamb, 2004; Lewis and Lamb, 2003). Accordingly, it is important to attend to the gender-specific needs of parents in designing strategies to recruit and retain them in prevention programs related to their families and children (Pruett et al., 2017).

Cross-national interventions further attest to the critical importance of attention to gender-specific needs of parents. Randomized trials with families affected by HIV indicated that across countries (South Africa, Thailand, and the United States), men were more likely to respond to stress with flight-or-flight responses and women with tending and befriending (Rotheram-Borus et al., 2011). Accordingly, there have been efforts to design interventions to accommodate these gender differences in both delivery formats and activities. Community-based "mentor mothers," for example, were most beneficial for mothers seeking help via interventions, whereas men were more likely to be engaged via group activities, such as sports or vocational training. Similarly, Cabrera et al. (2015) note that fathers may be more willing to participate in a "game of basketball" than the "morning coffee" that many early childhood programs offer, and they recommend running support groups for "fathers" rather than just for "parents," sending the message that the role of a father is valued and is supported, independent of support to mothers.

In their review of existing programs for fathers, Pruett and colleagues (2017) indicate that whereas it is generally more difficult to engage fathers than mothers in preventive intervention programs, there are some avenues that seem promising. These include efforts to recruit fathers along with mothers via couples' work in early childhood (i.e., while the father is still involved with the mother and child before any possible estrangement, as it is much more difficult to engage fathers when strife has entered the inter-parent relationship). Pruett et al. (2017) also suggest focused efforts to make the facilities themselves more "father friendly" (e.g., by addressing implicit biases of staff that fathers will intrinsically be uninvolved and portraying pictures of fathers with babies in the program facilities). At the most basic level, other approaches would be to highlight in the media those men who are positive role models of fatherhood early in life and even bring such individuals to high schools to talk with young men on this topic, well before they become fathers.

Davison et al. (2019) examine strategies for and barriers to father engagement in early obesity prevention during the child's first 1,000 days of life. The review finds that although obesity prevention programs have great potential to engage fathers, there are a number of micro- and macro-level barriers that hinder access and participation. Applying a policy, systems, and environmental perspective, the authors recommend the following strategies to enhance father engagement: integrate father-engagement standards into national practice guidelines (e.g., American Academy of Pediatrics, American College of Obstetricians and Gynecologists), develop educational and marketing materials (e.g., pamphlets) specific to fathers, and partner with local father advocacy organizations to identify new strategies to engage fathers. Other research has homed in on preconception (Kotelchuck and Lu, 2017) and pediatric care (Yogman and Garfield, 2016) as important platforms for engaging fathers.

What is clear is that speaking about promoting good parenting in gender-neutral terms will likely be a disservice to both fathers and mothers. The literature clearly delineates what mothers need most centrally to function well as mothers (again, aside from basic necessities for physical survival): authentic connections with and support from others in their everyday lives. Relationship-based strategies that are highly effective, such as those in home visiting programs for new mothers, will not necessarily generalize to new fathers, paving the way to their enhanced mental health, positive fathering behaviors, and attachment to the child. For example, in low-income African American families, mothers responded well to the tend and befriend approach; however, the recruitment of biological fathers was more likely through opportunities for enhanced earnings to support their families (Jackson, 2015). Much more work is needed, therefore, on ascertaining how best to engage fathers and retain them in prevention and intervention programs.

It is important to note that the National Institutes of Health (NIH) changed their policies about gender inclusion around the 1990s, when there was a concerted move to include women in intervention trials. The NIH Office of Research on Women's Health was formed in 1990

> in response to congressional, scientific and advocacy concerns that a lack of systemic and consistent inclusion of women in NIH-supported clinical research could result in clinical decisions being made about health care for women based solely on findings from studies of men—without any evidence that they were applicable to women. (Mazure and Jones, 2015)

As researchers and practitioners think of how best to promote the well-being of young children via effective support for their primary caregivers, it would be prudent to avoid presuming that we can simply transfer program strategies and procedures from mothers to fathers. Although instances where a father is solely responsible for the child are not as common, this in no way obviates the need for understanding the most effective paths to reach and benefit these fathers. One evidence-based program that provides an avenue to reach fathers along with mothers is the Family Check-Up (FCU) program (see Box 4-6 for a description of FCU as a promising model).

Reviews of past national-level efforts targeting fathers further attest to the importance of further work in this area. As Lu and colleagues (2010) have noted, many fathers in the United States face substantial barriers to staying involved in their children's lives, and this is especially the case for many low-income fathers and men of color. These barriers operate at multiple levels, including intrapersonal (e.g., poor knowledge, attitudes and behaviors toward parenting) and interpersonal (e.g., strained relationship with the mother or maternal grandmother), neighborhoods and communities (e.g., high unemployment and incarceration rates, which influence social norms), cultural or societal (e.g., popular cultural perceptions of black fathers as expendable and irresponsible, racial stratification and institutionalized racism), policy (e.g., the "marriage penalty" within Earned Income Tax Credit [EITC] and Temporary Assistance for Needy Families [TANF], child support enforcement), and even historic (slavery and forced family separation among African Americans

---

BOX 4-6
Family Check-Up (FCU) Program: Promising Model[a]

The FCU is a strengths-based intervention that reduces children's problem behaviors by improving parenting and family management practices. Stretching back over 20 years, the FCU integrates assessment with motivation-enhancement strategies to tailor intervention goals to meet the unique needs of each family and increase family engagement. It has been implemented in a variety of settings, including public school systems, American Indian tribal communities, publicly funded health centers, hospitals, and community mental health centers. Any professional who provides services to families with children can use the FCU.

Using a strengths-based, ecological, adaptive framework, the FCU focuses on children ages 2 through 17. It is based on a family-centered model derived from "basic research on social development and intervention science" (Dishion and Kavanagh, 2003, p. 3) and differs from traditional family-centered approaches by emphasizing methods to promote a family's motivation to change (Shaw et al., 2009). By providing parents with the tools that they need to manage their children's behaviors effectively and to build a strong and positive relationship with their children, the FCU addresses the social environment as a social determinant of health. The program is multisector, engaging state research institutions, professional caregivers, mental health professionals and institutions, public schools, the Institute of Education Sciences, and the National Institutes of Health. Several studies have shown that the FCU is effective in achieving positive outcomes for families. For example, outcome data suggest that compared with the children of families who never participated in the FCU, children of families that did participate have fewer behavior and emotional problems, better emotion regulation, increased school readiness, and decreased risk for obesity (Brennan et al., 2013; Dishion et al., 2008, 2014; Lunkenheimer et al., 2008; McEachern et al., 2013; Shaw et al., 2006, 2009).

---

[a] The committee used selection criteria to identify examples of promising models highlighted in this report (see Appendix A for a list of the criteria). These examples all apply developmental science and aim to advance health equity during the preconception through early childhood periods.
SOURCES: ASU Reach Institute, 2018; The Center for Parents & Children, n.d.

---

and forced removal of American Indians from their land) (Lu et al., 2010). Life course factors, such as ACEs or the absence of the father's father growing up, can also influence father involvement. As discussed in the next section, institutionalized racism against men of color leads to higher rates of incarceration that precludes many fathers from being present in their children's lives, establishing healthy relationships, and providing the necessary support to the mother.

In recognition of both the importance of fathers for child development, and the challenges fathers face, Congress has authorized and funded grants for fatherhood programs for more than a decade. Evaluation of four federally funded Responsible Fatherhood programs from 2011 to 2018 has yielded mixed results (Avellar et al., 2019). All four programs consisted primarily of group-based workshops covering topics such as the meaning of fatherhood, child development, co-parenting, finding and retaining employment, and even personal development topics, such as coping with stress, responding to discrimination, problem solving, self-sufficiency, and goal planning. Participation in the programs resulted in improved parenting, specifically their self-reported nurturing behavior and engagement in age-appropriate activities with children, but not in-person contact, financial support, co-parenting, earnings, or socio-emotional and mental well-being (Avellar et al., 2019).

One possible explanation for the mixed results is that most extant fatherhood programs still do too little, too late. Men's capacity to support and nurture others needs to be cultivated over their entire life course, not only after they become fathers (Lu et al., 2010). This includes their capacity to form stable, positive relationships; as discussed throughout this report, this depends on the presence of a stable, nurturing relationship with a caregiver during their own early childhood. Thus, future research on father involvement needs to take a more integrative life course approach, studying how boys become men, men become fathers, and how we as a society can better nurture the development of fatherhood across the life course.

Conclusion 4-3: There is an urgent need to develop interventions well suited for fathers and other male caregivers; existing approaches that are developed for and tested with women cannot be assumed to generalize to other caregivers, with equal effectiveness, in the successful recruitment, retention, and support of men and fathers who take care of young children in prevention programs.

Future fatherhood programs also need to go beyond affecting individual knowledge, attitudes, and behaviors toward changing the family, neighborhood, social, and cultural contexts of fatherhood. Public policy changes to remove barriers—such as the "marriage penalty" within EITC and TANF, making child support more "father friendly" by calculating payment based on actual earnings, adjusting and forgiving arrearages, and allowing a greater amount of the child support payment to be passed through to the child—can go a long way toward strengthening father involvement. Micro- and macroeconomic policies to reduce poverty and strengthen fathers' capacity to contribute financially to the family can also help. Most importantly, fatherhood initiatives, if they are going to succeed in advancing health equity, need to have a core objective that addresses institutionalized racism in employment, education, housing, health care, criminal justice, and other systems that keep many low-income fathers and men of color from living out their true potentials in our society.

> **Recommendation 4-1: Federal, state, and local agencies, along with private foundations and philanthropies that invest in research, should include in their portfolios research on the development of preventive interventions that target fathers and other male caregivers. Special attention should be given to the recruitment, retention, and support of men and fathers parenting young children from underserved populations.**

The Role of Culture as Context

Anthropological perspectives on the study of children's development, pioneered by Margaret Mead, John and Beatrice Whiting, Robert A. Levine, and others, emphasize the importance of the cultural context that embeds children, families, and institutions that are important determinants of children's development. Subsequent elaborations by Super and Harkness (1986) labeled these influences as the "developmental niche." The developmental niche consists of "(1) the physical and social settings in which the child lives [micro systems in Bronfenbrenner's (1979) work], (2) the culturally regulated practices of child care and child rearing [that exist in all microsystems, including family, education, and health care settings], and (3) the psychology of the caretakers" (p. 552). They expand as follows:

> Regularities in the subsystems, as well as thematic continuities from one culturally defined developmental stage to the next, provide material from which the child abstracts the social, affective, and cognitive rules of the culture, much as the rules of grammar are abstracted from the regularities of the speech environment. The three components of the developmental niche form the cultural context of child development. (Bronfenbrenner, 1979, p. 552)

More recent formulations have refined these initial theoretical postulates to articulate more specifically how culture permeates the settings that children navigate and how they impinge on development. Rogoff (2003), Vygotski (1978), and Weisner (2002) describe culture as embedded in daily routines and interactions by which the child is enculturated into patterns of behavior, language/communication, and cognitions. A recent revision of Bronfenbrenner's bio-ecological model emphasizes how settings or microsystems through social interactions, daily routines, space, and other resource allocations enact on a daily basis cultural belief systems that may or may not align on behalf of the children's development (Vélez-Agosto et al., 2017). Service providers and caregivers need to be cognizant that practices that may be perceived or interpreted as harmful by other groups are embedded within a complex cultural system with its own deeply embedded logic. (See the section on Cultural Considerations for Subgroups for specific examples.) For that reason, cultural differences need to be accepted, incorporated, or renegotiated as part of interventions and educational efforts. Traditional cultural practices, as unfamiliar as they might seem for some, might be sources of strengths and resilience.

Subgroup Differences

Although there are universal processes of development that point out the importance of the quality of intimate family relationships for early child development, there can also be powerful influences that are largely unique to particular contexts; these potent *within-group* processes can affect children in both positive and negative ways. Considering the former, for example, specific processes have been identified as strengths or natural coping mechanisms that foster resilience within particular racial or ethnic groups, such as familism and respect for family obligations among Latinos and other collective-oriented cultures and effective family racial/ethnic socialization. Familism and family obligations provide the bases for family members to be involved in crisis management and the daily needs of mothers and children. Racial socialization provides children of color with an age-appropriate understanding of how racism operates and instills strengths and coping mechanisms based on positive and strong ethnic pride and identity. At the same time, these family contexts can place unique demands on children and families and lead to obstacles if they are not understood or accepted or are undermined by the majority culture; unintentionally, they might contribute to the emergence of health disparities very early in life.

This section describes subgroups in which there are specific, unique risk and protective factors that can affect the quality of parent–child relationships and the child's development; these need to be taken into account as interventions are designed to address health disparities. It should be emphasized here that ensuing discussions of subgroups does not imply that "all are the same" within them. There is invariably great heterogeneity between individuals and families within each subgroup, and it is important to recognize this, particularly in the design and implementation of interventions. Furthermore, while there may be unique risk and protective factors ascribed to these groups, the existing intervention research does not provide one-size-fits-all approaches to guide programs and policies working to serve these subgroups. These subgroups can differ from mainstream groups due to a variety of reasons, including

- Differential access to critical health-promoting resources (e.g., families not having access to safe housing and neighborhoods, preventive care, appropriate educational opportunities);
- Cultural differences due to language (e.g., non-English speakers in a monolingual English environment), religious background (e.g., Muslims), or recent migration;

BOX 4-7
Children of Same-Sex Parents

In the past two decades, developmental researchers have provided a wealth of evidence that children of same-sex parents show patterns of adjustment that are comparable to those of heterosexual parents. Pioneered by Charlotte Patterson in the 1990s in response to heterosexist and homophobic questions in psychology, judicial opinions, and popular stereotypes, this burgeoning research in child development has shown that it is the quality of parent–child relationships, rather than having same- versus different-sex parents, that is critical for children's adjustment (e.g., Wainright and Patterson, 2008; Wainright et al., 2004). A meta-analysis of 19 studies confirmed that children raised by same-sex parents have patterns of adjustment that are just as healthy as those of their counterparts raised by heterosexual parents (Crowl et al., 2008).

- Chronic stress (e.g., groups in poverty struggling to meet basic needs, such as shelter and health care, and those facing excessive pressures to achieve, usually in well-educated affluent communities); and
- Discrimination (e.g., racial or ethnic discrimination, homophobia, or discrimination against gender-atypical people [see Box 4-7 and the section on lesbian, gay, bisexual, transgender, queer [LGBTQ] youth and families]).

Children Living in Poverty: Meeting Basic Needs

As noted earlier, the most fundamental needs in Maslow's hierarchy are related to physical survival; when parents struggle to have their basic human needs met—for shelter, food, and health care—all in the family are at risk. Parents who are preoccupied by fulfilling basic needs for themselves and their children inevitably find it challenging to attend to their children's emotional, behavioral, and educational needs. Living in poverty is stressful on parents and can compromise the quality of their parenting behaviors, the evolving parent–child relationship, and the well-being of their developing children.

As discussed in Chapter 3, one of the most studied and documented factors that affects children adversely is living in poverty (Evans, 2004). Beyond physical survival, chronic poverty places children at risk because the physiological, safety, relational, self-esteem, and self-actualization needs—including those of the parents and the child—are all jeopardized; all of these need to be minimally fulfilled to prevent health disparities.

Low socioeconomic status (SES) and parental education are associated with limited access and use of critical health-promoting resources, and they contribute to psychological distress and physical health disparities. Research has consistently shown that poverty creates living conditions that negatively affect parenting and the mother–child relationship. The daily stresses associated with living in poverty lead to higher incidence of maternal depression, which, as noted earlier, is linked with a poorer quality of mother-infant interaction (Jackson, 2000; Taylor and Conger, 2017). Similarly, poverty has been linked to less capacity for parenting in a consistent and loving way, because it creates high levels of psychological distress that interfere with successful parenting (Conger and Conger, 2002; McLoyd, 1990). Families living in poverty with young children represent one of the most at-risk populations for health disparities, and programs and policies targeting them (see Chapter 6 for more on economic, food, and housing security) within a prevention and early intervention framework should be a priority for our nation.

Cultural Considerations for Subgroups

Other groups whose family relations might be at risk are those whose cultural background (i.e., lack of familiarity or congruency with the dominant North American culture and language) limits their access to critical health-promoting resources or can become an obstacle as they operate with daily practices and routines that are different from that dominant culture. For example, a limited grasp of the English language might impede a parent's consideration of high-quality early intervention or preschool programs (Moss and Puma, 1995). They might also espouse different family constellations (e.g., where grandmothers are very involved in caretaking); these other adults might interfere with their family operations, as might external influences, such as educators or health care providers.

Differences in acculturation among family members can also be sources of risk and resilience for families of immigrant backgrounds or members of other nondominant cultures. It has been observed that as children acculturate more than their parents (i.e., become more familiar with dominant North American culture and language), there is more conflict between parents and children (Schwartz et al., 2012). In addition, children might assume parenting tasks, such as taking on adult roles, negotiating school systems, and communicating with other officials for services (e.g., driver's licenses and bank accounts) for their parents.

The evidence on the effects of these added responsibilities on the children's development, so-called family obligations or brokering, is mixed: in some contexts, they might be burdensome, while in others they seem to be protective (Dorner et al., 2008; Fuligni and Pedersen, 2002). When taken to extremes and in developmentally inappropriate ways, however, taking on these roles is unhealthy for children. In recent years, the increased number of parental deportations and separation of parents and children at the southern U.S. border has led to an increasing number of children of immigrant background being traumatized and pushed into developmentally inappropriate parenting roles, which will lead to increasing relationship disturbances and subsequent health disparities (Bouza et al., 2018).

In other instances, traditional cultural practices that are appropriate in their original context clash with mainstream North American institutions, and these cultural practices inadvertently place children in at-risk pathways and contribute to problems in family relationships. As an example, many societies (i.e., Japanese, Korean) do not use direct verbal communications with infants and young children. Yamamoto and Li (2011) have shown that some preschools make Asian American students feel inadequate because their quietness, a desirable trait in their home culture, is considered a "problem" in the preschool environment. By contrast, acknowledging and fostering bicultural competencies in families, children, and service providers offers a good foundation for fostering early development in diverse populations (Ho, 2015; Padilla, 2008).

Finally, as presented in Chapter 3, discriminatory practices by systems, institutions, and the population at large can affect family relationships. Cultural mistrust from years of oppression from dominant groups, such as those experienced by African Americans, American Indians/Alaska Natives (AIs/ANs), and immigrants of various races and nationalities in this country, might interfere with family functioning. Cultural mistrust can be transmitted intergenerationally, as promoting mistrust has been identified as a particular type of ethnic racial socialization practice (Hughes et al., 2006). These attitudes permeate relationships with others, including with family members and health care providers (Moseley et al., 2007). Mothers and other main caregivers from other cultural backgrounds might not only have problems accessing supports from mainstream institutions but also experience family conflicts because the experiences of parents and children with mainstream institutions might differ. Although these factors can be listed individually, multiple factors are present in many individuals, families, neighborhoods, and regions (e.g., rural versus urban). This is why theoretical frameworks have emphasized the multiplicity of factors that are usually present in creating health disparities (García Coll et al., 1996). Moreover, new theories of intersectionality refer to those processes as differential access to power and as exclusion from benefits and assets and the existence of oppression and privilege at many societal levels (Bowleg, 2012; Brown et al., 2016;

Hankivsky and Christoffersen, 2008). Among the strongest factors associated with health disparities are gender, SES, and race (Becares and Priest, 2015; NASEM, 2017; Williams et al., 2010). In many instances, these factors are multiplicative, not additive, throughout childhood and adulthood.

At the same time, the protective factors that are unique for these populations need to be considered. The "immigrant paradox" refers to the findings that across physical and mental health and in educational and occupational outcomes, children and adults of immigrant backgrounds outperform native-born children, in spite of having been poorer and less acculturated to the dominant North American culture (García Coll and Marks, 2012). This phenomenon is poorly understood: it is unclear if motivational factors impel first and second generations to excel; if acculturation to poverty and its association with detrimental lifestyles and choices place subsequent generations at risk; or if discrimination and racism is more obvious to subsequent generations, and therefore its pernicious effects influence subsequent generations more.

Regardless, the traditional notion of rapid acculturation and complete assimilation as the successful model for incorporating immigrants has been questioned based on this evidence, and models of biculturalism and promotion of ethnic pride (Umaña-Taylor et al., 2014) are suggested as alternatives for successful incorporation. Finally, studies point out that state- and country-level policies that support families of immigrant background lead to fewer health disparities in youth (Filindra et al., 2011; Marks et al., 2018).

Children in Foster Care and Children with Incarcerated Parents

As discussed in the previous sections, a healthy (positive) relationship with main caregivers is one of the basic cornerstones of children's development and is necessary to prevent many health disparities. There are populations that, for a variety of reasons, lack the stability and quality of parenting needed to promote their children's development. Children in foster care and whose parents have been incarcerated often have multiple stressful life events before removal from parental care (Leve et al., 2012; Murray et al., 2012). The actual parental incarceration or loss of child custody is usually preceded by involvement with illegal activities and/or parental substance abuse, unstable housing, domestic violence, and/or child neglect or abuse. These children might be exposed to extreme stress, particularly during the prenatal period, when the in-utero child should be especially targeted at the first indication of any family relational difficulties.

Children in foster care Children in foster care are overrepresented as a group in terms of health disparities (Goemans et al., 2015, 2016;

Leloux-Opmeer et al., 2016; Leve et al., 2012). In most instances, these children's parents have lost or given up their parental rights because they cannot provide their children with stable, healthy relationships and other critical health-promoting resources needed for their well-being. However, children from certain racial and ethnic populations are disproportionately represented in the child welfare system. For example, AI/AN families are twice as likely to be investigated as the national population of families, and cases are twice as likely to be substantiated, with AI/AN children three times as likely to be placed in foster care as the national population of children (Hill, 2007) (see Table 4-1 for data on this disproportionality).

TABLE 4-1 Disproportionate Foster Care of AI/AN Children: 15 States with the Highest Rates

State	Disproportionality Rate[a] 2014	Percent of Children Who Are AI/AN	Percent of Children in Foster Care Who Are AI/AN
Minnesota	17.0	1.4%	23.9%
Nebraska	8.4	1.1%	9.3%
Idaho	5.2	1.2%	6.0%
Iowa	4.8	0.3%	1.7%
Wisconsin	4.8	1.1%	5.1%
Washington	4.3	1.5%	6.3%
Oregon	4.0	1.2%	4.9%
Montana	3.9	9.5%	36.9%
North Dakota	3.0	8.1%	31.4%
South Dakota	3.7	12.9%	47.9%
Alaska	2.6	17.8%	46.6%
Utah	2.5	0.9%	2.3%
New Hampshire	2.3	0.2%	0.5%
California	2.0	0.4%	0.8%
North Carolina	2.0	1.2%	2.4%
Massachusetts	1.2	0.2%	0.2%
Maine	1.1	0.8%	0.9%

[a] Data are sourced from Woods, S., and A. Summers. 2016. *Technical assistance bulletin: Disproportionality rates for children of color in foster care (Fiscal Year 2014).* Reno, NV: National Council of Juvenile and Family Court Judges.
SOURCE: NICWA, 2017.

Disruptions in attachment and other regulatory processes are consistently found in this population (Barone et al., 2017; Goemans et al., 2016; Leloux-Opmeer et al., 2016; Vasileva and Petermann, 2018). However, it has been found that foster care does not ameliorate these problems and actually might lead to more negative adaptive functioning after 1 year in such placement (Goemans et al., 2015).

Policies and practices of parental removal and replacement need to be carefully implemented. The stability of nurturing and supportive relationships, as described earlier in this chapter, is a crucial consideration for these populations (Jones Harden, 2004). If parents are unavailable or incapable of providing such conditions, placement with other family members, foster parents, or adoption is advisable, but only if these substitute parents can, in turn, provide stability and responsive parenting. That means that the quality and timing of care provided by family substitutes, including foster and/or kinship care and/or adoption or the reunification with the original biological family, has to be carefully planned and implemented to avoid re-traumatizing children through their interactions with these systems (Font et al., 2018).

In terms of supportive policies, the passage of the Family First Prevention Services Act in 2018 provides an opportunity to advance evidence-based child welfare policies through the investment of federal funds in children at risk for foster care, in foster family homes, or in qualified residential treatment programs or other special settings.[3] Most notably, the legislation provides support for programs and practices to keep children with their families safely (e.g., allowing states to use Title IV-E funds to prevent children's entry into foster care) (NCSL, 2019).

Children with incarcerated parents Incarceration is more prevalent in marginalized populations, adding to these populations' multiple risks for poor health outcomes. Analysis of incarceration rates shows much higher rates in low-income, minority populations (Acker et al., 2019; Wildeman and Wang, 2017). It has been widely documented that discriminatory policies and practices in the definitions of crimes, arrests, sentencing, and incarceration practices lead to an overrepresentation of low-income and minority populations, which has resulted in widespread incarceration within these communities (Acker et al., 2019; NRC, 2014). These higher rates not only affect the developing mother–child relationship but also disrupt the networks of support for parents frequently found in other family or neighborhood members.

---

[3] H.R.253—Family First Prevention Services Act of 2017.

Research clearly demonstrates the negative effects of parental incarceration on the child (Christian, 2009; Wildeman and Wang, 2017). Parental incarceration usually leads to family financial and housing instability and to more mental disorders and physical health problems in the partner (the parent who stays behind), which in turn is associated with higher incidence of child abuse and neglect (Acker et al., 2019). Various studies, including a meta-analysis, show that parental incarceration is associated with higher risks of children's antisocial behaviors, learning disabilities, and behavioral problems (Murray et al., 2012; Turney, 2014). Long-term educational, occupational, and physical and mental health outcomes as well as criminal behaviors are all related to parental incarceration (Acker et al., 2019).

Given the importance of attachment to the primary caregiver, maternal incarceration is believed to be more detrimental for young children than paternal incarceration and is a serious risk factor for future psychopathology (Murray and Murray, 2010; Parke and Clarke-Stewart, 2001; Shlafer and Poehlmann, 2010). This is concerning, given that almost 80 percent of incarcerated women are mothers (McCambell, 2005). For that reason, policies and practices that ensure adequate access and visitation to the incarcerated parent and promote healthy attachments is seen as a fundamental need and right of the child(ren) left behind (UNM, 2011).

LGBTQ Parents and Children

The parents and children that do not conform to normative gender expression and sexual orientation schemas of society (the LGBTQ community) are also placed at risk by contextual circumstances. The current cultural, religious, and political climate in the United States is divided on the acceptance and approval of these behaviors. Although research indicates that same-sex parents have been found to raise children with similar developmental outcomes as those of opposite-sex parents (see Box 4-7), about one-third of the population still expects negative impacts on children (Drake, 2013).

From an equity perspective, the LGBTQ community has historically gained rights for families through legislation and court precedence, such as the Supreme Court decision to uphold same-sex marriage as a constitutional right in 2015.[4] This landmark court case was instrumental in securing marital benefits (e.g., financial, social) for same-sex couples and their children. As of 2016, 20 states and Washington, DC, had enacted legislation that prohibits discrimination based on sexual orientation and gender identity or expression in employment, housing, and

---

[4] *Obergefell v. Hodges,* 576 U.S. (2015).

public accommodations—all of which are critical to promoting healthy development for children.

Even with such laws and policies, members of these populations are often subjected to discriminatory acts and microaggressions (IOM, 2011). Some have to "hide" their orientation and expressions from family, friends, and co-workers, which sometimes leads to the adoption of high-risk behaviors, such as unprotected sex, or internalizing disorders, such as depression, self-injurious behavior, and anxiety (IOM, 2011). Others may passively accept or actively repudiate discriminatory acts, exclusions, verbal and physical aggressions, and microaggressions as they express and adopt these less normative behaviors. These varied reactions to homophobia and discrimination can be associated with high levels of chronic stress and contribute to long-lasting health disparities (IOM, 2011).

While sexual orientation and gender identity may be more salient during adolescence, there is evidence to suggest that LGBTQ children demonstrate their inclinations to gender-atypical behaviors and same-sex orientation quite early (Rae et al., 2019). Many parents identify cross-dressing, toy preferences, and identification with heroes/heroines as displaying these preferences as early as the infancy and toddler years. As the typical puberty age has dropped, the issues that used to arise later in adolescence (i.e., identity, dating) are moving into childhood.

The LGBTQ population of children and youth is overrepresented in the adoption of risky behaviors and psychopathology. The 2011 Institute of Medicine report *The Health of Lesbian, Gay, Bisexual, and Transgender People* (IOM, 2011) identified the following key findings from the literature about LGBTQ youth during childhood and adolescence:

- LGBTQ youth are at increased risk for suicidal ideation and attempts and depression.
- Rates of smoking, alcohol consumption, and substance use may be higher among LGBTQ than heterosexual youth.
- The homeless youth population contains a disproportionate number of LGBTQ youth. Some research suggests that young transgender women are also at significant risk for homelessness.
- LGBTQ youth report experiencing elevated levels of violence, victimization, and harassment compared with heterosexual and non-gender-variant youth.
- Families and schools appear to be two possible focal points for intervention research.

These findings are corroborated by data from the Youth Risk Behavior Survey, which identify LGBTQ youth as being at risk for bullying, intimate partner violence (IPV), and sexual assault (CDC, 2017).

Children in High-Achieving Schools

As noted at the outset of this section, the standouts in groups of children and families exposed to high levels of chronic stress include those at both extremes of SES. Evidence of the challenges facing children and families in poverty, summarized here, have been reviewed extensively in the literature, with studies burgeoning around publication of the landmark Special Issue of *Child Development* on poverty more than 20 years ago (Brooks-Gunn and Duncan, 1997; Elder, 2018; Huston et al., 1994). By contrast, the evidence showing that youth in high-achieving contexts are an at-risk population is nascent, and the findings are counterintuitive for most. Extant evidence of adjustment difficulties among these children is presented here, followed by consideration of why this subgroup might merit attention in this particular report, which is focused on family-based prevention for children known to be at risk given life adversities.

With regard to the existing evidence on children of well-educated, relatively affluent parents, studies using varied samples and methods have converged in indicating relatively high levels of adjustment problems, likely linked with long-standing, ubiquitous pressures to excel at academics and extracurricular activities. Studies of students attending high-achieving schools (HASs) (public and independent; day and boarding; in different parts of the country) have consistently determined that they show rates of clinically significant problems, notably depression, anxiety, rule-breaking, and substance use, at rates that are (a) much higher than national norms and (b) sometimes higher than those in urban poverty (the latter is particularly true for substance misuse; see Luthar and Kumar, 2018; Luthar et al., 2013). Two large-scale analyses of national datasets in Norway and the United States (Coley et al., 2018; Lund et al., 2017) have confirmed a U-shaped association between community-level affluence and students' adjustment problems; in fact, students at more affluent schools had the highest levels of substance use.

In a recent longitudinal study spanning 50 years, Gollner et al. (2018) showed that students at a HAS had *poorer* outcomes decades later than their counterparts at middle-achievement schools. The authors said that constant social comparisons among a population of largely talented students were likely implicated in this result, which led to lower educational expectations of the self. Similarly, a collection of three studies involving 5th- to 10th-graders in Germany (Pekrun et al., 2019) showed that in all three schools, being in a high-achieving context had negative links with self-concept and emotions, and conversely, being in less HASs was better for self-concept and emotion.

Over time, accumulating evidence on this population has led to global statements about the high levels of risk among these youth. Almost a decade ago, Koplewicz et al. (2009) referred to their problems as "an epidemic." A 2018 report on adolescent wellness, released by the Robert Wood Johnson Foundation, noted the following as the most critical "high-risk" environments: exposure to poverty, trauma, discrimination/ racism, and high pressure to achieve, usually found in relatively affluent communities (Geisz and Nakashian, 2018).

Importantly, risks can be further exacerbated for vulnerable populations in HAS settings. Recent research has shown that African American boys in relatively high SES communities reported significantly higher depression and substance abuse, probably as a result of greater discrimination/racism in their communities—likely dominated by white families (Assari and Caldwell, 2018; Assari et al., 2018a,b; Lewis and Van Dyke, 2018). There is value, therefore, in considering issues of racial socialization for children of color who have the "double jeopardy" of having few children who look like them in their schools, neighborhoods, and communities.

With regard to why this subgroup of children and families might be relevant for this report on early childhood and equities in adaptation, two factors are relevant; one has to do with "sleeper effects" and the other with the need for early prevention. With regard to the first issue (as has been discussed earlier), the charge of this committee is not just to prevent problems that are manifested in early childhood—temper tantrums or bed-wetting—but, equally, those whose seeds are sown in early childhood and then "incubate" and become evident by early adolescence. It is clear that the prevention of problems among HAS youth (and other youth who suffer poor outcomes due to various types of adversity) cannot start when they are already teens; by then, a great deal of damage has already been done. Instead, what is needed is attention to these issues among parents when the children are still young. In fact, there are recent suggestions that the effects of high-achieving environments can be seen as early as preschool (Pekrun et al., 2019).

Second, there is a great deal of preventive potential in working with families in these settings toward raising awareness of the nature of risks and potential problems. Unlike low-income communities where an influx of resources is often needed for prevention, in this case, dissemination of accumulated evidence from science, with associated recommendations (Luthar et al., 2013), can be helpful. It is particularly important for parents to (a) understand the level and seriousness of adjustment problems that researchers have recurrently documented in HASs and (b) be vigilant in their own homes, starting from early childhood, against being overly invested in the child's "resume-building" (Gollner et al., 2018; Luthar and Kumar, 2018; Pekrun et al., 2019).

It is also critical to note that just as children in high-achieving contexts can be vulnerable, so can their mothers (who are, again, as in most contexts, their primary caregivers). Panel studies over time have shown that well-educated mothers have shown substantial increases in hours spent on activities related to their children, with increases greater than those among well-educated fathers and less well-educated mothers or fathers (Kalil et al., 2012; Ramey and Ramey, 2010). In terms of sheer hours, therefore, this group can be especially stretched thin and chronically stressed. Cross-disciplinary studies have established other factors that can challenge their well-being, including the "invisible labor" involved in being responsible for overseeing the schedules and activities of everyone in the household (see Ciciolla and Luthar, 2019; Lareau and Weininger, 2008; Yavorsky et al., 2015).

A 2019 study showing increases in depression over the past decade in the high-income groups, and among women in particular, provides additional testimony to the seriousness of these issues (Twenge et al., 2019). Changes over time were examined for four cohorts/generations and considering four groups of family incomes. The findings showed that cohort increases in serious psychological distress were the largest in the highest income group. Among adolescents, time period increases in rates of a major depressive episode were the largest in the highest income group and smallest in the lowest income group; among adults, the cohort increase in suicidal ideation was largest and smallest in the highest and lowest income groups, respectively. The authors concluded that "with the exception of adult MDE [major depressive episodes] and suicide attempts, the cohort increases were the largest and most consistently seen among those with the highest income" (Twenge et al., 2019, p. 10). Additionally, among adults, the increases in mood disorder indicators and all suicide related variables (suicidal thoughts, plans, and attempts) were consistently higher among women than men.

The evidence on youth and families in high-achieving contexts was reviewed above in some detail because this is a newly identified at-risk group, encompassing at least 20–25 percent of the U.S. population (e.g., Twenge et al., 2019). Additionally, despite the seriousness of the problems that are increasingly documented, there remains reluctance to afford attention to them in research and policy (Geisz and Nakashian, 2018).

In addition to HAS families, there are other such groups that are increasingly being identified as showing high vulnerability relative to norms, such as subgroups based on sexual identity and preference. Questions on both of these dimensions are now arising among children at younger and younger ages (often well before adolescence), creating stress and confusion for the child as well as the parents. Children who identify as neither male nor female but rather as "nonbinary" show elevated rates of anxiety, depression, and other psychological difficulties, as do children who identify not as heterosexual but as lesbian, gay, bisexual, or questioning. Regarding transgender youth, considerations of gender reassignment are also now coming up in many families well before adolescence. All of these subgroups will need concerted attention in the years ahead in terms of understanding how best to help both children and parents effectively negotiate these issues at home and outside it, such as in the children's peer groups.

Youth from Asian backgrounds are yet another illustration of a group that is potentially vulnerable but rarely included in discussions of children at risk. These children are often thought of as both privileged and "model minorities" (e.g., Lee et al., 2009; Ngo and Lee, 2007), but in fact, many U.S. families of Asian origin actually live in low-SES households. Furthermore, issues of discrimination arguably affect Asian youth just as they do other racial and ethnic minorities. At the same time, Asians are not considered as an ethnic minority group in discussions of discrimination, prejudice, and stereotype (Wong and Halgin, 2006) the way that youth from African American, Latino, or AI/AN backgrounds are. It is important to emphasize that this is not a zero-sum game; research and policy attention to the needs and challenges of Asian Americans by no means implies detracting from the very real and well-documented challenges faced by other ethnic minority groups in the United States.

In addition to including such neglected subgroups in discussions of those needing attention to prevention, more attention to risk processes that were not an issue at the time that *From Neurons to Neighborhoods* (NRC and IOM, 2000) was released is also warranted, and social media is critical in this regard. In discussions of why there continue to be increases in children's depression since the early 2000s, social media is often noted as a major factor (Hoge et al., 2017). Yet, there remain several questions about which aspects of social media use are truly damaging to children's mental health. Possibilities range from the amount of time spent on social media to spreading rumors about others, being the victim of bullying, "sexting" and accessing pornography, and constant social comparisons or feeling "less than" others. In Chapter 3, there is a section devoted to the problem of bullying even among young children; clearly, there is a lot of work that still remains to reduce this major risk process—and, now, to also disentangle and address the new challenges introduced by the widespread use of social media from young ages onward. As Weisz et al. (2019) note, the nature of childhood disorders may be changing faster than our treatments are:

> Threats to youth mental health are becoming more diverse and multiform. . . . Current threats encompass pressures to excel as well as new pressures to excel in increasingly competitive academic and social

environments, images conveyed via advertising and social media that could make anyone feel inadequate, risks of harm via text messages and cyberbullying, and even fear of being gunned down at school. (Weisz et al., 2019, p. 233)

To summarize, as policy makers and prevention scientists think about groups of young children and caregivers whose life circumstances are likely to place them at high risk for adjustment problems, the needs of all families need to be taken into consideration. Low levels of maternal education, coexisting with poverty and often single motherhood, clearly spell risks for adjustment problems and parenting difficulties among mothers, as noted earlier. At the same time, there are other groups that are increasingly being identified as requiring attention in future prevention efforts, including children and parents in extremely fast-paced, stressful, competitive communities, and sexual minority youth. Similarly, there are new risk processes that have arisen in the past couple of decades that potentially have strong negative effects on children and merit concerted attention in future research and policy when considering what should and should not be prioritized in preventive interventions.

In conclusion, psychologists, educators, and other health professionals need to work with groups of families that are especially vulnerable due to exposure to high levels of stress or adversity, with efforts beginning from preconception onward. These efforts will involve harnessing protective processes, and minimizing risk factors, in interventions that have a sound basis in developmental theory, science, and cumulative research evidence; have shown promising results in prior prevention studies; and are pragmatic (i.e., can feasibly be taken to large scale in the real world).

Conclusion 4-4: Specific subgroups of children have unique needs and challenges when adjusting to adversity. Careful attention to potent subculture-specific processes need to be considered in working with subgroups well known to face serious inequities in relation to mental health—including families experiencing chronic poverty; immigrants; lesbian, gay, bisexual, transgender, queer (LGBTQ) children and LGBTQ parents; and those where children are separated from parents due to incarceration or foster care. Among the groups more recently identified as being at high risk for chronic stress are children and parents, particularly mothers, in high-achieving, relatively affluent communities.

Recommendation 4-2: Federal, state, local, tribal, and territorial agencies, along with private foundations and philanthropies that invest in research, should include in their portfolios research on the development of interventions that are culturally

sensitive and tailored to meet the needs of subgroups of children known to be vulnerable, such as those living in chronic poverty, children from immigrant backgrounds, children in foster care, and children with incarcerated parents.

In addition to addressing major goals relevant for children in general (e.g., fostering caregiver well-being and minimizing maltreatment), programs need to include components that specifically address unique, powerful risk and protective processes within these subgroups of children. As discussed above, it cannot be assumed that evidence-based interventions and promising models developed in specific populations will work in other contexts. The validity and adaptability of interventions need to be empirically tested in groups that differ greatly in the sources of chronic stress and cultural backgrounds.

INTERVENTIONS TO PROMOTE RELATIONAL SUPPORTS AND CAREGIVER WELL-BEING

As developmental scientists have emphasized the critical importance of relational supports for the well-being of mothers and thus, their parenting, intervention trials have shown strong benefits of relational interventions. Indeed, the core components of several effective interventions suggest that over and above learning particular skills, it is improvements in mothers' overall well-being, within the context of supportive relationships, that are the most critical "engine" underlying the positive changes. To illustrate, the Incredible Years intervention by Webster-Stratton and colleagues (2001) targets children's school readiness and parenting skills while helping parents to cope with personal problems; parents are able to form valuable support networks with "buddies" from parent groups (Borden et al., 2010). Ammerman and colleagues' (2005) Every Child Succeeds program for depressed mothers provides in-home cognitive behavior therapy and a supportive home visiting component. A cardinal component in Dozier's Attachment and Biobehavioral Catch-up (ABC) is consistent respect, warmth, and support displayed by project staff or therapists to participating mothers (Dozier et al., 2005).

This section focuses on interventions with the strongest evidence base to foster healthy child development through supporting caregivers. First, there is a discussion of the evidence on home visiting, a well-established model for providing services to children and families, and the following section describes a range of interventions that have shown promise. The committee presents these as opportunities to use the science to drive action on caregiver and child well-being; however, the presentation of these interventions does not indicate prioritization of one over another.

Different populations will require varying interventions based on their needs and context, in addition to specific tailoring to meet these unique needs depending on the population.

Home Visiting Programs

One of the earliest program models built around the notion of supporting caregivers is home visiting. Home visiting programs in the United States focus on promoting child health and development by providing parenting support and other child-centered services in the home (e.g., developmental screenings and referrals to services and treatment) to at-risk families from the prenatal stage through age 6 (HRSA, n.d.). One of the primary goals of home visiting is to improve child health and educational outcomes. Home visiting programs have provided services to families in the United States since the late 1800s (Minkovitz et al., 2016), but the 2010 federal Maternal, Infant, and Early Childhood Home Visiting (MIECHV) program led to the expansion and supported standardization of home visiting implementation and evaluation. In fiscal year 2018, the MIECHV program served approximately 150,000 parents and children in 76,000 families across all 50 states; Washington, DC; 5 territories; and 23 tribal and urban AI/AN communities, providing nearly 1 million home visits annually and 5.2 million home visits between 2012 and 2018 (HRSA, n.d.). By law, state and territory awardees have to spend the majority of their MIECHV program grants to implement evidence-based home visiting models, with up to 25 percent of funding available to implement promising approaches that will undergo rigorous evaluation.[5] Tribal home visiting programs are encouraged to select evidence-based home visiting curricula, but as the research evidence is limited, this is not a program requirement. Most tribal home visiting programs chose to implement evidence-based curricula with cultural adaptations developed with intensive community input and engagement, which enhanced family engagement and retention (Pratt and Chapman, n.d.). Home visiting services may also receive support from many other federal, state, and local public and private sources.

This section summarizes the evidence on home visiting, highlighting a few exemplar programs. Given the multidisciplinary and cross-sector nature of this topic, the chapters later in the report will discuss home visiting with respect to specific levers in certain domains to enhance or support such programs. (See Chapters 5 and 7 for more on the role of the health system and of ECE, respectively.)

---

[5] For more information see https://mchb.hrsa.gov/maternal-child-health-initiatives/home-visiting-overview (accessed June 8, 2019).

Summary of the Evidence on Home Visiting Programs

A growing body of evidence suggests that home visiting by a nurse, a social worker, or an early educator during pregnancy and in the first years of a child's life improves a whole host of child and family outcomes, including promotion of maternal and child health, prevention of child abuse and neglect, positive parenting, child development, and school readiness. The positive impact continues well into adolescence and early adulthood. For example, in a 19-year follow-up of a randomized controlled trial (RCT), Eckenrode et al. (2010) found that relative to the comparison group, girls in the pregnancy and infancy nurse-visited group were 58 percent less likely to have been arrested and 43 percent less likely to have been convicted. Nurse-visited girls born to unmarried and low-income mothers also had fewer children and less Medicaid use.

One meta-analysis examined the impact of 18 implementation factors (including staff selection, training, supervision, and fidelity monitoring) and four study characteristics (publication type, target population, study design, comparison group) in predicting program outcomes (Casillas et al., 2016). The greatest program effects were found to be on increased positive parenting and reduced likelihood of maltreatment; the former had the largest effects. The programs were significantly less effective for children's health and behavior. Furthermore, provision of high-quality supervision and fidelity monitoring were key factors associated with beneficial outcomes. Programs serving families with one or more risk factors had significantly greater effect sizes compared to programs serving all families.

Avellar and Supplee (2013) reviewed the research on home visiting, and nearly 9 out of 12 programs (of the 32 reviewed) that met evidence-based criteria also showed favorable effects on children's social-emotional development or behavioral problems. Five programs showed one or more favorable effects on cognitive development, and five showed improvements in reductions in some aspect of child maltreatment (only six of the programs assessed maltreatment).

Another meta-analysis examined the effect of home visiting on six outcomes: birth outcomes, parenting behavior and skills, maternal life course, child cognitive outcomes, child physical health, and child maltreatment (Filene et al., 2013). Mean effect sizes were significant and positive for three of the six outcome domains: maternal life course outcomes, child cognitive outcomes, and parent behaviors and skills (Filene et al., 2013). Effect sizes for birth outcomes were significantly larger for programs that used nonprofessional home visitors, matched clients and home visitors on race and/or ethnicity, or included problem solving.

Effect sizes were larger for parent behaviors and skills programs that addressed parental substance use and taught parents developmental norms and appropriate expectations, discipline and behavior management techniques, and responsive and sensitive parenting practices. Improved child maltreatment outcomes were associated with problem solving and teaching parents how to select alternative caregivers for children. The effects on children's cognition were better in programs that taught parents responsive and sensitive parenting practices or "required parents to role-play or practice skills during home visits. Using professional home visitors was a significant predictor of better child physical health outcomes, as was teaching discipline and behavior management techniques" (Filene et al., 2013, p. S104).

Following a review of the research literature in 2018 (Sama-Miller et al., 2018), the Home Visiting Evidence of Effectiveness project, established by the Administration for Children and Families (ACF) in the U.S. Department of Health and Human Services, identified 20 home visiting models as meeting criteria of effectiveness to recommend for state-based home visitation programs (OPRE, 2018). Based on the available high- or moderate-quality studies, the review showed that most of these programs have multiple favorable effects with sustained impact, with Healthy Families America and the Nurse-Family Partnership (NFP) showing favorable impact across the greatest breadth of outcomes. Most models had favorable impacts on primary measures of child development, school readiness, and positive parenting practices; none of the models, however, showed impacts on a primary measure of reductions in juvenile delinquency, family violence, and crime (Sama-Miller et al., 2018).

A national evaluation of the effectiveness of the MIECHV program from 2012 to 2017, based on random assignment of families, found statistically significant positive effects in 4 out of 12 confirmatory outcomes: the quality of the home environment, the frequency of psychological aggression toward the child, the number of Medicaid-paid child emergency department (ED) visits, and child behavior problems (Michalopoulos et al., 2019). Most estimated effects are similar to but somewhat smaller than the average found in past studies of individual home visiting models. Differences in effects among the evidence-based models are generally consistent with the models' focuses. For example, Parents as Teachers produced the largest increase in parental supportiveness, and NFP produced the largest reduction in ED visits for children (Michalopoulos et al., 2019).

Potential to Reduce Disparities

The field of home visiting research continues to expand, with researchers identifying measurement frameworks (West et al., 2018) and factors contributing to implementation and replication (Paulsell et al., 2014). The state and tribal MIECHV recipients are required to implement rigorous program evaluations, which also help inform best practices and identify model programs and approaches and support the development and implementation of cultural adaptations necessary to ensure program retention, engagement, and cultural fit (Denmark et al., 2018; Hiratsuka et al., 2018). While the evidence remains limited for significant improvements in the reduction of health disparities, some studies have demonstrated that home visiting resulted in improved outcomes and so offered savings in terms of a return on investment of $2–$4 for every dollar spent (Cannon et al., 2017).

Among nondepressed mothers or families without multiple Child Protective Services (CPS) reports prior to study enrollment, home visiting was associated with a significantly lower likelihood of CPS report recidivism. These results indicate potential for home visiting to prevent maltreatment recidivism but, importantly, suggest that home visiting approaches, with weekly in-home visits by a trained home visitor, is warranted for mothers exhibiting significant depressive symptoms or families with extensive CPS histories (Jonson-Reid et al., 2018). However, among 220 low-income home visiting enrollees in a regional setting, mothers who experienced maltreatment in childhood had a heightened risk for membership in the mild and moderate-severe depression subgroup trajectories (Teeters et al., 2016). Mothers reporting higher social support saw a significant reduction in the risk of experiencing either mild or moderate-severe depression subgroup trajectories, while mothers reporting an increased belief in having control over one's life (i.e., locus of control) also saw a significantly reduced risk for assignment in either the mild or moderate-severe subgroups. Moreover, the depression score of mothers experiencing moderate to high depression was not significantly lower while enrolled in home visiting, though the depression scores for mothers at the minimal and mild levels of depression were significantly lower over time (Teeters et al., 2016). These results suggest that the effect of home visiting may also depend on maternal depression level, demonstrating that tailoring home visiting curricula to best fit maternal risk factors may be warranted.

Exemplar Programs and Promising Practices

The NFP home visiting curriculum has demonstrated multiple positive outcomes, including a reduction in domestic violence reports (Eckenrode et al., 2017). Mothers receiving visits from nurse home visitors had fewer health care encounters for injuries and higher ratings of the home environment and parent's reports of caregiving (Kitzman et al., 1997; Macmillan et al., 2009; Olds et al., 1997; Zielinski et al., 2009). NFP is the only home visiting program to have statistically significant positive effects over time on substantiated cases of child maltreatment.

Healthy Families New York, a Healthy Families America–accredited home visiting program, has demonstrated positive effects for fathers' participation. Families with father participation were more than four times as likely to be retained, and engaged fathers were more likely to live at home with the child and to remain emotionally involved at 6 months (McGinnis et al., 2018).

The Family Spirit home visiting intervention is the only program that has demonstrated efficacy in American Indian communities. To date, it has only been implemented in three rural, tribal communities in the Southwest. Nevertheless, Family Spirit has seen that high-risk mothers had significantly greater parenting knowledge (effect size = 0.42) and parental locus of control (effect size = 0.17), fewer depressive symptoms (effect size = 0.16) and externalizing problems (effect size = 0.14), and lower past-month use of marijuana (odds ratio [OR] = 0.65) and illegal drugs (OR = 0.67). Moreover, children in Family Spirit had fewer externalizing (effect size = 0.23), internalizing (effect size = 0.23), and dysregulation (effect size = 0.27) problems (Barlow et al., 2015).

Culture is embedded across many important components of parenting, and it has only recently been actively integrated into home visiting services. However, few culturally specific home visiting curricula have sufficient evidence to be deemed evidence-based practices. Some are considered promising, with some positive quasi-experimental support for program, family, and child outcomes. For example, *Kūlia I Ka Nu'u* works with families with children 2.5–5 years old using a Montessori approach with Native Hawaiian culture to support parents in building their child's school readiness and school success (Yoshimoto et al., 2014). Parent educators help families learn more about Native Hawaiian values and practices and incorporate these cultural values into the curriculum, which includes literacy, math, art, social studies, and science. *Kūlia I Ka Nu'u* is unique to the island of O'ahu. *Pūlama I NāKeiki* (PINK) provides services to Native Hawaiian families prenatally to 3 years of age. PINK supports families in identifying and learning more about cultural traditions and how strengthening cultural knowledge contributes to family life. Parent educators provide culturally based information about prenatal health, childbirth, child development, and child rearing (Yoshimoto et al., 2014).

Expanding the Impact of Home Visiting

To maximize the impact of effective home visiting programs, there is a need to expand their reach by scaling them to larger and different populations; currently, only 40 percent of U.S. counties provide home visiting services, with 13 states offering home visiting in 75 percent of counties and 10 states providing it in 10 or fewer counties (NHVRC, 2018). In 2017, more than 300,000 families received home visiting services, though the National Home Visiting Resource Center estimates that about 18 million additional families could benefit but were not being reached (NHVRC, 2018). The MIECHV program was reauthorized in 2018 at a funding level of $400 million annually through 2022 (Sandstrom, 2019). To address remaining unmet needs, the federal program needs to be funded at a much higher level in the next reauthorization. States can further expand support for evidence-based home visiting services through state general funds, Medicaid financing, or braiding of different funding streams (Johnson, 2019). Presently, 20 states are using Medicaid to expand state capacity and reduce unmet needs for home visiting services, including universal home visiting, such as in Oregon and Washington State. Many states are using a Medicaid State Plan Amendment to support home visiting services under targeted case management benefit; other states, such as Maryland and South Carolina, had made home visiting demonstration or pilot projects part of a larger Medicaid 1115 or 1915(b) waiver. South Carolina is braiding approximately $17 million in philanthropic investments with $13 million in Medicaid funding through a 1115 waiver to finance a pay-for-success approach. Under this approach, private (and public) funders provide up-front capital to expand social services through a "social impact bond"; the government pays for all or part of the program only if it measurably improves the lives of participants (Johnson, 2019). South Carolina has committed an additional $7.5 million in payment if independent evaluators find positive results from expanded home visiting services (Johnson, 2019).

Scaling up requires more than simple replication of an effective home visiting model to reproduce positive effects. It entails the careful consideration and balance of fidelity, spread, and tailoring models for local adaptation. To support fidelity in the home visiting field, Paulsell et al. (2014) argue that two conditions need to be met: (1) research on efficacy, effectiveness, and dissemination need to document challenges that threaten fidelity; and (2) the field needs to standardize measurement and improve understanding of valid and reliable fidelity measures within and across models. While model fidelity is an important mediator of program success, home visiting implementation requires flexibility to tailor the program to the needs and/or assets of the community or population being served. This is especially critical when applying an equity approach, so that all children and families receive the services that they need. One strategy may be for the MIECHV program to work with model developers in identifying core program elements across models, while allowing state grantees to choose additional elements from various models to enhance and tailor the core program to the differential needs and vulnerabilities of individual families and communities. Additionally, others have proposed proportionate universalism—a tiered approach where every new parent in a community receives at least one home visit, while the quantity and intensity of follow-up services are adjusted to the needs and assets of high-risk families, to improve program cost-effectiveness (Marmot et al., 2010). (See the section on Synthesizing the Evidence for Conclusion 4-5 on applying a tiered approach to services.) Most importantly, as the committee discusses in Chapter 5, home visiting must not become yet another siloed prenatal and early childhood service. Future evidence-based home visiting programs need to continue to partner with, coordinate, colocate with, and expand the reach and impact of other ECE programs and the future redesigned advanced medical home. Home visiting can thus serve as a linchpin between health care, social services, and early childhood education.

Lastly, the relatively modest impact of the MIECHV program demonstrated in the national evaluation has been observed in other early childhood programs that scaled up from RCTs to population-wide interventions (Center on the Developing Child at Harvard University, 2016). Studies that focus on average effects may mask wide variation in impacts if they do not or cannot account for the differential susceptibilities of individuals, families, or communities. Often, RCTs cannot easily be adjusted, adapted, or enhanced after randomization (see Chapter 1 for a discussion about the limitations of RCTs). Future home visiting and ECE research needs to move beyond searching for one-size-fits-all solutions to define more precisely which intervention works best for which patients or populations under what circumstances.

Researchers, program leaders, and policy makers should focus on expanding the concept of precision home visiting that advances which programs and activities are best for which family, in which communities, and for what outcomes.

Recommendation 4-3: To strengthen and expand the impact of evidence-based home visiting programs:

- **Federal policy makers should expand the Maternal, Infant, and Early Childhood Home Visiting Program.**
- **The Health Resources and Services Administration (HRSA) and the Administration for Children and Families (ACF) should work with program developers to increase flexibility for states and communities, to tailor the program to the needs and/or assets of the community or population being served.**
- **Federal, state, local, tribal, and territorial agencies overseeing program implementation should continue to strengthen programmatic coordination and policy alignment between home visiting, other early care and education programs, and medical homes.**

State policy makers should further expand support for evidence-based home visiting services through general funds, Medicaid, and braiding of multiple funding streams. HRSA and ACF should continue to ensure program effectiveness and accountability of the expanded program. Expansion of home visiting programs should be done in conjunction with the expansion of other public investments and services.

Given the resources needed to provide high-quality home visiting, cost is an important consideration. Yarnoff et al. (2019) developed and piloted a tool to standardize the collection of home visiting data, in addition to assessing program costs for 45 local implementing agencies that participate in MIECHV. The study reported an average cost per family served of $12,556 for agencies serving less than 100 families, versus $7,117 for agencies serving more than 100 families.[6] Burwick et al. (2014) conducted a cost analysis for 25 implementing agencies and found that the average estimated annual cost to operate a home visiting program was $580,972.[7] Costs varied drastically from program to program, ranging from $206,426 to $1,207,054. Estimating and comparing costs of home visiting programs—and by extension, of expanding them—can be difficult for a number of reasons. As noted above, program costs vary, and this could be attributable to the services offered, duration, transportation costs—particularly in rural and/or tribal communities—and family and agency characteristics (Burwick et al., 2014; Yarnoff et al., 2019). Further research is needed to understand how to expand home visiting programs cost effectively, and a tiered approach would provide tailored services based on family needs (see Conclusion 4-5 for more on a tiered approach). Finally, strengthening programmatic coordination and alignment across sectors, as indicated in the recommendation, could potentially reduce costs.

Other Evidence-Based Programs Focusing on Mothers

Outside of home visiting, perhaps the first program to explicitly target mothers' well-being is Lieberman's Infant Parent Psychotherapy (IPP), designed with the recognition that a critical prerequisite in working with mothers at high risk for maltreating their infants is attention to the women's own psychological needs. The program has been expanded for

---

[6] The study authors calculated cost of the program per family by dividing total program costs by the average monthly number of families served by the agency and then calculated weighted mean cost per family served as the sum of costs across all agencies divided by the sum of families served.

[7] The cost analysis was conducted using "the 'ingredient' or resource cost method, which involved itemizing the types of resources (or ingredients) needed to provide services, gathering information on the types and value of resources used by each agency during the study period, and aggregating costs to estimate total program costs" (Burwick et al., 2014, p. xii).

work with mothers and toddlers (Toddler Parent Psychotherapy [TPP]), and therapeutic strategies combine cognitive behavioral, psychodynamic, and social learning theories. A cardinal ingredient, however, is high empathy and support for the mother, with recognition that "the most effective interventions are not spoken but rather enacted through the therapist's empathic attitude and behavior toward the mother as well as the baby" (Lieberman and Zeanah, 1999, p. 556). A number of studies have now documented the benefits of IPP and TPP, implemented with mothers across diverse settings (see Lieberman et al., 2011).

Another program with a strong emphasis on respect, warmth, and support by intervention staff to participating mothers is Dozier's ABC. In this program, goals are to target insecure early attachments by intervention services to foster caregivers' positive qualities, including responsiveness, nurturance, and their own attachment states of mind (Dozier et al., 2002). The program has been refined and tested in RCTs for more than 20 years. Results show that those receiving the intervention showed significant gains compared to control groups, which included better quality of attachment between mothers and children and improved self-regulation in both (Bernard et al., 2015; Bick and Dozier, 2013; Dozier et al., 2002). See Box 4-8 for more on the ABC program as an example of a promising model.

Another program with focused attention on the well-being of mothers is the Relational Psychotherapy Mothers' Group (RPMG) intervention (Luthar and Suchman, 2000), developed for mothers at risk for maltreating their children—specifically, low-income women with histories of substance abuse. As with IPP and ABC, core therapeutic components in RPMG include a strong emphasis on empathy, genuineness, and warmth and using insight-oriented approaches to improve parenting skills and efficacy. There were two major differences between RPMG and programs for mother–child dyads, both related to potential for scaling up. The first was the choice of a group format rather than individual sessions, thus potentially reaching more women for 1 hour of clinicians' time. Second, RPMG was designed for mothers of children from birth through adolescence, with developmental issues addressed as part of the program, again allowing for inclusion of a wide range of women. Results of two clinical trials showed benefits of RPMG. Compared to treatment as usual in their methadone clinics, mothers who received the 24-week intervention showed lower risk for child maltreatment—by mothers' and children's reports—and better personal adjustment as well as both mothers' and children's reports of child maladjustment and on mothers' drug use via urinalyses (Luthar and Suchman, 2000). At 6 months posttreatment, RPMG recipients continued to be at an advantage, although the magnitude of group differences was reduced. In the second trial, RPMG was compared to relapse prevention therapy (RPT). RPMG mothers again fared better

BOX 4-8
Attachment and Biobehavioral Catch-Up
(ABC) Program: A Promising Model[a]

Developed in 1994, the ABC Intervention is an internationally available training program for caregivers of infants and toddlers through early adolescence, including high-risk birth parents and caregivers of young children in foster care, kinship care, and adoptive care. Parent coaches conduct 10 weekly home visits, approximately 60 minutes each. The model is designed to help caregivers provide nurturance even when children do not appear to need it, mutually responsive interactions in which caregivers follow children's lead, and nonfrightening care. Parent coaches provide immediate feedback on the caregivers' interaction with the child to help the caregivers attend to the target behaviors. The model also incorporates homework and video feedback.

While the original version included children from 6 to 48 months old, the model has been updated to include two different versions: (1) infants (6–24 months) and (2) toddlers (24–48 months). The model is based on attachment theory and stress neurobiology, and it addresses the social and physical environments by helping caregivers sensitively respond to children's behavioral signals, enhancing children's behavioral and regulatory capacities, and fostering the development of secure attachments between children and their caregivers. The model was developed by academic researchers and continues to be evaluated by them, though it has expanded significantly since its origin. ABC has partnered with state agencies, community-based nonprofits, or religiously affiliated funds. The National Institutes of Health also funds many of their research projects. Infant ABC coaches are trained intensively and supervised for 1 year, while toddler ABC coaches have to receive additional training afterward. The project originated at the University of Delaware, and certified ABC parent coaches are currently available across the United States in communities in Delaware, Hawaii, Idaho, Kansas, Kentucky, Louisiana, Maryland, Michigan, Minnesota, New York, North Carolina, North Dakota, Ohio, Oklahoma, and Pennsylvania. Internationally, ABC coaches are available in Australia, Germany, Norway, Russia, South Africa, and Sweden.

The program was designed to address inequities in social environments that affect children exposed to trauma in early childhood. Positive interactive experiences can stimulate healthy development of the central nervous system, foster a positive sense of self, and help maltreated children learn to accurately interpret and respond to emotional, environmental, and social cues. Four independent randomized controlled trials (RCTs) support the efficacy of ABC and suggest that it is effective in improving attachment and helping regulate both biology and behavior in at-risk children (see, for example, Bernard et al., 2015; Lind et al., 2014). In addition to findings from these RCTs, researchers have also found evidence to support ABC's efficacy through dissemination studies with pre- and postintervention assessments.

---

[a] The committee used selection criteria to identify examples of promising models highlighted in this report (see Appendix A for a list of the criteria). These examples all apply developmental science and aim to advance health equity during the preconception through early childhood periods.

SOURCES: ACF, 2018; Attachment Biobehavioral Catch-Up, 2017.

than RPT mothers at posttreatment per mothers' self-reports, children's reports, and urinalyses (Luthar et al., 2007). But again, at 6 months of follow-up, they lost many of their gains.

These findings collectively indicate that even after external interventions are completed, it is critical to ensure continuity in supports for mothers who are vulnerable to depression and other mental illness. Similar messages have emerged from Olds et al.'s (2007) widely used, efficacious program, NFP, which provides regular home visits for low-income, single mothers by a warm, supportive nurse. These home visits begin in the prenatal months and continue through the babies' second birthdays. Yet, as Golden and colleagues (2011) underscore, mothers' needs for help are not necessarily resolved when children reach 2 years old. In fact, mothers who have received this program report widespread, continuing depression in their communities, with many women desiring and needing support from others who can be reliable sources of caring over time.

In view of this accumulated work, therefore, one critical challenge for those working with vulnerable mothers is to ascertain how these mothers might continue to receive support even when time-limited supportive interventions cease, and in this regard, peer-based interventions are promising. Specifically, there is potential value in groups run by "graduates" of supportive programs who receive subsequent training and supervision in facilitating groups for peers (see Bryan and Arkowitz, 2015). Reportedly, this strategy has been used successfully with mothers who themselves had experienced perinatal depression, who regularly met with other women who were currently depressed. Bryan and Arkowitz (2015) conducted a meta-analytic review and found that peer-administered interventions (PAIs) produced substantial reductions in symptoms of depression. The magnitude of beneficial changes over time was significantly greater than those in no treatment conditions and was also comparable to non-peer-administered interventions. Interestingly, PAIs that were administered purely by peers were more effective than those that also involved a professional in the treatment, in a secondary role.

In future efforts to use such peer-based groups for mothers, some have suggested drawing on a type of model (not the intervention itself) that has been used extensively for decades and with minimal costs: the 12-step model (see Luthar et al., 2015). Community-based meetings in this program, specifically Alcoholics Anonymous, benefit more than 1.3 million Americans, and its benefits can be equal to or even greater than those of professional interventions (Kelly et al., 2012). A major "active ingredient" in this program, again, is ongoing access to dependable, authentic supports; members speak of unconditional acceptance with others sharing similar challenges and their ability to reach out to others when in distress. In the future, there could be value in using such community-based groups to promote resilience in at-risk mothers. Sustaining the type of supportive connections that mothers came to depend on in the active phase of relational interventions might be possible with continued weekly meetings (Luthar, 2015).

This has been a recurrent theme in prevention and policy: scientists increasingly urge the use of networks that already exist in communities, bringing them to bear in interventions that become self-sustaining over time (Luthar, 2015). To illustrate, within affordable housing complexes, Antonucci and colleagues (2014) described programs that focused on creating mutually supportive networks among residents. Kazdin and Rabbitt (2013) described several low-cost, feasible, and effective interventions using lay people (rather than professional therapists), including hair stylists in beauty salons, trained to assess depression and to provide appropriate referrals. Hofmann and Hayes (2019) underscored the potential value of training paraprofessionals in the specific procedures that highly trained clinicians have identified as being most promising in engendering improved mental health.

An alternative approach is to deliberately foster women's connections with reliable others in their everyday lives over the duration of a formal, relational intervention. This was the strategy used in an RCT of the Authentic Connections (AC) Groups program at the Mayo Clinic, tested with mothers who were health providers—a professional group at high risk for depression, burnout, and even suicide compared to norms. From the start of the 3-month program through the end, there was a focused, concerted effort to have women reach out to their "go-to committees" in their personal lives; thus, authentic connections were forged both within the groups and outside of them in the mothers' everyday lives. In comparison with a control group (given 1 hour of freed time over 3 months to attend groups, as were intervention mothers), AC Groups women showed significantly greater gains across multiple adjustment indexes ranging from depression and self-compassion to lowered burnout at work and decreased levels of cortisol (Luthar et al., 2017). Moreover, effect sizes across outcomes were generally in the moderate range, and gains were still stronger 3 months after the intervention program was over (partial eta squares of 0.08–0.19; median, 0.16; according to Cohen [1988], partial eta squares correspond to the following effect sizes in the real world: 0.02 is small; 0.13 is medium; and 0.26 is large).

The success of these in-person AC Groups led to efforts to conduct them in a virtual format, via videoconferencing, to achieve potentially wider and easier dissemination (Luthar et al., in press). Results of this study indicated the successful completion of five different virtual groups (3–6 women each, for a total of 23), with the sample involving mostly mothers, most with advanced (graduate) degrees and almost all in high-pressure careers. As with the in-person version, the 3-month program had zero dropouts. Participants' mean ratings of the groups' effectiveness were 9.6 of 10, and the "Net Promoter Score" (percent of promoters subtracting percent of detractors) fell in the exceptionally high range (Luthar et al., in press). Open-ended responses emphasized participants' appreciation of access to robust, authentic connections with other caring women (which endured well after the program was completed). Given the low cost and ease of access—from mothers' own workplaces, homes, or even while traveling—such virtual groups might be considered a useful model to be explored further in future work with mothers (indeed, the use of virtual connections have been increasingly emphasized; see Hofmann and Hayes, 2019; Weisz et al., 2019).

In concluding this section on interventions, the literature reviewed suggests the value of a tiered approach to psychological interventions for mothers at risk due to their life adversities, along with their children, and as early as possible—preferably prenatally. All approaches involve ensuring strong, dependable supports for the mother or other primary caregiver. At the broadest level of interventions, there is particular promise in those that bring together mothers in communities or virtually to provide such mutual, ongoing support. For women needing greater psychological help, time-limited, evidence-based group therapies emphasizing connections and mutual support and making maximal use of existing resources would be useful. The most intensive level would be one-on-one interventions, such as those involving home visiting or work with mother–child dyads to enhance strong attachment quality. Given the critical need to support caregiver well-being and to prevent child maltreatment (see Conclusions 4-1 and 4-2), in addition to the review of high-quality interventions that are offered in community settings for families, the committee offers the following recommendation to support the development and implementation of such interventions.

> **Recommendation 4-4: Policy makers at the federal, state, local, territorial, and tribal levels and philanthropic organizations should support the creation and implementation of programs that ensure families have access to high-quality, cost-effective, local community-based programs that support the psychosocial well-being of the primary adult caregivers and contribute to building resilience and reducing family stress.**

Measures to Be Used

In concluding this section, there is consideration of measures that should be included in evaluating results of large-scale preventive interventions targeting young children and their mothers. At a minimum, there should be brief assessments of the mothers' depressive symptoms, stress, feelings of rejection to the child, any involvement with CPS, and IPV, as well as the degree to which they have positive, buffering relationships in their lives. Possible measures include the 20-item Zung Self-Rating Depression Scale (Zung, 1965), 10-item Perceived Stress Scale-10 (Cohen et al., 1983), and 10-item subscale on parental undifferentiated rejection from the Parental Acceptance-Rejection Questionnaire (Rohner et al., 1980). For supportive relationships, potential measures might include the Satisfaction with Friends subscale (four items from the Inventory of Parent Experiences; Crnic, 1983) and two single items that have consistently shown significant, robust links with multiple aspects of mothers' well-being: "Do you feel seen and loved for the person you are, at your inner core?" and "When you are deeply distressed, do you feel comforted in the ways you need?" (Ciciolla and Luthar, 2019; Luthar and Ciciolla, 2015). Finally, if any studies propose additional expensive assessments to inform future interventions (such as biomarkers as mediators, moderators, or outcomes), researchers need to explain how the findings from these will be applied not only in laboratory-based RCTs but also in large-scale interventions reaching vulnerable children and families in their own homes, schools, and community settings. Given the need to identify individuals at risk for early adversity and toxic stress, the committee offers the following recommendation to close a gap in the system. Furthermore, screening requires alignment with available services for children and families (see Chapters 5 and 8 for more on screening and alignment with services).

Recommendation 4-5: Health care providers who care for pregnant women and children should routinely track levels of individual health and social risk among mothers and children over time, using periodic assessments via a short set of scientifically validated measures.

SYNTHESIZING THE EVIDENCE

To summarize, major conclusions deriving from this chapter include the following. Promoting resilience in childhood rests, first, on ensuring the well-being of children's primary caregivers—usually, their mothers—and this requires the mothers' ongoing access to strong, supportive relationships, beyond meeting basic needs for survival. Maltreatment is of utmost importance among the various parenting behaviors that should be targeted in preventive interventions; minimizing neglect and abuse by caregivers and others needs to be a top priority. Gender specificity is advised in interventions for parents, with separate delineation of how mothers and fathers each are most effectively recruited, retained, and helped in interventions. When considering children who need preventive interventions, there are several subgroups whose unique challenges need to be considered. These include subgroups that have been extensively documented in past research to be at risk—such as children in chronic poverty, those separated from their parents, and recent immigrants—and those shown more recently as contending with high stress and distress, such as children and families in high-achieving communities and youth who are in the minority based on gender identification and sexual orientation.

As future interventions for mothers and children are taken to large scale, it will be useful to employ a tiered approach with the intensiveness of services increasing with the level of the mother's distress. At a fundamental level, universal, supportive interventions for mothers from pregnancy onward are needed. This includes using existing resources for supportive group-based interventions (e.g., organized in their own communities, such as in preschools or schools) that are, where possible, led by peers and/or accessed virtually. Universal interventions also need to include at least one home visit after birth to ascertain if mother and child have the supports they need, and, if difficulties are found, to provide connections to local resources for the family.

Conclusion 4-5: A tiered approach is needed for families known to be at risk due to their life adversities, with appropriate investment of resources to expand delivery of promising cost-effective programs and assessments via scientifically sound measures of critical constructs. This includes the need for

- *Universal, supportive interventions for mothers and*
- *More resource-intensive programs.*

To promote these first-level, universal programs, federal, state, and local agencies overseeing program implementation could develop and monitor community-based support groups for mothers within existing programs, such as the MIECHV program, Head Start, Early Head Start, and Special Supplemental Nutrition Program for Women, Infants, and Children. Care providers within these programs require appropriate referral sources for mothers and children who need intensive, one-on-one care (e.g., through home visiting). Enhanced coverage by major insurance providers for programs offering group-based care, support, and therapeutic interventions for mothers is also necessary (see Chapter 5 for more on health care needs for this population).

To identify mothers who might need more intensive services, a brief battery of questionnaires should be used as a screening tool. Specifically, measures of maternal stress and depression (described in this chapter) should be routinely administered at prenatal and pediatric "well-baby" visits. Those mothers who manifest high distress will need referrals to programs that offer evidence-based therapeutic interventions. Intensive programs for mothers in distress can be for groups or individuals. Programs that are short term and involve groups of women, such as AC Groups or the Mental health Outreach for Mothers (MOMS) Partnership, can help to maximize both reach and cost-effectiveness. (See Box 4-9 for information on the MOMS Partnership as a promising model.)

BOX 4-9
MOMS Partnership: A Promising Model[a]

Based in New Haven, Connecticut, the MOMS Partnership is an evidence-based, community-driven initiative that offers mental health and trauma-related services and parenting and job readiness programs to single mothers in at-risk neighborhoods (Center on the Developing Child, 2019). The program recruits participants by "meeting" mothers at locations they frequent (i.e., grocery stores, laundromats, shelters, community colleges, libraries, and nail and hair salons) (White et al., 2018).The program's mission is "to reduce depressive symptoms and increase social and economic mobility among overburdened, under-resourced mothers, thereby strengthening generations of families to flourish and succeed" (MOMS Partnership, n.d.-c).

Beginning in 2010 and in partnership with mothers and community partners, the program has conducted surveys to identify and understand the needs of pregnant women, parents, other caregivers, and families in the community (Smith, 2018). Findings from more than 4,000 interviews have directly informed the design of the program. The program delivers a "bundle" of local services, including those to build skills (e.g., for stress management and work success), community mental health ambassadors, referrals to local services and resources, and social networks and support (Smith, 2018).

The program has demonstrated promising initial outcomes, including findings from a 2012–2016 randomized controlled trial in New Haven public housing and multigenerational outcomes from two quasi-experimental studies (Smith, 2018). Evaluation of the program has shown that at completion, 76 percent of participants have fewer depressive symptoms and participants experience a 67 percent decrease in parenting stress (MOMS Partnership, n.d.-a).

Beginning in 2019, the MOMS Partnership will replicate its program in Washington, DC, through a partnership with the DC Department of Human Services and via DC's Temporary Assistance for Needy Families (TANF) program (Clayton et al., 2018; MOMS Partnership, n.d.-b). The MOMS Partnership has also collaborated with Vermont Reach Up, that state's TANF program, to replicate the program in Vermont by 2020.

---

[a] The committee used selection criteria to identify examples of promising models highlighted in this report (see Appendix A for a list of the criteria). These examples all apply developmental science and aim to advance health equity during the preconception through early childhood periods.

Where necessary, mothers in serious distress need to be referred to more resource intensive, one-on-one programs, such as ABC and Infant/Toddler Parent Psychotherapy. Home visiting, with concurrent referrals to available supports as needed—formal and informal—should exist within the community. Ideally, all types of intensive services would be coordinated with the pediatricians' offices in a team-based approach to providing care (see more on team-based approaches in the health care setting in Chapter 5).

It will be critical to allocate resources to monitoring the quality of interventions delivered. All intervention programs need to be culturally sensitive, be adapted to community needs, have clear procedures for the selection and training of clinicians, and have mechanisms in place to ensure fidelity and quality of services. Support is needed for programs across tier levels of delivery, universal and intensive. Furthermore, taking an ecological perspective on promoting caregiver well-being and attachment would require supportive policies that facilitate healthy social connections and family cohesion during these critical years of early life. For example, paid parental leave following the birth of a child is one policy that has evidence for shaping child and family outcomes (AEI-Brookings Working Group on Paid Family Leave, 2017). (See Chapter 6 for a full discussion and Recommendation 6-1 on implementing paid leave.)

Finally, in evaluating the effectiveness of programs for at-risk mothers and their children, measures need to focus on those maternal dimensions that are known to strongly affect the mother–child relationship and hence child well-being. This would include measures of maternal depression and stress, feelings of rejection or hostility to the child, available support for mothers, and any contact with CPS. These assessments should be a routine part of prenatal, postnatal, and pediatric visits, along with other physical health indexes that are assessed and recorded. Careful, balanced consideration of all of these aspects of intervention design, delivery, and measurement—with all of the investment of resources called for by each aspect—is critical to move toward meaningfully increasing equity in well-being, considering America's most vulnerable children and families.

REFERENCES

ACF (Administration for Children and Families). 2018. *Implementing Attachment and Biobehavioral Catch-up intervention.* https://homvee.acf.hhs.gov/Implementation/3/Attachment-and-Biobehavioral-Catch-Up-ABC--Intervention-Model-Overview/51 (accessed January 11, 2019).

Acker, J., P. Braveman, E. Arkin, L. Leviton, J. Parsons, and G. Hobor. 2019. *Mass incarceration threatens health equity in America.* Princeton, NJ: Robert Wood Johnson Foundation.

Adams, T. R., E. D. Handley, J. T. Manly, D. Cicchetti, and S. L. Toth. 2019. Intimate partner violence as a mechanism underlying the intergenerational transmission of maltreatment among economically disadvantaged mothers and their adolescent daughters. *Development & Psychopathology* 31(1):83–93.

AEI-Brookings Working Group on Paid Family Leave. 2017. *Paid family and medical leave: An issue whose time has come.* Washington, DC: The Brookings Institution.

Ammerman, R. T., F. W. Putnam, J. Stevens, L. J. Holleb, A. L. Novak, and J. B. Van Ginkel. 2005. In-home cognitive behavior therapy for depression: An adapted treatment for first time mothers in home visitation. *Best Practices in Mental Health* 1:1–14.

Antonucci, T. C., K. J. Ajrouch, and K. S. Birditt. 2014. The convoy model: Explaining social relations from a multidisciplinary perspective. *Gerontologist* 54(1):82–92.

Assari, S., and C. H. Caldwell. 2018. High risk of depression in high-income African American boys. *Journal of Racial and Ethnic Health Disparities* 5(4):808–819.

Assari, S., F. X. Gibbons, and R. L. Simons. 2018a. Perceived discrimination among black youth: An 18-year longitudinal study. *Behavioral Sciences* 8(5).

Assari, S., B. Preiser, M. M. Lankarani, and C. H. Caldwell. 2018b. Subjective socioeconomic status moderates the association between discrimination and depression in African American youth. *Brain Sciences* 8(4).

ASU (Arizona State University) Reach Institute. 2018. *Family check-up for providers.* https://reachinstitute.asu.edu/family-check-up/agencies (accessed May 2, 2019).

Attachment Biobehavioral Catch-Up. 2017. *The Attachment Biobehavioral Catch-up (ABC) program.* http://www.abcintervention.org/about (accessed January 11, 2019).

Avellar, S. A., and L. H. Supplee. 2013. Effectiveness of home visiting in improving child health and reducing child maltreatment. *Pediatrics* 132:S90–S99.

Avellar, S., R. Covington, Q. Moore, A. Patnaik, and A. Wu. 2019. *Effects of four responsible fatherhood programs for low income fathers: Evidence from the parents and children together evaluation.* OPRE Report 2019-05. Washington, DC: Office of Planning, Research, and Evaluation, Administration for Children and Families, U.S. Department of Health and Human Services.

Balaji, A. B., A. H. Claussen, D. C. Smith, S. N. Visser, M. J. Morales, and R. Perou. 2007. Social support networks and maternal mental health and well-being. *Journal of Women's Health (Larchmt)* 16(10):1386–1396.

Barlow, A., B. Mullany, N. Neault, N. Goklish, T. Billy, R. Hastings, S. Lorenzo, C. Kee, K. Lake, C. Redmond, A. Carter, and J. T. Walkup. 2015. Paraprofessional-delivered home-visiting intervention for American Indian teen mothers and children: 3-year outcomes from a randomized controlled trial. *American Journal of Psychiatry* 172(2):154–162.

Barlow, K., and B. L. Chapin. 2010. The practice of mothering: An introduction. *Ethos* 38(4):324–338.

Barone, L., F. Lionetti, and J. Green. 2017. A matter of attachment? How adoptive parents foster post-institutionalized children's social and emotional adjustment. *Attachment & Human Development* 19(4):323–339.

Baumeister, R. F., E. Bratslavsky, C. Finkenauer, and K. D. Vohs. 2001. Bad is stronger than good. *Review of General Psychology* 5(4):323–370.

Becares, L., and N. Priest. 2015. Understanding the influence of race/ethnicity, gender, and class on inequalities in academic and non-academic outcomes among eighth-grade students: Findings from an intersectionality approach. *PLoS ONE* 10(10):e0141363.

Bernard, K., R. Simons, and M. Dozier. 2015. Effects of an attachment-based intervention on child protective services—referred mothers' event-related potentials to children's emotions. *Child Development* 86(6):1673–1684.

Bick, J., and M. Dozier. 2013. The effectiveness of an attachment-based intervention in promoting foster mothers' sensitivity toward foster infants. *Infant Mental Health Journal* 34(2):95–103.

Bloch, J. R., D. A. Webb, L. Mathews, E. F. Dennis, I. M. Bennett, and J. F. Culhane. 2010. Beyond marital status: The quality of the mother-father relationship and its influence on reproductive health behaviors and outcomes among unmarried low income pregnant women. *Maternal & Child Health Journal* 14(5):726–734.

Bolger, K. E., and C. J. Patterson. 2003. Sequelae of child maltreatment: Vulnerability and resilience. In *Resilience and vulnerability: Adaptation in the context of childhood adversities,* edited by S. S. Luthar. New York: Cambridge University Press. Pp. 156–181.

Borden, L. A., T. R. Schultz, K. C. Herman, and C. M. Brooks. 2010. The Incredible Years parent training program: Promoting resilience through evidence-based prevention groups. *Group Dynamics: Theory, Research, and Practice* 14(3):230–241.

Bouza, J., D. E. Camacho-Thompson, G. Carlo, X. Franco, C. García Coll, L. C. Halgunseth, A. Marks, G. Livas Stein, C. Suarez-Orozco, and R. M. B. White. 2018. *The science is clear: Separating families has long-term damaging psychological and health consequences for children, families, and communities.* Washington, DC: Society for Research in Child Development.

Bowleg, L. 2012. The problem with the phrase women and minorities: Intersectionality—an important theoretical framework for public health. *American Journal of Public Health* 102(7):1267–1273.

Brennan, L. M., E. C. Shelleby, D. S. Shaw, F. Gardner, T. J. Dishion, and M. Wilson. 2013. Indirect effects of the Family Check-up on school-age academic achievement through improvements in parenting in early childhood. *Journal of Educational Psychology* 105(3):762.

Bronfenbrenner, U. 1979. *The ecology of human development: Experiments by nature and design.* London, UK: Harvard University Press.

Brooks-Gunn, J., and G. J. Duncan. 1997. The effects of poverty on children. *The Future of Children* 7(2):55–71.

Brown, T. H., L. J. Richardson, T. W. Hargrove, and C. S. Thomas. 2016. Using multiple-hierarchy stratification and life course approaches to understand health inequalities: The intersecting consequences of race, gender, SES, and age. *Journal of Health and Social Behavior* 57(2):200–222.

Bryan, A. E., and H. Arkowitz. 2015. Meta-analysis of the effects of peer-administered psychosocial interventions on symptoms of depression. *American Journal of Community Psychology* 55(3–4):455–471.

Burwick, A., H. Zaveri, L. Shang, K. Boller, D. Daro, and D. A. Strong. 2014. *Costs of early childhood home visiting: An analysis of programs implemented in the supporting evidence-based home visiting to prevent child maltreatment initiative.* Princeton, NJ: Mathematica Policy Research, Inc.

Cabrera, N. J., J. D. Shannon, and C. S. Tamis-LeMonda. 2007. Fathers' influence on their children's cognitive and emotional development: From toddlers to pre-K. *Applied Developmental Science* 11(4):208–213.

Cabrera, N. J., H. E. Fitzgerald, R. H. Bradley, and L. Roggman. 2014. The ecology of father-child relationships: An expanded model. *Journal of Family Theory and Review* 6:336–354.

Cabrera, N. J., L. Torres, R. Dion, and S. Baumgartner. 2015. *H-pact: A descriptive study of responsible fatherhood programs serving hispanic men.* OPRE report 2015-112. Washington, DC: Office of Planning, Research and Evaluation, Administration for Children and Families, U.S. Department of Health and Human Services.

Cannon, J. S., M. R. Kilburn, L. A. Karoly, T. Mattox, A. N. Muchow, and M. Buenaventura. 2017. *Investing early: Taking stock of outcomes and economic returns from early childhood programs.* Santa Monica, CA: RAND Corporation.

Casey, B. J., A. Galvan, and L. H. Somerville. 2016. Beyond simple models of adolescence to an integrated circuit-based account: A commentary. *Developmental Cognitive Neuroscience* 17:128–130.

Casillas, K. L., A. Fauchier, B. T. Derkash, and E. F. Garrido. 2016. Implementation of evidence-based home visiting programs aimed at reducing child maltreatment: A meta-analytic review. *Child Abuse & Neglect* 53:64–80.

CDC (Centers for Disease Control and Prevention). 2014. *Understanding Child Maltreatment.* https://www.cdc.gov/violenceprevention/pdf/cm-factsheet--2013.pdf (accessed April 2, 2019).

CDC. 2017. *LGBT youth*. https://www.cdc.gov/lgbthealth/youth.htm (accessed June 14, 2019).

Center on the Developing Child at Harvard University. 2010. *The foundations of lifelong health are built in early childhood*. Cambridge, MA: Harvard University.

Center on the Developing Child at Harvard University. 2011. *Building the brain's "air traffic control" system: How early experiences shape the development of executive function: Working paper no. 11*. Cambridge, MA: Harvard University.

Center on the Developing Child at Harvard University. 2016. *From best practices to breakthrough impacts: A science-based approach to building a more promising future for young children and families*. Cambridge, MA: Harvard University.

Center on the Developing Child at Harvard University. 2019. *MOMS partnership*. https://developingchild.harvard.edu/innovation-application/innovation-in-action/moms (accessed June 10, 2019).

Christian, S. 2009. *Children of incarcerated parents*. Washington, DC: National Conference of State Legislatures.

Cicchetti, D. 2010. Resilience under conditions of extreme stress: A multilevel perspective. *World Psychiatry* 9(3):145–154.

Cicchetti, D. 2013. Annual research review: Resilient functioning in maltreated children—past, present, and future perspectives. *Journal of Child Psychology and Psychiatry* 54(4):402–422.

Cicchetti, D., and R. Rizley. 1981. Developmental perspectives on the etiology, intergenerational transmission, and sequelae of child maltreatment. *New Directions for Child and Adolescent Development* 11:31–55.

Cicchetti, D., and S. L. Toth. 2015. Child maltreatment. In *Handbook of child psychology and developmental science: Socioemotional process*, 7th ed. Vol. 3, edited by M. E. Lamb and R. M. Lerner. Hoboken, NJ: John Wiley & Sons.

Cicchetti, D., and S. L. Toth. 2016. Child maltreatment and developmental psychopathology: A multilevel perspective. In *Developmental psychopathology: Maladaptation and psychopathology*, 3rd ed. Vol. 3, edited by D. Cicchetti. Hoboken, NJ: John Wiley & Sons.

Cicchetti, D., F. A. Rogosch, and S. L. Toth. 2006. Fostering secure attachment in infants in maltreating families through preventive interventions. *Development and Psychopathology* 18(3):623–649.

Ciciolla, L., and S. S. Luthar. 2019. Invisible household labor and ramifications for adjustment: Mothers as captains of households. *Sex Roles* 1–20.

Clayton, A., L. Callinan, K. Klem, and M. Smith. 2018. *Embracing 2-gen: Findings from the District of Columbia's TANF survey*. New Haven, CT: Yale School of Medicine.

Cohen, J. 1988. *Statistical power analysis for the behavioral sciences*, 2nd ed. New York: Academic Press.

Cohen, S., T. Kamarck, and R. Mermelstein. 1983. A global measure of perceived stress. *Journal of Health and Social Behavior* 24(4):385–396.

Coley, R. L., J. Sims, E. Dearing, and B. Spielvogel. 2018. Locating economic risks for adolescent mental and behavioral health: Poverty and affluence in families, neighborhoods, and schools. *Child Development* 89(2):360–369.

Conger, R. D., and K. J. Conger. 2002. Resilience in Midwestern families: Selected findings from the first decade of a prospective, longitudinal study. *Journal of Marriage and Family* 64:361–373.

Crnic, K. 1983. *Inventory of parent experiences*. University Park, PA: The Pennsylvania State University, Department of Psychology.

Crowl, A., A. Soyeon, and J. Baker. 2008. A meta-analysis of developmental outcomes for children of same-sex and heterosexual parents. *Journal of GLBT Family Studies* 4(3):385–407.

Dahl, R. E. 2004. Adolescent brain development: A period of vulnerabilities and opportunities. Keynote address. *Annals of the New York Academy of Sciences* 1021:1–22.

Davison, K. K., A. Gavarkovs, B. McBride, M. Kotelchuck, R. Levy, and E. M. Taveras. 2019. Engaging fathers in early obesity prevention during the first 1,000 days: Policy, systems, and environmental change strategies. *Obesity (Silver Spring)* 27(4):525–533.

Denmark, N., K. Peplinski, M. Sparr, J. Labiner-Wolfe, S. Zaid, P. Gupta, and K. M. Miller. 2018. Introduction to the special issue on taking home visiting to scale: Findings from the maternal, infant, and early childhood home visiting program state-led evaluations. *Maternal and Child Health Journal* 22(Suppl 1):1–2.

Dishion, T. J., and K. Kavanagh. 2003. *Intervening in adolescent problem behavior: A family-centered approach.* New York: Guilford Press.

Dishion, T. J., D. Shaw, A. Connell, F. Gardner, C. Weaver, and M. Wilson. 2008. The family check-up with high-risk indigent families: Preventing problem behavior by increasing parents' positive behavior support in early childhood. *Child Development* 79(5):1395–1414.

Dishion, T. J., L. M. Brennan, D. S. Shaw, A. D. McEachern, M. N. Wilson, and B. Jo. 2014. Prevention of problem behavior through annual family check-ups in early childhood: Intervention effects from home to early elementary school. *Journal of Abnormal Child Psychology* 42(3):343–354.

Domitrovich, C. E., J. A. Durlak, K. C. Staley, and R. P. Weissberg. 2017. Social-emotional competence: An essential factor for promoting positive adjustment and reducing risk in school children. *Child Development* 88(2):408–416.

Dong, M., W. H. Giles, V. J. Felitti, S. R. Dube, J. E. Williams, D. P. Chapman, and R. F. Anda. 2004. Insights into causal pathways for ischemic heart disease: Adverse childhood experiences study. *Circulation* 110(13):1761–1766.

Dorner, L. M., M. F. Orellana, and R. Jiménez. 2008. "It's one of those things that you do to help the family": Language brokering and the development of immigrant adolescents. *Journal of Adolescent Research* 23(5):515–543.

Dozier, M., D. Dozier, and M. Manni. 2002. Recognizing the special needs of infants' and toddlers' foster parents: Development of a relational intervention. *Zero to Three Bulletin* 22:7–13.

Dozier, M., O. Lindhiem, and J. Ackerman. 2005. Attachment and Biobehavioral Catch-up: An intervention targeting empirically identified needs of foster infants. In *Duke series in child development and public policy. Enhancing early attachments: Theory, research, intervention, and policy,* edited by L. J. Berlin, Y. Ziv, L. Amaya-Jackson, and M. T. Greenberg. New York: Guilford Press.

Drake, B. 2013. *Fewer Americans have negative views of more gays raising children.* https://www.pewresearch.org/fact-tank/2013/06/25/fewer-americans-have-negative-views-of-more-gays-raising-children (accessed April 19, 2019).

Dube, S. R., D. Fairweather, W. S. Pearson, V. J. Felitti, R. F. Anda, and J. B. Croft. 2009. Cumulative childhood stress and autoimmune diseases in adults. *Psychosomatic Medicine* 71(2):243–250.

Dudley, K. J., X. Li, M. S. Kobor, T. E. Kippin, and T. W. Bredy. 2011. Epigenetic mechanisms mediating vulnerability and resilience to psychiatric disorders. *Neuroscience and Biobehavioral Reviews* 35(7):1544–1551.

Eckenrode, J., M. Campa, D. W. Luckey, C. R. Henderson, Jr., R. Cole, H. Kitzman, E. Anson, K. Sidora-Arcoleo, J. Powers, and D. Olds. 2010. Long-term effects of prenatal and infancy nurse home visitation on the life course of youths: 19-year follow-up of a randomized trial. *Archives of Pediatric & Adolescent Medicine* 164(1):9–15.

Eckenrode, J., M. I. Campa, P. A. Morris, C. R. Henderson, Jr., K. E. Bolger, H. Kitzman, and D. L. Olds. 2017. The prevention of child maltreatment through the Nurse Family Partnership program: Mediating effects in a long-term follow-up study. *Child Maltreatment* 22(2):92–99.

Elder, G. H. 2018. *Children of the Great Depression.* New York: Routledge.

Evans, G. W. 2004. The environment of childhood poverty. *American Psychologist* 59(2):77–92.

Filene, J. H., J. W. Kaminski, L. A. Valle, and P. Cachat. 2013. Components associated with home visiting program outcomes: A meta-analysis. *Pediatrics* 132(Suppl 2):S100–S109.

Filindra, A., D. Blanding, and C. G. Coll. 2011. The power of context: State-level policies and politics and the educational performance of the children of immigrants in the United States. *Harvard Educational Review* 81(3):407–438.

Font, S. A., K. Sattler, and E. Gershoff. 2018. Measurement and correlates of foster care placement moves. *Child and Youth Services Review* 91:248–258.

Fredrickson, B. L., and M. F. Losada. 2005. Positive affect and the complex dynamics of human flourishing. *The American Psychologist* 60(7):678–686.

Fuligni, A. J., and S. Pedersen. 2002. Family obligation and the transition to young adulthood. *Developmental Psychology* 38(5):856–868.

Gallagher, M., and R. J. Nelson. 2003. *Handbook of psychology, biological psychology (Volume 3)*. Hoboken, NJ: John Wiley & Sons, Inc.

García Coll, C. T., and A. K. Marks. 2012. *The immigrant paradox in children and adolescents: Is becoming American a developmental risk?* Washington, DC: American Psychological Association.

García Coll, C., G. Lamberty, R. Jenkins, H. P. McAdoo, K. Crnic, B. H. Wasik, and H. Vazquez Garcia. 1996. An integrative model for the study of developmental competencies in minority children. *Child Development* 67(5):1891–1914.

Geisz, M. B., and M. Nakashian. 2018. *Adolescent wellness: Current perspectives and future opportunities in research, policy, and practice*. Princeton, NJ: Robert Wood Johnson Foundation.

Giurgescu, C., L. Fahmy, J. Slaughter-Acey, A. Nowak, C. Caldwell, and D. P. Misra. 2018. Can support from the father of the baby buffer the adverse effects of depressive symptoms on risk of preterm birth in black families? *AIMS Public Health* 5(1):89–98.

Goemans, A., M. van Geel, and P. Vedder. 2015. Over three decades of longitudinal research on the development of foster children: A meta-analysis. *Child Abuse & Neglect* 42:121–134.

Goemans, A., M. van Geel, M. van Beem, and P. Vedder. 2016. Developmental outcomes of foster children: A meta-analytic comparison with children from the general population and children at risk who remained at home. *Child Maltreatment* 21(3):198–217.

Golden, O., A. Hawkins, and W. Bearsdlee. 2011. *Home visiting and maternal depression: Seizing the opportunities to help mothers and young children*. Washington, DC: The Urban Institute.

Gollner, R., R. I. Damian, B. Nagengast, B. W. Roberts, and U. Trautwein. 2018. It's not only who you are but who you are with: High school composition and individuals' attainment over the life course. *Psychological Science* 29(11):1785–1796.

Goodman, S. H., and J. Garber. 2017. Evidence-based interventions for depressed mothers and their young children. *Child Development* 88(2):368–377.

Grusec, J. E., and M. Davidov. 2010. Integrating different perspectives on socialization theory and research: A domain-specific approach. *Child Development* 81(3):687–709.

Hammock, E. A. D., and P. Levitt. 2006. The discipline of neurobehavioral development: The emerging interface of processes that build circuits and skills. *Human Development* 49(5):294–309.

Hamoudi, A., D. W. Murray, L. Sorensen, and A. Fontaine. 2015. *Self-regulation and toxic stress: A review of ecological, biological, and developmental studies of self-regulation and stress*. OPRE report #2015-30. Washington, DC: U.S. Department of Health and Human Services, Administration for Children and Families, Office of Planning, Research and Evaluation.

Hankivsky, O., and A. Christoffersen. 2008. Intersectionality and the determinants of health: A Canadian perspective. *Critical Public Health* 18(3):271–283.

Harold, G. T., L. D. Leve, and R. Sellers. 2017. How can genetically informed research help inform the next generation of interparental and parenting interventions? *Child Development* 88(2):446–458.

Hill, R. B. 2007. *An analysis of racial-ethnic disproportionality and disparity at the national state and county levels.* Casey-CSSP Alliance for Racial Equity in Child Welfare.

Hiratsuka, V. Y., M. E. Parker, J. Sanchez, R. Riley, D. Heath, J. C. Chomo, M. Beltangady, and M. Sarche. 2018. Cultural adaptations of evidence-based home-visitation models in tribal communities. *Infant Mental Health Journal* 39(3):265–275.

Ho, J. 2015. Bicultural children: What parents and teachers should know. *Childhood Education* 91(1):35–40.

Hofmann, S. G., and S. C. Hayes. 2019. The future of intervention science: Process-based therapy. *Clinical Psychological Science: A Journal of the Association for Psychological Science* 7(1):37–50.

Hoge, E., D. Bickham, and J. Cantor. 2017. Digital media, anxiety, and depression in children. *Pediatrics* 140(S2):S76–S80.

Hrdy, S. B. 1999. *Mother nature: A history of mothers, infants, and natural selection.* New York: The Ballantine Publishing Group.

Hrdy, S. B. 2011. *Mothers and others: The evolutionary origins of mutual understanding.* Cambridge, MA: Harvard University Press.

HRSA (Health Resources and Services Administration). n.d. *The maternal, infant, and early childhood home visiting program: Partnering with parents to help children succeed.* https://mchb.hrsa.gov/sites/default/files/mchb/MaternalChildHealthInitiatives/HomeVisiting/pdf/programbrief.pdf (accessed August 13, 2018).

Hughes, D., J. Rodriguez, E. P. Smith, D. J. Johnson, H. C. Stevenson, and P. Spicer. 2006. Parents' ethnic-racial socialization practices: A review of research and directions for future study. *Developmental Psychology* 42(5):747–770.

Huston, A. C., V. C. McLoyd, and C. García Coll. 1994. Children and poverty: Issues in contemporary research. *Child Development* 65(2):275–282.

IOM (Institute of Medicine). 2011. *The health of lesbian, gay, bisexual, and transgender people: Building a foundation for better understanding.* Washington, DC: The National Academies Press.

Jackson, A. 2015. Strategies for supporting low-income and welfare-dependent parents of young children. In *Parenting Matters: Supporting Parents of Children Ages 0–8, Appendix A. Public Information-Gathering Session Agenda, meeting 2, panel: Addressing the Needs of Specific Populations.* National Academies of Sciences, Engineering, and Medicine. Washington, DC: The National Academies Press. P. 397.

Jackson, A. P. 2000. Maternal self-efficacy and children's influence on stress and parenting among single black mothers in poverty. *Journal of Family Issues* 21(1):3–16.

Johnson, K. 2019. *Medicaid and home visiting: The state of states' approaches.* https://ccf.georgetown.edu/wp-content/uploads/2019/01/Medicaid-and-Home-Visiting.pdf (accessed March 20, 2019).

Jolly, S., K. A. Griffith, R. DeCastro, A. Stewart, P. Ubel, and R. Jagsi. 2014. Gender differences in time spent on parenting and domestic responsibilities by high-achieving young physician-researchers. *Annals of Internal Medicine* 160(5):344–353.

Jones, T. L., and R. J. Prinz. 2005. Potential roles of parental self-efficacy in parent and child adjustment: A review. *Clinical Psychology Review* 25(3):341–363.

Jones Harden, B. 2004. Safety and stability for foster children: A developmental perspective. *The Future of Children* 14(1):31–47.

Jonson-Reid, M., B. Drake, J. N. Constantino, M. Tandon, L. Pons, P. Kohl, S. Roesch, E. Wideman, A. Dunnigan, and W. Auslander. 2018. A randomized trial of home visitation for CPS-involved families: The moderating impact of maternal depression and CPS history. *Child Maltreatment* 23(3):281–293.

Kalil, A., R. Ryan, and M. Corey. 2012. Diverging destinies: Maternal education and the developmental gradient in time with children. *Demography* 49(4):1361–1383.

Kalmakis, K.A., and G. E. Chandler. 2015. Health consequences of adverse childhood experiences: A systematic review. *Journal of the American Association of Nurse Practitioners* 27(8):457–465.

Kaufman, J. S., and E. Ziegler. 1987. Do abused children become abusive parents? *American Journal of Orthopsychiatry* 57(2):186–192.

Kazdin, A. E., and S. M. Rabbitt. 2013. Novel models for delivering mental health services and reducing the burdens of mental illness. *Clinical Psychological Science* 1(2):170–191.

Kelly, J. F., B. Hoeppner, R. L. Stout, and M. Pagano. 2012. Determining the relative importance of the mechanisms of behavior change within Alcoholics Anonymous: A multiple mediator analysis. *Addiction* 107(2):289–299.

Kitzman, H., D. L. Olds, D. R. J. Henderson, C. A. Hanks, R. Cole, R. Tatelbaum, and K. Barnard. 1997. Effects of home visitation by nurses on pregnancy outcomes, childhood injuries, and repeated childbearing: A randomized controlled trial. *JAMA* 278(8):644–652.

Knitzer, J. 2000. Early childhood mental health services: A policy and systems development perspective. In *Handbook of early childhood intervention*, 2nd ed., edited by J. P. Shonkoff and S. J. Meisels. Cambridge, MA: Cambridge University Press. Pp. 416–438.

Koplewicz, H. S., A. Gurian, and K. Williams. 2009. The era of affluence and its discontents. *Journal of the American Academy of Child and Adolescent Psychiatry* 48(11):1053–1055.

Kopp, C. 2013. *Becoming female: Perspectives on development*. New York: Springer. Pp. 313–332.

Kotelchuck, M., and M. Lu. 2017. Father's role in preconception health. *Maternal and Child Health Journal* 21(11):2025–2039.

Lamb, M. E. 2004. *The role of the father in child development*. New York: Wiley.

Lareau, A., and E. B. Weininger. 2008. Time, work, and family life: Reconceptualizing gendered time patterns through the case of children's organized activities. *Sociological Forum* 23:419–454.

Lee, S., H. S. Juon, G. Martinez, C. E. Hsu, E. S. Robinson, J. Bawa, and G. X. Ma. 2009. Model minority at risk: Expressed needs of mental health by Asian American young adults. *Journal of Community Health* 34(2):144–152.

Lee, S. J., C. A. Taylor, and J. L. Bellamy. 2012. Paternal depression and risk for child neglect in father-involved families of young children. *Child Abuse and Neglect* 36(5):461–469.

Leloux-Opmeer, H., C. Kuiper, H. Swaab, and E. Scholte. 2016. Characteristics of children in foster care, family-style group care, and residential care: A scoping review. *Journal of Child and Family Studies* 25:2357–2371.

Lerner, R. M., and W. F. Overton. 2017. Reduction to absurdity: Why epigenetics invalidates all models involving genetic reduction. *Human Development* 60(2–3):107–123.

Leve, L. D., G. T. Harold, P. Chamberlain, J. A. Landsverk, P. A. Fisher, and P. Vostanis. 2012. Practitioner review: Children in foster care—vulnerabilities and evidence-based interventions that promote resilience processes. *Journal of Child Psychology and Psychiatry* 53(12):1197–1211.

Lewis, C., and M. E. Lamb. 2003. Fathers' influences on children's development: The evidence from two-parent families. *European Journal of Psychology of Education* 18(2):211–228.

Lewis, T. T., and M. E. Van Dyke. 2018. Discrimination and the health of African Americans: The potential importance of intersectionalities. *Current Directions in Psychological Science* 27(3):176–182.

Lieberman, A. F., and C. H. Zeanah. 1999. Contributions of attachment theory to infant-parent psychotherapy and other interventions with infants and young children. In *Handbook of attachment*, edited by J. Cassidy and P. R. Shaver. New York: Guilford Press. Pp. 555–574.

Lieberman, A. F., E. Padron, P. Van Horn, and W. W. Harris. 2005. Angels in the nursery: The intergenerational transmission of benevolent parental influences. *Infant Mental Health Journal* 26(6):504–520.

Lieberman, A. F., A. Chu, P. Van Horn, and W. W. Harris. 2011. Trauma in early childhood: Empirical evidence and clinical implications. *Development and Psychopathology* 23(2):397–410.

Lind, T., K. Bernard, E. Ross, and M. Dozier. 2014. Intervention effects on negative affect of CPS-referred children: Results of a randomized clinical trial. *Child Abuse & Neglect* 38(9):1459–1467.

Lino, M., K. Kuczynski, N. Rodriguez, and T. Schap. 2017. *Expenditures on children by families, 2015.* Miscellaneous publication no. 1528-2015. Alexandria, VA: U.S. Department of Agriculture, Center for Nutrition Policy & Promotion.

Lu, M. C., L. Jones, M. J. Bond, K. Wright, M. Pumpuang, M. Maidenberg, D. Jones, C. Garfield, and D. L. Rowley. 2010. Where is the F in MCH? Father involvement in African American Families. *Ethnicity and Disease* 20:S2–S49.

Lund, T. J., E. Dearing, and H. D. Zachrisson. 2017. Is affluence a risk for adolescents in Norway? *Journal of Research on Adolescence* 27(3):628–643.

Lunkenheimer, E. S., T. J. Dishion, D. S. Shaw, A. M. Connell, F. Gardner, M. N. Wilson, and E. M. Skuban. 2008. Collateral benefits of the Family Check-up on early childhood school readiness: Indirect effects of parents' positive behavior support. *Developmental Psychology* 44(6):1737–1752.

Luthar, S. S. 2015. Mothering mothers. *Research in Human Development* 12(3–4):295–303.

Luthar, S. S., and L. Ciciolla. 2015. Who mothers mommy? Factors that contribute to mothers' well-being. *Developmental Psychology* 51(12):1812–1823.

Luthar, S. S., and N. Eisenberg. 2017. Resilient adaptation among at-risk children: Harnessing science toward maximizing salutary environments. *Child Development* 88(2):337–349.

Luthar, S. S., and N. L. Kumar. 2018. Youth in high-achieving schools: Challenges to mental health and directions for evidence-based interventions. In *Handbook of school-based mental health promotion*, edited by A. W. Leschied, D. H. Saklofske, and G. L. Flett. Pp. 441–458.

Luthar, S. S., and C. C. Sexton. 2007. Maternal drug abuse versus maternal depression: Vulnerability and resilience among school-age and adolescent offspring. *Development and Psychopathology* 19(1):205–225.

Luthar, S. S., and N. E. Suchman. 2000. Relational psychotherapy mothers' group: A developmentally informed intervention for at-risk mothers. *Development and Psychopathology* 12(2):235–253.

Luthar, S. S., N. E. Suchman, and M. Altomare. 2007. Relational psychotherapy mothers' group: A randomized clinical trial for substance abusing mothers. *Development and Psychopathology* 19(1):243–261.

Luthar, S. S., S. H. Barkin, and E. J. Crossman. 2013. "I can, therefore I must": Fragility in the upper-middle classes. *Development and Psychopathology* 25(4 Pt. 2):1529–1549.

Luthar, S., E. J. Crossman, and P. J. Small. 2015. Resilience and adversity. In *Handbook of child psychology and developmental science*, 7th ed., Vol. 3, edited by R. M. Lerner and M. E. Lamb. New York: Wiley. Pp. 247–286.

Luthar, S. S., A. Curlee, S. J. Tye, J. C. Engelman, and C. M. Stonnington. 2017. Fostering resilience among mothers under stress: "Authentic connections groups" for medical professionals. *Women's Health Issues* 27(3):382–390.

Luthar, S. S., N. L. Kumar, and R. Benoit. In press. Authentic connections virtual groups: Fostering resilience among mothers in high-stress settings. *Development and Psychopathology.*

Macmillan, H. L., C. N. Wathen, J. Barlow, D. M. Fergusson, J. M. Leventhal, and H. N. Taussig. 2009. Interventions to prevent child maltreatment and associated impairment. *The Lancet* 373(9659):250–266.

Marks, A. K., J. L. McKenna, and C. García Coll. 2018. National immigration receiving contexts: A critical aspect of native-born, immigrant, and refugee youth well-being. *European Psychologist* 23(1):6–20.

Marmot, M., J. Allen, P. Goldblatt, T. Boyce, D. McNeish, and M. Grady. 2010. *Fair society, healthy lives: Strategic review of health inequalities in England post-2010*. The Marmot Review. http://www.instituteofhealthequity.org/resources-reports/fair-society-healthy-lives-the-marmot-review/fair-society-healthy-lives-full-report-pdf.pdf (accessed August 25, 2019).

Maslow, A. H. 1943. A theory of human motivation. *Psychological Review* 50(4):370–396.

Masten, A. S. 2014. Global perspectives on resilience in children and youth. *Child Development* 85(1):6–20.

Mazure, C. M., and D. P. Jones. 2015. Twenty years and still counting: Including women as participants and studying sex and gender in biomedical research. *BMC Women's Health* 15:94.

McCambell, S. W. 2005. *Gender-responsive strategies—for women offenders*. Washington, DC: U.S. Department of Justice.

McEachern, A. D., G. M. Fosco, T. J. Dishion, D. S. Shaw, M. N. Wilson, and F. Gardner. 2013. Collateral benefits of the Family Check-up in early childhood: Primary caregivers' social support and relationship satisfaction. *Journal of Family Psychology* 27(2):271–281.

McGinnis, S., E. Lee, K. Kirkland, C. Smith, C. Miranda-Julian, and R. Greene. 2018. Engaging at-risk fathers in home visiting services: Effects on program retention and father involvement. *Child & Adolescent Social Work Journal* 36(2):189–200.

McLeod, S. 2018. *Maslow's Hierarchy of Needs*. https://www.simplypsychology.org/maslow. html (accessed January 24, 2019).

McLoyd, V. C. 1990. The impact of economic hardship on black families and children: Psychological distress, parenting, and socioemotional development. *Child Development* 61:311–346.

Michalopoulos, C., K. Faucetta, C. J. Hill, X. A. Portilla, L. Burrell, H. Lee, A. Dugggan, and V. Knox. 2019. *Impacts on family outcomes of evidence-based early childhood home visiting-results from the Mother and Infant Home Visiting Program Evaluation*. Washington, DC: U.S. Department of Health and Human Services, Administration for Children and Families, Office of Planning, Research and Evaluation.

Minkovitz, C. S., K. M. O'Neill, and A. K. Duggan. 2016. Home visiting: A service strategy to reduce poverty and mitigate its consequences. *Academic Pediatrics* 16(Suppl 3):S105–S111.

Modecki, K. L., M. J. Zimmer-Gembeck, and N. Guerra. 2017. Emotion regulation, coping, and decision making: Three linked skills for preventing externalizing problems in adolescence. *Child Development* 88(2):417–426.

MOMS (Mental health Outreach for Mothers) Partnership. n.d.-a. *Impact*. https://medicine. yale.edu/psychiatry/moms/impact (accessed June 10, 2019).

MOMS Partnership. n.d.-b. *Where we're going*. https://medicine.yale.edu/psychiatry/moms/where/where.aspx (accessed June 10, 2019).

MOMS Partnership. n.d.-c. *Who we are*. https://medicine.yale.edu/psychiatry/moms/are/who.aspx (accessed January 28, 2019).

Morris, A. S., L. R. Robinson, J. Hays-Grudo, A. H. Claussen, S. A. Hartwig, and A. E. Treat. 2017. Targeting parenting in early childhood: A public health approach to improve outcomes for children living in poverty. *Child Development* 88(2):388–397.

Moseley, K. L., G. L. Freed, C. M. Bullard, and S. D. Goold. 2007. Measuring African-American parent's cultural mistrust while in a healthcare setting. *Journal of the Medical Association* 99(1):15–21.

Moss, M., and M. Puma. 1995. *Prospects: The congressionally mandated study of educational growth and opportunity. First year report on language minority and limited English proficient students*. Washington, DC: U.S. Department of Education, Office of Bilingual Education and Minority Languages Affairs.

Murgatroyd, C., and D. Spengler. 2011. Epigenetics of early child development. *Frontiers in Psychiatry* 2:16.

Murray, J., and L. Murray. 2010. Parental incarceration, attachment and child psychopathology. *Attachment & Human Development* 12(4):289–309.

Murray, J., D. P. Farrington, and I. Sekol. 2012. Children's antisocial behavior, mental health, drug use, and educational performance after parental incarceration: A systematic review and meta-analysis. *Psychological Bulletin* 138(2):175–210.

NASEM (National Academies of Sciences, Engineering, and Medicine). 2016. *Parenting matters: Supporting parents of children ages 0–8.* Washington, DC: The National Academies Press.

NASEM. 2017. *Communities in action: Pathways to health equity.* Washington, DC: The National Academies Press.

National Partnership for Women & Families. 2018. *Raising expectations: A state-by-state analysis of laws that help working family caregivers.* Washington, DC: National Partnership for Women & Families.

National Scientific Council on the Developing Child. 2004. *Young children develop in an environment of relationships (working paper 1).* Cambridge, MA: Center on the Developing Child at Harvard University.

National Scientific Council on the Developing Child. 2010. *Early experiences can alter gene expression and affect long-term development.* Working paper no. 10. Cambridge, MA: Center on the Developing Child at Harvard University.

NCSL (National Conference of State Legislators). 2019. *Family First Prevention Services Act.* http://www.ncsl.org/research/human-services/family-first-prevention-services-act-ffpsa.aspx (accessed June 4, 2019).

Ngo, B., and S. J. Lee. 2007. Complicating the image of model minority success: A review of southeast Asian American education. *Review of Educational Research* 77(4):415–453.

NHVRC (National Home Visiting Resource Center). 2018. *2018 home visiting yearbook.* https://www.nhvrc.org/wp-content/uploads/NHVRC_Yearbook_2018_FINAL.pdf (accessed March 20, 2019).

NICWA (National Indian Child Welfare Association). 2017. *What is disproportionality in child welfare?* https://www.nicwa.org/wp-content/uploads/2017/09/Disproportionality-Table.pdf (accessed June 4, 2019).

NRC (National Research Council). 2014. *The growth of incarceration in the United States: Exploring causes and consequences.* Washington, DC: The National Academies Press.

NRC and IOM. 2000. *From neurons to neighborhoods: The science of early childhood development.* Washington, DC: National Academy Press.

Olds, D. L., J. Eckenrode, C. R. Henderson, Jr., H. Kitzman, J. Powers, R. Cole, and D. Luckey. 1997. Long-term effects of home visitation on maternal life course and child abuse and neglect: 15-year follow-up of a randomized trial. *JAMA* 278(8):637–643.

Olds, D. L., H. Kitzman, C. Hanks, R. Cole, E. Anson, K. Sidora-Arcoleo, D. W. Luckey, C. R. Henderson, Jr., J. Holmberg, R. A. Tutt, A. J. Stevenson, and J. Bondy. 2007. Effects of nurse home visiting on maternal and child functioning: Age-9 follow-up of a randomized trial. *Pediatrics* 120(4):e832–e845.

OPRE (Office of Planning, Research and Evaluation). 2018. *Home visiting models reviewing evidence of effectiveness.* https://homvee.acf.hhs.gov/homevee_executive_summary_brief.pdf#Brief1 (accessed July 15, 2019).

Padilla, A. 2008. Developmental processes related to intergenerational transmission of culture. In *Cultural transmission: Psychological, developmental, social, and methodological aspects,* edited by U. E. Schonpflug. Cambridge, MA: Cambridge University Press. Pp. 185–211.

Parke, R. D., and K. A. Clarke-Stewart. 2001. *Effects of parental incarceration on young children.* Bethesda, MD: Office of the Assistant Secretary for Planning and Evaluation.

Paulsell, D., P. Del Grosso, and L. Supplee. 2014. Supporting replication and scale-up of evidence-based home visiting programs: Assessing the implementation knowledge base. *American Journal of Public Health* 104(9):1624–1632.

Pears, K. C., and D. M. Capaldi. 2001. Intergenerational transmission of abuse: A two-generational prospective study of an at-risk sample. *Child Abuse & Neglect* 25(11):1439–1461.

Pekrun, R., K. Murayama, H. W. Marsh, T. Goetz, and A. C. Frenzel. 2019. Happy fish in little ponds: Testing a reference group model of achievement and emotion. *Journal of Personality and Social Psychology* 117(1):166–185.

Phares, V., E. Lopez, S. Fields, D. Kamboukos, and A. M. Duhig. 2005. Are fathers involved in pediatric psychology research and treatment? *Journal of Pediatric Psychology* 30(8):631–643.

Plant, D. T., E. D. Barker, C. S. Waters, S. Pawlby, and C. M. Pariante. 2013. Intergenerational transmission of maltreatment and psychopathology: The role of antenatal depression. *Psychological Medicine* 43(3):519–528.

Plantin, L., A. A. Olukoya, and P. Ny. 2011. Positive health outcomes of fathers' involvement in pregnancy and childbirth paternal support: A scope study literature review. *Fathering* 9(1):87–102.

Pratt, J., and R. Chapman. n.d. *Culture, collaboration, and innovation: How tribal home visiting programs are working to improve outcomes for children, families, and communities.* https://www.acf.hhs.gov/sites/default/files/ecd/4478_thv_culture_collaboration_and_innovation_synthesis_report_final.pdf (accessed June 5, 2019).

Pruett, M. K., K. Pruett, C. P. Cowan, and P. A. Cowan. 2017. Enhancing father involvement in low-income families: A couples group approach to preventive intervention. *Child Development* 88(2):398–407.

Purewal, S. K., M. Bucci, L. G. Wang, K. Koita, S. S. Marques, D. Oh, and N. B. Harris. 2016. Screening for adverse childhood experiences (ACEs) in an integrated pediatric care model. *Zero to Three* 36(3):10–17.

Rae, J. R., S. Gulgoz, L. Durwood, M. DeMeules, R. Lowe, G. Lindquist, and K. R. Olson. 2019. Predicting early-childhood gender transitions. *Psychological Science* 30(5):669–681.

Rahman, A., P. J. Surkan, C. E. Cayetano, P. Rwagatare, and K. E. Dickson. 2013. Grand challenges: Integrating maternal mental health into maternal and child health programmes. *PLoS Medicine* 10(5):e1001442.

Ramey, G., and V. A. Ramey. 2010. The rug rat race. *Brookings Papers on Economic Activity* 41(1):129–199.

Reis, H. T., W. A. Collins, and E. Berscheid. 2000. The relationship context of human behavior and development. *Psychological Bulletin* 126(6):844–872.

Reynolds, A. J., S. R. Ou, C. F. Mondi, and M. Hayakawa. 2017. Processes of early childhood interventions to adult well-being. *Child Development* 88(2):378–387.

Rogoff, B. 2003. *The cultural nature of human development.* New York: Oxford University Press.

Rohner, E. C., R. P. Rohner, and S. Roll. 1980. Perceived parental acceptance-rejection and children's reported behavioral dispositions: A comparative and intracultural study of American and Mexican children. *Journal of Cross-Cultural Psychology* 11(2):213–231.

Rotheram-Borus, M. J., J. A. Stein, and Y. Y. Lin. 2001. Impact of parent death and an intervention on the adjustment of adolescents whose parents have HIV/AIDS. *Journal of Consulting and Clinical Psychology* 69(5):763–773.

Rotheram-Borus, M. J., D. Swendeman, S. J. Lee, L. Li, B. Amani, and M. Nartey. 2011. Interventions for families affected by HIV. *Translational Behavioral Medicine* 1(2):313–326.

Rutter, M. 1987. Psychosocial resilience and protective mechanisms. *The American Journal of Orthopsychiatry* 57(3):316–331.

Sama-Miller, E., L. Akers, A. Mraz-Esposito, M. Zukiewicz, S. Avellar, D. Paulsell, and P. Del Grosso. 2018. *Home visiting evidence of effectiveness review: Executive summary.* OPRE Report #2017-58. Washington, DC: U.S. Department of Health and Human Services.

Sampson, R. J., and J. H. Laub. 2003. Desistance from crime over the life course. In *Handbook of the life course*. Boston, MA: Springer.

Sandstrom, H. 2019. *Early childhood home visiting programs and health*. Health Affairs Health Policy Brief, April 25, 2019.

Schwartz, S. J., J. B. Unger, S. E. Des Rosiers, S. Huang, L. Baezconde-Garbanati, E. I. Lorenzo-Blanco, J. A. Villamar, D. W. Soto, M. Pattarroyo, and J. Szapocznik. 2012. Substance use and sexual behavior among recent Hispanic immigrant adolescents: Effects of parent-adolescent differential acculturation and communication. *Drug and Alcohol Dependence* 125(Suppl 1):S26–S34.

Schwebel, D. C., and C. M. Brezausek. 2010. How do mothers and fathers influence pediatric injury risk in middle childhood? *Journal of Pediatric Psychology* 35(8):806–813.

Seifer, R. 2003. Young children with mentally ill parents: Resilient developmental systems. In *Resilience and vulnerability: Adaptation in the context of childhood adversities*, edited by S. S. Luthar. New York: Cambridge University Press. Pp. 29–49.

Shaw, D. S., T. J. Dishion, L. Supplee, F. Gardner, and K. Arnds. 2006. Randomized trial of a family-centered approach to the prevention of early conduct problems: 2–year effects of the Family Check-up in early childhood. *Journal of Consulting and Clinical Psychology* 74(1):1–9.

Shaw, D. S., A. Connell, T. J. Dishion, M. N. Wilson, and F. Gardner. 2009. Improvements in maternal depression as a mediator of intervention effects on early childhood problem behavior. *Development and Psychopathology* 21(2):417–439.

Shlafer, R. J., and J. Poehlmann. 2010. Attachment and caregiving relationships in families affected by parental incarceration. *Attachment & Human Development* 12(4):395–415.

Smith, J. D., S. M. St. George, and G. Prado. 2017. Family-centered positive behavior support interventions in early childhood to prevent obesity. *Child Development* 88(2):427–435.

Smith, M. 2018. PowerPoint presentation to the Committee on Applying Neurobiological and Socio-Behavioral Sciences from Prenatal Through Early Childhood Development: A Health Equity Approach. Washington, DC. August 6, 2018. http://nationalacademies. org/hmd/~/media/Files/Agendas/Activity%20Files/Children/Prenatal-Early%20 Childhood%20Development/2018-AUG-06/2-4%20Smith%20-%20updated.pdf (accessed June 10, 2019).

Sparks, E. A., and R. F. Baumeister. 2008. If bad is stronger than good, why focus on human strength. *Positive Psychology: Exploring the Best in People* 1:55–79.

Sroufe, L. A., B. Egeland, E. A. Carlson, and W. A. Collins. 2005. *The development of the person: The Minnesota study of risk and adaptation from birth to adulthood*. New York: Guilford Press.

Steen, M., S. Downe, N. Bamford, and L. Edozien. 2012. Not-patient and not-visitor: A meta-synthesis fathers' encounters with pregnancy, birth and maternity care. *Midwifery* 28(4):362–371.

Super, C. M., and S. Harkness. 1986. The developmental niche: A conceptualization at the interface of child and culture. *International Journal of Behavioral Development* 9:545–569.

Taylor, Z. E., and R. D. Conger. 2017. Promoting strengths and resilience in single-mother families. *Child Development* 88(2):350–358.

Teeters, A. R., R. T. Ammerman, C. E. Shenk, N. K. Goyal, A. T. Folger, F. W. Putnam, and J. B. Van Ginkel. 2016. Predictors of maternal depressive symptom trajectories over the first 18 months in home visiting. *American Journal of Orthopsychiatry* 86(4):415–424.

Teitler, J. O. 2001. Father involvement, child health, and maternal health behavior. *Children and Youth Services Review* 23(4/5):403–425.

The Center for Parents & Children. n.d. *The family check-up*. https://www.cpc.pitt.edu/intervention-models/the-family-check-up (accessed May 2, 2019).

Toth, S. L., J. A. Gravener-Davis, D. J. Guild, and D. Cicchetti. 2013. Relational interventions for child maltreatment: Past, present, and future perspectives. *Development & Psychopathology* 25:1601–1607.

Toth, S. L., C. L. M. Petrenko, J. A. Gravener-Davis, and E. D. Handley. 2016. Advances in prevention science: A developmental psychopathology perspective. In *Developmental psychopathology*, edited by D. Cicchetti. New York: Wiley.

Turney, K. 2014. Stress proliferation across generations? Examining the relationship between parental incarceration and childhood health. *Journal of Health and Social Behavior* 55(3):302–319.

Twenge, J. M., A. B. Cooper, T. E. Joiner, M. E. Duffy, and S. G. Binau. 2019. Age, period, and cohort trends in mood disorder indicators and suicide-related outcomes in a nationally representative dataset, 2005–2017. *Journal of Abnormal Psychology* 128(3):185–199.

Umaña-Taylor, A. J., S. M. Quintana, R. M. Lee, W. E. Cross, D. Rivas-Drake, S. Schwartz, M. Syed, T. Yip, E. Seaton, and ERI Study Group. 2014. Ethnic and racial identity during adolescence and into young adulthood: An integrated conceptualization. *Child Development* 85(1):21–39.

UNM (University of New Mexico). 2011. Connecting children with incarcerated parents. *Child Protection Best Practices Bulletin*. Pp. 1–6.

Valentino, K. 2017. Relational interventions for maltreated children. *Child Development* 88(2):359–367.

Vasileva, M., and F. Petermann. 2018. Attachment, development, and mental health in abused and neglected preschool children in foster care: A meta-analysis. *Trauma, Violence, & Abuse* 19(4):443–458.

Vélez-Agosto, N. M., J. G. Soto-Crespo, M. Vizcarrondo-Oppenheimer, S. Vega-Molina, and C. García Coll. 2017. Bronfenbrenner's bioecological theory revision: Moving culture from the macro into the micro. *Perspectives on Psychological Science* 12(5):900–910.

Vogel, C. A., R. H. Bradley, H. H. Raikes, K. Boller, and J. K. Shears. 2006. Relation between father connectedness and child outcomes. *Parenting: Science & Practice* 6(2):189–209.

Vygotsky, L. S. 1978. *Mind in society*. Cambridge, MA: Harvard University Press.

Wainright, J. L., and C. J. Patterson. 2008. Peer relations among adolescents with female same-sex parents. *Developmental Psychology* 44(1):117–126.

Wainright, J. L., S. T. Russell, and C. J. Patterson. 2004. Psychosocial adjustment, school outcomes, and romantic relationships of adolescents with same-sex parents. *Child Development* 75(6):1886–1898.

Webster-Stratton, C., M. J. Reid, and M. Hammond. 2001. Preventing conduct problems, promoting social competence: A parent and teacher training partnership in Head Start. *Journal of Clinical Child Psychology* 30(3):283–302.

Weisner, T. S. 2002. Ecocultural understanding of children's developmental pathways. *Human Development* 45(4):275–281.

Weisz, J. R., S. Kuppens, M. Y. Ng, R. A. Vaughn-Coaxum, A. M. Ugueto, D. Eckshtain, and K. A. Corteselli. 2019. Are psychotherapies for young people growing stronger? Tracking trends over time for youth anxiety, depression, attention-deficit/hyperactivity disorder, and conduct problems. *Perspectives on Psychological Science* 14(2):216–237.

West, A., A. K. Duggan, K. Gruss, and C. S. Minkovitz. 2018. Creating a measurement framework for service coordination in maternal and early childhood home visiting: An evidence-informed, expert process. *Children and Youth Services Review* 89:289–297.

White, R., A. Mosle, and M. Sims. 2018. *States leading the way: Practical solutions that lift up children and families*. Washington, DC: The Aspen Institute.

Wildeman, C., and E. A. Wang. 2017. Mass incarceration, public health, and widening inequality in the USA. *The Lancet* 389(10077):1464–1474.

Williams, D. R., S. A. Mohammed, J. Leavell, and C. Collins. 2010. Race, socioeconomic status, and health: Complexities, ongoing challenges, and research opportunities. *Annals of the New York Academy of Sciences* 1186:69–101.

Wing, R., A. Gjelsvik, M. Nocera, and E. L. McQuaid. 2015. Association between adverse childhood experiences in the home and pediatric asthma. *Annals of Allergy, Asthma and Immunology* 114(5):379–384.

Wise, P. H. 2009. Confronting social disparities in child health: A critical appraisal of life-course science and research. *Pediatrics* 124(Suppl 3):S203–S211.

Wong, F., and R. Halgin. 2006. The "model minority": Bane or blessing for Asian Americans? *Journal of Multicultural Counseling and Development* 34(1):38–49.

Yamamoto, Y., and J. Li. 2011. *Is being quiet a virtue or a problem? Implications of a study on Chinese immigrant children in the U.S.* https://www.childresearch.net/papers/multi/2011_01.html (accessed May 2, 2019).

Yarnoff, B., O. Khavjou, C. Bradley, J. Leis, J. Filene, A. Honeycutt, R. Herzfeldt-Kamprath, and K. Peplinski. 2019. Standardized cost estimates for home visiting: Pilot study of the home visiting budget assistance tool (HV-BAT). *Maternal and Child Health Journal* 23(4):470–478.

Yates, T. M., B. Egeland, and A. Sroufe. 2003. Rethinking resilience. In *Resilience and vulnerability: Adaptation in the context of childhood adversities,* edited by S. S. Luthar. New York: Cambridge University Press.

Yavorsky, J. E., C. M. Dush, and S. J. Schoppe-Sullivan. 2015. The production of inequality: The gender division of labor across the transition to parenthood. *Journal of Marriage and the Family* 77(3):662–679.

Yogman, M., and C. F. Garfield. 2016. Fathers' roles in the care and development of their children: The role of pediatricians. *Pediatrics* 138(1):e20161128.

Yoshimoto, D. K., N. T. Robertson, and D. K. Hayes. 2014. Insights in public health: The Hawai'i home visiting network: Evidence-based home visiting services in Hawai'i. *Hawai'i Journal of Medicine & Public Health: A Journal of Asia Pacific Medicine & Public Health* 73(5):155–160.

Zeanah, C. H., and P. D. Zeanah. 1989. Intergenerational transmission of maltreatment: Insights from attachment theory and research. *Psychiatry* 52(2):177–196.

Zielinski, D. S., J. Eckenrode, and D. L. Olds. 2009. Nurse home visitation and the prevention of child maltreatment: Impact on the timing of official reports. *Development and Psychopathology* 21(2):441–453.

Zung, W. W. 1965. A self-rating depression scale. *Archives of General Psychiatry* 12(1):63–70.

5

Leveraging the Health Care System to Improve Outcomes and Promote Health Equity

INTRODUCTION

Significant differences in health status among women, infants, and children and inadequate response to the role of early life stressors on life course health indicate a need for an important transformation of the U.S. health care system and its delivery of preconception, prenatal, postpartum, and pediatric care, which are the focus of this chapter (see Box 5-1 for an overview of the chapter). Changes are urgently needed to better address health disparities, including those by race/ethnicity and socioeconomic status (SES) (see Chapter 1 for a more detailed discussion of disparities). For example, the most recent statistics on maternal and infant mortality and other birth outcomes (see Box 5-2) highlight significant disparities and demonstrate the urgency of changes to the health care system to more rapidly and effectively address and reverse concerning trends. As the evidence in this report demonstrates, much chronic disease and disability among adults has origins in infancy and childhood. Furthermore, changing needs of the population, with growing diversity and greater understanding of the health impacts of social determinants of health (SDOH), also signal the need for major changes throughout the health care system.

As detailed in this chapter, the current health care system often delivers limited, episodic, inequitable, and fragmented services. It focuses on clinical medical care, which recognizes the myriad of social factors that affect health outcomes but often addresses such factors in fragmented and variable ways. The health care system serves as one platform, along

BOX 5-1
Chapter in Brief: Leveraging the Health Care System

This chapter discusses opportunities to leverage the health care system in supporting healthy early childhood development, with a focus on improving access to health care services, improving quality of care, improving the organization and financing of care, and transforming the content of health care to address the social, economic, cultural, and environmental determinants of health. The chapter also addresses ways to apply a life course perspective and new knowledge about child development, including the effects of adversity, trauma, and the toxic stress response, to address needs, challenges, and strategies for the health care system in the preconception, prenatal, postpartum, and early childhood periods at the practice, policy, and systems levels.

Chapter conclusions in brief:

- The current health care system focuses mainly on clinical goals and addresses the multiple determinants of health in fragmented and highly variable ways. Despite the high quality of clinical care, the health status of America's children and young families is far worse than in comparable developed countries. U.S. health care provides only limited attention to integration of health care for the whole family across the life course, integration of mental and behavioral health with the rest of health care, or integration of health care within community systems to better support children and families.
- Although health insurance coverage has grown substantially in the past few decades, mainly through Medicaid expansions and other insurance enhancements, access remains a problem for many families with young children, who experience numerous barriers to obtaining health care services in addition to lack of health insurance coverage. Further efforts are

with public health and other sectors, to address the social determinants that underlie many health inequities. To better address inequities, it is necessary to transform the organization, delivery, and financing of health care to incorporate community-focused teams and integration across multiple sectors to address the SDOH, poverty, mental and behavioral health (MBH), chronic disease, disparities, adversity, and family well-being. Achieving these goals will require ensuring access to care, focusing and improving quality of care, changing the organization and financing of health care, and strengthening the content of health care.

Based on available evidence and existing resources, the committee identified three domains as important for focusing on preconception, prenatal, and early childhood interventions: health care systems and services (Chapter 5), healthy living conditions (Chapter 6), and early care and education (Chapter 7) (for the committee's conceptual model, see Figure 1-9). This chapter focuses on health care systems and services, needed to address financial and nonfinancial barriers to care and to ensure that all families have access to adequate preconception, prenatal, postpartum, and pediatric care.

- Promising strategies can improve quality of preconception, prenatal, and child health care, such as developing and implementing new measures, including for adversity and social determinants, along with efforts to strengthen the training of the health care workforce to better understand diversity and implicit bias and to address equity in health care.
- Programs that build on home visiting, referrals to community partners, and integrated community efforts have enhanced outcomes for children and families. New technologies have expanded care and access, increased understanding of the social determinants, and improved communication about health and chronic disease. New payment arrangements can accelerate the transformation of health services to programs to support families and population health.

Chapter recommendations in brief:

- Increase access to preconception, prenatal, postpartum, and pediatric health care.
- Expand accountability and improve quality of preconception through pediatric care.
- Adopt policies and practices that improve the organization, financing, and integration of care systems from preconception through pediatric care, with a focus on the caregiver and child together as the unit of care and collaboration with community-based services.
- Transform preconception, prenatal, postpartum, and pediatric health care to address the root causes of poor health and well-being, including social determinants.

including preventive care and clinical care delivery systems, and also emphasizes critical links and opportunities for alignment with other partners in the health care system and in other sectors in the community.

The health care sector is positioned to play a crucial role in advancing health equity by providing care and services during the preconception, prenatal, postpartum, and early childhood periods. Preconception, prenatal, and pediatric care provide a point of entry into the health care system for women and men, as well as children, especially those in the first few years of life. However, the current health care system organizational fragmentation and the episodic delivery of health care services, coupled with institutional and systemic disadvantage, have resulted in significant disparities in access to and use of health care services. Health care that is well organized, accessible over time, high quality, universally available, and effectively integrated for all people could provide continuous access to a wide variety of resources and services and decrease disparities in

BOX 5-2
Health and Health Services Disparities
for Women, Infants, and Children

Maternal mortality—Maternal mortality in the United States increased from 7.2 deaths per 100,000 live births in 1987 to 17.2 deaths per 100,000 live births in 2015 (CDC, 2019c). There are large racial disparities as well—as of 2010, black women were three to four times more likely to die from a pregnancy-related complication than non-Hispanic white women (Creanga et al., 2015).

Infant mortality—In 2016, infant mortality rates were 11.4 per 1,000 live births for non-Hispanic black infants, 9.4 per 1,000 live births for American Indian/Alaska Native infants, 7.4 per 1,000 live births for Native Hawaiian or other Pacific Islander infants, 5.0 per 1,000 live births for Hispanic infants, 4.9 per 1,000 live births for non-Hispanic white infants, and 3.6 per 1,000 live births for Asian infants (CDC, 2019b).

Low birth weight—In 2016, low birth weight rates in the United States were 13.7 percent for non-Hispanic black women and 7.0 percent for non-Hispanic white women (Martin et al., 2018). In the same year, rates among Hispanic subgroups ranged from 9.5 percent for Puerto Rican women to 6.9 percent for Mexican women (Martin et al., 2018). In 2013, rates among Asian and Pacific Islander subgroups were 10.6 percent for Asian Indian women, 9.4 percent for Filipino women, and 5.9 percent for Chinese women (Child Trends, 2015).

Preterm birth—In 2016, preterm birth rates were 13.8 percent among non-Hispanic black mothers and 8.63 percent among non-Hispanic Asian mothers. For Hispanic subgroups, rates ranged from 11.0 percent for Puerto Rican mothers to 9.1 percent for Central and South American mothers (Martin et al., 2018).

Prenatal care—In 2006, the rate of women who received prenatal care in the first trimester was 58 percent for black and Hispanic women and 76 percent for white women (69 percent of women overall received prenatal care) (Bryant et al., 2010).

Health insurance—In 2016, 55.4 percent of black children and 56.8 percent of Hispanic children were covered by public insurance, compared to 31.9 percent of non-Hispanic white children and 26.8 percent of Asian children (Child Trends, n.d.; U.S. Census Bureau, 2017). In the same year, black and Hispanic children made up 20 and 37 percent, respectively, of all children covered by Medicaid and the Children's Health Insurance Program, yet they were 14 and 25 percent, respectively, of all children (Brooks and Wagnerman, 2018). In 2017, 4.9 percent of black children and 7.7 percent of Hispanic children were uninsured, compared with 4.3 percent of non-Hispanic white children and 4.6 percent of Asian children (Berchick et al., 2018).

Health status—In 2011–2012, 5.0 percent of Hispanic children interviewed in Spanish (3.6 percent of Hispanic children interviewed in English) and 3.6 percent of non-Hispanic black children had poor or fair health, compared to 2.7 percent of non-Hispanic white children (Pastor et al., 2015). In addition, children and youth receiving Supplemental Security Income payments for severe disability are disproportionately black and Latino (NASEM, 2015).

use of health care services. Given that recognizing risk factors (biological, social, and environmental) as early as possible is fundamental to addressing health inequities, universal access to health care services is a critical component to decreasing and eliminating health inequities (Veugelers and Yip, 2003).

Although health care plays an integral role, the health care sector alone cannot meaningfully address health inequities, nor is it the primary actor or leader. Cross-sectoral and multidisciplinary collaboration is essential for decreasing health inequities. As discussed in Chapter 1, the United States spends more on health care than any other country, yet has some of the worst outcomes and gravest disparities. Despite significant improvements in the last century, troubling trends have persisted and worsened in the current century (e.g., life expectancy has decreased, and maternal mortality rates have increased [see Box 5-2]) (CDC, 2019c; Murphy et al., 2018). Although children and youth represented about 45 percent of the Medicaid population in 2013, they received only about 19 percent of Medicaid expenditures (MACPAC, 2018). In addition, about 95 percent of U.S. spending on health is related to treatment and medical services; only about 5 percent is allocated to population-level health improvement and prevention (McGinnis et al., 2002). The United States spends the highest percentage of its gross domestic product on health care services among all nations but has poor health outcomes in many areas, including neonatal and maternal mortality, deaths from injuries, and rates of substance use. Improving health outcomes requires more rapid learning regarding interventions that work and those that do not, focusing investment in effective interventions and their deployment, and more equitable allocation of resources to other sectors outside of health care. As Steuerle and Isaacs (2014) document, federal spending on programs to support children and families has faced immense budgetary pressures as health care spending has increased.

The committee embraced the life course approach, which emphasizes the impact of an individual's experiences throughout a lifetime—and across generations—on health outcomes (see Chapter 3). Given the multigenerational impacts of toxic stress, food and housing instability, chronic disease, and parental ill health on the health of children, all family members need access to health care services across the life course. Thus, this chapter highlights the many ways in which our current system represents a patchwork of services offered at different times in life (e.g., little or no continuity, intermittent insurance coverage, poor access to providers, eligibility for services for short periods of time) and how U.S. health care needs to be redesigned and rebuilt on a firmer foundation of care across the life course with added boosters during life junctures most critical to a child's health. This chapter covers health care services delivered and

received during the preconception, prenatal, postpartum, and early childhood periods—junctures at which well-timed services can boost the odds
for good health across the life course.

This chapter generally focuses on health care provided by physicians, although there are many other practitioners that play an important
role in the health care system during these life periods, such as nurses,
nurse practitioners, nurse-midwives, doulas, social workers, specialized
therapists, and mental health practitioners. However, given the scope of
this report, the committee could not cover all of these in great detail. In
addition, there are a number of forthcoming National Academies reports
on topics related to this chapter, including the roles of other important
practitioners. These include studies on the future of nursing 2020–2030,
which has a focus on reducing health disparities and producing a culture
of health[1]; assessing health outcomes by birth settings[2]; and integrating social needs care into the delivery of health care to improve the
nation's health.[3] Finally, the 2019 National Academies report *The Promise
of Adolescence: Realizing Opportunity for All Youth* (NASEM, 2019) covers
topics not included here, such as sexual and reproductive health care for
adolescents—including unintended pregnancy.

The health care system as a whole is robust and frequently interacts with children and their families by providing a nearly universal
touchpoint with all women and children from the prenatal period to
age 3, making it an important system through which to address health
inequities. However, it is important to note that the health care system
is not the main vehicle through which change should occur to address
the SDOH, nor is it where additional funds should be funneled to do so.
Rather, the health care system needs to be better leveraged to not only
provide medical care but also address the SDOH (including barriers to
access other than health insurance, such as lack of or inadequate transportation to medical visits, cost-sharing, and lack of culturally competent
services) (Woolf, 2019). However, as noted above and described in detail
below, the health care system does need to change to more systematically
address the upstream causes of poor health and health inequities. To do
so, the health care sector needs to engage and partner with other sectors to
actively address the SDOH and find common solutions to meet the needs

---

[1] For more information, see http://www.nationalacademies.org/hmd/Activities/
Workforce/futureofnursing2030.aspx (accessed April 5, 2019).

[2] For more information, see https://sites.nationalacademies.org/DBASSE/BCYF/
Research_Issues_in_the_Assessment_of_Birth_Settings/index.htm (accessed April 5, 2019).

[3] For more information, see http://nationalacademies.org/hmd/activities/healthservices/
integratingsocialneedscareintothedeliveryofhealthcaretoimprovethenationshealth.aspx (accessed April 5, 2019).

of children and families (see Recommendations 8-1 and 8-5 in Chapter 8 for more on the need for cross-sector approaches and integration of care to advance health equity).

This chapter includes an introduction to the history and current content of preconception, prenatal, postpartum, and pediatric health care and sections describing efforts to improve access, quality, and innovative delivery/financing of better health care during these critical and sensitive periods of life. As noted above, the life course perspective illustrates that health care from preconception through early childhood is a continuum of care that needs to take place across the life-span and take into account intergenerational effects. Thus, as this chapter discusses, an integrated health care system, which will require addressing a multitude of structural, professional, practical, and cultural barriers, is necessary to accelerate improvement in health care services, with the ultimate goal of improving health outcomes and decreasing health inequities.

BACKGROUND AND CURRENT CHARACTERISTICS OF HEALTH CARE

Preconception Care

A primary goal of preconception care is to improve the health of men and women during their reproductive years, especially shortly before conceiving a child. The Centers for Disease Control and Prevention (CDC) defines preconception care as "a set of interventions that aim to identify and modify biomedical, behavioral, and social risks to a woman's health or pregnancy outcome through prevention and management" (Johnson et al., 2006). As discussed in Chapter 2, preconception health is important not only for pregnancy outcomes but also for the lifelong health of children and even the health of the next generation (*The Lancet*, 2018). Disparities in preconception health can thus set up intergenerational transmission of health disparities. Using data from the Behavioral Risk Factor Surveillance System, 2013–2015, and Pregnancy Risk Assessment Monitoring System, 2013–2014, Robbins et al. (2018) found significant disparities in nine preconception health indicators by race/ethnicity, age, and insurance status (see Tables 5-1 and 5-2). They found that among older women (35–44 years), non-Hispanic black women, uninsured women, and those residing in southern states, prevalence estimates of risk factor indicators were generally highest and prevalence estimates of health-promoting indicators were generally lowest.

Advancing health equity in birth and child health outcomes begins with reducing preconception health disparities. For decades, preconception care has been proposed as a key population-level strategy for

TABLE 5-1 Prevalence of Preconception Health Indicators Among Nonpregnant Reproductive-Aged Women (18–44 years), by Age Group, Race/Ethnicity, and Insurance—Behavioral Risk Factor Surveillance System, United States, 2013–2015[a]

Characteristic	Depression[b] (2014–2015) % (95% CI)	Diabetes[b,c] (2014–2015) % (95% CI)	Hypertension[b,c,d] (2013, 2015) % (95% CI)	Current Cigarette Smoking[e] (2014–2015) % (95% CI)	Normal Weight[f] (2014–2015) % (95% CI)	Recommended Physical Activity[d,g] (2013, 2015) % (95% CI)
Age group (years)[h]						
18–24	19.2 (18.4–20.1)	1.0 (0.8–1.2)	5.0 (4.5–5.4)	13.4 (12.7–14.1)	57.0 (55.9–58.2)	53.3 (52.1–54.4)
25–34	22.6 (22.0–23.3)	2.4 (2.1–2.7)	9.2 (8.7–9.7)	19.5 (18.9–20.1)	42.7 (41.8–43.5)	49.7 (48.9–50.6)
35–44	23.1 (22.5–23.7)	5.3 (4.9–5.6)	17.0 (16.4–17.6)	16.8 (16.3–17.4)	37.9 (37.2–38.7)	49.0 (48.2–49.8)
Race/ethnicity[h]						
White	27.0 (26.5–27.6)	2.6 (2.4–2.8)	10.2 (9.8–10.5)	21.1 (20.6–21.6)	49.0 (48.3–49.6)	53.8 (53.2–54.4)
Black	16.2 (15.1–17.2)	4.5 (4.0–5.1)	18.3 (17.3–19.3)	15.6 (14.5–16.7)	30.0 (28.6–31.5)	42.8 (41.3–44.3)
Hispanic	15.5 (14.6–16.4)	3.6 (3.2–4.1)	9.5 (8.7–10.3)	8.9 (8.2–9.6)	37.2 (35.9–38.6)	46.0 (44.6–47.4)
Other	14.8 (13.6–16.1)	2.4 (1.9–2.8)	8.0 (7.1–9.0)	11.3 (10.3–12.4)	57.6 (55.6–59.6)	50.3 (48.2–52.4)

Insurance[i,j]

Yes	22.3 (21.8–22.7)	3.1 (2.9–3.2)	10.8 (10.5–11.2)	16.1 (15.7–16.5)	46.1 (45.6–46.7)	51.8 (51.2–52.4)
No	20.3 (19.2–21.3)	3.2 (2.8–3.6)	11.5 (10.8–12.2)	21.0 (20.0–22.0)	38.6 (37.2–40.0)	44.0 (42.7–45.3)
Overall	**21.9 (21.5–22.3)**	**3.1 (2.9–3.2)**	**10.9 (10.6–11.2)**	**16.9 (16.5–17.2)**	**44.9 (44.4–45.5)**	**50.4 (49.9–50.9)**

NOTE: CI = confidence interval.

[a] For indicators relying on annual standard core questions (i.e., questions that are asked annually by all states), estimates are based on 2014–2015 data. For indicators that are based on the biannual rotating core survey, CDC combined years 2013 and 2015; includes 50 U.S. states and the District of Columbia. Data self-reported by women aged 18–44 years.

[b] Self-report of ever having been told by a health care provider that they have the condition.

[c] Excluded if occurring only during pregnancy.

[d] Hypertension and physical activity questions are included as part of the biannual rotating core that is administered in odd years; therefore, 2013 and 2015 data were used.

[e] Defined as smoking 100 or more cigarettes in a lifetime and currently smoking cigarettes every day or some days at the time of the interview.

[f] Normal weight was defined as having a body mass index of 18.5–24.9 kg/m^2 as determined by self-reported weight and height.

[g] Participation in enough moderate and/or vigorous physical activity in a usual week was defined as meeting the U.S. Department of Health and Human Services recommended levels of aerobic physical activity. Respondents were classified as meeting recommendations if they reported at least 150 minutes per week of moderate-intensity activity, at least 75 minutes per week of vigorous-intensity activity, or a combination of moderate-intensity and vigorous-intensity activity (where vigorous activity minutes are multiplied by two) totaling at least 150 minutes per week.

[h] In chi-square tests, differences by age and by race/ethnicity are significant at $p < 0.05$ for all indicators.

[i] Defined as having any kind of health care coverage, including prepaid plans such as health maintenance organizations or government plans such as Medicare or Indian Health Service.

[j] In chi-square tests, differences by insurance are significant at $p < 0.05$ for all indicators except diabetes and hypertension.

SOURCE: Robbins et al., 2018.

TABLE 5-2 Prevalence of Preconception Health Indicators Among Reproductive-Aged Women (aged 18–44 years) with a Recent Live Birth, by Age Group, Race/Ethnicity, and Insurance—Pregnancy Risk Assessment Monitoring System, United States, 2013–2014[a]

Characteristic	Recent Unwanted Pregnancy[b] % (95% CI)	Pregnancy Multivitamin Use[c] % (95% CI)	Postpartum Use of Effective Contraception[d] % (95% CI)
Age group (years)[e]			
18–24	6.4 (5.8–7.1)	17.9 (17.0–18.9)	64.9 (63.6–66.2)
25–34	4.9 (4.6–5.3)	37.4 (36.6–38.2)	55.1 (54.3–55.9)
35–44	9.8 (8.9–10.8)	45.4 (43.8–46.9)	50.6 (49.0–52.3)
Race/ethnicity[e]			
White	5.0 (4.6–5.4)	37.8 (37.1–38.6)	56.8 (55.9–57.6)
Black	11.6 (10.4–12.8)	21.6 (20.2–23.2)	64.9 (63.1–66.7)
Hispanic	6.4 (5.6–7.3)	26.2 (24.8–27.7)	59.3 (57.5–61.0)
Other	6.0 (5.2–6.8)	31.7 (30.1–33.4)	44.6 (42.8–46.5)
Prepregnancy insurance[f,g]			
Yes	5.8 (5.5–6.1)	37.4 (36.7–38.1)	56.7 (56.0–57.4)
No	7.3 (6.6–8.1)	17.1 (16.0–18.2)	57.9 (56.4–59.5)
Overall	**6.1 (5.8–6.4)**	**33.6 (33.0–34.2)**	**56.9 (56.3–57.6)**

NOTE: CI = confidence interval.

[a] Includes Alabama, Alaska, Arkansas, Colorado, Delaware, Georgia, Hawaii, Illinois, Iowa, Maine, Maryland, Massachusetts, Michigan, Minnesota, Missouri, Nebraska, New Hampshire, New Jersey, New Mexico, New York, New York City, Oklahoma, Oregon, Pennsylvania, Rhode Island, Tennessee, Utah, Vermont, Washington, West Virginia, Wisconsin, and Wyoming. Data self-reported by women aged 18–44 years who recently had a live birth.

[b] Defined as a pregnancy among women who reported that just before they got pregnant with their most recent live-born infant, they did not want to be pregnant then or at any time in the future.

[c] Defined as taking a multivitamin, prenatal vitamin, or folic acid supplement every day of the month before pregnancy.

[d] Includes male or female sterilization, implant, intrauterine device, injectable, pill, patch, or ring.

[e] In chi-square tests, differences by age and by race/ethnicity are significant at $p < 0.05$ for all indicators.

[f] Defined as having private, Medicaid, other government plans such as TRICARE, military health care, Indian Health Service or tribal, and other kinds of health insurance during the month before pregnancy.

[g] In chi-square tests, differences by insurance are significant at $p < 0.05$ for all indicators except postpartum use of effective contraception.

SOURCE: Robbins et al., 2018.

improving birth outcomes. Clinical recommendations have been developed regarding the key components of preconception care, which include addressing primarily undiagnosed, untreated, or poorly controlled medical conditions; immunization history; medication and radiation exposure in early pregnancy; nutritional issues; family history and genetic risk; tobacco and substance use and other high-risk behaviors; occupational and environmental exposures; family planning and reproduction life plans; social issues; and mental health issues (Jack et al., 2008). Men could also benefit from preconception care, although the content of care is less well defined for them (Frey et al., 2008).

The evidence base supporting a range of services for preconception care as critical to child health has been well documented and includes folic acid supplementation; appropriate management of hyperglycemia; rubella, influenza, and hepatitis vaccination; a low phenylalanine diet; and provision of antiretroviral medications to reduce the risk for mother-to-child HIV transmission (Johnson et al., 2006; Korenbrot et al., 2002). Yet, several recent reviews regarding the most effective health care structures to ensure translating this science into action have found mixed results. Burgess et al. reviewed nine studies and found that fertility intention screening was associated with improved knowledge related to healthier pregnancy but not increased provision of new contraception services for those not desiring pregnancy (Burgess et al., 2018). Lassi et al. (2014) reviewed 161 studies and found evidence of effectiveness for preconception care in improving outcomes for women with diabetes, epilepsy, phenylketonuria (PKU), and depression. Hemsing et al. (2017) reviewed 29 preconception interventions and found that the majority of interventions offered assessment or screening followed by brief intervention or counseling. Overall, these interventions demonstrated improvements in at least some of the outcomes measured (Hemsing et al., 2017). However, several other systematic reviews failed to find conclusive evidence of improved pregnancy outcomes associated with the following types of preconception care: routine prepregnancy health promotion (Whitworth and Dowswell, 2009), genetic risk assessment (Hussein et al., 2018), preconception care for diabetic women (Tieu et al., 2017b), interconception care for women with a history of gestational diabetes (Tieu et al., 2017a), preconception health and programs for women who are overweight or obese (Opray et al., 2015), preconception lifestyle advice for people with subfertility (Anderson et al., 2010), and preconception care in the primary care setting (Hussein et al., 2016). This could be largely due to a lack of randomized controlled trials (RCTs) or poor study quality, but this may also reflect the limits of preconception care services as they are currently conceived, organized, and delivered.

Currently, the content of preconception care is too ill defined and limited, its access is too restricted and episodic, its quality is too

disparate and inequitable, and its organization and delivery are too fragmented and siloed to fully deliver on its promise as an intergenerational
equalizer of population health (Verbiest et al., 2016). The timing of preconception care has been identified as a major limitation contributing to
the health care system's failures in achieving optimal delivery of preconception care. Preconception care is commonly regarded as a single
prepregnancy checkup a few months before the couple attempts to conceive. The timing of such an approach, however, could miss nearly half
of all pregnancies, which are unplanned (Finer and Zolna, 2016), and
approximately 37 percent of all births in the United States, which are
unintended at the time of conception (Mosher et al., 2012). Moreover,
such an approach may be appropriate to address certain risk factors (e.g.,
folic acid supplementation, low phenylalanine diet, or cessation of certain
teratogenic exposures) but may be too late to address others. For example,
preconception counseling 3 months before pregnancy may be timely to
avoid ingesting methylmercury, which has a half-life of 50 days (CDC,
2016), but too late to reduce the bioaccumulation of dioxins and dioxin-
like compounds (DLCs), which have a half-life of 7–8 years (IOM, 2003).
DLCs are lipophilic and bioaccumulate in animal fat; hence, the Institute
of Medicine recommended that girls and young women drink low-fat or
skim milk instead of whole milk and eat foods lower in animal fat years
before they become pregnant (IOM, 2003). Switching to low-fat milk
and/or a low-fat diet a few months before pregnancy would do little to
reduce fetal exposure to DLCs. Furthermore, to expect preconception care
to reverse allostatic load (the cumulative physiological toll from chronic
stress) in a single visit may be asking too much. Thus, rather than considering preconception care as a single prepregnancy checkup, it needs
to be re-conceptualized, tested, and integrated into health care services
delivered consistently, continuously, and comprehensively for women
(and men) across the life course.

Another limit of preconception care, as commonly practiced, is its
narrow clinical focus. While its benefits in reducing certain biomedical or behavioral risks (e.g., folate deficiency, PKU, smoking) have been
well documented, these are often not the major drivers of disparities
in birth and child health outcomes. Preconception care could have a
greater impact in advancing health equity if it is better set up to optimize
management of chronic conditions, such as hypertension, diabetes, and
obesity, that disproportionately affect low-income women and women
of color; yet, for many women, the lack of access to and the episodic
nature of preconception care limit its effectiveness as a population-wide
strategy for advancing equity in preconception health. Preconception care
offers an important opportunity for addressing MBH issues, but in many
underresourced communities, a positive screen is often not backed up by

available referral services, such as cognitive behavioral therapy, alcohol rehabilitation, tobacco cessation counseling and referral, substance use treatment, or trauma-informed care (TIC). Most importantly, preconception care is presently ill equipped to address many social determinants of preconception health, such as food insecurity, housing instability, occupational or environmental exposures, or intimate partner violence. This is not a flaw of preconception care per se but of the larger U.S. health care system, which is poorly designed to tackle the SDOH; nonetheless, preconception care represents an important missed opportunity for advancing health equity, with its prevailing narrow focus on fixing biomedical and behavioral risks.

The evidence base regarding the effectiveness of preconception care is also limited by the relative dearth of research on which preconception interventions succeed in advancing health equity in birth and child health outcomes. For example, despite increasing recognition of the health impact of maternal allostatic load on not only birth and child health outcomes but also the developmental origins of health and disease, there has been a paucity of intervention research on what can be done during preconception care to reduce maternal allostatic load. Similarly, little is known on how preconception care might reduce the risk of aberrant placentation, epigenetic reprogramming, and neuroendocrine, immune-inflammatory, and metabolic dysregulation, which could contribute to disparities in birth outcomes and lifelong health.

Approaches to incorporate reproductive life planning discussions into routine visits for women of child-bearing age (e.g., asking every woman of reproductive age at every routine visit whether she would like to become pregnant at some point and, if so, when that might be [Callegari et al., 2017])—have led to increased delivery of preconception care services prior to pregnancy. However, these strategies have been criticized for focusing too much on reproductive *choice* and not enough on reproductive *justice*. The maternalism inherent in the traditional concept of preconception care (as narrowly defined by the current health care system) has been criticized by some for promoting the trope of "women as reproductive vessels" (Waggoner, 2013). Others have argued that preconception care (and contraceptive care) is limited by a primary focus on changing individual behaviors instead of the historical and social contexts of those behaviors and on promoting reproductive choice instead of broader reproductive access, especially for communities of color. This reality gave rise to the reproductive justice movement in the 1990s, which focused on a woman's right to *have* a child or *not* to have a child and explicitly recognized that, while pregnancy intention and choice are important, many women do not have the requisite resources to access the essential tools to control their own reproductive destiny. These include, but are not limited to, reliable birth control, adoption, abortion, and paid maternity leave. Reproductive justice activists have maintained that

> reproductive safety and dignity depended on having the resources to get good medical care and decent housing, to have a job that pays a living wage, to live without police harassment, to live free of racism in a physically healthy environment—all of these (and other) conditions of life were fundamental conditions for reproductive dignity and safety— reproductive justice—along with legal contraception and abortion. (Ross and Solinger, 2017, p. 56)

Pregnancy intention is key to promoting good maternal, neonatal, and childhood health outcomes (Hall et al., 2017), but the decision to have a child does not occur in a vacuum. It is rooted in the environmental, socioeconomic, and political world in which a woman and her family live. A discussion of preconception care is incomplete if it is not centered in the broader context of U.S. history, which included concerted efforts to encourage some women to reproduce while going to great lengths to make sure other women did not. Such distinctions were often based on race, class, and/or immigration status, with a paternalistic presumption that some women were inherently fit to be mothers while others were not. Notable examples of public policies influencing the reproductive status of women in this country include the eugenics movement, forced sterilization campaigns, and welfare programs penalizing women for having a man in the home or having children (Kluchin, 2009; Ross and Solinger, 2017; Stern, 2005). As an example, in the 1970s, many low-income women and women of color, including Puerto Rican, African American, Chicano, and American Indian/Alaska Native (AI/AN) women, experienced mass forced sterilization. AI/AN women suffered particularly serious abuse from federal policies that enabled AI/AN children to be taken from their families in addition to numerous violations of reproductive rights (Torpy, 2000). These examples underscore that there is much more at play than personal reproductive choice when a woman makes the decision of whether to have children and emphasize how the health care system can best support all women and families equitably in making this important decision.

Prenatal and Postpartum Care

For decades, the delivery of prenatal care has been a cornerstone of the U.S. strategy to reduce infant mortality and perinatal disparities (Alexander and Kotelchuck, 2001; Lu et al., 2003, 2010). The primary focus of prenatal care has shifted over time from focusing on medical intervention to providing more comprehensive intervention and prevention with public health approaches (Lu and Lu, 2008; Lu et al., 2010). Prenatal care originated from research conducted in early 20th-century England by John W. Ballantyne, who proposed that "to prevent fetal abnormalities and reduce maternal, fetal, and neonatal deaths, medical supervision for pregnant women should be provided throughout pregnancy rather than only during labor" (Lu and Lu, 2008, p. 592). In the United States, prenatal care began with a program of nurse home visiting to pregnant women by Mrs. William Lowell Putnam at the Boston Lying-In Hospital in 1901, which led to the establishment of an outpatient clinic in 1911 that provided prenatal visits consisting of history and physical examination, blood pressure measurement, and urinalysis (Lu and Lu, 2008). From the beginning, the content of prenatal care was influenced by concerns about toxemia (preeclampsia), which was diagnosed by high blood pressure and excess protein in the urine. Such concerns also contributed to establishing the timing and frequency of prenatal visits (Lu and Lu, 2008).

Several studies (Eisner et al., 1979; Gortmaker, 1979; Greenberg, 1983; IOM, 1973; Taffel, 1978) published in the 1970s found a significant association between no prenatal care and the incidence of low birth weight (LBW), a leading cause of infant mortality and perinatal disparities. Citing these studies, an IOM report concluded that the "overwhelming weight of the evidence is that prenatal care reduces low birthweight" (IOM, 1985, p. 146) and promoted prenatal care as a key population-wide public health intervention for improving birth outcomes in the United States. In 1986, the U.S. Public Health Service assembled an expert panel to assess the content of prenatal care. In its 1989 report, the expert panel identified three basic components of prenatal care: (1) early and continuing risk assessment, (2) health promotion, and (3) medical and psychosocial interventions and follow-up (NIH, 1989). Soon thereafter, Congress enacted a series of legislative initiatives that incrementally expanded Medicaid eligibility to low-income pregnant women and children independent of their welfare status. Many states then further expanded Medicaid eligibility and streamlined the process of enrollment into prenatal care (Handler et al., 2011). Arguments for expansion of access to prenatal care were bolstered by cost-effectiveness analyses, which suggested that savings could be achieved by reducing LBW, though the cost savings may have been overstated (Huntington and Connell, 1994).

In part stemming from these national and state policies, the adoption of timely and adequate prenatal care has increased substantially over the past few decades (Kogan et al., 1998; Martin et al., 2002; Piper et al., 1994). This increase, however, did not lead to an immediate reduction in LBW or disparities in birth outcomes. While many reasons could have contributed to the persistent poor outcomes (Alexander and Slay, 2002), some began to question the effectiveness of prenatal care as a population-wide strategy for improving birth outcomes. Two reviews published in 1995 raised concerns regarding the validity of the evidence used to support the benefit of prenatal care (Alexander and Korenbrot, 1995; Fiscella, 1995). Citing problems with inconsistent results, insufficient adjustment for prematurity bias, and inadequate control for the effect of critical confounders and potential selection bias in earlier studies, Fiscella concluded that "current evidence does not satisfy the criteria necessary to establish that prenatal care definitely improves birth outcomes" (Fiscella, 1995, p. 475). Alexander and Korenbrot (1995) also concluded from their systematic review that "[t]here is little done during the standard prenatal care visit that could be expected to reduce low birth weight" (Alexander and Korenbrot, 1995, p. 113). Lu et al. (2003) concluded from a review of the *content* of prenatal care in 2003 that neither preterm birth nor intrauterine growth restriction—the twin constituents of LBW—can be effectively prevented by prenatal care in its present form. They contended that "[p]reventing LBW will require reconceptualization of prenatal care as part of a longitudinally and contextually integrated strategy to promote optimal development of women's reproductive health not only during pregnancy, but over the life course" (Lu et al., 2003, p. 362).

These critiques led to a dampening of enthusiasm for prenatal care and a search for alternative strategies, such as bolstering preconception care services, to improve birth and child health outcomes in the United States. It should be noted, however, that most extant studies examined prenatal care in a limited form, addressing primarily clinical risk factors for pregnancy complications rather than what truly matters to both maternal (and paternal) health and the developmental origins of the child's future health. They also focused on a few birth outcomes rather than examining a broader array of health and developmental outcomes for children and families (Lu et al., 2010). While there is great evidence that pregnancy is a critical life event and a sensitive period for healthy child development, experts still disagree about how the health care system should effectively organize and deliver prenatal care.

Later in this chapter, the committee calls for a redesign of prenatal care to improve access, content, quality, delivery, and financing. Access can be improved with outreach, care coordination, and technology. Content could be expanded to include more detailed assessment, education, and management of psychosocial and environmental risks. Quality improvement efforts could address implicit bias and unequal treatment. Most importantly, this committee calls for a transformation of the organization and delivery of prenatal care to achieve greater vertical, horizontal, and longitudinal integration, including greater linkages to community services and women's health across the life course. This report does not address health systems redesign to better support childbirth in the United States, as it is the subject of an ongoing study by another National Academies committee.[4]

---

[4] See https://sites.nationalacademies.org/DBASSE/BCYF/Research_Issues_in_the_ Assessment_of_Birth_Settings/index.htm (accessed July 26, 2019).

Postpartum Care

The postpartum period marks the time after delivery when maternal physiology returns to the nonpregnant state. This period, often referred to as the "fourth trimester," is generally considered to last 6–8 weeks (ACOG, 2018b). Many traditional cultures prescribe 30–40 days of rest and recovery (ACOG, 2018b), such as zuò yuè zi ("doing the month") in China and Taiwan (Pillsbury et al., 1978), a 21-day period of rest called sam chil il in Korea (Dennis et al., 2007; Park and Dimigen, 1995), la cuarentena (which also means quarantine and comes from cuarenta, the word for 40 in Spanish) in Latin America, and lying-in, which gave rise to the establishment of lying-in hospitals in England and the United States during the 20th century (Eberhard-Gran et al., 2010). In many cultures, the woman and her newborn are surrounded by family and community members who offer instrumental emotional support during this period. In the United States, however, many women have to navigate the postpartum transition on their own with little formal or informal support, wrestling with lack of sleep, fatigue, pain, stress, breastfeeding difficulties, and new onset or exacerbation of preexisting health and social issues, such as postpartum depression, substance dependence, intimate partner violence, and other concerns (ACOG, 2018b).

Postpartum care provides an opportunity to address these issues, but for many U.S. women, it is often limited to a single 6-week postpartum visit, and some women receive no postpartum care at all. In the Listening to Mothers III Survey, one-third of respondents reported attending one postpartum office visit, while 1 in 10 mothers reported not having a visit (Declercq et al., 2013). Among the latter group, "I felt fine and didn't need to go" (42 percent), "I felt that I had already completed all of my maternity care" (18 percent), "too hard to get to office" (12 percent), and "didn't have insurance" (7 percent) were the most common reasons given for not having a visit (Declercq et al., 2013, p. ix). Nonattendance is greater among certain groups, including low-income women, Medicaid insurance holders, and those with inadequate prenatal care (DiBari et al., 2014). One recent study of Medicaid deliveries in California found that only half of all women and one-third of African American women attended a postpartum visit (Thiel de Bocanegra et al., 2017).

Even for women who receive postpartum care, the typical 6-week postpartum visit may be too late to address some early onset issues and too limited to address other late onset or persistent problems. For example, more than half of postpartum strokes occur within 10 days of discharge (Too et al., 2018) and 17.5 percent of pregnancy-related deaths occur between 43 and 365 days postpartum, often as a result of cardiomyopathy or mental health conditions (Building U.S. Capacity to Review and Prevent Maternal Deaths, 2018), which a 6-week postpartum visit may be ill equipped to prevent. Rather than an arbitrary "6-week" check, in 2018, the American College of Obstetricians and Gynecologists (ACOG) called for a reconceptualization of postpartum care as an ongoing process, the timing of which should be individualized and woman centered (ACOG, 2018b). ACOG recommends that all women have contact with their obstetric care providers within the first 3 weeks postpartum. Women with hypertensive disorders of pregnancy should be seen no later than 7–10 days postpartum, and women with severe hypertension should be seen within 72 hours (ACOG, 2018b). ACOG recommends that this initial assessment should be followed up with ongoing care as needed, concluding with a comprehensive postpartum visit no later than 12 weeks after birth.

ACOG also recommends that the comprehensive postpartum visit include a full assessment of physical, social, and psychological well-being, including the following domains: mood and emotional well-being; infant care and feeding; sexuality, contraception, and birth spacing; sleep and fatigue; physical recovery from birth; chronic disease management; and health maintenance (ACOG, 2018b). In practice, however, providing comprehensive postpartum care is disincentivized by prevailing health care financing practices, whereby the postpartum visit is bundled with the rest of obstetrical care, for which providers receive a global payment with no additional reimbursement for postpartum care. To deliver comprehensive postpartum care, ACOG also recommends an interprofessional postpartum care team, which consists of the primary maternity care provider, infant health care provider, primary care provider, and specialty consultants, as well as a care coordinator or case manager, lactation support provider, home visitor, and family and friends (ACOG, 2018b). Presently, the care settings where many women receive postpartum care preclude such interprofessional approaches, and transforming the organization and delivery of postpartum care in the absence of additional reimbursement will likely be challenging. Lastly, ACOG recommends that the postpartum care team help facilitate transition to ongoing well-woman care (ACOG, 2018b). This is especially important for women who have chronic health conditions or have experienced a pregnancy complication, given growing research suggesting that pregnancy may be a window to a woman's future health outlook. For example, women with pregnancies complicated by preterm birth, gestational diabetes, or hypertensive disorders of pregnancy have a higher lifetime risk of maternal cardiometabolic disease (Dassanayake et al., 2019). However, for many low-income women, especially in states without Medicaid expansion, access to ongoing well-woman care becomes limited upon termination of their Medicaid coverage at 60 days postpartum.

Recognizing the importance of the postpartum period as a critical time for a woman and her infant that sets the stage for their long-term health and well-being, this committee calls for a redesign of postpartum care to improve access, content, quality, delivery, and financing to better leverage its potential for advancing health equity. As will be discussed later in the chapter, access could be enhanced by colocation of maternal and infant services; greater use of home visiting, doula services, community health workers, and mHealth technology; and increased access to paid family and medical leave. Expanded care is needed to more holistically address not only clinical issues but also psychosocial and environmental concerns, with greater attention to social determinants of maternal, child, and family health and well-being. Quality could be improved by promoting quality measurement and continuous quality improvement (CQI), supporting workforce training, and, as discussed throughout the chapter, addressing implicit bias and unequal treatment along the care continuum. Organization and delivery of care could be strengthened through care coordination, systems integration, and interprofessional teamwork. To support this redesign, the committee calls for developing and testing innovative financing models, including pay-for-performance and pay-for-outcomes, unbundling postpartum care from global payment, and extending Medicaid coverage for 1 year postpartum.

Pediatric Care

The goal of pediatric care is to provide services to children and families that will improve their health status and functioning. Usual services include brief clinical encounters ("checkups") beginning in the hospital immediately after birth and continuing through childhood and adolescence, with decreasing visit frequency. Typical services have traditionally included providing regular immunizations, monitoring growth and development and nutrition, advising parents on common aspects of child development, and managing common illnesses and injuries. Child health care has a focus on prevention and includes regular screening for a wide range of conditions, including drowning risk, lead exposure, anemia, adversity, hunger, and infectious diseases, as well as child behavior and development.

Much of the work in pediatric well-child care grew from early efforts of the U.S. Children's Bureau and then the growth of public health departments in the states (Lesser, 1965). The U.S. Children's Bureau emphasized early nutrition and safe milk for babies and checked feeding and weight gain. With the development of immunizations to protect children (and communities) from dangerous infectious diseases, many state health departments developed immunization clinics. The 1921 Sheppard-Towner Act[5] led to substantial federal investment in well-child health programs.

---

[5] Also known as the National Maternity and Infancy Protection Act or the Promotion of the Welfare and Hygiene of Maternity and Infancy Act, the Sheppard-Towner Act provided states with federal funding to develop programs that would increase education of prenatal and infant care. The Act was passed in an effort to decrease the high rates of infant mortality in the United Sates. See https://embryo.asu.edu/pages/sheppard-towner-maternity-and-infancy-protection-act-1921 (accessed April 19, 2019).

The American Medical Association (AMA) opposed the Act as government intrusion into health care, leading to the departure of pediatricians from the AMA and the formation of the American Academy of Pediatrics (AAP) (Baker, 1994). With the growth of the AAP, pediatricians (many of whom had worked in the public well-child clinics) increasingly integrated the elements of well-child care into their practices, ultimately overshadowing public service programs (Baker, 1994). Thus, much of pediatric well-child care grew from notions of improving child nutrition and weight gain and preventing serious infections (e.g., diphtheria, tetanus, polio). Many of those acute infections have disappeared (although immunizations remain critically important) and have been replaced with epidemics of chronic diseases in pediatric populations. Where less than 2 percent of children in 1960 had a serious chronic condition that interfered on a daily basis with their usual activities (e.g., school and play), by 2010, more than 8 percent had such conditions, representing a 400 percent growth in these conditions (Halfon et al., 2012; Houtrow et al., 2014; Newacheck et al., 1986; Perrin et al., 2014). These high rates of chronic conditions mainly reflect greater numbers of children with obesity, asthma, neurodevelopmental conditions (especially autism spectrum disorders [ASDs]), and mental health conditions. While rates of mental health conditions increase with child age, one in six or more children ages 2–8 have diagnosed mental, behavioral, or developmental conditions (CDC, 2019a). Children with chronic medical conditions also have higher rates of mental and behavioral conditions than similar children without chronic conditions (Perrin et al., 2019).

These growing rates have led health care providers for children to recognize the importance of behavioral health in all aspects of pediatric care—the interaction of physical and mental/behavioral health and their common coexistence, along with the increasing rates of MBH conditions in children and adolescents. Initially codified in some of the Rochester child health studies more than a half century ago (Haggerty et al., 1975), this interest has grown into active work by several professional groups to build capacity and competence in behavioral health into the well-child experience (AAP, 2018; Foy and AAP Task Force on Mental Health, 2010). MBH accounts for a large proportion of visits in pediatric primary care and complicates care for most chronic conditions.

Screening is a key step in prevention and an integral part of pediatric care. Given the brief time available in a child health supervision visit, pediatric clinicians cannot do all of the recommended screening, so they make choices for their practices, based in part on the characteristics of their patient population. Generally, child health practitioners (e.g., pediatricians, family physicians, family nurse practitioners, physician assistants) choose screening instruments that are brief, easily scored and interpreted, and able to identify conditions that have moderate prevalence or saliency in their practice communities (AAP, 2016). Most child health professionals screen for growth and development, including behavioral issues and developmental delays, and for certain conditions that early treatment may ameliorate, including ASD. AAP has codified much of child and adolescent preventive care in its document *Bright Futures*, and the Patient Protection and Affordable Care Act (ACA) included *Bright Futures* as the basis for pediatric preventive care (AAP, 2016).

The high rates and persistence of poverty among America's children have led many groups to address this problem. To address food insecurity, AAP and the Food Research & Action Center (FRAC) developed a toolkit for pediatricians that includes a validated, AAP-recommended two-question screening tool called The Hunger Vital Sign™ (AAP and FRAC, 2017). In addition, AAP, recognizing that poverty affects so many aspects of child health and development and essentially all types of clinical problems, joined these efforts by making poverty a major segment of its Agenda for Children (AAP, n.d.-a). All pediatricians face the consequences of child poverty in their practices. Children with leukemia and other serious conditions experience higher mortality, and poverty affects all children's ability to adhere to medication and treatment (Mishra et al., 2011). Low-income children have higher rates of most chronic conditions and typically have more severe cases (WHO, n.d.). Poverty affects parents' resources to care for their children's illnesses and limits access to many treatment services. AAP has educated pediatricians about poverty and what they can do in their practices (AAP Council on Community Pediatrics, 2016), and pediatricians increasingly screen for poverty and other SDOH, particularly checking for access to day care, home and neighborhood safety, hunger, and housing, especially along with partnering community agencies (Garg et al., 2015; Shekarchi et al., 2018).

Furthermore, pediatricians have provided much leadership in the development of life course sciences, theory, and practice, in part because of their perspective based in the dynamics of child development in the context of families and communities, along with their recognition of the early childhood antecedents of many long-term health and mental health conditions (Halfon, 2012; Halfon and Hochstein, 2002).

Over the past few decades, there has been significant growth in diversity in the pediatric population without similar diversification of the pediatrics workforce (AAP Committee on Pediatric Workforce, 2013). Recognition of disparities has driven pediatric efforts to address equity and ensure equal access to services and treatment. Efforts to transition into team care and use telehealth mechanisms reflect in part the recognition that such changes will help pediatricians more effectively work on issues of poverty in their patients and communities. These changes acknowledge that enhancing pediatric practice with personnel who are knowledgeable and skillful in helping families access a breadth of community services will help address disparities.

Pediatric care in the United States is organized across a variety of small and large practices, federally qualified health centers (FQHCs), and hospital-based programs (for general and specialty care). Increasingly, smaller, community-based practices have merged to become larger, multi-site practices, some limited to the care of children and youth, while others are multispecialty programs offering a larger range of services to a population of all ages. Many children's hospitals have hospital-based primary care programs and/or organized relationships or networks with primary care practices in their surrounding communities. Both safety net hospitals and FQHCs more often serve a large, low-income, Medicaid-insured population (Nath et al., 2016) with overrepresentation of black and Latino children and youth (Georgetown University Center for Children and Families, 2017, 2018). Pediatricians have pioneered the concept of the medical home, an organized central place to coordinate all of the health care needs of a patient or family. In recent years, this notion has spread among many other physician groups, especially family medicine and internal medicine. Expanded visions of the medical home increasingly embrace characteristics of community-based, comprehensive care (Ader et al., 2015; Bair-Merritt et al., 2015; Homer et al., 2008; Patient-Centered Primary Care Collaborative, n.d.; Stille et al., 2010). Medical homes have helped efforts, especially in family medicine and pediatrics, to move to a whole-family, whole-child approach. Routine screening in pediatric care for parental mental health (especially postpartum depression) and other risks (e.g., smoking, firearms) and inclusion of parent training programs in pediatric programs are examples of ways that clinical care has become more family focused.

The distribution of subspecialists—physicians who care for more complex and usually chronic conditions—differs for children and adults. Adult-treating subspecialists are widely distributed, but subspecialists for children are mainly centralized in hospitals that care for large numbers of children and youth. This distribution leads to different problems with access for young children and families. These children's hospital programs, some freestanding and others part of larger general hospitals, provide the majority of health care for children with highly specialized needs—the groups with complex medical conditions and rarer childhood conditions. The substantial numbers of children and youth with chronic and complex health conditions, especially those with less common chronic conditions, need regular access to specialized pediatric care (e.g., specialized surgeons or pediatric cardiology).

Conclusion 5-1: The current health care system focuses mainly on clinical goals and addresses the multiple other determinants of health in fragmented and highly variable ways. Despite the high quality of clinical care, the health status of America's children and young families is far worse than in comparable developed countries. U.S. health care provides only limited attention to integration of health care for the whole family, health care across the life course, or integration of mental and behavioral health with the rest of health care.

The need for the integration of health care and the whole-family approach is discussed in more detail later in the chapter.

IMPROVING ACCESS TO HEALTH CARE SERVICES

To realize the full potential of health care services, people need access to regular primary and preventive care across the life course. The nation will be best served by a health care system that guarantees all people universal access to high-quality health care across the life course and in which preconception, prenatal, and pediatric care represent a series of well-timed, more intense encounters with a broader array of services ("boosters") during critical junctures in life. Cramming a life course worth of health care into a single preconception visit (or even a few visits) a few months before attempting to conceive will do little to advance equity in birth outcomes or children's health. Similarly, prenatal and pediatric care that is primarily based on episodic, short visits to a medical clinic or office for a narrow range of clinical services scheduled when convenient for health care systems and providers is not enough to reverse the trend of centuries of inequitable health care treatment and outcomes experienced by our nation's children.

Health Insurance Is Necessary But Not Sufficient

Health insurance is a major facilitator to ensuring access to health care services; lack of insurance coverage is a significant barrier (Bailey et al., 2016; Choi et al., 2011; DeVoe et al., 2010, 2012a; Howell and Kenney, 2012; IOM, 2002; Sommers et al., 2015, 2017a; Tumin et al., 2019; Wallace and Sommers, 2016; Wherry et al., 2016). A Commonwealth Fund report found that insured women were significantly more likely than uninsured women to receive cancer screenings and other preventive services and to have a regular source of care (Gunja et al., 2017) (see Figure 5-1). Even for those with a usual source of care, health insurance improves access to more comprehensive services (DeVoe et al., 2008c, 2012a). For children, health insurance substantially improves health care access and use (IOM, 1998). The large majority of children and youth in the United States (about 95 percent) have health insurance coverage, with about 30 to 40 percent

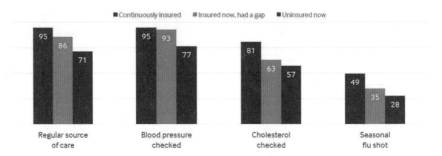

FIGURE 5-1 Percent of women ages 19–64 with a regular source of care and receiving preventive services by insurance status.
NOTES: "Continuously insured" refers to women who were insured for the full year up to and on the survey field date; "Insured now, had a gap" refers to women who were insured at the time of the survey but were uninsured at any point during the year before the survey field date; "Uninsured now" refers to women who reported being uninsured at the time of the survey. Respondents were asked if they had their blood pressure checked within the past 2 years (in past year if has hypertension or high blood pressure); had their cholesterol checked in the past 5 years (in past year if has hypertension, heart disease, or high cholesterol); and had their seasonal flu shot within the past 12 months. Data are sourced from the Commonwealth Fund Biennial Health Insurance Survey (2016).
SOURCE: Gunja et al., 2017.

of it from public sources: Medicaid and the Children's Health Insurance Program (CHIP) (Alker and Pham, 2018; Cornachione et al., 2016). The small percentage of children and youth without health insurance use fewer health care services and fare much worse on measures of health and health care quality (DeVoe et al., 2008a,b, 2010, 2012b).

Although studies of health insurance interventions are usually natural experiments, the Oregon Health Insurance Experiment, in which a 2008 lottery extended Medicaid to selected residents, represented a rare opportunity to assess the impact of insurance coverage through a randomized study design (James, 2015). Findings from the experiment confirm the well-documented associations between an individual's health insurance and access to health care and the causal link between a parent having access to insurance and a child gaining coverage (Bailey et al., 2016; DeVoe et al., 2015b,c; Gold et al., 2014; Hatch et al., 2016; Marino et al., 2016; O'Malley et al., 2016). Efforts to achieve expanded coverage in Massachusetts and several other states also led to similar landmark studies showing the importance of health insurance as a facilitator of health care access (Finkelstein et al., 2012; Smith and Chien, 2019).

Shortly after Oregon's insurance expansions and related efforts to achieve expanded coverage in Massachusetts and elsewhere, the ACA increased access to health insurance coverage nationally to millions of Americans through a combination of Medicaid expansions, private insurance reforms, and premium tax credits and subsidies through new "exchange" plans. After the ACA, the percentage of uninsured women decreased from 20 percent (19 million) in 2010 to 11 percent (11 million) in 2016 (Gunja et al., 2017). Low-income women and women of color have made particularly large gains. Women ages 19–64 earning less than 200 percent of the federal poverty level (FPL) who are uninsured fell from 25 percent in 2010 to 16 percent in 2016 for black women, 49 percent in 2010 to 32 percent in 2016 for Latina women, and 34 percent in 2010 to 18 percent in 2016 overall (see Figure 5-2). For children and youth, the ACA also led to the lowest rates of child uninsurance in U.S. history. While some of the insurance gains for pediatric populations reflected new eligibility under the ACA, most gains resulted from newly insured parents learning of their children's eligibility for existing programs (particularly

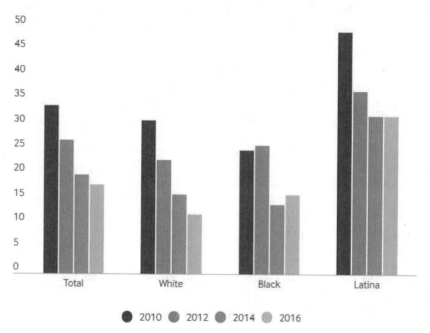

FIGURE 5-2 Percent of women ages 19–64 who are uninsured and earn less than 200 percent of the federal poverty level.
NOTES: Income levels are for a family of four in 2016. Rates are for those who were uninsured at the time of the survey. Data are sourced from the Commonwealth Fund Biennial Health Insurance Survey (2010, 2012, 2014, 2016).
SOURCE: Gunja et al., 2017.

Medicaid and CHIP) (Garrett and Gangopadhyaya, 2015), reconfirming that insurance is a family affair (DeVoe et al., 2008b, 2009, 2011a, 2015a,c,d; Dubay and Kenney, 2003; IOM, 2002; Yamauchi et al., 2013).

Prior to the ACA expansions, insurance coverage was not accessible to many low-income women of child-bearing age unless they became pregnant. Even after becoming pregnant, some women experienced long delays to obtain coverage, and some were unable to access care until the second or third trimester (see Table 5-3). CDC reported that in 2009, the percentage of women who were uninsured decreased from 23.4 percent in the month before pregnancy to 1.5 percent at the time of delivery, while Medicaid coverage increased from 16.6 percent in the month before pregnancy to 43.9 percent at delivery (D'Angelo et al., 2015). Even with the recent gains in access to coverage before and during a pregnancy, more than one in five (21.3 percent) American women who gave birth in 2016 began prenatal care after the first trimester; 4.6 percent began care in the third trimester; and 1.6 percent received no care at all. In all, approximately 15 percent of American women received inadequate prenatal care. Moreover, there are significant racial/ethnic, socioeconomic, and geographic disparities in prenatal care use (Osterman and Martin, 2018).

In addition to access to coverage, the ACA further improved access to essential care for women, especially preconception care, by mandating coverage for women's preventive services, including all Food and Drug Administration–approved contraceptive methods and counseling and at least one well-woman preventive care visit per year with no cost-sharing (HRSA, 2018; Women's Preventive Services Initiative, n.d.). Preconception care is also covered under well-woman preventive visits (Women's Preventive Services Initiative, n.d.). Additionally, the law mandated coverage for essential health benefits (EHBs), including maternity care and mental health services. The ACA prohibited gender rating (charging women a higher premium than men) and banned lifetime caps on benefits and exclusions based on preexisting conditions, which protected access for women with chronic conditions. A Commonwealth Fund report found that between 2010 and 2016, the percent of women ages 19–64 with health conditions who found it very difficult or impossible to find coverage they needed in the individual market decreased by nearly half, while those who said they were not getting care because of costs (did not fill prescription, skipped recommended test or treatment, had a medical problem but did not seek primary or specialty care) decreased from 48 percent to 38 percent (Gunja et al., 2017). Several other studies have also shown similar improvements (Angier et al., 2015, 2017, 2019a; Heintzman et al., 2017; Hoopes et al., 2016; Huguet et al., 2017, 2018; Sommers et al., 2016, 2017b).

Presently, it is unclear what affects recent efforts to deregulate the ACA, such as the repeal of the individual mandate, proposed extension

TABLE 5-3 Trimester That Prenatal Care Began, by Selected Characteristics: United States, 2016

| | Timing of PNC | | | | |
| | | | | Late or No PNC[a] | |
Selected Characteristic	First Trimester	Second Trimester	Total Percent	Late PNC[b]	No PNC
Total	77.1	16.7	6.2	4.6	1.6
Age of Mother					
Under 20	61.2	27.6	11.2	8.3	2.9
Under 15	36.7	37.6	25.7	19.2	6.5
15–19	61.5	27.5	11.0	8.2	2.9
20–24	70.3	21.7	8.0	5.9	2.1
25–29	77.8	16.3	6.0	4.4	1.5
30–34	82.1	13.1	4.8	3.6	1.2
35–39	81.7	13.5	4.8	3.6	1.2
40 and over	78.4	16.0	5.6	4.1	1.5
Race and Hispanic Origin					
Non-Hispanic, single-race:					
White	82.3	13.4	4.3	3.3	1.1
Black	66.5	23.5	10.0	7.0	3.0
American Indian or Alaska Native	63.0	24.5	12.5	9.2	3.3
Asian	80.6	14.0	5.4	4.6	0.8
Asian Indian	83.4	12.1	4.6	3.9	0.7
Chinese	81.2	11.4	7.4	6.9	0.5
Filipino	82.8	13.4	3.8	3.0	0.8
Japanese	85.5	10.5	4.0	3.2	0.8
Korean	85.3	10.6	4.1	3.4	0.7
Vietnamese	80.2	15.3	4.5	3.3	1.2
Other Asian	71.7	22.0	6.3	5.0	1.3
Native Hawaiian or Other Pacific Islander	51.9	28.9	19.2	14.2	5.0
Hawaiian	69.9	20.5	9.6	6.0	3.6
Guamanian	72.1	21.4	6.6	5.0	1.6
Samoan	56.9	29.1	14.0	10.4	3.6
Other Pacific Islander	43.8	31.3	24.8	18.4	6.4

continued

TABLE 5-3 Continued

	Timing of PNC			Late or No PNC[a]	
Selected Characteristic	First Trimester	Second Trimester	Total Percent	Late PNC[b]	No PNC
Hispanic	72.0	20.3	7.7	5.6	2.1
Mexican	71.4	20.6	8.0	5.7	2.3
Puerto Rican	76.2	18.1	5.7	4.3	1.4
Cuban	82.0	14.1	3.8	2.9	0.9
Central or South American	68.1	22.7	9.2	6.9	2.2
Other and unknown Hispanic	74.3	18.8	6.8	5.1	1.7
Live-Birth Order					
1st birth	79.0	15.3	5.7	4.4	1.3
2nd birth	80.1	14.8	5.1	3.9	1.2
3rd birth	75.8	18.0	6.2	4.6	1.6
4th birth or higher	66.2	23.8	10.0	6.7	3.3
Educational Attainment[c,d]					
Less than high school	62.7	26.1	11.2	7.5	3.7
High school	73.4	19.5	7.2	5.0	2.2
Some college[e]	80.2	15.1	4.7	3.5	1.2
Bachelor's degree or higher	87.6	9.1	3.3	2.8	0.5
Source of Payment for the Delivery					
Medicaid	68.1	23.3	8.6	6.4	2.2
Private insurance	87.0	10.3	2.7	2.1	0.6
Self-pay	54.8	25.4	19.8	13.2	6.6
Other[f]	75.0	16.8	8.2	5.8	2.3

NOTES: PNC = prenatal care. Chi-squared test statistics for each variable by trimester prenatal care began were statistically significant ($p < 0.05$). Data are sourced from the National Center for Health Statistics National Vital Statistics System.

 [a] PNC that began in the third trimester and no PNC.
 [b] PNC that began in the third trimester.
 [c] Excludes women under age 25.
 [d] Significantly increasing trend in first trimester PNC by educational attainment ($p < 0.05$).
 [e] Includes associate's degree.
 [f] Includes Indian Health Service, CHAMPUS (Civilian Health and Medical Program of the Uniformed Services) or TRICARE, other government (federal, state, or local), and charity.
SOURCE: Osterman and Martin, 2018.

of short-term coverage policies (which do not have to comply with many ACA consumer protections) (Keith, 2018), state waiver for EHBs, and religious and moral exemptions from contraceptive coverage mandates, will have on access to primary and preventive services for both men and women. It is likely that, as with prior policies that scaled back insurance access, these repeal efforts will negatively impact access to and use of recommended primary and preventive care services (Carlson et al., 2006; DeVoe et al., 2012a; Solotaroff et al., 2005; Tumin et al., 2019).

As demonstrated above, Medicaid is an important source of insurance coverage and facilitator of basic access to women's health care services, particularly for low-income women. In 2014, Medicaid provided more than 25 million low-income women with health and long-term care coverage (Kaiser Family Foundation, 2017), approximately two-thirds of them between ages 19 and 49. Medicaid is particularly important for low-income women and women of color. While overall 1 in 5 women of reproductive age (20 percent) were enrolled in Medicaid in 2015, 27 percent of Hispanic women, 31 percent of African American women, and nearly half (48 percent) of low-income women in the United States were enrolled (Sonfield, 2017). Expansion of Medicaid coverage for pregnant women in the 1990s led to significant increases in access to and use of prenatal care; today, Medicaid covers nearly half of all births in the United States (Kaiser Family Foundation, 2017). For nonpregnant women, the ACA legislation extended Medicaid eligibility to all individuals with household incomes up to 138 percent of the FPL; however, a 2012 Supreme Court ruling in *National Federation of Independent Business v. Sebelius* made Medicaid expansion optional for states, resulting in inconsistent coverage policies across the country (Kaiser Family Foundation, 2017). As of May 2019, 36 states and Washington, DC, have expanded Medicaid; 14 states have not (Kaiser Family Foundation, 2019). Overall, the rate of uninsurance among low-income women of reproductive age decreased by 13.2 percentage points due to the ACA Medicaid expansions (Johnston et al., 2018). A recent study found that from 2011 to 2016, states that expanded Medicaid showed significant improvements in black-white disparities in preterm, very preterm, LBW, and very LBW rates compared to states that did not (Brown et al., 2019). Studies have shown that in states that expanded Medicaid, disparities by race and ethnicity in the rates of insurance coverage and access to care have narrowed more than in states that have not (Artiga et al., 2019; Hayes et al., 2017).

Medicaid and CHIP finance health insurance for nearly 50 percent of U.S. children and youth. Children and youth with public insurance have about the same rates of use and quality of care as those with commercial insurance (DeVoe et al., 2011b,c), although those data do not account for the higher rates of chronic conditions and disability among publicly insured children. Although most U.S. children and youth currently have health insurance, children who are low income or from racial and ethnic minority populations face problems with lack of access to ongoing, comprehensive health care services (McCormick et al., 2001; Weinick and Krauss, 2000). Children and youth with public insurance (Medicaid and CHIP) disproportionately include black and Latino populations (Georgetown University Center for Children and Families, 2017, 2018).

Medicaid demonstration waivers have shown promise in allowing states to test new approaches in Medicaid that differ from federal program rules (Musumeci et al., 2018) in order to expand and broaden access to coverage for populations that have traditionally not been eligible for Medicaid. For example, 27 states have established limited-scope Medicaid family planning programs through waivers to extend access to family planning services to uninsured women who do not qualify for full Medicaid coverage. This includes low-income women whose incomes are not low enough or who have lost Medicaid eligibility after giving birth (Kaiser Family Foundation, 2017). Additionally, Louisiana has added an interpregnancy component to their Medicaid waiver to provide interconception care for low-income, high-risk women who had an adverse birth outcome (ASTHO, 2013). Medicaid waivers have also helped children and youth with special health care needs access a number of treatment services in home and community settings. The original Medicaid waiver was for an Iowa child who had Medicaid coverage while hospitalized (because her parents' income was not considered for inpatient eligibility) but would lose it if she came home with multiple and complex needed services. The waiver allowed hospital care to be substituted with home care (Perrin et al., 1993).

Other Medicaid demonstration waivers have been proposed that could negatively impact eligibility, enrollment, and benefits, including work and reporting requirements, coverage lock-outs, premium cost-sharing, restrictions on presumptive eligibility and retroactive coverage, and time limits on coverage (Flowers and Accius, 2019). The impact of these waivers on access to preconception, prenatal, and pediatric health care services is still being studied; however, similar policies making Medicaid eligibility more restrictive in the past (e.g., proof of citizenship requirements) have had negative effects on access to care (Angus and Devoe, 2010; Bauer et al., 2011; Hatch et al., 2014). Arkansas has seen thousands of working-age adults, including many with dependent children at home, lose Medicaid benefits, along with no growth in job participation (Rudowitz et al., 2019; Sommers et al., 2019). However, federal courts struck down Arkansas' work requirement for expanded Medicaid coverage in March 2019. Recent reports indicate the first increase in rates of uninsurance among children in a decade, in part reflecting new restrictions on parents' access (Alker and Pham, 2018).

Many Factors Affect Access to Health Care Services

A complex array of factors beyond insurance coverage influence preconception, prenatal, and pediatric care use (Heaman et al., 2014; Kalmuss and Fennelly, 1990). Some of these factors include the complexity of household needs and social challenges (e.g., child care, transportation, addictions, lack of support), caregiver qualities (lack of time, negative behaviors), health system barriers (shortage of providers), and program/service characteristics (distance, long waits, short visits). Such barriers (particularly transportation to health care facilities, ability to pay for needed treatments, taking time from work for health care appointments, and costs related to housing and food) may take priority over health care for families.

Regarding access to prenatal care, a study of 246 African American women residing in Washington, DC, identified psychosocial stress, substance use, child care problems, negative attitudes toward pregnancy and prenatal care, insurance/financial constraints, and nonparticipation in the Special Supplemental Nutrition Program for Women, Infants, and Children (WIC) program as key determinants of lower than recommended rates of prenatal care use (Johnson et al., 2007). Another study of low-income African American women in Milwaukee, Wisconsin, identified structural barriers to prenatal care, such as transportation and insurance; negative or ambivalent attitudes toward prenatal care, perceived poor quality of care, and unintended pregnancy; and psychosocial stressors, such as overall life stress and chaos (Mazul et al., 2017).

Children and youth with special health care needs (SHCN) represent a population that experiences unique access challenges. A sizable percentage of U.S. children (10–20 percent or more, depending on the definition; about 11.4 percent of children ages 0–5 and 22.7 percent of children ages 6–11) have SHCN (HHS, 2015; NASEM, 2018) and their needs depend on the severity and prevalence of the condition. Most children and youth with more common conditions (asthma, obesity, mental health conditions, and neurodevelopmental conditions) receive the bulk of their care in community pediatric settings, including hospital outpatient clinics. Children and youth with more severe and less common conditions get a large part of their care from specialized pediatric hospitals (Perrin et al., 2014). Many households have difficulty gaining access to specialized care because most subspecialists are found in centralized children's hospitals, which may be distant from their homes. Children insured by Medicaid, who are disproportionately black or Latino (Georgetown University

Center for Children and Families, 2017, 2018), particularly experience problems in accessing subspecialists (Bisgaier and Rhodes, 2011). Furthermore, narrow insurance networks may not include all needed specialists, creating barriers to needed subspecialty care.

Ensuring access to quality health care requires addressing both financial and nonfinancial barriers. Lu et al. (2010) identified a number of promising strategies to increase financial and nonfinancial access to timely care, including policy initiatives to promote innovative care models, support outreach and care coordination, and increase provider participation in Medicaid-funded care. State Medicaid agencies have increasingly relied on managed care organizations (private-sector companies that contract with Medicaid to manage the program) to implement and manage Medicaid programs. Currently, about 80 percent of Medicaid recipients receive care through a managed care arrangement (MACPAC, 2016). Many managed care organizations have experimented with new programs or financing, although there are few consistent patterns (Institute for Medicaid Innovation, n.d.). It is also not yet apparent whether this trend has had a significant impact on reducing health disparities. Another example is Oregon's coordinated care organization (CCO) model, implemented in 2012 and designed to improve the coordination of care for the state's Medicaid beneficiaries. In the state, CCOs cover a distinct geographic area and have broad budgeting authority for Medicaid and CHIP funding within that area, along with incentives to improve quality and broaden attention to social determinants of care in part through active collaboration with schools and community agencies (Oregon Health Authority, 2018; Stecker, 2013). CCOs led to significant increases in early prenatal care initiation and a reduction in disparities across insurance types but no difference in overall prenatal care adequacy (Muoto et al., 2016).

Regarding access to postpartum care, colocating postpartum and well-baby care has been suggested as a strategy for improving access (Stuebe et al., 2019). Colocating care could reduce transportation, child care, medical leave, and other barriers and facilitate care coordination for issues that require joint assessment and management of both mother and infant, such as breastfeeding (Stuebe et al., 2019). Greater use of home visitors, doulas, and community health workers can also help improve access (Hans et al., 2018). Providing culturally congruent care to women of color can increase breastfeeding and reduce perinatal disparities (Kozhimannil et al., 2013), but only three states currently provide Medicaid coverage for doula services (Stuebe et al., 2019). Leveraging mHealth technology, such as text messaging, remote blood pressure monitoring, and telehealth, can also improve postpartum follow-up (ACOG, 2018b; CMS Maternal & Infant Health Initiative, 2015). Presently, nearly one-quarter of women return to work within 10 days postpartum, and nearly half return to work within 40 days postpartum (Klerman et al., 2014); expanding paid family and medical leave could also increase access to and use of postpartum care (Rossin-Slater and Uniat, 2019) (see Chapter 6 for a discussion on paid family leave). Because many health and psychosocial issues persist or emerge beyond 60 days postpartum, some experts have called for extending Medicaid coverage for at least 12 months postpartum, especially in Medicaid nonexpansion states (Stuebe et al., 2019).

For nearly three decades, state Title V programs have played an important role in increasing access to and use of timely prenatal care and other family health care services through outreach and coordination by (1) facilitating partnerships among agencies that provide direct services to pregnant women; (2) helping to ensure that maternal and child health professionals in WIC, Head Start, and other public programs provide pregnant women with accurate and current information on coverage in their state; (3) increasing access to presumptive Medicaid eligibility, which provides pregnant women with access to immediate prenatal care; and (4) increasing continuity of coverage for low-income women who become pregnant (Association of Maternal & Child Health Programs, 2016). State and federal Maternal and Child Health Programs (Title V) have had even longer histories of involvement with very young children, following earlier Children's Bureau programs for safe milk and infant nutrition (Lesser, 1965). At least 30 percent of federal support for state programs has been allocated for well-child programs, and at least 30 percent goes to programs for children with SHCN (formerly the Crippled Children's Service) (HRSA, 2019, n.d.). As with women's health, state programs have helped to facilitate partnerships across key agencies, improve knowledge of the health status of children and youth in the state, and link households with other agencies, especially Medicaid and the U.S. Social Security Administration (for Supplemental Security Income [SSI] coverage).

Recent growth of community acute care clinics—some operated by pharmacy chains and others by larger hospitals—have offered new community-based access to health care. These centers offer immediate and convenient care for (generally minor) acute conditions. The centers offer variable connections to children's and families' ongoing primary care; in several communities, such centers have worked to share medical records and referral information with ongoing primary care programs (Conners et al., 2017). Acute care centers, at times collaborating with telehealth companies, can offer immediate and convenient services. For example, a parent of a sick child can call from home (or work), reach a health care clinician, describe symptoms, and efficiently receive advice. Nonetheless, most innovative walk-in clinics, acute care centers, and commercial telehealth models have focused on middle-income communities and less on low-income areas. Thus, there is no evidence that they reduce disparities.

Improving Access to Needed Health Care

Based on its review of the evidence in the sections above, the committee concludes:

Conclusion 5-2: Although health insurance coverage has grown substantially in the past few decades, mainly through Medicaid expansions and other insurance enhancements, access remains a problem for many families with young children, who experience numerous barriers to obtaining health care services in addition to lack of health insurance coverage. Multiple agencies, especially the Maternal and Child Health Bureau, have worked to diminish barriers to care. Further efforts are needed to address financial and nonfinancial barriers to care and to ensure that all families have access to adequate preconception, prenatal, postpartum, and pediatric care.

To address the issues identified related to access to care, the committee recommends:

Recommendation 5-1: The U.S. Department of Health and Human Services, state, tribal, and territorial Medicaid agencies, public and private payers, and state and federal policy makers should adopt policies and practices that ensure universal access to high-quality health care across the life course. This includes

- **Increasing access to patient- and family-centered care,**
- **Ensuring access to preventive services and essential health benefits, and**
- **Increasing culturally and linguistically appropriate outreach and services.**

Achieving this recommendation requires

- **Increasing access to patient- and family-centered care.** Specific actions include integrating services longitudinally, vertically, and horizontally to increase entry points to care for children and families; incorporating enabling services to facilitate access to care; expanding attention to whole family needs in clinical care; and overcoming household challenges, such as transportation and child care needs. (See the sections that follow for discussion on the need to integrate health care services across the life course.)
- **Supporting comprehensive access across the life course.** Expand comprehensive supports for health across the life course. Programs should increase awareness of and access to family planning services and general preventive health services that keep parents healthy and promote positive attachments essential to early life development.

- **Protecting access to benefits.** Ensure continuous coverage and access for all men, women, and children. Coverage should include child and family preventive services and EHBs, with a prohibition against lifetime benefit caps and preexisting condition exclusions.
- **Actively promoting inclusion in coverage and care.** Promote culturally and linguistically appropriate outreach and services as well as increased diversity in the health care workforce.
- **Systematic application of measures.** For example, adoption of a measure to assess disparities in timely and adequate access to well-woman care, prenatal, and pediatric care as a national performance measure by the Title V Maternal and Child Health Block Grant.

PROMOTING QUALITY OF CARE

Quality health care is timely, equitable, safe, patient centered, efficient, and effective (IOM, 2001). Equitable care means care that does not vary in quality because of demographic characteristics, such as sex, ethnicity, geographic location, or SES (IOM, 2001). For populations who have access to health care services, the quality of the care they receive is not always safe and is often not equitable. Regarding preconception care, a survey of more than 800 women of reproductive age found that more than 1 in 4 (27 percent) were prescribed a medication with a potential teratogen (a potential cause of birth defects). Of these women, 43 percent received no counseling from their provider regarding the teratogenicity of the medication or the need for contraception (Schwarz et al., 2013). A recent review of 31 studies (Goossens, 2018) identified multiple barriers to high-quality preconception care at the provider level (unfavorable attitude and lack of knowledge of preconception care, not working in a medical discipline or clinical setting that provides maternity care, lack of clarity on the responsibility for providing preconception care) and the client level (not contacting a health care provider in the preconception stage, negative attitude, and lack of knowledge of preconception care). Limited resources (e.g., lack of time, tools, guidelines, and reimbursement) were frequently reported at the organizational and societal levels. Disparities are well documented in prenatal and pediatric care across similar domains.

Performance Measurement and Quality Improvement Efforts

Performance measurement is a common strategy currently being employed by state and local governments, payers, hospital accreditation bodies, and professional organizations to improve health care quality. It is often linked to change strategies—public reporting and pay-for-performance (Berwick et al., 2003; Chassin, 2002; Hibbard et al., 2005; IOM, 2006; Lindenauer et al., 2007; Millenson, 2004). Public reporting fosters interest in quality on the part of physicians and hospital leaders, perhaps by appealing to their professional ethos or creating market advantages (Lindenauer et al., 2014; Marshall et al., 2000). Pay-for-performance programs are intended to enhance the business case for quality improvement (QI) by rewarding excellence and reversing what have been described as perverse financial incentives that can deter providers and hospitals from investing in QI efforts (Dudley et al., 1998; Epstein et al., 2004; Millenson, 2004).

To date, the National Quality Forum has endorsed 18 perinatal and reproductive measures, none of which addresses ambulatory[6] preconception or prenatal care (NQF, 2016). The only prenatal and postpartum care performance measures currently in use are the two Healthcare Effectiveness Data and Information Set measures on the rates of first trimester prenatal care and postpartum visits (NCQA, 2018).

There are more measures specific to the quality of child health care that address some of the main aspects of well-child care (e.g., immunizations, regular visits, screening, developmental assessment). The reauthorization of CHIP in 2009 provided the first major support for quality measurement in public health insurance programs for children and youth and led to substantial growth in pediatric care measures and ongoing efforts to expand and refine these measures (AHRQ, 2018; Perrin, 2012). Measures have generally focused on children without chronic conditions, with the exception of high-prevalence conditions (especially asthma), and quality-of-care measures for children with disability are much more limited (Perrin, 2012). Medicaid publishes and updates a quality measure set for children (Medicaid, n.d.). Several groups have catalogued children's quality measures (Beal et al., 2004), and the AAP and the National Initiative for Children's Health Quality, among others, have pursued consensus on best child health quality measures (Adirim et al., 2017).

The Collaborative Improvement and Innovation Network (CoIIN) is an example of a model aimed at improving maternal and child health that combines both CQI and collaborative learning to address infant mortality and perinatal disparities. The CoIIN was launched in 2012 in 13 southern U.S. states (Public Health Regions IV and VI), with early success leading to a national expansion of the program to other states. The CoIIN brought together state teams of clinical and public health leaders and policy makers to implement evidence-based and promising strategies, supported by virtual shared workspace, CQI experts, and a data dashboard that provided real-time data to drive real-time improvements (Ghandour et al., 2017). Between 2011 and 2014, early elective delivery at less than 39 weeks decreased by 22 percent versus 14 percent in other regions, smoking cessation during pregnancy increased by 7 percent

---

[6] Ambulatory care is care provided by health care professionals in outpatient settings (AHRQ, n.d.-a).

versus 2 percent, and back sleep position increased by 5 percent versus 2 percent. Preterm birth decreased by 4 percent, twice that observed in other regions, but infant mortality reductions did not differ significantly (Hirai et al., 2018b). The CoIIN is particularly notable in its application of CQI methodologies, which have largely been limited to clinical settings, to drive improvements in population-level perinatal outcomes.

While these efforts have improved adherence to standardized care processes, inequitable care remains pervasive throughout the system. Inequitable care is care that does not address the unique challenges and vulnerabilities made relevant by differential life experiences based on social characteristics, such as gender, ethnicity, language preference, geographic location, and SES (IOM, 2001). For example, a major component of preventive health care is culturally and linguistically sensitive and literacy-appropriate health education to promote behavioral changes. Thus, an office or clinic visit is only the prelude to fully completing the care. To fully attain the effects of care, an individual or family needs to take that education to the home and follow through with it (e.g., eat more healthy foods). If the social environment in the community or home does not have the resources to support these behavioral changes (insufficient income or no neighborhood stores to purchase healthy foods), the care plan remains unfulfilled, and the effectiveness of the care remains limited, despite the practitioners' best intentions (Lu et al., 2010).

Multiple studies of the implementation of quality measures indicate substantial improvement in attention to specific processes in the delivery of health care services (e.g., increasing screening rates, testing for harmful side effects of treatment). Increasingly, payers have assessed quality of care (e.g., screening and immunization rates) and offer financial incentives to achieve quality thresholds. These incentives have improved processes linked to better health outcomes; further research is needed to determine their impact on health outcomes directly and on disparities. Often, these assessments are done at a population level and do not highlight disparities or account for practices caring for populations with different characteristics. Thus, in addition to traditional methods to assess performance and QI, there are a number of other areas that are receiving increased attention in efforts to attain equitable health care practices, including developing new metrics and measurement methods to account for child development and well-being in the context of an intersectional and multidimensional view of health and health equity and enhanced workforce education and training (including training to recognize and address implicit bias).

Development of New Metrics and Measurement Methods

Growing recognition of MBH concerns among children and youth has led to the development of newer measures of developmental and behavioral screening (including social and emotional screening), treatment, and outcomes, including measures of follow-up for medications used to treat some pediatric mental health conditions. Few measures routinely collected today address the SDOH. Furthermore, toxic stress and its precipitants, including many social determinants, such as adverse childhood experiences (ACEs), housing instability, food insecurity, or poverty and racism, are inadequately assessed in health care settings. Substantial evidence notes that much adult chronic disease has its origins in childhood and adolescence, often associated with the SDOH discussed throughout this report (Marmot et al., 2001). (See also the discussion of the Perry Preschool and Abcedarian Projects in Chapter 7.) The majority of adult mental health conditions originate in childhood or adolescence. An emerging body of research also suggests that some chronic childhood and adult diseases have a fetal origin (Barker, 1995, 2003, 2004; Calkins and Devaskar, 2011; de Boo and Harding, 2006; Kimm, 2004; Skogen and Overland, 2012) and that factors such as maternal and paternal stress, nutrition and physical activities, and occupational and environmental exposures may play a critical role in epigenetic modification and developmental programming of future health and disease. Information regarding these risks is not routinely collected, monitored, or reported during standard preconception or prenatal care visits, nor would this be feasible in a brief office visit. Until recently, pediatric care providers were not routinely screening for ACEs; however, the AAP released two policy statements and conducted substantial practitioner education, which bolstered rates of attention in community practice (Kerker et al., 2016; Szilagyi et al., 2016). Even having clear standards for screening does not ensure that all child health practitioners screen for all relevant issues. A recent paper using parent reports found that, nationally, 37 percent of children received developmental screening with a validated tool (Hirai et al., 2018a). Another study, based on physician report, indicated that more than 80 percent of pediatricians reported using one or more formal tools to screen for autism, with 88 percent screening at 18 months and 74 percent screening at 24 months (Coury et al., 2017).

Several national initiatives have begun to advance primary care clinicians' understanding of ACEs and toxic stress and their capacities and competencies to identify and respond to risk factors for toxic stress and other adversities, such as the Trauma-Informed Primary Care Initiative, a partnership between the National Council for Behavioral Health and Kaiser Permanente[7]; the National Pediatric Practice Community on ACEs, an initiative of the Center for Youth Wellness[8]; the Trauma-Informed Care

---

[7] For more information, see https://www.thenationalcouncil.org/trauma-informed-primary-care-initiative-learning-community (accessed April 29, 2019).
[8] For more information, see https://nppcaces.org (accessed April 29, 2019).

Implementation Resource Center,[9] developed by the Center for Health Care Strategies; and other initiatives (APA and AAP, 2017; APA Task Force on Childhood Poverty, 2013). AAP has recommended regular screening for precipitants of toxic stress (Garner et al., 2012), and several professional organizations have compiled tools and resources to support clinicians in screening for social determinants (including risk factors for toxic stress), maternal depression, and early child development, such as the AAP Screening & Technical Assistance Resource Center and the American Academy of Family Physicians's Center for Diversity and Health Equity (AAP, 2010; Gleason et al., 2016; Sege and Amaya-Jackson, 2017).[10] Many other professional organizations are also issuing similar statements and recommendations; for example, the American Heart Association has called for upstream identification and mitigation of ACEs as a risk factor for cardiometabolic disease (NASEM, 2015; Suglia et al., 2018).

As the science advances regarding contributors to child health equity, new measures that capture the SDOH, including indicators of cumulative adversity and family issues that may impact health and development, have become available. The development of these measures is well under way, addressing such issues as household hunger, lack of money for utilities, difficulty finding jobs, need for child care, or housing problems (AAP, n.d.-b; Arthur et al., 2018; Center for Youth Wellness, n.d.; Ellis, 2001; Garg et al., 2015; Gottlieb et al., 2016). The substantial increased attention to screening and identification of the SDOH and adversity in early childhood has led to much consideration of how child and family health care services might prioritize screening centered on the SDOH. However, many different screening tools exist for the SDOH, with little consensus or guidelines on which ones are most appropriate or effective in different health care settings or contexts (Morone, 2017; Pai et al., 2016). Early studies show promising results with screening and intervention, and most of this work has been done in primary care practices, especially those that care for children and families (Angier et al., 2019b; Bazemore et al., 2016; Cottrell et al., 2018; DeVoe et al., 2016). There are a number of scientists actively engaged in building the evidence for SDOH screening and referral (e.g., which tools to use, how to screen, when to screen, how to incorporate technology). Providers will typically screen more when they can refer to programs that can address child and family needs. Where resources are limited, they are less likely to try to identify problems (Garg et al., 2016).

---

[9] For more information, see https://www.chcs.org/resource/trauma-informed-care-implementation-resource-center (accessed July 17, 2019).

[10] For more information on the American Academy of Family Physicians (AAFP) Center for Diversity and Health Equity, see https://www.aafp.org/patient-care/social-determinants-of-health/everyone-project/cdhe.html (accessed April 29, 2019). For more information on AAFP's "EveryONE Project" to advance health equity in every community, see https://www.aafp.org/patient-care/social-determinants-of-health/everyone-project.html (accessed April 29, 2019).

With the increased recognition of the need to expand risk assessment for ACEs, the development of evidence-based, effective strategies for early and continuing assessments of ACEs and other social and environmental determinants will be a key ingredient in transforming the delivery and measurement of preconception, prenatal, and pediatric care. In addition, there is an urgent need to develop biomedical measures to detect and treat toxic stress.

Interest has grown in measuring broader outcomes that may reflect more than health care, such as school readiness at age 5 (Jones et al., 2015) or a new composite measure of being healthy and ready to learn (Child Trends, 2018; Ghandour et al., 2018). These broader measures recognize the importance of cross-sector collaboration to keep children healthy and the health sector's role in helping children and their families access other needed resources (housing, food, and other supports) to help improve these outcomes.

As new metrics are developed, there is growing recognition that quality measurement is multidimensional and can be impacted by the clinical and social complexity of patients, families, and populations. For example, providers caring for patient populations in at-risk contexts are sometimes held accountable for achieving similar gains in quality metrics as providers in affluent communities without adjustment for patient complexity, putting them at risk for financial loss. Misaligned financial incentives can perpetuate disparities in health care access for underserved populations and fail to recognize quality initiatives that are reducing disparities (or exacerbating them) for certain subgroups if all members of the population are not starting at the same baseline or improving at the same rate. Efforts are currently under way to create adequate adjustments for traditional measures (NCQA, n.d.), although developing adjustments for diverse child populations has been difficult (Kuhlthau et al., 2005).

Enhanced Workforce Education and Training

Workforce development and training is another important strategy for improving the quality of health care. The increased attention to identifying and addressing social, economic, and environmental factors adversely impacting the health of children and families has led to enhanced curricula in the training programs for child and family health care providers. These additional components strengthen the emphasis on learning about the social and community aspects of care for patients and families, implicit bias and unequal treatment, and how to more effectively collaborate with community organizations to improve care and outcomes. This education variably addresses adversity, biases, and disparities, with increasing attention to such issues as food and housing insecurity and the importance of screening for ACEs and recognizing microaggressions.

Advancing health equity requires sustained commitment and resources to increase the diversity and representativeness of our health care workforce. The next generation of health care providers also needs to be better equipped with knowledge, skills, and tools to address MBH issues, ameliorate toxic stress, and provide TIC. This training requires explicit curricula on how to recognize and eliminate implicit bias and unequal treatment in health care. The future workforce needs to develop competencies in team-based care, working across disciplines and sectors to tackle the social and environmental determinants of health.

Transforming the health care system to provide culturally competent care is critical to advancing health equity. It is crucial that the health care workforce receive education and training in cultural competence. Betancourt et al. (2003) define a culturally competent health care system as "one that acknowledges and incorporates—at all levels—the importance of culture, assessment of cross-cultural relations, vigilance toward the dynamics that result from cultural differences, expansion of cultural knowledge, and adaptation of services to meet culturally unique needs" (Betancourt et al., 2003, p. 294). The importance of culturally competent care is also relevant to efforts to increase patient- and family-centered care, as "cultural competence enhances the ability of health systems and providers to address individual patients' preferences and goals" (Saha et al., 2008). The wide diversity of household backgrounds—cultural, racial, ethnic, and linguistic—and the expected demographic changes that will result in successively more diverse future generations make it important that the health care system have the capacity to understand and respond to cultural variations in health practices and understanding (see Box 5-3 on the role of doulas and Box 5-4 on the role of nurse-midwives and midwives in prenatal and postnatal care and culturally appropriate care). Although more providers entering the workforce have had cultural training and speak languages other than English than a generation ago, many households still face difficulties accessing culturally responsive and linguistically appropriate care. Access to such subspecialty care may be particularly challenging, especially for diagnostic and long-term care services that address cultural and language needs. For example, young children with ASD often need specialized therapists who work intensively on communication with the child and between the child and family. A Spanish-speaking family, however, can find it difficult to identify a Spanish-speaking therapist (Dabney et al., 2015).

Ensuring equity calls for strategies to diminish cultural and linguistic barriers through training and increased recruitment of health care providers from culturally diverse communities. It also requires explicit training on eliminating implicit bias and unequal treatment in health care. Unequal preconception, prenatal, and pediatric care based on race, ethnicity, and SES has been well documented (Brett et al., 1994; Kogan et al., 1994;

BOX 5-3
The Role of Doulas in Advancing Health Equity

A doula is "a trained professional who provides continuous physical, emotional, and informational support to a mother before, during, and shortly after childbirth to help her achieve the healthiest, most satisfying experience possible" (DONA International, n.d.). Doulas receive training on providing support during birth and/or the postpartum periods but do not perform medical or clinical tasks. For information on midwives, who receive medical and clinical training, see Box 5-4.

Evidence suggests that supportive care and services from doulas improves maternal and infant outcomes in the prenatal through postpartum periods. A joint consensus statement from the American College of Obstetricians and Gynecologists and the Society for Maternal-Fetal Medicine stated that "one of the most effective tools to improve labor and delivery outcomes is the continuous presence of support personnel, such as a doula" (Caughey et al., 2014). Similarly, a 2017 Cochrane systematic review of 26 studies found that women who received continuous support during childbirth, including from doulas, had improved maternal and infant outcomes (Bohren et al., 2017).

Importantly, doulas of color can provide culturally appropriate support to women of color that is sensitive to the historical injustices experienced by people of color within the health care system. Doulas can help to bridge the divide between patients and their health care providers by assisting patients with health literacy and social support, thus improving both access to health care services and the quality of care (Kozhimannil et al., 2016). Providing such care is critically important to address the significant disparities in pregnancy outcomes in women of color, particularly African American women, in the United States.

Increasing access to culturally sensitive supports for women of color, such as doula care, is essential for decreasing health inequities. However, women of color are often least likely to have access to such care and services because doulas are rarely covered by insurance (Thich, 2016). An approach to increase access to doula care is a community-based doula program, which emerging evidence has found to be effective in improving health outcomes for women of color. Administered by the Health Resources and Services Administration and Maternal and Child Health Bureau, the Community-Based Doula Program is a model that provides culturally appropriate peer-to-peer support based on the life course approach during the perinatal and early postpartum periods. The program serves women and families in communities with high levels of health and social needs (the majority of participants are black or Hispanic, and a small number are from tribal communities), and the program's community-based doulas "are of and from the communities being served" (HealthConnect One, 2014). Data findings of the program include rates of breastfeeding, including breastfeeding duration, that are higher than those documented by the Centers for Disease Control and Prevention's Pregnancy Risk Assessment and Monitoring System (PRAMS) and breastfeeding goals of Healthy People 2020, as well as caesarean section rates that are lower than those documented by PRAMS.

BOX 5-4
The Role of Midwives in Advancing Health Equity

Midwives, defined here as certified nurse-midwives, certified midwives, and midwives whose education and licensure meet the International Confederation of Midwives Global Standards for Midwifery Education (AAP Committee on Fetus and Newborn and ACOG Committee on Obstetric Practice, 2017), are health care professionals who provide low-risk women with services that include primary care; gynecologic and family planning services; care during the preconception, pregnancy, childbirth, and postpartum periods; and care of the healthy newborn during the first 28 days of life (American College of Nurse-Midwives, 2012). Medicare and Medicaid reimburse for care provided by midwives in all U.S. states, and private insurance reimburses for their services in most states (American College of Nurse-Midwives, 2012).

The midwifery model of care tends to allow more time for patient interactions, with a holistic approach to health behavior education (Palmer et al., 2010; Vonderheid et al., 2007). In addition, African American women participating in CenteringPregnancy, a form of group prenatal care predominantly facilitated by midwives (see Box 5-5 for more information), have a significantly reduced preterm birth rate (Carter et al., 2016; Ickovics et al., 2007; Picklesimer et al., 2012).

Full integration of midwives into the health care system may provide an opportunity to both improve pregnancy outcomes and reduce health disparities. A recent study by Vedam et al. (2018) measured midwifery and health care integration with the Midwifery Integration Scoring System (MISS) and found an association between states with higher MISS scores and lower rates of infant mortality (including by race), cesarean section, preterm birth, and low birth weight infants than states with lower MISS scores.

Kotelchuck et al., 1997). In a randomized trial of 524 providers who were shown videos depicting patients of varying sociodemographic characteristics, providers were more likely to recommend levonorgestrel intrauterine contraception for low-SES Latina and African American women than low-SES white women (Dehlendorf et al., 2010). Patients from low-SES backgrounds were judged to be significantly more likely than patients from high-SES backgrounds to have a sexually transmitted infection and/or an unintended pregnancy and were also judged to be less knowledgeable. An analysis of data from the National Maternal and Infant Health Survey demonstrated that black women were less likely than white women to receive advice from their prenatal care providers about smoking cessation and alcohol use (Kogan et al., 1994). Stereotyping and implicit bias on the part of health care providers are factors that may play a role (ACOG, 2015). Advancing health equity in birth and child health outcomes will require addressing implicit bias and unequal treatment in health care (see Chapters 7 and 8 for more on implicit bias training).

Most existing training programs offer some, albeit limited, exposure to training in cultural diversity and how culture influences health care and behaviors. In a few settings, clinicians in training learn skills in team care, although integrated training programs are rare. Case Western Reserve University is starting a new program where medical students, nursing students, and others will train together in a new multischool training and research building. All of these areas (cultural and linguistic diversity, the SDOH, MBH, and team experience) merit increased attention in medical training in general and in pediatrics specifically.

There is increased recognition that health care providers need to be not only well versed in medical interventions to treat illness but effective advocates in addressing the broader factors contributing to unequal access to services and treatment and impacting efforts to achieve health equity.

Improving Quality of Care

Based on its review of the evidence the committee concludes:

Conclusion 5-3: Strategies to improve the quality of preconception, prenatal, and child health care have included developing and implementing new measures, including for adversity and social determinants, along with efforts to strengthen the training of the health care workforce to better understand diversity and implicit bias and to address equity in health care.

To improve the quality of care provided in the preconception through early childhood periods, the committee recommends:

Recommendation 5-2: To expand accountability and improve the quality of preconception, prenatal, postpartum, and pediatric care,

- **Public and private payers should include new metrics of child and family health and well-being that assess quality using a holistic view of health and health equity. Federal, state, and other agencies, along with private foundations and philanthropies that invest in research, should support the development and implementation of new measures of accountability, including key drivers of health, such as social determinants, along with measuring variations by key subgroups to determine disparities;**
- **Public and private payers, including the Health Resources and Services Administration's (HRSA's) Bureau of Primary Care and Maternal and Child Health Bureau, Centers for Disease Control and Prevention, Centers for Medicare & Medicaid Services (CMS), and perinatal and pediatric quality**

collaboratives, should expand the use of continuous quality improvement, learning communities, payment for performance, and other strategies to enhance accountability; and
- Health care–related workforce development entities should expand efforts to increase diversity, inclusion, and equity in the health care workforce, including diversity-intensive outreach, mentoring, networking, and leadership development for underrepresented faculty and trainees.

Workforce development (bullet 3) will need to be addressed by several entities, including the Accreditation Council for Graduate Medical Education and specialty boards, professional schools, training programs, funders of graduate education in health professions (CMS, HRSA, and others), and teaching hospitals, including children's hospitals. Metrics for accountability include

- **Social determinants and risk measures:** Measures that reflect whether risks were identified early and whether families received needed help, with key drivers of health inequities that lie beyond traditional clinical purview but profoundly impact their health, such as housing instability, food security, and exposure to adversity or trauma.
- **Cross-sector developmental measures:** Measures that move beyond common indicators of child development, such as immunizations and management of acute infections or common chronic conditions, to address an expanded set of clinical indicators crucial for children and caretakers, including MBH. Measures should reflect healthy life course development, such as language at age 3, school readiness at age 5, reading proficiency at age 8, and high school graduation rates, as well as indicators of concern (need for special education, substance use, executive functioning, major behavior disorders).
- **Disparities as explicit measurement domains:** Measures that hold providers accountable not just for delivering services but also for improving outcomes and closing gaps in outcomes among key populations or subgroups. Quality measures should be adjusted for the social and clinical complexity of patient populations.

INNOVATIVE DELIVERY MODELS AND FINANCING CARE

Most preconception, prenatal, postpartum, and pediatric care is delivered through face-to-face office visits. For many families, but especially low-income families, this often requires taking unpaid leave from work, arranging child care and transportation, and waiting an hour or two for a 5- to 30-minute visit (Lewis et al., 2017). Preconception care is usually one short visit, with no consistency in what is accomplished during that visit, and a large percentage of families do not even receive this minimal level of care (Poels et al., 2016). Current prenatal care guidelines continue to recommend 14 or more prenatal visits during pregnancy, despite a lack of evidence supporting this number. Most visits consist of a spot blood pressure check and urine dip, a cursory auscultation of fetal heart tone and fundal height measurement, and a hurried conversation with a provider who, despite best intentions, often does not have sufficient time or training to educate patients about self-care let alone address their psychosocial concerns or occupational and environmental exposures (Lu, 2019). Similarly, postpartum care is usually one short visit (two after cesarean delivery), which consists of a cursory review of problems, a pelvic exam, and an often hurried discussion of contraceptive options, if the latter happens at all. Pediatric care also focuses on assessment of common issues, along with immunizations and other preventive services, in short office visits with limited time for extensive screening and counseling. Nonetheless, the multiple scheduled health supervision visits during the prenatal and early childhood periods can serve to connect families with trusted health advisors. For young children who have frequent pediatric care visits in the first years of life, health care provides a main entry point to health and many other services that can support the promotion of health for preschool children and their families (Garg et al., 2015; Patient-Centered Primary Care Collaborative, n.d.; Stille et al., 2010). In most communities, the current configuration of services does not take full advantage of this opportunity for maximizing collaborations across sectors and implementing concurrent interventions to strengthen children and families.

Concerns regarding increasing health care costs, health care provider availability, dissatisfaction with wait times, and the minimal opportunity for education and support associated with the individual care model have given rise to interest in alternative models of care. For children, a system of care designed to prevent and treat common infectious diseases faces a population whose health reflects infections less than noninfectious chronic conditions. Growing epidemics of nonfatal chronic conditions, especially MBH conditions (Halfon et al., 2012; Houtrow et al., 2014), much greater understanding of the SDOH, increasing diversity in the sociocultural makeup of the U.S. population, and the tremendous growth in the science of early childhood development all call for new strategies and structures for delivering and financing preconception, prenatal, and pediatric care, including efforts to address inequities (Perrin and Dewitt, 2011). Social, economic, and environmental determinants of health generally affect the health of children and families more than usual medical treatments, and traditional ways of delivering health care have relatively limited impact on early childhood growth, development, and health.

Some innovative ideas being tested in prenatal and well-baby care are group visits, multidisciplinary teams, strategies to link health care with other community resources, and increased use of new technologies (see section on the use of technology below).

Group Visits

Group visits and innovative designs that bring patients with similar needs together for health care encounters (face to face or virtually) increase the time available for the educational component of the encounter, improve efficiency, and reduce repetition (ACOG, 2018a). The group visit model is being tested for prenatal care because group visits are designed to enhance patient education while providing opportunities for social support and retaining the risk screening and physical assessment of individual care (ACOG, 2018a). In some settings, the groups continue meeting for postpartum and/or newborn care sessions. This model is especially promising in the reconceptualization of postpartum care, which would move away from a single clinical encounter toward more comprehensive, ongoing support for the postpartum transition.

While initial observational studies (Thielen, 2012) and a large RCT (Ickovics et al., 2007) found significant improvement in perinatal outcomes in group visit models, a more recent Cochrane review (Catling et al., 2015) and a meta-analysis of 10 observational studies and 4 RCTs (Carter et al., 2016) found no significant difference in preterm birth, LBW, breastfeeding, or neonatal intensive care unit admissions. However, it should be noted that while there was no overall difference in outcomes between women in traditional and group prenatal care, black women in group prenatal care showed a 41 percent reduction in preterm births in the largest RCT (Ickovics et al., 2007) and the meta-analysis, respectively. CenteringPregnancy is a model of group prenatal care that has demonstrated some promising but mixed findings in improving maternal and birth outcomes, including decreasing disparities by race and ethnicity (see Box 5-5). CenteringParenting is a similar innovative model of group postpartum care that brings together a cohort of six to seven mother–infant dyads for 1 year postpartum (Bloomfield and Rising, 2013); its impact on outcomes remains to be established.

Father and Partner Involvement

As discussed in Chapter 4, fathers can play an important role in their children's development, and the health system could do better in engaging fathers' involvement. Several authors have suggested innovative approaches to strengthen engagement through preconception

---

BOX 5-5
CenteringPregnancy: A Promising Model[a]

CenteringPregnancy provides group prenatal care to women in a supportive, educational, and interactive environment. The model was developed and is implemented by the Centering Healthcare Institute, a Boston-based nonprofit started in the 1990s that works with health care providers to implement group care models (its three models are CenteringPregnancy, CenteringParenting, and CenteringDiabetes) in more than 585 locations, including large health systems, across the country.

The CenteringPregnancy group prenatal care model enables participants to spend more time with their provider and to learn, discuss with, and receive support from other pregnant women in a group environment (Centering Healthcare Institute, n.d.-b). In addition to each participant having individual time with their provider for physical health assessments, groups of 8–10 women due at about the same time participate in a curriculum of 10 90-minute or 2-hour sessions (in line with the recommended schedule of 10 prenatal visits) that include provider- and staff-facilitated information sharing and discussion about health and nutrition, childbirth preparation, stress reduction, labor and delivery, breastfeeding, relationships, and parenting (Centering Healthcare Institute, n.d.-b). Participants are active in their own care by taking their own weight and blood pressure and recording their own health data, and they are women of varying age, race/ethnicity, and socioeconomic background (Centering Healthcare Institute, n.d.-b). The program aims for participants to form meaningful and supportive relationships with other participants, many of whom continue their participation with CenteringParenting's model of family-centered well-child care (Centering Healthcare Institute, n.d.-a).

Research shows that CenteringPregnancy has led to improved birth outcomes, including significantly lower risk of preterm birth, low birth weight (LBW) or very

---

(Kotelchuck and Lu, 2017), prenatal (CPIPO, 2010), postpartum, and pediatric care (Yogman and Garfield, 2016), though evidence of effectiveness is still lacking. Kotelchuck and Lu (2017) proposed a research agenda for advancing the father's role in preconception health, focusing on three priority domains: increasing the basic epidemiology and risk factor knowledge base; implementing and evaluating men's preconception health/fatherhood interventions (addressing clinical health care, psychological resiliency/maturation, and the SDOH); and fostering more fatherhood health policy and advocacy research. The Commission on Paternal Involvement in Pregnancy Outcomes (CPIPO) proposed 40 research, practice, and policy recommendations for strengthening fathers' engagement, including the development of "father-friendly" hospital settings, practices, and policies (CPIPO, 2010). CPIPO also called out the importance of developing more effective methods of recruitment and retention of men in communities with high levels of poor pregnancy outcomes in research. Similarly, Yogman and Garfield (2016) pointed out the important role of

LBW infants, infants who are small for gestational size, and fetal death (Chen et al., 2017; Cunningham et al., 2019; Gareau et al., 2016; Ickovics et al., 2016; Tanner-Smith et al., 2014). Ickovics et al. (2007) also found that participants were less likely to have poorer-quality prenatal care, were more knowledgeable and better prepared for childbirth, had greater satisfaction with their care, and were more likely to breastfeed than those receiving individual care (Ickovics et al., 2007). In addition, Gareau et al. (2016) estimate that South Carolina saved nearly $2.3 million with a $1.7 million investment in implementing the model, which achieved an average savings of $22,667 for every premature birth prevented, $29,627 for decreasing the rate of LBW, and $27,249 for decreasing the risk of a neonatal intensive care unit stay.

The model has also been shown to decrease disparities in birth outcomes by race and ethnicity. Picklesimer et al. (2012) found decreased disparities in the risk of preterm birth for black women relative to white and Hispanic women who participated in the program (Picklesimer et al., 2012). In addition, Ikovics et al. (2007) found that black women who participated had the largest decreases in preterm birth (Ickovics et al., 2007).

Some studies and reviews have found no or mixed evidence of changes in the risk of preterm birth, LBW, prenatal care costs, and delivery between group and prenatal care (Carter et al., 2016; Catling et al., 2015; Ickovics et al., 2007; Tanner-Smith et al., 2014). However, the authors of two reviews note that further research is needed due to the small number of studies and participants and the lack of high-quality studies (Carter et al., 2016; Catling et al., 2015).

---

[a] The committee used selection criteria to identify examples of promising models highlighted in this report (see Appendix A for a list of the criteria). These examples all apply developmental science and aim to advance health equity during the preconception through early childhood periods.

child health providers in supporting and encouraging father involvement, with special attention to fathers' involvement across childhood ages and the influence of fathers' physical and mental health on their children. Given the growing diversity of families, similar attention is needed to engaging partners of all types across the health system.

Multidisciplinary Teams

Another growing innovation is the sharp increase in multidisciplinary teams delivering care to children and families, including team members from sectors other than health care. Teams in primary care and obstetrical care settings take diverse forms, but they all reflect a dedicated move from care provided by physicians alone to much greater involvement of nonphysician providers in ongoing care (Halfon et al., 2014). Team care has grown from early models of physician–nurse practitioner collaboration dating back half a century. Many subspecialty programs, for adults and children, have long had teams providing care, with substantial documentation of their effectiveness (Katkin et al., 2017; Lahiri et al., 2016). Typical elements of a primary care team address (1) chronic care management (especially for the high-prevalence conditions other than mental health)—often with a nurse or nurse practitioner having main responsibilities, (2) mental and behavioral health—often through a colocated mental health professional (see below), (3) linking families with community resources (e.g., through a staff member knowledgeable about community benefits and resources or through medical–legal partnerships [MLPs]), and (4) helping families assess readiness for becoming parents and building their child-raising skills (e.g., programs to plan for parenthood, parenting programs in health care offices, connecting with home visiting programs, or encouraging families to read to children at an early age). Over the past few decades, nurses have played increasingly broad roles, including prevention and care management. Few teams include all these components, but the growth of team care has addressed all of them in different models.

Models that incorporate evidence supporting teams in health care settings to develop multidisciplinary care coordination programs involving families, social workers, paraprofessionals or peer workers, and community partners have evolved over time to help families of high-risk children be more proactive at managing health risks (Van Cleave et al., 2015). Programs such as the Parent-focused Redesign for Encounters, Newborns to Toddlers (PARENT) have used health educator coaches for parents to deliver well-child care that incorporates social risk screening and referral, with developmental and behavioral assessments (Coker et al., 2016). Efforts to use team-based care (coupled with telehealth mechanisms) in part reflect the recognition that such changes will help to more effectively address the many factors contributing to the health of patients and communities. These changes recognize that enhancing health care practices with personnel who are knowledgeable and skillful in helping families access a breadth of community services will address disparities.

Integrating mental health and behavioral health services into primary care is a widespread innovation that usually involves having a mental health professional (e.g., a master's level psychologist, social worker, or psychiatric nurse specialist) colocated in the practice (Ader et al., 2015; Stancin and Perrin, 2014; Team Up for Children, n.d.). One such program embeds mental health workers in several community health center pediatric practices so that they can see patients jointly or transfer them easily and immediately.[11] These personnel both see patients directly and help to train the primary care practitioners to hone their own mental health skills. In another model that has experienced much growth (now in more than 30 states), primary

---

[11] For more information, see https://www.teamupforchildren.org (accessed May 9, 2019).

care clinicians can access telephone backup services that support their in-office care of mental health problems (Sarvet et al., 2010; Straus and Sarvet, 2014). Occasionally, backup providers will see patients directly for one to two visits, although the majority of services provided are either directly to the primary care provider or by referral to community resources for ongoing mental health care (e.g., community cognitive behavioral therapy providers).[12] Most studies of programs that integrate behavioral health care services into primary care to address the increased prevalence of mental health diagnoses, early childhood developmental conditions, and substance use disorders in families have shown substantial promise (AHRQ, n.d.-b; Balasubramanian et al., 2017; Kwan and Nease, 2013).

Embedded programs that directly address the SDOH focus on having onsite professional social workers or other staff who provide in-person services or navigation to families (Fierman et al., 2016) or who help families find needed community resources. Several established programs do this kind of work, including the following (see also Box 5-6 for information on another initiative, Pediatrics Supporting Parents):

- The Health Leads program uses patient advocates to meet with families, guide them to community resources, and integrate SDOH care into the routines of clinical care (Garg et al., 2012). It has been shown to improve child health outcomes in a randomized trial (Gottlieb et al., 2016).
- Reach Out and Read is a practic-embedded program in pediatric care settings encouraging parent–child interaction and literacy development and has been shown to result in higher language proficiency in at-risk children (Mendelsohn et al., 2001).
- The PARENT program uses coaches for parents to expand the capacity of providers to address family social risks. An RCT of the program showed improvements in use of developmental screening and other preventive care and reduced emergency department (ED) visits early in life (Coker et al., 2016).
- HealthySteps (with sites in more than 20 states; Washington, DC; and Puerto Rico [Zero to Three, n.d.-a]) combines practice-based services using early child educators or nurses with early childhood training with community linkages focused on newborn care, safety, and developmental issues. This program has shown some evidence for impacts on parent–child communication (Minkovitz et al., 2007) (see Box 5-8 for more on HealthySteps).
- MLPs assist families with the legal challenges that often go hand-in-hand with unmet needs related to social determinants and have been shown to improve subjective well-being and positive

---

[12] The 21st Century Cures Act and expansion of phone backup programs.

BOX 5-6
Identifying Strategies to Support Parents in Clinical Settings

Pediatrics Supporting Parents is a multiphase initiative supported by a consortium of foundations that is exploring opportunities in the context of pediatric well-child visits to promote children's healthy social and emotional development.

Phase 1: The Center for the Study of Social Policy (CSSP) has identified evidence-informed, scalable strategies to improve social and emotional health, the parent–child bond, and parental mental health (an important mediator of social-emotional development and the parent–child bond) during well-child visits. This includes a study of how strategies may differ with respect to pediatric practice or community settings.

Phase 2: The National Institute for Children's Health Quality has assessed the findings from CSSP and uses them to inform a learning community of pediatric primary care practices who will pilot the strategies and make recommendations for scaling them up at a national level.

Based on the findings from the report *Promoting Young Children's (Ages 0–3) Socioemotional Development in Primary Care* (NICHQ, 2016), this initiative has adopted the framework of four "design elements" of strategies to engage parents: (1) assessment, (2) education, (3) modeling, and (4) connection (NICHQ, 2016). The initiative's theory of change identifies these design elements as contributors to the primary outcomes of interest (i.e., social-emotional health, parent–child bond, parental mental health).

CSSP employed a multistep approach and applied a robust set of criteria (see Appendix C of CSSP, 2018, for more information) to identify 13 evidence-informed and promising programs to explore further through site visits. The organizing framework for these programs identified 10 important areas of strategy:

1. Anticipatory guidance
2. Screening, connection, and access
3. Health-related resources
4. Curriculum-based courses for parents/caregivers
5. Observations
6. Group well-child visits
7. Mental health consultation
8. Physician extenders
9. Home visiting
10. Trainings/child quality improvement

SOURCE: CSSP, 2018.

---

impact health care use (Klein et al., 2013; Sandel et al., 2010) (see Chapter 6 for more information on MLPs).

- Help Me Grow is a coalition of 28 states, communities, and individuals invested in ambitious and resourceful early childhood systems that optimally serve all families and children.

It is designed to help states and communities leverage existing resources to identify children in at-risk environments, link families to community-based services, and help families support healthy development of their children, including through child health provider outreach (Help Me Grow, 2017).

- Filming Interactions to Nurture Development (FIND) is a video coaching program that aims to strengthen positive interactions between caregivers and children to reinforce developmentally supportive interactions, or what is known as "serve and return." Early evaluation studies show participation in the FIND Fathers project was associated with improvements in parenting stress, father involvement, and child behavior problems; other evaluations are ongoing (Center on the Developing Child at Harvard University, n.d.).

The growth of teams also supports expanded attention to social, economic, and environmental determinants of health among children and families. Team-based care helps practices encourage families to share information more effectively, as different team members focus on different aspects of a family's health and health determinants. Strong community knowledge and linkages help these efforts succeed, and some practices embed community health workers and other laypeople with lived experience, community expertise, and inherent trust among community members. Here too the value of team-based community-oriented care has many advantages over traditional physician-centered practice. Community health workers know community resources (e.g., housing, food, employment) and can assist families in getting the help they need (e.g., resources to find improved housing for a child with asthma who wheezes because of mold in her apartment instead of repeated ED visits for nebulizer treatments).

Enhanced Services to Identify and Address Social, Economic, and Environmental Determinants of Health

There has been increased recognition of the impact of adverse social, economic, and environmental determinants on health outcomes over the past several decades. Federal and state public health efforts have moved to enhance care to better identify and address these factors (Lu et al., 2010). For prenatal care, enhanced care models have been designed to deliver coordinated, augmented, enabling, enriched, comprehensive, or "wraparound" prenatal care services—particularly for low-income populations. Enhanced prenatal care typically refers to routine prenatal care visits combined with ancillary services that may entail outreach efforts, counseling about WIC, case management, social work, psychosocial counseling, social support, health promotion/education, transportation, home visiting, and follow-up services to facilitate the ongoing use of the prenatal services offered (Alexander and Kotelchuck, 2001). The Comprehensive Perinatal Service Program enhances prenatal care with nutrition counseling, social services, and health education (Korenbrot et al., 1995). Most federally funded Healthy Start programs enhance prenatal care with care coordination, case management, and home visiting (Badura et al., 2008). In his systematic review of three types of enhanced prenatal care—home visiting programs, comprehensive care programs, and preterm prevention programs—Fiscella (1995) failed to find conclusive evidence of effectiveness of enhanced prenatal care for preventing adverse birth outcomes. It should be noted, however, that Fiscella examined the impact of enhanced prenatal care on only three immediate birth outcomes—perinatal death, LBW, and preterm birth; the impact of enhanced prenatal care on other short- and long-term health outcomes for children and families remains largely unexplored. A study of the Illinois Family Case Management program, another enhanced prenatal care program, did find that participation resulted in a lower LBW rate (Silva et al., 2006).

Health care providers have explored three basic approaches to the challenge of meeting social needs outside of their practices: (1) home visiting programs connected to the practice, (2) screening for risks and referring to community programs, and (3) community-level interventions.

Home Visiting Programs Connected to the Practice

Home visiting has a long history of effective programs for young families (based on early experiments in Ithaca, New York, and Hawaii); nurses or other trained personnel make home visits for young families, in some cases during pregnancy, and in all cases in the first few years of a child's life. For a more detailed discussion of home visiting, see Chapter 4. Some programs are closely integrated with health care providers; others work independently but share information. The Nurse-Family Partnership program has shown evidence of reducing child abuse and neglect (Macmillan et al., 2009) with home visiting, for example. Some of the targeted programs that focus on specific needs, such as child abuse, child neglect, or LBW babies, have improved health outcomes in high-risk families (Avellar and Supplee, 2013; Radcliffe et al., 2013; Rushton et al., 2015). In the past few years, Congress has supported growth in home visiting programs by allocating new funds to allow for expanding the programs and the households covered. For an example of a community-based nurse home visiting program that has demonstrated promising findings in improving the health and well-being of children and their families, see Box 5-7.

BOX 5-7
Family Connects Durham: A Promising Model[a]

Family Connects Durham (formerly Durham Connects) is a nurse home visit-ing program offered at no cost to families of newborns in Durham County, North Carolina. The program serves all families with newborns regardless of income or socioeconomic status (SES), and its mission is to "increase child well-being by bridging the gap between parent needs and community resources" (Center for Child & Family Health, n.d.). First implemented in 2008, the program was devel-oped by the Duke Endowment and the founding director of the Duke Center for Child and Family Policy, Kenneth Dodge, in conjunction with community partners with the goal to prevent child maltreatment and support all children and families in Durham, regardless of SES, with a model that could be replicated in other commu-nities. The program maintains a commitment to community engagement through its Community Advisory Board, which includes representation from local agencies and is a collaborative effort of the Center for Child & Family Health, Duke Center for Child and Family Policy, Durham County Department of Health, and Durham County Department of Social Services. In addition to local grants, the program's funders include the Duke Endowment, Durham County Government, and United Way of the Greater Triangle.

A registered nurse with clinical and/community health experience typically visits about 3 weeks (but up to 12 weeks) postpartum to provide a weight and health check for the newborn and ensure that the mother is recovering from childbirth. Nurses may also provide information and community-based resources on topics such as breastfeeding, child care, postpartum depression, and social isolation. Families may be contacted 1 month after the home visit to ensure that the commu-nity resources and supports discussed during the visit were obtained. In addition, pediatricians, obstetricians, and family practitioners within the community partner with the program to share information and improve patient care. The program has Spanish-speaking nurses and matches families with nurses who speak their preferred language whenever possible. Nurses neither request nor report families' U.S. residency status.

In two randomized controlled trials, Dodge et al. found that by the time the infant was 6 or 12 months old, families who received a nurse home visit through the program had greater community connections, better use of higher-quality child care, higher-quality parenting behaviors, enhanced home environments, improved mother mental health, and reduced emergency medical care for infants (Dodge et al., 2013, 2014). Furthermore, it is estimated that cities of similar size to Durham that average about 3,187 births per year could save about $6.7 million in commu-nity health care costs during the first 2 years of an infant's life if $2.2 million was invested each year in nurse home visiting (i.e., it is estimated that the program saves $3.02 in emergency health care costs for every $1 it spends) (Center for Child and Family Health, n.d.).

---

[a] The committee used selection criteria to identify examples of promising models high-lighted in this report (see Appendix A for a list of the criteria). These examples all apply developmental science and aim to advance health equity during the preconception through early childhood periods.

Screening in the Practice and Referral to a Community Partner

WE CARE, a program based in pediatric primary care and serving low-income families, combines a screening tool and referrals to community resources for at-risk families who want assistance with social needs; the results from RCTs showed that families in the program were more likely to connect to social determinants resources, had fewer unaddressed needs, were more likely to be employed, and were less likely to live in a shelter at follow-up compared to those not in the program (Garg et al., 2007, 2015). Other pediatric-based "screen and refer" programs, relying on either trained family specialists or volunteer community navigators, have shown similarly promising impacts on outcomes such as connection to social needs, increased immunization rates, and reduced early life ED use in randomized studies (Gottlieb et al., 2016; Sege et al., 2015). A range of more focused pediatric-based programs addressing specific social needs through screening and intervention have also shown promising results in high-quality studies, including programs focused on improving habitability for children with asthma (Krieger et al., 2005), the Safe Environment for Every Kid program focused on reducing intrafamily stress/violence and improving food security (Dubowitz et al., 2011, 2012; Feigelman et al., 2011), clinic-based referrals to Head Start (Silverstein et al., 2004), and StreetCred, which helps families get benefits they are eligible for (e.g., nutrition programs, Earned Income Tax Credit, SSI) (Marcil et al., 2018). Programs have also successfully deployed community health workers to do home assessments and education, and results indicated reduced asthma triggers among children (Campbell et al., 2015; Williams et al., 2006). Other community collaboration models compile resource directories and connect people to publicly available benefits, including Temporary Assistance for Needy Families or the Supplemental Nutrition Assistance Program, as well as to community resources or private programs that can assist at-risk families (Henize et al., 2015).

Primary care providers have worked in this space for some time, with a growing body of evidence around effective programs and interventions. Several state Medicaid agencies have also begun to test promising models to incentivize providers in their efforts to address SDOH (including early detection of adversity and trauma experienced by children and their caregivers), greater integration with other community providers, and MBH integration (Van Buren, 2018). These innovative efforts together promise ways to strengthen preconception, prenatal, and pediatric care, help it move to team care and improve use of new technologies, and strengthen integration with other community services to enhance child health and well-being. North Carolina has developed an ambitious Early Childhood Action Plan, which has goals such as healthy children who are safe and nurtured, learning, and ready to succeed (NCDHHS, n.d.).

The plan builds on the science of early childhood and brain development and aims to address health equity. New York's First Thousand Days program includes statewide early home visiting, expansion of the Centering-Pregnancy program (see Box 5-5), a requirement that managed care plans must have a child-specific quality agenda, and data system development to enhance cross-sector collaboration (United Hospital Fund, 2018).

Community-Level Interventions

Lastly, addressing the SDOH needs to encompass improved, collaborative systems for addressing medical and psychosocial risk factors at not only the individual child/family level but also the community level. Community-based parent support programs can provide resources through parent and child play groups, parenting information and support classes, and connecting families to medical or child care services (Trivette and Dunst, 2014). (For more information on supports for parents and caregivers, see Chapter 4.) The goal of these programs is to improve the health, well-being, and development of children by improving parents' caregiving skills and providing parents with adequate social supports and services (Goodson, 2014). Such programs are most effective when they are "family-centered as opposed to professionally-centered" and "capacity-building as opposed to dependency forming" (Trivette and Dunst, 2014). In pediatrics, family-centered care is care that is "based on the understanding that the family is the child's primary source of strength and support and that the child's and family's perspectives and information are important in clinical decision making" (AAP Committee on Hospital Care, 2003, p. 691). Family-centered care can lead to improved child health and behavioral outcomes (Dunst and Trivette, 2009; Dunst et al., 2007; Kuo et al., 2012), and it is vital that community-based programs connect families to medical services where family-centered care is standard.

The 2016 National Academies report *Parenting Matters: Supporting Parents of Children Ages 0–8* describes specific elements of effective programs, which include (1) parents as partners, (2) tailoring interventions to parent and child needs, (3) service integration and interagency collaborative care, (4) peer support, (5) trauma-informed services, (6) cultural relevance, and (7) inclusion of fathers (NASEM, 2016). HealthySteps is a community-based pediatric primary care model that prioritizes the role of parents and caregivers as active participants in the care of their children (see Box 5-8 for more information on HealthySteps). Several initiatives have effectively coordinated health, social services, family support, and educational services, such as the Harlem Children's Zone (Harlem Children's Zone, n.d.) and the multisite Best Babies Zone initiative (Best Babies Zone, n.d.). A 2017 National Academies report, *Communities in*

BOX 5-8
HealthySteps: A Promising Model[a]

HealthySteps is a team-based, family-centered pediatric primary care model that aims to improve the health, well-being, and school readiness of infants and toddlers in low-income families. The cornerstone of the model is a child development professional, known as a HealthySteps Specialist (HSS), who connects with families during well-child visits as part of the primary care team. The HSS supports families by coordinating care and screenings, offering guidance and referrals to local agencies and programs (e.g., MBH services for maternal depression, food banks and legal clinics for food and housing insecurity), and providing on-demand aid, including through electronic communication and home visiting, between primary care visits. Infants are enrolled in the program at their newborn visit (or as early as possible before their 6-month visit), and families may continue in the program until the 3-year-old well-child visit at most sites and until the child is 5 years old at some sites (MacLaughlin et al., 2017). The program is a national network of more than 140 pediatric and family practice sites in 20 states; Washington, DC; and Puerto Rico (Zero to Three, n.d.-a) that has served more than 37,000 children ages 0–3, including refugee children (Buchholz et al., 2016).

The program was analyzed through a 15-site national evaluation in 2003 (Guyer et al., 2003), and several single-site evaluations have also taken place. Findings from the evaluations suggest that the model can help to achieve improved outcomes in child health and development, breastfeeding and early nutrition, connections to resources, child safety, parenting knowledge and practices, parent and physician satisfaction, maternal depression, and early literary and school readiness (Zero to Three, 2017). For example, Minkovitz et al. (2007) conducted interviews with mothers when their children were 5.5 years of age and found that families who participated in the program were more satisfied with their care, more likely to remain at their original practice, less likely to use severe discipline, more likely to report concerns with their children's behavior, and more likely to have their children read books. Such findings indicate that the program's positive effects, while modest, may continue after the intervention has ended. Further evaluation of the program's recent innovations and for specific outcomes is ongoing (Zero to Three, n.d.-b).

---

[a] The committee used selection criteria to identify examples of promising models highlighted in this report (see Appendix A for a list of the criteria). These examples all apply developmental science and aim to advance health equity during the preconception through early childhood periods.

Action: Pathways to Health Equity, documents several such place-based, community-level initiatives.

In addition to knowing the community to better direct patients to resources, health care institutions can treat surrounding neighborhoods as "patients" and intervene more directly in the SDOH. In one such case study, the Healthy Neighborhoods, Healthy Families Initiative, a pediatric center invested in a multifaceted housing intervention in the surrounding neighborhood and significantly improved vacancy rates, though the health impacts on children in the area are still being evaluated (Kelleher et al., 2018). Similarly, a community health center in Wisconsin partnered with urban planners to integrate health into sustainable land-use planning practices in an effort to shape overall community health outcomes (McAvoy et al., 2004). Health systems have also begun to participate in larger cross-sector efforts and partnerships predicated on the principles of collective impact, such as Accountable Communities of Health (ACH), which bring together a wide range of partners from across sectors to collectively address the SDOH. These efforts are nascent, however, and high-quality evidence on the health impacts of the ACH model or similar initiatives is not yet available. CMS recently released a request for proposals to address similar opportunities at the child health level, with a strong emphasis on MBH and building community coalitions to improve outcomes based on social determinants criteria (CMS, 2019).

Another promising example is the redesign of the federal Healthy Start program in 2015 to place greater emphasis on improving women's health before and between pregnancies and across the life course, strengthening families, increasing father engagement, and addressing the SDOH through the collective impact model (whereby Healthy Start grantees serve as the backbone organizations in facilitating coordination and collaboration with social services, housing, economic and community development, and other nonhealth sectors to prevent infant mortality in the community). Results from more rigorous evaluation of the Healthy Start program are expected to be available in 2019 (NICHQ, n.d.).

Embracing New Technologies

Technological advances may help to transform the model of brief, episodic visits in a busy practice, especially in underresourced settings, by improving communication and care in several ways. A health care system redesign that better leverages eHealth technologies and social networking in innovative ways can enable more effective health promotion than current short visits. With many technological opportunities emerging to implement such a redesign, an important consideration is that machine learning algorithms may suffer from the same biases reflected in the data on which they are built, such that their use in health care may inadvertently perpetuate and even exacerbate existing health disparities (Char et al., 2018; Gianfrancesco et al., 2018). Research is needed to identify strategies to minimize such biases as new technologies are implemented more widely in health care and other sectors (Turner Lee, 2018).

Increasingly, health care providers are experimenting with telehealth strategies to augment their services and make them more accessible and convenient for families (Burke et al., 2015). Most used and studied in the area of providing mental health services remotely, telehealth has expanded substantially in the management of many chronic diseases of children and adults. New technologies allow better home and community monitoring of chronic disease and assessing symptoms and clinical signs over phone and video. Increased use of technological innovations might also improve access before and during pregnancy (Lu et al., 2010). Telehealth has been proposed as a way to help overcome many of the access barriers described earlier; women could be connected to their providers or specialists at any-time from anywhere. In addition, mHealth could make health promotion more accessible using simple mobile phone functions. Instead of bringing children and families to care, future research, practice, and policy initia-tives to increase access should work on leveraging technological innova-tions to bring care to people in their homes and communities.

Technological innovations, data sciences, and design thinking could be leveraged to redesign care around the needs of children and families and not just provider or clinic schedules. Technologies such as wearables, sensors, and lab-on-a-chip hold potential if they are proven to reliably and more continuously collect high-quality data that lead to improved care, better patient experiences, and more equitable health outcomes. Such data, collected from the comfort of a woman's own home throughout her pregnancy, may include not only information on blood pressure or urine protein but also nutrition and physical activities, stress and sleep, and occupational, environmental, and other exposures that affect preg-nancy outcomes and developmental origins of health and disease. With remote home monitoring, it is possible to continuously transmit data to the Cloud, which, with the aid of artificial intelligence and machine learning, could be used to improve predictive analytics. For preconcep-tion and prenatal care, these enhanced data might help triage women to different levels and components of care (e.g., routine follow-up, a call from a health educator, a home visitor, or an urgent appointment with a specialist). Instead of adhering to a uniform schedule, this approach might enable the frequency and content of preconception and prenatal visits to be determined by the specific changing needs and risks of each woman. Much work in childhood chronic disease, especially ASD and inflammatory bowel disease, similarly uses remote data to inform the need for office visits, rather than relying on routine follow-up periods. Linking these data with genomic, proteomic, metabolomic, psychosocial, and environmental data might help create a more precise risk profile that could inform the design of more personalized and precise interventions.

New health care technologies can also enhance other communications between health care providers and their patients and markedly change the character and components of regular care if these are high quality and well focused on characteristics most valued by households (Olson et al., 2018). Texting has been used to encourage healthy behaviors or advise on routine care (e.g., developmentally specific infant care advice, such as text4baby) (Evans et al., 2012). Texting has also improved low-income mothers' adherence to immunizations for their children (Hofstetter et al., 2015; Stockwell et al., 2012).

In addition, new and emerging technologies could play an important role in decreasing health inequities. Digital tools that leverage artificial intelligence and machine learning have the capacity to better identify social risk factors and improve systems of referral and follow-up for patients when used with care and appropriate data sources (Padarthy et al., 2019). Advanced technological systems can help collect social risk screening data without relying so heavily on the point of care encounter, such as using patient-accessible electronic health records to pre-collect screening data in advance of clinical encounters. Indeed, not all screening needs to take place in clinical offices or at visits at all—electronic practice gateways allow families to respond to questionnaires before or after visits, and texting can help encourage their participation. Head Start and other early childhood sites can also screen, and data sharing across communities can expedite care and response. In addition to ambulatory settings, some health systems have also implemented screening within EDs and trauma centers, especially around issues of violence and trauma, but evidence on the effectiveness of screening within those settings is still preliminary (Juillard et al., 2016; Smith et al., 2013).

Health information technology (IT) can be used in a variety of other ways to augment health care services (e.g., promote patient education, assist with care coordination). Health IT in health care settings can also be used to support provider decision making and reduce errors. For example, reminders generated by electronic medical records can be used to encourage prenatal providers to prescribe progesterone to eligible patients with a documented history of spontaneous preterm delivery, to tell pediatric care providers about overdue immunizations, or to prompt follow-up on abnormal lab results, which can sometimes be missed in busy, understaffed clinics, especially in underresourced communities. Health education materials are accessible on the Internet and through smartphone apps. For example, pregnant patients can find information about self-care on websites such as the U.S. Department of Agriculture's ChooseMyPlate.gov,[13] which provides useful tools for nutritional self-assessment and education to pregnant women. Parents can access a variety of parenting resources and guidance regarding health and wellness for early childhood. Health IT can also help link clients to needed services, such as the Healthy City website,[14] which maps community services in

---

[13] For more information, see https://www.choosemyplate.gov/nutritional-needs-during pregnancy (accessed May 9, 2019).

[14] For more information, see http://www.healthycity.org (accessed May 9, 2019).

Los Angeles County down to the zip code and Census tract level using geographic information system technology.

Financing to Support Innovation

Payment arrangements for most health care services, from both public and private (mainly employer-sponsored health insurance) sources, rely on fee-for-service mechanisms where payment reflects the number of services provided (e.g., health supervision visits, acute care visits, vaccinations) and covers only specified services. Fee-for-service arrangements provide few incentives for many of the changes that are critical for preparing health care providers to better deliver services to meet the needs of children, youth, and families, especially attention to mental/behavioral health, addressing the SDOH, building community links, and incorporating telehealth. Traditional payment focuses on services, rather than on improving the health of populations. While providers recognize the many factors influencing health in prenatal and early childhood, traditional payment strategies maximize the numbers of patients per hour, often resulting in less time spent with each patient, without providing support for the longer visits needed by some households (e.g., those facing housing or economic insecurity). Many health providers are already experimenting with new organizational structures to address changing needs and better respond to the main influences on health outcomes and well-being. Practices increasingly face the need to manage chronic conditions, address MBH, respond to cultural and linguistic diversity, and help with poverty and other SDOH, including efforts to address inequities in care and outcomes. These views reflect growing attention to child and family health in a holistic way. Health care providers are embracing team-based care models and new technologies (Katkin et al., 2017). Yet, current financing models prevent many health care providers from practicing in multidisciplinary teams; integrating health services with other community services; placing more emphasis on population health strategies; using technologies to enhance communication, assess risk, and extend care; and tailoring services to address equity and disparities.

Optimizing care and support for postpartum families will also require policy changes. Presently, many insurers bundle reimbursement for prenatal care, delivery, and a single postpartum visit into one global fee, creating a disincentive for providers to provide comprehensive postpartum care or see patients more than once. Many women lose their pregnancy-related Medicaid coverage at 60 days postpartum. Payers often do not recognize the care provided to parents in pediatric and family medicine care settings. Thus, changes in the scope of postpartum care would require changes to reimbursement policies that support postpartum care as an ongoing process, rather than an isolated visit, such as unbundling from global obstetrics payment, pay-for-performance, and extension of Medicaid coverage for at least 12 months postpartum.

Public and private payers in the past few years have shown interest in moving to alternative payment mechanisms, where providers increasingly take (financial) responsibility for a specified population. These arrangements can provide very different incentives for the organization and provision of health care services. For example, they allow more care to take place out of office through the expanded use of telemedicine and lowering use of high-cost services of limited value (Berwick et al., 2008; Dzau et al., 2017; Wong et al., 2018). The growth of accountable care organizations (ACOs) follows this interest in changing incentives to improve care. Several children's hospitals have developed ACOs (Makni et al., 2015; Perrin et al., 2017), although most of the growth in ACOs has come from large multispecialty programs with a main emphasis on practice transformation and cost savings for older populations.

As noted previously, Medicaid plays a major role in insuring children, youth, and pregnant women, and, increasingly, young parents. Its success and persistence are critical to the health of these populations, and Medicaid program enhancements generally implementing the changes in organization and financing described in this chapter will improve health and health inequities. As also noted above, children's hospitals (including organized children's health programs in general hospitals) provide most of the subspecialty care for children and youth with more complex and less common health conditions. Insofar as many children have public health insurance—with even higher rates among children with chronic health conditions—children's hospitals rely substantially on public financing. This reliance, however, puts these institutions at financial risk, as Medicaid generally pays much less than Medicare or private payers do for the same service. Although rates vary greatly among the states, on average, Medicaid pays at about two-thirds of the Medicare rates (Biener and Selden, 2017).

Substantial moves to capitated or population health payments will greatly enhance the needed changes in health care arrangements. Here, too, several state Medicaid programs have innovated in their programs for children and youth. New York has focused on value-based payments, including efforts to define value measures for children and develop incentives to reward value improvements (NY Department of Health, 2017), based in large part on a careful analysis of value-based payment strategies for children (Bailit Health, 2016). Colorado has developed a Healthy Families Checklist, setting standards for Medicaid, strengthening eligibility opportunities for Medicaid, expanding benefits to include care coordination, and changing payment policy to support delivery system

BOX 5-9
How Population Payments Can Enhance
Use of New Technology

A 6-year-old girl in 1st grade complains of an earache. New technology allows a trained layperson to take a picture of the girl's ear membrane and send it to the child's health care provider. Paying physicians for the number of visits they carry out provides an incentive to have the child (with a parent) come for an office visit to determine whether she has an ear infection. Physicians who no longer receive compensation for each visit but are instead reimbursed based on the needs of the patient population can examine the eardrum remotely and decide whether the child has an infection—potentially saving a trip to the office for both child and parent.

design (Ascend at The Aspen Institute, 2018). Massachusetts has reframed its Medicaid program as an ACO, emphasizing MBH integration, the SDOH, and long-term supports and services (MA Executive Office of HHS, 2017). The committee supports health care payment reform efforts that promote value-based care, tie payment to population health outcomes rather than service delivery, and incentivize strategies that better address prevention and health equity. (See Box 5-9 for more on population health payments.)

Organization and Integration of Health Care Services

Based on its review of the evidence, the committee concludes:

Conclusion 5-4: Recent efforts to transform health care to address social determinants, early adversity, and mental and behavioral health integration and to develop community-based health care teams have increasingly addressed the changing needs of young families and children. Programs that build on home visiting, referrals to community partners, and integrated community efforts have enhanced outcomes for children and families. New technologies have expanded care and access, improved understanding of the social determinants, and improved communication about health and chronic disease. New payment arrangements can accelerate the transformation of health services to programs to support families and population health.

To advance the integration of health care services in an organization, the committee recommends:

Recommendation 5-3: The U.S. Department of Health and Human Services, state, tribal, and territorial government Medicaid

agencies, health systems leaders, and state and federal policy makers should adopt policies and practices that improve the organization and integration of care systems, including promoting multidisciplinary team-based care models that focus on integrating preconception, prenatal, and postpartum care with a whole-family focus, development of new practice and payment models that incentivize health creation and improve service delivery, and structures that more tangibly connect health care delivery systems to other partners outside of the health care sector.

Achieving this recommendation requires the following:

- **Spread multidisciplinary team-based care models in community settings.** Promote the adoption and spread of multigenerational, team-based care models that support patients with a mix of traditional clinical professionals, such as doctors, nurses, social workers, and pharmacists, with mental health professionals, as well as community health workers or peer support specialists. Team activities include chronic disease management, integrated MBH, family support in early childhood, including access to parent training, and referral/connection to needed community services (housing, food, etc.).
- **Develop more integrated models for preconception, prenatal, and postpartum care delivery modes.** Models and interventions should allow women to engage in a continuum of services on their preferred terms, including culturally and linguistically appropriate service models, multigenerational care, approaches that employ home or community-based service delivery for women who prefer those settings, or programs that use new technologies and work to intentionally incorporate a woman's existing social support networks into her prenatal and postnatal care plan.
- **Adopt and spread integrated, whole-family and family-centered care models.** The best models give providers the ability to address the health of individuals and families comprehensively, including clinical health, integrated with MBH and health-related social determinants. Expanded child and family health models include assessment of family strengths and needs and strategies to address them, moving beyond individual care.
- **Develop and use new technologies that improve care and improve accessibility.** Advances include remote monitoring, as well as technologies to enhance ongoing communication, such as texting, virtual visits, and data sharing.
- **Align payment reform with health creation rather than service delivery.** Payment should promote value-based care and

tie payment to population health outcomes rather than service delivery. Payment should incentivize strategies that address health creation and health equity and include comprehensive, coordinated, community-engaged care.

- **Develop cross-sector collaboration at systems levels to address the intersection of drivers across the health continuum.** Programs should seek collective impact or similar cross-sector efforts, such as ACH and other place-based initiatives, that aim to align health care, public health, social services, housing, education, and other sectors around aligned goals and common strategies. Shared governance structures should promote collaboration, including investment in administrative infrastructure and backbone organizations to manage collaboratives, thereby ensuring the flow of information and funding across sectors, and other strategies for sharing efforts and savings.

THE FUTURE OF PRECONCEPTION THROUGH PEDIATRIC CARE

Vision: To advance health equity, reduce health disparities, and improve birth and child health outcomes, the committee calls for a health care system that ensures access for all to high-quality health care across the life course. Transformation of preconception, prenatal, postpartum, and pediatric care will address early childhood sensitive and key life periods by including attention to the root causes of poor health (e.g., access to safe housing, high-quality education, food security), early adversity, and equity. The system will respond to the needs of children and their families holistically and through team-based care and by connecting them with community resources and integrating services across the life course. Ensuring appropriate preconception, prenatal, postpartum, and pediatric care will have long-lasting effects on the health and well-being of our nation's children.

> **Recommendation 5-4: Transform preconception, prenatal, postpartum, and pediatric care to address the root causes of poor health and well-being—the social, economic, environmental, and cultural determinants of health and early adversity—and to align with the work of other sectors addressing health equity.**
>
> **The U.S. Department of Health and Human Services should convene an expert panel to reconceptualize the content and delivery of care, identify the specific changes needed, develop a blueprint for this transformation, and implement a plan to monitor and revise the blueprint over time.**

Implementation of this recommendation will require

- An update of clinical care guidelines and standards by the Women's Preventive Services Initiative, *Bright Futures*, American College of Obstetricians and Gynecologists, American Academy of Pediatrics, American Academy of Family Physicians, and others actively developing clinical care guidelines and standards to include this new content of care;
- Medical accreditation bodies, relevant programs, and agencies to develop performance monitoring and quality improvement based on this new content of care;
- Clinical care educational authorities, such as the Accreditation Council for Graduate Medical Education, to develop curricula, training, experiences, and competencies based on the updated guidelines; and
- Public and private payers to cover services reflecting this new content of care.

This work should take place within a larger framework of social and reproductive justice and include diverse voices, especially from communities most affected by adverse birth and child health outcomes. To expand the content of preconception to pediatric care to address key drivers of health inequities better, specific actions include

- **Recognize the impact of both adverse and enriching experiences across the life course and cumulative effects on health and well-being.** Address transitions between care providers and move from disjointed episodic care to an integrated continuum of longitudinal health care designed to optimize health production across the life course.
- **Include trauma assessment and response as an integral part of care.** Expand practice capabilities to screen for and respond to trauma and early life adversities as part of the standard of care for all families. Advance the biomedical detection and treatment of toxic stress in clinical practice, including during the development of methods for early detection and implementation of evidence-based interventions such as connections to community resources designed to help address the effects of trauma. (See Recommendation 8-2 in Chapter 8 for more on screening and rapid assessment.)
- **Change the content of clinical training to include social determinants of health, MBH integration, and early adversity.** Expand training, care protocols, and workflows to address the SDOH as a routine part of clinical best practices, especially in early life. To accomplish this, curricula and related training experiences need to

be expanded to include competency-based training on screening and mitigation of early adversity, providing TIC, addressing the SDOH, and reducing implicit bias and unequal treatment in health care. Progress toward objectives and training outcomes should be benchmarked. (See Recommendation 8-3 in Chapter 8 on TIC.)

- **Implement an equitable whole-child, whole-family, multi-generational approach.** Expand clinical best practice to address the child and parents in an integrated, whole-family view of health that includes children, parents, and other caregivers. Train clinicians in ways that enhance the equitable delivery of care, including culturally competent caregiving and family-centered care that includes families and caregivers as partners in their own and their children's care. Clinicians and clinical staff should have ongoing training and accountability in areas of implicit bias and equity in evaluation and treatment.

CONCLUSION

Applying the science of early development to transform preconception, prenatal, postpartum, and pediatric care has the potential to advance health equity. To better meet the needs of the populations receiving this care, the access, quality, and content of clinical care need to be addressed. This will require the health care system to be an active partner with other sectors and communities who are leading the way to address the root causes of health inequities—the social, economic, environmental, and cultural determinants of health.

REFERENCES

AAP (American Academy of Pediatrics). 2010. Enhancing pediatric mental health care: Report from the American Academy of Pediatrics Task Force on Mental Health. *Pediatrics* 125(Suppl 3):S69–S74.

AAP. 2016. *Bright Futures: Guidelines for supervision of infants, children, and adolescents*, 4th ed. Elk Grove Village, IL: American Academy of Pediatrics.

AAP. 2018. *Blueprint for children. 2018 update: Achievements in child health advocacy.* Washington, DC: American Academy of Pediatrics.

AAP. n.d.-a. *AAP agenda for children.* https://www.aap.org/en-us/about-the-aap/aap-facts/AAP-Agenda-for-Children-Strategic-Plan/Pages/AAP-Agenda-for-Children-Strategic-Plan.aspx (accessed June 4, 2019).

AAP. n.d.-b. *Screening tools.* https://screeningtime.org/star-center/#/screening-tools#top (accessed April 16, 2019).

AAP and FRAC (Food Research & Action Center). 2017. *Addressing food insecurity: A toolkit for pediatricians.* Washington, DC: American Academy of Pediatrics and Food Research & Action Center.

AAP Committee on Fetus and Newborn and ACOG (American College of Obstetricians and Gynecologists) Committee on Obstetric Practice. 2017. In *Guidelines for perinatal care,*

8th ed., edited by S. J. Kilpatrick, L.-A. Papile, and G. A. Macones. Elk Grove Village, IL, and Washington, DC: American Academy of Pediatrics and American College of Obstetricians and Gynecologists.

AAP Committee on Hospital Care. 2003. Family-centered care and the pediatrician's role. *Pediatrics* 112(3 Pt. 1):691–697.

AAP Committee on Pediatric Workforce. 2013. Enhancing pediatric workforce diversity and providing culturally effective pediatric care: Implications for practice, education, and policy making. *Pediatrics* 132(4):e1105–e1116.

AAP Council on Community Pediatrics. 2016. Poverty and child health in the United States. *Pediatrics* 137(4).

ACOG (American College of Obstetricians and Gynecologists). 2015. Committee opinion no. 649: Racial and ethnic disparities in obstetrics and gynecology. *Obstetrics & Gynecology* 126:e130–e134.

ACOG. 2018a. Committee opinion no. 731: Group prenatal care. *Obstetrics & Gynecology* 131(3):e104–e108.

ACOG. 2018b. Committee opinion no. 736: Optimizing postpartum care. *Obstetrics & Gynecology* 131(5):e140–e150.

Ader, J., C. J. Stille, D. Keller, B. F. Miller, M. S. Barr, and J. M. Perrin. 2015. The medical home and integrated behavioral health: Advancing the policy agenda. *Pediatrics* 135(5):909–917.

Adirim, T., K. Meade, K. Mistry, Council on Quality Improvement and Patient Safety, and Committee on Practice and Ambulatory Management. 2017. A new era in quality measurement: The development and application of quality measures. *Pediatrics* 139(1):e20163442.

AHRQ (Agency for Healthcare Research and Quality). 2018. *All PQMP measures.* https://www.ahrq.gov/pqmp/measures/all-pqmp-measures.html (accessed April 30, 2019).

AHRQ. n.d.-a. *Ambulatory care.* https://www.ahrq.gov/professionals/quality-patient-safety/quality-resources/tools/ambulatory-care/index.html (accessed July 17, 2019).

AHRQ. n.d.-b. *The Academy: Integrating behavioral health and primary care. Literature collection.* https://integrationacademy.ahrq.gov/products/literature-collection (accessed June 12, 2019).

Alexander, G. R., and C. C. Korenbrot. 1995. The role of prenatal care in preventing low birth weight. *The Future of Children* 5(1):103–120.

Alexander, G. R., and M. Kotelchuck. 2001. Assessing the role and effectiveness of prenatal care: History, challenges, and directions for future research. *Public Health Reports* 116(4):306–316.

Alexander, G. R., and M. Slay. 2002. Prematurity at birth: Trends, racial disparities, and epidemiology. *Mental Retardation and Developmental Disabilities Research Reviews* 8(4):215–220.

Alker, J., and O. Pham. 2018. *Nation's progress on children's health coverage reverses course.* Washington, DC: Georgetown University Health Policy Institute, Center for Children and Families.

American College of Nurse-Midwives. 2012. *Midwifery: Evidence-based practice.* http://www.midwife.org/acnm/files/cclibraryfiles/filename/000000002128/midwifery%20evidence-based%20practice%20issue%20brief%20finalmay%202012.pdf (accessed July 19, 2019).

Anderson, K., R. J. Norman, and P. Middleton. 2010. Preconception lifestyle advice for people with subfertility. *Cochrane Database of Systematic Reviews* 4:CD008189.

Angier, H., M. Hoopes, R. Gold, S. R. Bailey, E. K. Cottrell, J. Heintzman, M. Marino, and J. E. DeVoe. 2015. An early look at rates of uninsured safety net clinic visits after the Affordable Care Act. *Annals of Family Medicine* 13(1):10–16.

Angier, H., M. Hoopes, M. Marino, N. Huguet, E. A. Jacobs, J. Heintzman, H. Holderness, C. M. Hood, and J. E. DeVoe. 2017. Uninsured primary care visit disparities under the Affordable Care Act. *Annals of Family Medicine* 15(5):434–442.

Angier, H., D. Ezekiel-Herrera, M. Marino, M. Hoopes, E. A. Jacobs, J. E. DeVoe, and N. Huguet. 2019a. Racial/ethnic disparities in health insurance and differences in visit type for a population of patients with diabetes after Medicaid expansion. *Journal of Health Care for the Poor and Underserved* 30(1):116–130.

Angier, H., E. A. Jacobs, N. Huguet, S. Likumahuwa-Ackman, S. Robert, and J. E. DeVoe. 2019b. Progress towards using community context with clinical data in primary care. *Family Medicine and Community Health* 7(1):e000028.

Angus, L., and J. Devoe. 2010. Evidence that the citizenship mandate curtailed participation in Oregon's Medicaid family planning program. *Health Affairs* 29(4):690–698.

APA (American Psychological Association) and AAP (American Academy of Pediatrics). 2017. *US child poverty curriculum.* https://www.aap.org/en-us/advocacy-and-policy/aap-health-initiatives/CPTI/Pages/U-S-Child-Poverty-Curriculum.aspx (accessed May 20, 2019).

APA Task Force on Childhood Poverty. 2013. *A strategic road-map: Committed to bringing the voice of pediatricians to the most important problem facing children in the US today.* http://www.academicpeds.org/taskforces/pdfs/StrategicRoadMap_ver3.pdf (accessed May 20, 2019).

Arthur, K. C., B. A. Lucenko, I. V. Sharkova, J. Xing, and R. Mangione-Smith. 2018. Using state administrative data to identify social complexity risk factors for children. *Annals of Family Medicine* 16(1):62–69.

Artiga, S., K. Orgera, and A. Damico. 2019. *Changes in health care coverage by race and ethnicity since implementation of the ACA, 2013–2017. Issue brief.* San Francisco, CA: Kaiser Family Foundation.

Ascend at The Aspen Institute. 2018. *Healthy families checklist.* https://ascend.aspeninstitute.org/resources/medicaid-checklist (accessed May 11, 2019).

Association of Maternal & Child Health Programs. 2016. *Opportunities to optimize access to prenatal care through health transformation.* Washington, DC: Association of Maternal & Child Health Programs.

ASTHO (Association of State and Territorial Health Officials). 2013. *Preconception care fact sheet.* Arlington, VA: Association of State and Territorial Health Officials.

Avellar, S. A., and L. H. Supplee. 2013. Effectiveness of home visiting in improving child health and reducing child maltreatment. *Pediatrics* 132:S90–S99.

Badura, M., K. Johnson, K. Hench, and M. Reyes. 2008. Healthy Start: Lessons learned on interconception care. *Women's Health Issues* 18(Suppl 6):S61–S66.

Bailey, S. R., M. Marino, M. Hoopes, J. Heintzman, R. Gold, H. Angier, J. P. O'Malley, and J. E. DeVoe. 2016. Healthcare utilization after a Children's Health Insurance Program expansion in Oregon. *Maternal and Child Health Journal* 20(5):946–954.

Bailit Health. 2016. *Value-based payment models for Medicaid child health services.* Needham, MA: Bailit Health.

Bair-Merritt, M. H., M. Mandal, A. Garg, and T. L. Cheng. 2015. Addressing psychosocial adversity within the patient-centered medical home: Expert-created measurable standards. *The Journal of Primary Prevention* 36(4):213–225.

Baker, J. P. 1994. Women and the invention of well child care. *Pediatrics* 94(4 Pt. 1):527–531.

Balasubramanian, B. A., D. J. Cohen, K. K. Jetelina, L. M. Dickinson, M. Davis, R. Gunn, K. Gowen, F. V. deGruy, 3rd, B. F. Miller, and L. A. Green. 2017. Outcomes of integrated behavioral health with primary care. *Journal of the American Board of Family Medicine* 30(2):130–139.

Barker, D. J. P. 1995. The fetal and infant origins of disease. *European Journal of Clinical Investigation* 25(7):457–463.

Barker, D. J. P. 2003. The developmental origins of adult disease. *European Journal of Epidemiology* 18(8):733–736.

Barker, D. J. P. 2004. The developmental origins of adult disease. *Journal of the American College of Nutrition* 23(Suppl 6):S588–S595.

Bauer, J., L. Angus, N. Fischler, K. D. Rosenberg, T. F. Gipson, and J. Devoe. 2011. The impact of citizenship documentation requirements on access to Medicaid for pregnant women in Oregon. *Maternal and Child Health Journal* 15(6):753–758.

Bazemore, A. W., E. K. Cottrell, R. Gold, L. S. Hughes, R. L. Phillips, H. Angier, T. E. Burdick, M. A. Carrozza, and J. E. DeVoe. 2016. "Community vital signs": Incorporating geo-coded social determinants into electronic records to promote patient and population health. *Journal of the American Medical Informatics Association* 23(2):407–412.

Beal, A. C., J. P. Co, D. Dougherty, T. Jorsling, J. Kam, J. Perrin, and R. H. Palmer. 2004. Quality measures for children's health care. *Pediatrics* 113(1 Pt. 2):199–209.

Berchick, E. R., E. Hood, and J. C. Barnett. 2018. *Current Population Reports, P60-264. Health insurance coverage in the United States: 2017.* Washington, DC: U.S. Government Printing Office.

Berwick, D. M., B. James, and M. J. Coye. 2003. Connections between quality measurement and improvement. *Medical Care* 41(Suppl 1):I30–I38.

Berwick, D. M., T. W. Nolan, and J. Whittington. 2008. The triple aim: Care, health, and cost. *Health Affairs* 27(3):759–769.

Best Babies Zone. n.d. *About us.* http://www.bestbabieszone.org/About-Us-2016 (accessed June 20, 2019).

Betancourt, J. R., A. R. Green, J. E. Carrillo, and O. Ananeh-Firempong, 2nd. 2003. Defining cultural competence: A practical framework for addressing racial/ethnic disparities in health and health care. *Public Health Reports* 118(4):293–302.

Biener, A. I., and T. M. Selden. 2017. Public and private payments for physician office visits. *Health Affairs* 36(12):2160–2164.

Bisgaier, J., and K. V. Rhodes. 2011. Auditing access to specialty care for children with public insurance. *New England Journal of Medicine* 364(24):2324–2333.

Bloomfield, J., and S. S. Rising. 2013. CenteringParenting: An innovative dyad model for group mother-infant care. *Journal of Midwifery & Women's Health* 58(6):683–689.

Bohren, M. A., G. J. Hofmeyr, C. Sakala, R. K. Fukuzawa, and A. Cuthbert. 2017. Continuous support for women during childbirth. *Cochrane Database of Systematic Reviews* 7:CD003766.

Brett, K. M., K. C. Schoendorf, and J. L. Kiely. 1994. Differences between black and white women in the use of prenatal care technologies. *American Journal of Obstetrics and Gynecology* 170(1):41–46.

Brooks, T., and K. Wagnerman. 2018. *Snapshot of children's coverage by race and ethnicity.* Washington, DC: Georgetown University Health Policy Institute.

Brown, C. C., J. E. Moore, H. C. Felix, M. K. Stewart, T. M. Bird, C. L. Lowery, and J. M. Tilford. 2019. Association of state Medicaid expansion status with low birth weight and preterm birth. *JAMA: Journal of the American Medical Association* 321(16):1598–1609.

Bryant, A. S., A. Worjoloh, A. B. Caughey, and A. E. Washington. 2010. Racial/ethnic disparities in obstetric outcomes and care: Prevalence and determinants. *American Journal of Obstetrics and Gynecology* 202(4):335–343.

Buchholz, M., C. Fischer, K. L. Margolis, and A. Talmi. 2016. Early childhood behavioral health integration in pediatric primary care: Serving refugee families in the Healthy Steps Program. *Zero to Three* 36(6):4–10.

Building U.S. Capacity to Review and Prevent Maternal Deaths. 2018. *Report from nine maternal mortality review committees.* https://reviewtoaction.org/Report_from_Nine_MMRCs (accessed June 13, 2019).

Burgess, C. K., P. A. Henning, W. V. Norman, M. G. Manze, and H. E. Jones. 2018. A systematic review of the effect of reproductive intention screening in primary care settings on reproductive health outcomes. *Family Practice* 35(2):122–131.

Burke, B. L., Jr., R. W. Hall, and the Section on Telehealth Care. 2015. Telemedicine: Pediatric applications. *Pediatrics* 136(1):e293–e308.

Calkins, K., and S. U. Devaskar. 2011. Fetal origins of adult disease. *Current Problems in Pediatric and Adolescent Health Care* 41(6):158–176.

Callegari, L. S., A. R. Aiken, C. Dehlendorf, P. Cason, and S. Borrero. 2017. Addressing potential pitfalls of reproductive life planning with patient-centered counseling. *American Journal of Obstetrics and Gynecology* 216(2):129–134.

Campbell, J. D., M. Brooks, P. Hosokawa, J. Robinson, L. Song, and J. Krieger. 2015. Community health worker home visits for Medicaid-enrolled children with asthma: Effects on asthma outcomes and costs. *American Journal of Public Health* 105(11):2366–2372.

Carlson, M. J., J. DeVoe, and B. J. Wright. 2006. Short-term impacts of coverage loss in a Medicaid population: Early results from a prospective cohort study of the Oregon Health Plan. *Annals of Family Medicine* 4(5):391–398.

Carter, E. B., L. A. Temming, J. Akin, S. Fowler, G. A. Macones, G. A. Colditz, and M. G. Tuuli. 2016. Group prenatal care compared with traditional prenatal care: A systematic review and meta-analysis. *Obstetrics & Gynecology* 128(3):551–561.

Catling, C. J., N. Medley, M. Foureur, C. Ryan, N. Leap, A. Teate, and C. S. Homer. 2015. Group versus conventional antenatal care for women. *Cochrane Database of Systematic Reviews* 2:CD007622.

Caughey, A. B., A. G. Cahill, J. M. Guise, and D. J. Rouse. 2014. Safe prevention of the primary cesarean delivery. *American Journal of Obstetrics & Gynecology* 210(3):179–193.

CDC (Centers for Disease Control and Prevention). 2016. *Biomonitoring summary: Mercury.* https://www.cdc.gov/biomonitoring/mercury_biomonitoringsummary.html (accessed March 26, 2019).

CDC. 2019a. *Data and statistics on children's mental health.* https://www.cdc.gov/childrensmentalhealth/data.html (accessed June 5, 2019).

CDC. 2019b. *Infant mortality.* https://www.cdc.gov/reproductivehealth/maternalinfanthealth/infantmortality.htm (accessed July 13, 2018).

CDC. 2019c. *Pregnancy mortality surveillance system.* https://www.cdc.gov/reproductivehealth/maternalinfanthealth/pregnancy-mortality-surveillance-system.htm (accessed July 16, 2019).

Center for Child & Family Health. n.d. *Family connects Durham.* https://www.ccfhnc.org/programs/family-connects-durham (accessed May 9, 2019).

Center for Youth Wellness. n.d. *Center for Youth Wellness ACEQ & user guide.* https://centerforyouthwellness.org/cyw-aceq (accessed April 16, 2019).

Center on the Developing Child at Harvard University. n.d. *FIND: Filming Interactions to Nurture Development.* https://developingchild.harvard.edu/innovation-application/innovation-in-action/find (accessed May 9, 2019).

Centering Healthcare Institute. n.d.-a. *CenteringParenting.* https://www.centeringhealthcare.org/what-we-do/centering-parenting (accessed May 9, 2019).

Centering Healthcare Institute. n.d.-b. *CenteringPregnancy.* https://www.centeringhealthcare.org/what-we-do/centering-pregnancy (accessed July 17, 2019).

Char, D. S., N. H. Shah, and D. Magnus. 2018. Implementing machine learning in health care—addressing ethical challenges. *New England Journal of Medicine* 378(11):981–983.

Chassin, M. R. 2002. Achieving and sustaining improved quality: Lessons from New York State and cardiac surgery. *Health Affairs* 21(4):40–51.

Chen, L., A. H. Crockett, S. Covington-Kolb, E. Heberlein, L. Zhang, and X. Sun. 2017. Centering and Racial Disparities (CRADLE study): Rationale and design of a randomized controlled trial of CenteringPregnancy and birth outcomes. *BMC Pregnancy and Childbirth* 17(1):118.

Child Trends. 2015. *Low and very low birthweight infants.* Bethesda, MD: Child Trends.

Child Trends. 2018. *Kindergarten Readiness National Outcome Measure.* https://www. childtrends.org/project/kindergarten-readiness-national-outcome-measure (accessed April 29, 2019).

Child Trends. n.d. *Health care coverage for children.* https://www.childtrends.org/indicators/ health-care-coverage (accessed April 18, 2019).

Choi, M., B. D. Sommers, and J. M. McWilliams. 2011. Children's health insurance and access to care during and after the CHIP expansion period. *Journal of Health Care for the Poor and Underserved* 22(2):576–589.

CMS (Centers for Medicare & Medicaid Services). 2019. *Integrated Care for Kids (InCK) model.* https://innovation.cms.gov/initiatives/integrated-care-for-kids-model (accessed April 16, 2019).

CMS Maternal & Infant Health Initiative. 2015. *Resources on strategies to improve postpartum care among Medicaid and CHIP populations.* https://www.medicaid.gov/medicaid/ quality-of-care/downloads/strategies-to-improve-postpartum-care.pdf (accessed July 19, 2019).

Coker, T. R., S. Chacon, M. N. Elliott, Y. Bruno, T. Chavis, C. Biely, C. D. Bethell, S. Contreras, N. A. Mimila, J. Mercado, and P. J. Chung. 2016. A parent coach model for well-child care among low-income children: A randomized controlled trial. *Pediatrics* 137(3):e20153013.

Conners, G. P., S. J. Kressly, J. M. Perrin, J. E. Richerson, and U. M. Sankrithi. 2017. Non-emergency acute care: When it's not the medical home. *Pediatrics* 139(5):e20170629.

Cornachione, E., R. Rudowitz, and S. Artiga. 2016. *Children's health coverage: The role of Medicaid and CHIP and issues for the future.* Menlo Park, CA: Kaiser Family Foundation.

Cottrell, E. K., R. Gold, S. Likumahuwa, H. Angier, N. Huguet, D. J. Cohen, K. D. Clark, L. M. Gottlieb, and J. E. DeVoe. 2018. Using health information technology to bring social determinants of health into primary care: A conceptual framework to guide research. *Journal of Health Care for the Poor and Underserved* 29(3):949–963.

Coury, D., A. Wolfe, P. H. Lipkin, B. Baer, S. L. Hyman, S. E. Levy, M. M. Macias, and B. Sisk. 2017. *Screening of young children for autism spectrum disorders: Results from a national survey of pediatricians.* Paper presented at Pediatric Academic Societies Annual Meeting, San Francisco, CA.

CPIPO (Commission on Paternal Involvement in Pregnancy Outcomes). 2010. *Commission outlook: Best and promising practices for improving research, policy and practice on paternal involvement in pregnancy outcomes.* Washington, DC: Joint Center for Political and Economic Studies.

Creanga, A. A., C. J. Berg, C. Syverson, K. Seed, F. C. Bruce, and W. M. Callaghan. 2015. Pregnancy-related mortality in the United States, 2006–2010. *Obstetrics & Gynecology* 125(1):5–12.

CSSP (Center for the Study of Social Policy). 2018. *Pediatrics Supporting Parents. Program analysis: Program and site selection process and results.* Washington, DC: Center for the Study of Social Policy.

Cunningham, S. D., J. B. Lewis, F. M. Shebl, L. M. Boyd, M. A. Robinson, S. A. Grilo, S. M. Lewis, A. L. Pruett, and J. R. Ickovics. 2019. An integrative model for the study of developmental competencies in minority children. *Journal of Women's Health* 28(1):17–22.

Dabney, K., L. McClarin, E. Romano, D. Fitzgerald, L. Bayne, P. Oceanic, A. L. Nettles, and L. Holmes, Jr. 2015. Cultural competence in pediatrics: Health care provider knowledge, awareness, and skills. *International Journal of Environmental Research and Public Health* 13(1):14.

D'Angelo, D. V., B. Le, M. E. O'Neil, L. Williams, I. B. Ahluwalia, L. L. Harrison, R. L. Floyd, and V. Grigorescu. 2015. Patterns of health insurance coverage around the time of pregnancy among women with live-born infants—Pregnancy Risk Assessment Monitoring System, 29 States, 2009. *MMWR Surveillance Summaries* 64(4):1–19.

Dassanayake, M., E. Langen, and M. B. Davis. 2019. Pregnancy complications as a window to future cardiovascular disease. *Cardiology in Review.* https://journals.lww.com/cardiologyinreview/Abstract/publishahead/Pregnancy_Complications_as_a_Window_to_Future.99700.aspx (accessed June 13, 2019).

de Boo, H. A., and J. E. Harding. 2006. The developmental origins of adult disease (Barker) hypothesis. *Australian and New Zealand Journal of Obstetrics and Gynaecology* 46(1):4–14.

Declercq, E. R., C. Sakala, M. P. Corry, S. Applebaum, and A. Herrlich. 2013. *Listening to Mothers III: New mothers speak out.* New York: Childbirth Connection.

Dehlendorf, C., R. Ruskin, K. Grumbach, E. Vittinghoff, K. Bibbins-Domingo, D. Schillinger, and J. Steinauer. 2010. Recommendations for intrauterine contraception: A randomized trial of the effects of patients' race/ethnicity and socioeconomic status. *American Journal of Obstetrics and Gynecology* 203(4):319.e311–319.e318.

Dennis, C.-L., K. Fung, S. Grigoriadis, G. E. Robinson, S. Romans, and L. Ross. 2007. Traditional postpartum practices and rituals: A qualitative systematic review. *Women's Health* 3(4):487–502.

DeVoe, J., A. Graham, H. Angier, A. Baez, and L. Krois. 2008a. Obtaining healthcare services for low-income children: A hierarchy of needs. *Journal of Health Care for the Poor and Underserved* 19(4):1192–1211.

DeVoe, J., L. Krois, T. Edlund, J. Smith, and N. Carlson. 2008b. Uninsurance among children whose parents are losing Medicaid coverage: Preliminary results from a statewide survey of Oregon families. *Health Services Research* 43(1 Pt. 2):401–418.

DeVoe, J. E., A. Graham, L. Krois, J. Smith, and G. L. Fairbrother. 2008c. "Mind the Gap" in children's health insurance coverage: Does the length of a child's coverage gap matter? *Ambulatory Pediatrics* 8(2):129–134.

DeVoe, J. E., C. J. Tillotson, and L. S. Wallace. 2009. Children's receipt of health care services and family health insurance patterns. *Annals of Family Medicine* 7(5):406–413.

DeVoe, J. E., M. Ray, L. Krois, and M. J. Carlson. 2010. Uncertain health insurance coverage and unmet children's health care needs. *Family Medicine* 42(2):121–132.

DeVoe, J. E., M. Ray, and A. Graham. 2011a. Public health insurance in Oregon: Under-enrollment of eligible children and parental confusion about children's enrollment status. *American Journal of Public Health* 101(5):891–898.

DeVoe, J. E., C. J. Tillotson, L. S. Wallace, S. Selph, A. Graham, and H. Angier. 2011b. Comparing types of health insurance for children: A public option versus a private option. *Medical Care* 49(9):818–827.

DeVoe, J. E., L. Wallace, S. Selph, N. Westfall, and S. Crocker. 2011c. Comparing type of health insurance among low-income children: A mixed-methods study from Oregon. *Maternal and Child Health Journal* 15(8):1238–1248.

DeVoe, J. E., C. J. Tillotson, L. S. Wallace, S. E. Lesko, and H. Angier. 2012a. The effects of health insurance and a usual source of care on a child's receipt of health care. *Journal of Pediatric Health Care* 26(5):e25–e35.

DeVoe, J. E., C. J. Tillotson, L. S. Wallace, S. E. Lesko, and N. Pandhi. 2012b. Is health insurance enough? A usual source of care may be more important to ensure a child receives preventive health counseling. *Maternal and Child Health Journal* 16(2):306–315.

DeVoe, J. E., C. Crawford, H. Angier, J. O'Malley, C. Gallia, M. Marino, and R. Gold. 2015a. The association between Medicaid coverage for children and parents persists: 2002–2010. *Maternal and Child Health Journal* 19(8):1766–1774.

DeVoe, J. E., M. Marino, H. Angier, J. P. O'Malley, C. Crawford, C. Nelson, C. J. Tillotson, S. R. Bailey, C. Gallia, and R. Gold. 2015b. Effect of expanding Medicaid for parents on children's health insurance coverage: Lessons from the Oregon experiment. *JAMA Pediatrics* 169(1):e143145.

DeVoe, J. E., M. Marino, R. Gold, M. J. Hoopes, S. Cowburn, J. P. O'Malley, J. Heintzman, C. Gallia, K. J. McConnell, C. A. Nelson, N. Huguet, and S. R. Bailey. 2015c. Community health center use after Oregon's randomized Medicaid experiment. *Annals of Family Medicine* 13(4):312–320.

DeVoe, J. E., C. J. Tillotson, H. Angier, and L. S. Wallace. 2015d. Predictors of children's health insurance coverage discontinuity in 1998 versus 2009: Parental coverage continuity plays a major role. *Maternal and Child Health Journal* 19(4):889–896.

DeVoe, J. E., A. W. Bazemore, E. K. Cottrell, S. Likumahuwa-Ackman, J. Grandmont, N. Spach, and R. Gold. 2016. Perspectives in primary care: A conceptual framework and path for integrating social determinants of health into primary care practice. *Annals of Family Medicine* 14(2):104–108.

DiBari, J. N., S. M. Yu, S. M. Chao, and M. C. Lu. 2014. Use of postpartum care: Predictors and barriers. *Journal of Pregnancy* 2014:530769.

Dodge, K. A., W. B. Goodman, R. A. Murphy, K. O'Donnell, and J. Sato. 2013. Randomized controlled trial of universal postnatal nurse home visiting: Impact on emergency care. *Pediatrics* 132(Suppl 2):S140–S146.

Dodge, K. A., W. B. Goodman, R. A. Murphy, K. O'Donnell, J. Sato, and S. Guptill. 2014. Implementation and randomized controlled trial evaluation of universal postnatal nurse home visiting. *American Journal of Public Health* 104(Suppl 1):S136–S143.

DONA International. n.d. *What is a doula?* https://www.dona.org/what-is-a-doula (accessed April 29, 2019).

Dubay, L., and G. Kenney. 2003. Expanding public health insurance to parents: Effects on children's coverage under Medicaid. *Health Services Research* 38(5):1283–1301.

Dubowitz, H., W. G. Lane, J. N. Semiatin, L. S. Magder, M. Venepally, and M. Jans. 2011. The Safe Environment for Every Kid model: Impact on pediatric primary care professionals. *Pediatrics* 127(4):e962–e970.

Dubowitz, H., W. G. Lane, J. N. Semiatin, and L. S. Magder. 2012. The SEEK model of pediatric primary care: Can child maltreatment be prevented in a low-risk population? *Academic Pediatrics* 12(4):259–268.

Dudley, R. A., R. H. Miller, T. Y. Korenbrot, and H. S. Luft. 1998. The impact of financial incentives on quality of health care. *The Milbank Quarterly* 76(4):511, 649–686.

Dunst, C. J., and C. M. Trivette. 2009. Meta-analytic structural equation modeling of the influences of family-centered care on parent and child psychological health. *International Journal of Pediatrics* 2009:576840.

Dunst, C. J., C. M. Trivette, and D. W. Hamby. 2007. Meta-analysis of family-centered helpgiving practices research. *Mental Retardation and Developmental Disabilities Research Reviews* 13(4):370–378.

Dzau, V. J., M. B. McClellan, J. M. McGinnis, S. P. Burke, M. J. Coye, A. Diaz, T. A. Daschle, W. H. Frist, M. Gaines, M. A. Hamburg, J. E. Henney, S. Kumanyika, M. O. Leavitt, R. M. Parker, L. G. Sandy, L. D. Schaeffer, G. D. Steele, Jr., P. Thompson, and E. Zerhouni. 2017. Vital directions for health and health care: Priorities from a National Academy of Medicine initiative. *JAMA* 317(14):1461–1470.

Eberhard-Gran, M., S. Garthus-Niegel, K. Garthus-Niegel, and A. Eskild. 2010. Postnatal care: A cross-cultural and historical perspective. *Archives of Women's Mental Health* 13(6):459–466.

Eisner, V., J. V. Brazie, M. W. Pratt, and A. C. Hexter. 1979. The risk of low birthweight. *American Journal of Public Health* 69(9):887–893.

Ellis, R. P. 2001. Formal risk adjustment by private employers. *Inquiry* 38(3):299–309.

Epstein, A. M., T. H. Lee, and M. B. Hamel. 2004. Paying physicians for high-quality care. *New England Journal of Medicine* 350(4):406–410.

Evans, W. D., J. L. Wallace, and J. Snider. 2012. Pilot evaluation of the Text4Baby mobile health program. *BMC Public Health* 12:1031.

Feigelman, S., H. Dubowitz, W. Lane, L. Grube, and J. Kim. 2011. Training pediatric residents in a primary care clinic to help address psychosocial problems and prevent child maltreatment. *Academic Pediatrics* 11(6):474–480.

Fierman, A. H., A. F. Beck, E. K. Chung, M. M. Tschudy, T. R. Coker, K. B. Mistry, B. Siegel, L. J. Chamberlain, K. Conroy, S. G. Federico, P. J. Flanagan, A. Garg, B. A. Gitterman, A. M. Grace, R. S. Gross, M. K. Hole, P. Klass, C. Kraft, A. Kuo, G. Lewis, K. S. Lobach, D. Long, C. T. Ma, M. Messito, D. Navsaria, K. R. Northrip, C. Osman, M. D. Sadof, A. B. Schickedanz, and J. Cox. 2016. Redesigning health care practices to address childhood poverty. *Academic Pediatrics* 16(Suppl 3):S136–S146.

Finer, L. B., and M. R. Zolna. 2016. Declines in unintended pregnancy in the United States, 2008–2011. *New England Journal of Medicine* 374(9):843–852.

Finkelstein, A., S. Taubman, B. Wright, M. Bernstein, J. Gruber, J. P. Newhouse, H. Allen, and K. Baicker. 2012. The Oregon Health Insurance Experiment: Evidence from the first year. *Quarterly Journal of Economics* 127(3):1057–1106.

Fiscella, K. 1995. Does prenatal care improve birth outcomes? A critical review. *Obstetrics & Gynecology* 85(3):468–479.

Flowers, L., and J. Accius. 2019. *The new Medicaid waivers: Coverage losses for beneficiaries, higher costs for states.* Washington, DC: AARP Public Policy Institute.

Foy, J. M., and AAP (American Academy of Pediatrics) Task Force on Mental Health. 2010. Enhancing pediatric mental health care: Report from the American Academy of Pediatrics Task Force on Mental Health. Introduction. *Pediatrics* 125(Suppl 3):S69–S74.

Frey, K. A., S. M. Navarro, M. Kotelchuck, and M. C. Lu. 2008. The clinical content of preconception care: Preconception care for men. *American Journal of Obstetrics and Gynecology* 199(6):S389–S395.

Gareau, S., A. Lopez-De Fede, B. L. Loudermilk, T. H. Cummings, J. W. Hardin, A. H. Picklesimer, E. Crouch, and S. Covington-Kolb. 2016. Group prenatal care results in Medicaid savings with better outcomes: A propensity score analysis of CenteringPregnancy participation in South Carolina. *Maternal and Child Health Journal* 20(7):1384–1393.

Garg, A., A. M. Butz, P. H. Dworkin, R. A. Lewis, R. E. Thompson, and J. R. Serwint. 2007. Improving the management of family psychosocial problems at low-income children's well-child care visits: The WE CARE Project. *Pediatrics* 120(3):547–558.

Garg, A., M. Marino, A. R. Vikani, and B. S. Solomon. 2012. Addressing families' unmet social needs within pediatric primary care: The Health Leads model. *Clinical Pediatrics* 51(12):1191–1193.

Garg, A., S. Toy, Y. Tripodis, M. Silverstein, and E. Freeman. 2015. Addressing social determinants of health at well child care visits: A cluster RCT. *Pediatrics* 135(2):e296–e304.

Garg, A., R. Boynton-Jarrett, and P. H. Dworkin. 2016. Avoiding the unintended consequences of screening for social determinants of health. *JAMA* 316(8):813–814.

Garner, A. S., J. P. Shonkoff, B. S. Siegel, M. I. Dobbins, M. F. Earls, L. McGuinn, J. Pascoe, and D. L. Wood. 2012. Early childhood adversity, toxic stress, and the role of the pediatrician: Translating developmental science into lifelong health. *Pediatrics* 129(1):e224–e231.

Garrett, B., and A. Gangopadhyaya. 2015. *Who gained health insurance coverage under the ACA, and where do they live?* Washington, DC: The Urban Institute.

Georgetown University Center for Children and Families. 2017. *Medicaid's role for children.* https://ccf.georgetown.edu/wp-content/uploads/2016/06/Medicaid-and-Children-update-Jan-2017-rev.pdf (accessed July 17, 2019).

Georgetown University Center for Children and Families. 2018. Snapshot of children's coverage by race and ethnicity. https://ccf.georgetown.edu/wp-content/uploads/2018/05/Kids-coverage-by-race-ethnicity-update-v2.pdf (accessed April 16, 2019).

Ghandour, R. M., K. Flaherty, A. Hirai, V. Lee, D. K. Walker, and M. C. Lu. 2017. Applying collaborative learning and quality improvement to public health: Lessons from the Collaborative Improvement and Innovation Network (CoIIN) to reduce infant mortality. *Maternal and Child Health Journal* 21(6):1318–1326.

Ghandour, R. M., K. Anderson Moore, K. Murphy, C. Bethell, J. Jones, R. Harwood, J. Buerlein, M. Kogan, and M. Lu. 2018. School readiness among U.S. children: Development of a pilot measure. *Child Indicators Research* 12(4):1389–1411.

Gianfrancesco, M. A., S. Tamang, J. Yazdany, and G. Schmajuk. 2018. Potential biases in machine learning algorithms using electronic health record data. *JAMA Internal Medicine* 178(11):1544–1547.

Gleason, M. M., E. Goldson, and M. W. Yogman. 2016. Addressing early childhood emotional and behavioral problems. *Pediatrics* 138(6):e20163025.

Gold, R., S. R. Bailey, J. P. O'Malley, M. J. Hoopes, S. Cowburn, M. Marino, J. Heintzman, C. Nelson, S. P. Fortmann, and J. E. DeVoe. 2014. Estimating demand for care after a Medicaid expansion: Lessons from Oregon. *The Journal of Ambulatory Care Management* 37(4):282–292.

Goodson, B. D. 2014. *Parent support programs and outcomes for children.* http://www.childencyclopedia.com/parenting-skills/according-experts/parent-support-programs-and-outcomes-children (accessed January 30, 2019).

Goossens, J. 2018. Barriers and facilitators to the provision of preconception care by healthcare providers: A systematic review. *International Journal of Nursing Studies* 87C:113–130.

Gortmaker, S. L. 1979. The effects of prenatal care upon the health of the newborn. *American Journal of Public Health* 69(7):653–660.

Gottlieb, L. M., D. Hessler, D. Long, E. Laves, A. R. Burns, A. Amaya, P. Sweeney, C. Schudel, and N. E. Adler. 2016. Effects of social needs screening and in-person service navigation on child health: A randomized clinical trial. *JAMA Pediatrics* 170(11):e162521.

Greenberg, R. S. 1983. The impact of prenatal care in different social groups. *American Journal of Obstetrics and Gynecology* 145(7):797–801.

Gunja, M. Z., S. R. Collins, M. M. Doty, and S. Beutel. 2017. *How the Affordable Care Act has helped women gain insurance and improved their ability to get health care.* https://www.commonwealthfund.org/publications/issue-briefs/2017/aug/how-affordable-care-act-has-helped-women-gain-insurance-and (accessed January 10, 2019).

Guyer, B., M. Barth, D. Bishai, M. Caughy, D. Burkom, and C. Tang. 2003. *Healthy Steps: The first three years: The Healthy Steps for Young Children Program National Evaluation.* Baltimore, MD: Johns Hopkins Bloomberg School of Public Health.

Haggerty, R. J., K. J. Roghmann, and I. B. Pless. 1975. *Child health and the community.* New York: John Wiley & Sons, Inc.

Halfon, N. 2012. Addressing health inequalities in the US: A life course health development approach. *Social Science & Medicine* 74(5):671–673.

Halfon, N., and M. Hochstein. 2002. Life course health development: An integrated framework for developing health policy & research. *The Milbank Quarterly* 80(3):433–479.

Halfon, N., A. Houtrow, K. Larson, and P. W. Newacheck. 2012. The changing landscape of disability in childhood. *The Future of Children* 22(1):13–42.

Halfon, N., P. Long, D. I. Chang, J. Hester, M. Inkelas, and A. Rodgers. 2014. Applying a 3.0 transformation framework to guide large-scale health system reform. *Health Affairs* 33(11):2003–2011.

Hall, J. A., L. Benton, A. Copas, and J. Stephenson. 2017. Pregnancy intention and pregnancy outcome: Systematic review and meta-analysis. *Maternal and Child Health Journal* 21(3):670–704.

Handler, A., J. Kennelly, and N. R. Peacock. 2011. *Reducing racial/ethnic disparities in reproductive and perinatal outcomes: The evidence from population-based interventions.* New York: Springer.

Hans, S. L., R. C. Edwards, and Y. Zhang. 2018. Randomized controlled trial of doula-home-visiting services: Impact on maternal and infant health. *Maternal and Child Health Journal* 22(Suppl 1):105–113.

Harlem Children's Zone. n.d. *Harlem Children's Zone.* https://hcz.org (accessed June 12, 2019).

Hatch, B. A., J. E. DeVoe, J. A. Lapidus, M. J. Carlson, and B. J. Wright. 2014. Citizenship documentation requirement for Medicaid eligibility: Effects on Oregon children. *Family Medicine* 46(4):267–275.

Hatch, B., S. R. Bailey, S. Cowburn, M. Marino, H. Angier, and J. E. DeVoe. 2016. Community health center utilization following the 2008 Medicaid expansion in Oregon: Implications for the Affordable Care Act. *American Journal of Public Health* 106(4):645–650.

Hayes, S. L., P. Riley, D. C. Radley, and D. McCarthy. 2017. *Reducing racial and ethnic disparities in access to care: Has the Affordable Care Act made a difference? Issue brief.* New York: The Commonwealth Fund.

HealthConnect One. 2014. *The perinatal revolution.* Chicago, IL: HealthConnect One.

Heaman, M. I., M. Moffatt, L. Elliott, W. Sword, M. E. Helewa, H. Morris, P. Gregory, L. Tjaden, and C. Cook. 2014. Barriers, motivators and facilitators related to prenatal care utilization among inner-city women in Winnipeg, Canada: A case-control study. *BMC Pregnancy and Childbirth* 14:227.

Heintzman, J., S. R. Bailey, J. DeVoe, S. Cowburn, T. Kapka, T. V. Duong, and M. Marino. 2017. In low-income Latino patients, post-Affordable Care Act insurance disparities may be reduced even more than broader national estimates: Evidence from Oregon. *Journal of Racial and Ethnic Health Disparities* 4(3):329–336.

Help Me Grow. 2017. *Building impact: 2017 annual report.* Hartford, CT: Connecticut Children's Medical Center.

Hemsing, N., L. Greaves, and N. Poole. 2017. Preconception health care interventions: A scoping review. *Sexual and Reproductive Healthcare* 14:24–32.

Henize, A. W., A. F. Beck, M. D. Klein, M. Adams, and R. S. Kahn. 2015. A road map to address the social determinants of health through community collaboration. *Pediatrics* 136(4):e993–e1001.

HHS (U.S. Department of Health and Human Services). 2015. *Child health USA 2014.* Rockville, MD: U.S. Department of Health and Human Services, Health Resources and Services Administration, Maternal and Child Health Bureau.

Hibbard, J. H., J. Stockard, and M. Tusler. 2005. Hospital performance reports: Impact on quality, market share, and reputation. *Health Affairs* 24(4):1150–1160.

Hirai, A. H., M. D. Kogan, V. Kandasamy, C. Reuland, and C. Bethell. 2018a. Prevalence and variation of developmental screening and surveillance in early childhood. *JAMA Pediatrics* 172(9):857–866.

Hirai, A. H., W. M. Sappenfield, R. M. Ghandour, S. Donahue, V. Lee, and M. C. Lu. 2018b. The Collaborative Improvement and Innovation Network (CoIIN) to Reduce Infant Mortality: An outcome evaluation from the US South, 2011 to 2014. *American Journal of Public Health* 108(6):815–821.

Hofstetter, A. M., N. DuRivage, C. Y. Vargas, S. Camargo, D. K. Vawdrey, A. Fisher, and M. S. Stockwell. 2015. Text message reminders for timely routine MMR vaccination: A randomized controlled trial. *Vaccine* 33(43):5741–5746.

Homer, C. J., K. Klatka, D. Romm, K. Kuhlthau, S. Bloom, P. Newacheck, J. Van Cleave, and J. M. Perrin. 2008. A review of the evidence for the medical home for children with special health care needs. *Pediatrics* 122(4):e922–e937.

Hoopes, M. J., H. Angier, R. Gold, S. R. Bailey, N. Huguet, M. Marino, and J. E. DeVoe. 2016. Utilization of community health centers in Medicaid expansion and nonexpansion states, 2013–2014. *The Journal of Ambulatory Care Management* 39(4):290–298.

Houtrow, A. J., K. Larson, L. M. Olson, P. W. Newacheck, and N. Halfon. 2014. Changing trends of childhood disability, 2001–2011. *Pediatrics* 134(3):530–538.

Howell, E. M., and G. M. Kenney. 2012. The impact of the Medicaid/CHIP expansions on children: A synthesis of the evidence. *Medical Care Research and Review* 69(4):372–396.

HRSA (Health Resources and Services Organization). 2018. *Women's preventive services guidelines.* https://www.hrsa.gov/womens-guidelines/index.html (accessed July 19, 2019).

HRSA. 2019. *Title V Maternal and Child Health Services Block Grant Program*. https://mchb. hrsa.gov/maternal-child-health-initiatives/title-v-maternal-and-child-health-services-block-grant-program (accessed April 29, 2019).

HRSA. n.d. *Understanding Title V of the Social Security Act*. Rockville, MD: U.S. Department of Health and Human Services.

Huguet, N., M. J. Hoopes, H. Angier, M. Marino, H. Holderness, and J. E. DeVoe. 2017. Medicaid expansion produces long-term impact on insurance coverage rates in community health centers. *Journal of Primary Care & Community Health* 8(4):206–212.

Huguet, N., R. Springer, M. Marino, H. Angier, M. Hoopes, H. Holderness, and J. E. DeVoe. 2018. The impact of the Affordable Care Act (ACA) Medicaid expansion on visit rates for diabetes in safety net health centers. *Journal of the American Board of Family Medicine* 31(6):905–916.

Huntington, J., and F. A. Connell. 1994. For every dollar spent—the cost-savings argument for prenatal care. *New England Journal of Medicine* 331(19):1303–1307.

Hussein, N., J. Kai, and N. Qureshi. 2016. The effects of preconception interventions on improving reproductive health and pregnancy outcomes in primary care: A systematic review. *European Journal of General Practice* 22(1):42–52.

Hussein, N., S. F. Weng, J. Kai, J. Kleijnen, and N. Qureshi. 2018. Preconception risk assessment for thalassaemia, sickle cell disease, cystic fibrosis and Tay-Sachs disease. *Cochrane Database of Systematic Reviews* 8:CD010849.

Ickovics, J. R., T. S. Kershaw, C. Westdahl, U. Magriples, Z. Massey, H. Reynolds, and S. S. Rising. 2007. Group prenatal care and perinatal outcomes: A randomized controlled trial. *Obstetrics & Gynecology* 110(2 Pt. 1):330–339.

Ickovics, J. R., V. Earnshaw, J. B. Lewis, T. S. Kershaw, U. Magriples, E. Stasko, S. S. Rising, A. Cassells, S. Cunningham, P. Bernstein, and J. N. Tobin. 2016. Cluster randomized controlled trial of group prenatal care: Perinatal outcomes among adolescents in New York City health centers. *American Journal of Public Health* 106(2):359–365.

Institute for Medicaid Innovation. n.d. *Best practices in Medicaid managed care*. https://www. medicaidinnovation.org/current-initiatives/best-practices (accessed June 20, 2019).

IOM (Institute of Medicine). 1973. *Infant death: An analysis by maternal risk and health care. Vol. 1 of Contrasts in Health Status*. Washington, DC: Institute of Medicine.

IOM. 1985. *Preventing low birthweight*. Washington, DC: National Academy Press.

IOM. 1998. *America's children: Health insurance and access to care*. Washington, DC: National Academy Press.

IOM. 2001. *Crossing the quality chasm: A new health system for the 21st century*. Washington, DC: National Academy Press.

IOM. 2002. *Health insurance is a family matter*. Washington, DC: The National Academies Press.

IOM. 2003. *Dioxins and dioxin-like compounds in the food supply: Strategies to decrease exposure*. Washington, DC: The National Academies Press.

IOM. 2006. *Performance measurement: Accelerating improvement*. Washington, DC: The National Academies Press.

Jack, B. W., H. Atrash, D. V. Coonrod, M. K. Moos, J. O'Donnell, and K. Johnson. 2008. The clinical content of preconception care: An overview and preparation of this supplement. *American Journal of Obstetrics and Gynecology* 199(6):S266–S279.

James, J. 2015. Health policy brief: The Oregon Health Insurance Experiment. *Health Affairs*, July 16.

Johnson, A. A., B. J. Hatcher, M. N. El-Khorazaty, R. A. Milligan, B. Bhaskar, M. F. Rodan, L. Richards, B. K. Wingrove, and H. A. Laryea. 2007. Determinants of inadequate prenatal care utilization by African American women. *Journal of Health Care for the Poor and Underserved* 18(3):620–636.

Johnson, K., S. F. Posner, J. Biermann, J. F. Cordero, H. K. Atrash, C. S. Parker, S. Boulet, and M. G. Curtis. 2006. Recommendations to improve preconception health and health care—United States: A report of the CDC/ATSDR Preconception Care Work Group and the Select Panel on Preconception Care. *Morbidity and Mortality Weekly Report Recommendations and Reports* 55(RR06):1–23.

Johnston, E. M., A. E. Strahan, P. Joski, A. L. Dunlop, and E. K. Adams. 2018. Impacts of the Affordable Care Act's Medicaid expansion on women of reproductive age: Differences by parental status and state policies. *Women's Health Issues* 28(2):122–129.

Jones, D. E., M. Greenberg, and M. Crowley. 2015. Early social-emotional functioning and public health: The relationship between kindergarten social competence and future wellness. *American Journal of Public Health* 105(11):2283–2290.

Juillard, C., L. Cooperman, I. Allen, R. Pirracchio, T. Henderson, R. Marquez, J. Orellana, M. Texada, and R. A. Dicker. 2016. A decade of hospital-based violence intervention: Benefits and shortcomings. *Journal of Trauma and Acute Care Surgery* 81(6):1156–1161.

Kaiser Family Foundation. 2017. *Medicaid's role for women. Fact sheet.* Kaiser Family Foundation, https://www.kff.org/womens-health-policy/fact-sheet/medicaids-role-for-women (accessed January 10, 2019).

Kaiser Family Foundation. 2019. *Status of state action on the Medicaid expansion decision.* https://www.kff.org/health-reform/state-indicator/state-activity-around-expanding-medicaid-under-the-affordable-care-act/?currentTimeframe=0&sortModel=%7B%22colId%22:%22Location%22,%22sort%22:%22asc%22%7D (accessed March 26, 2019).

Kalmuss, D., and K. Fennelly. 1990. Barriers to prenatal care among low-income women in New York City. *Family Planning Perspectives* 22(5):215–218, 231.

Katkin, J. P., S. J. Kressly, A. R. Edwards, J. M. Perrin, C. A. Kraft, J. E. Richerson, J. S. Tieder, and L. Wall. 2017. Guiding principles for team-based pediatric care. *Pediatrics* 140(2):e20171489.

Keith, K. 2018. Administration moves to liberalize rules on short-term, non-ACA-compliant coverage. *Health Affairs Blog.* https://www.healthaffairs.org/do/10.1377/hblog20180220.69087/full (accessed January 10, 2019).

Kelleher, K., J. Reece, and M. Sandel. 2018. The Healthy Neighborhood, Healthy Families initiative. *Pediatrics* 142(3):e20180261.

Kerker, B. D., A. Storfer-Isser, M. Szilagyi, R. E. Stein, A. S. Garner, K. G. O'Connor, K. E. Hoagwood, and S. M. Horwitz. 2016. Do pediatricians ask about adverse childhood experiences in pediatric primary care? *Academic Pediatrics* 16(2):154–160.

Kimm, S. Y. S. 2004. Fetal origins of adult disease: The Barker hypothesis revisited—2004. *Current Opinion in Endocrinology, Diabetes and Obesity* 11(4):192–196.

Klein, M. D., A. F. Beck, A. W. Henize, D. S. Parrish, E. E. Fink, and R. S. Kahn. 2013. Doctors and lawyers collaborating to HeLP children—outcomes from a successful partnership between professions. *Journal of Health Care for the Poor and Underserved* 24(3):1063–1073.

Klerman, J. A., K. Daley, and A. Pozniak. 2014. *Family and medical leave in 2012: Technical report.* Cambridge, MA: Abt Associates.

Kluchin, R. 2009. *Fit to be tied: Sterilization and reproductive rights in America, 1950–1980.* New Brunswick, NJ, and London, UK: Rutgers University Press.

Kogan, M. D., M. Kotelchuck, G. R. Alexander, and W. E. Johnson. 1994. Racial disparities in reported prenatal care advice from health care providers. *American Journal of Public Health* 84(1):82–88.

Kogan, M. D., J. A. Martin, G. R. Alexander, M. Kotelchuck, S. J. Ventura, and F. D. J. J. Frigoletto. 1998. The changing pattern of prenatal care utilization in the United States, 1981–1995, using different prenatal care indices. *JAMA* 279(20):1623–1628.

Korenbrot, C. C., A. Gill, Z. Clayson, and E. Patterson. 1995. Evaluation of California's statewide implementation of enhanced perinatal services as Medicaid benefits. *Public Health Reports* 110(2):125–133.

Korenbrot, C. C., A. Steinberg, C. Bender, and S. Newberry. 2002. Preconception care: A systematic review. *Maternal and Child Health Journal* 6(2):75–88.

Kotelchuck, M., and M. Lu. 2017. Father's role in preconception health. *Maternal and Child Health Journal* 21(11):2025–2039.

Kotelchuck, M., M. D. Kogan, G. R. Alexander, and B. W. Jack. 1997. The influence of site of care on the content of prenatal care for low-income women. *Maternal and Child Health Journal* 1(1):25–34.

Kozhimannil, K. B., L. B. Attanasio, R. R. Hardeman, and M. O'Brien. 2013. Doula care supports near-universal breastfeeding initiation among diverse, low-income women. *Journal of Midwifery & Women's Health* 58(4):378–382.

Kozhimannil, K. B., C. A. Vogelsang, R. R. Hardeman, and S. Prasad. 2016. Disrupting the pathways of social determinants of health: Doula support during pregnancy and childbirth. *Journal of the American Board of Family Medicine* 29(3):308–317.

Krieger, J. W., T. K. Takaro, L. Song, and M. Weaver. 2005. The Seattle-King County Healthy Homes Project: A randomized, controlled trial of a community health worker intervention to decrease exposure to indoor asthma triggers. *American Journal of Public Health* 95(4):652–659.

Kuhlthau, K., T. G. Ferris, R. B. Davis, J. M. Perrin, and L. I. Iezzoni. 2005. Pharmacy- and diagnosis-based risk adjustment for children with Medicaid. *Medical Care* 43(11):1155–1159.

Kuo, D. Z., A. J. Houtrow, P. Arango, K. A. Kuhlthau, J. M. Simmons, and J. M. Neff. 2012. Family-centered care: Current applications and future directions in pediatric health care. *Maternal and Child Health Journal* 16(2):297–305.

Kwan, B. M., and D. E. Nease, Jr. 2013. The state of the evidence for integrated behavioral health in primary care. In *Integrated behavioral health in primary care*, edited by M. Talen and A. Burke Valeras. New York: Springer. Pp. 65–98.

Lahiri, T., S. E. Hempstead, C. Brady, C. L. Cannon, K. Clark, M. E. Condren, M. F. Guill, R. P. Guillerman, C. G. Leone, K. Maguiness, L. Monchil, S. W. Powers, M. Rosenfeld, S. J. Schwarzenberg, C. L. Tompkins, E. T. Zemanick, and S. D. Davis. 2016. Clinical practice guidelines from the Cystic Fibrosis Foundation for preschoolers with cystic fibrosis. *Pediatrics* 137(4):e20151784.

Lassi, Z. S., A. M. Imam, S. V. Dean, and Z. A. Bhutta. 2014. Preconception care: Screening and management of chronic disease and promoting psychological health. *Reproductive Health* 11:S5.

Lesser, A. J. 1965. Closing the gaps in the nation's health services for mothers and children. *Bulletin of the New York Academy of Medicine* 41(12):1248–1254.

Lewis, C., M. K. Abrams, and S. Seervai. 2017. *Listening to low-income patients: obstacles to the care we need, when we need it.* https://www.commonwealthfund.org/blog/2017/listening-low-income-patients-obstacles-care-we-need-when-we-need-it (accessed July 19, 2019).

Lindenauer, P. K., D. Remus, S. Roman, M. B. Rothberg, E. M. Benjamin, A. Ma, and D. W. Bratzler. 2007. Public reporting and pay for performance in hospital quality improvement. *New England Journal of Medicine* 356(5):486–496.

Lindenauer, P. K., T. Lagu, J. S. Ross, P. S. Pekow, A. Shatz, N. Hannon, M. B. Rothberg, and E. M. Benjamin. 2014. Attitudes of hospital leaders toward publicly reported measures of health care quality. *JAMA Internal Medicine* 174(12):1904–1911.

Lu, M. C. 2019. The future of maternal and child health. *Maternal and Child Health Journal* 23(1):1–7.

Lu, M. C., and J. S. Lu. 2008. Prenatal care. In *Encyclopedia of infant and early childhood development*, Vol. 3, edited by M. M. Haith and J. B. Benson. Cambridge, MA: Academic Press. Pp. 591–604.

Lu, M. C., V. Tache, G. R. Alexander, M. Kotelchuck, and N. Halfon. 2003. Preventing low birth weight: Is prenatal care the answer? *The Journal of Maternal-Fetal & Neonatal Medicine* 13(6):362–380.

Lu, M. C., M. Kotelchuck, V. K. Hogan, K. Johnson, and C. Reyes. 2010. Innovative strategies to reduce disparities in the quality of prenatal care in underresourced settings. *Medical Care Research and Review* 67(Suppl):S198–S230.

MA (Massachusetts) Executive Office of HHS (U.S. Department of Health and Human Services). 2017. *MassHealth Delivery System Restructuring—Provider Overview.* Boston, MA: Commonwealth of Massachusetts.

MacLaughlin, S., L. Gillespie, and R. Parlakian. 2017. Using pediatric visits to support children and families: Ten positive outcomes from HealthySteps. *Zero to Three* 37(4):46–52.

Macmillan, H. L., C. N. Wathen, J. Barlow, D. M. Fergusson, J. M. Leventhal, and H. N. Taussig. 2009. Interventions to prevent child maltreatment and associated impairment. *The Lancet* 373(9659):250–266.

MACPAC (Medicaid and CHIP Payment and Access Commission). 2016. *Enrollment and spending on Medicaid managed care.* https://www.macpac.gov/subtopic/enrollment-and-spending-on-medicaid-managed-care (accessed April 16, 2019).

MACPAC. 2018. *MACStats: Medicaid and CHIP data book.* Washington, DC: Medicaid and CHIP Payment and Access Commission.

Makni, N., A. Rothenburger, and K. Kelleher. 2015. Survey of twelve children's hospital-based accountable care organizations. *Journal of Hospital Administration* 4(2):64–73.

Marcil, L. E., M. K. Hole, L. M. Wenren, M. S. Schuler, B. S. Zuckerman, and R. J. Vinci. 2018. Free tax services in pediatric clinics. *Pediatrics* 141(6):e20173608.

Marino, M., S. R. Bailey, R. Gold, M. J. Hoopes, J. P. O'Malley, N. Huguet, J. Heintzman, C. Gallia, K. J. McConnell, and J. E. DeVoe. 2016. Receipt of preventive services after Oregon's randomized Medicaid experiment. *American Journal of Preventive Medicine* 50(2):161–170.

Marmot, M., M. Shipley, E. Brunner, and H. Hemingway. 2001. Relative contribution of early life and adult socioeconomic factors to adult morbidity in the Whitehall II study. *Journal of Epidemiology and Community Health* 55(5):301–307.

Marshall, M. N., P. G. Shekelle, S. Leatherman, and R. H. Brook. 2000. Public disclosure of performance data: Learning from the US experience. *Quality in Health Care* 9(1):53–57.

Martin, J. A., B. E. Hamilton, S. J. Ventura, F. Menacker, M. M. Park, and P. D. Sutton. 2002. Births: Final data for 2001. *National Vital Statistics Reports* 51(2):1–102.

Martin, J. A., B. E. Hamilton, M. J. K. Osterman, A. K. Driscoll, and P. Drake. 2018. Births: Final data for 2016. *National Vital Statistics Reports* 67(1):1–55.

Mazul, M. C., T. C. Salm Ward, and E. M. Ngui. 2017. Anatomy of good prenatal care: Perspectives of low income African-American women on barriers and facilitators to prenatal care. *Journal of Racial and Ethnic Health Disparities* 4(1):79–86.

McAvoy, P. V., M. B. Driscoll, and B. J. Gramling. 2004. Integrating the environment, the economy, and community health: A community health center's initiative to link health benefits to smart growth. *American Journal of Public Health* 94(4):525–527.

McCormick, M. C., R. M. Weinick, A. Elixhauser, M. N. Stagnitti, J. Thompson, and L. Simpson. 2001. Annual report on access to and utilization of health care for children and youth in the United States—2000. *Ambulatory Pediatrics* 1(1):3–15.

McGinnis, J. M., P. Williams-Russo, and J. R. Knickman. 2002. The case for more active policy attention to health promotion. *Health Affairs* 21(2):78–93.

Medicaid. n.d. *Children's health care quality measures.* https://www.medicaid.gov/medicaid/quality-of-care/performance-measurement/child-core-set/index.html (accessed April 30, 2019).

Mendelsohn, A. L., L. N. Mogilner, B. P. Dreyer, J. A. Forman, S. C. Weinstein, M. Broderick, K. J. Cheng, T. Magloire, T. Moore, and C. Napier. 2001. The impact of a clinic-based literacy intervention on language development in inner-city preschool children. *Pediatrics* 107(1):130–134.

Millenson, M. L. 2004. Pay for performance: The best worst choice. *Quality and Safety in Health Care* 13(5):323–324.

Minkovitz, C. S., D. Strobino, K. B. Mistry, D. O. Scharfstein, H. Grason, W. Hou, N. Ialongo, and B. Guyer. 2007. Healthy Steps for Young Children: Sustained results at 5.5 years. *Pediatrics* 120(3):e658–e668.

Mishra, S. I., D. Gioia, S. Childress, B. Barnet, and R. L. Webster. 2011. Adherence to medication regimens among low-income patients with multiple comorbid chronic conditions. *Health & Social Work* 36(4):249–258.

Morone, J. 2017. An integrative review of social determinants of health assessment and screening tools used in pediatrics. *Journal of Pediatric Nursing* 37:22–28.

Mosher, W. D., J. Jones, and J. C. Abma. 2012. Intended and unintended births in the United States: 1982–2010. *National Health Statistics Reports* 55:1–28.

Muoto, I., J. Luck, J. Yoon, S. Bernell, and J. M. Snowden. 2016. Oregon's coordinated care organizations increased timely prenatal care initiation and decreased disparities. *Health Affairs* 35(9):1625–1632.

Murphy, S. L., J. Xu, K. D. Kocharek, and E. Arias. 2018. *Mortality in the United States, 2017. NCHS Data Brief No. 328.* Hyattsville, MD: U.S. Department of Health and Human Services, Centers for Disease Control and Prevention, National Center for Health Statistics.

Musumeci, M., R. Rudowitz, E. Hinton, L. Antonisse, and C. Hall. 2018. Section 1115 *Medicaid demonstration waivers: The current landscape of approved and pending waivers. Issue brief.* Kaiser Family Foundation. https://www.kff.org/medicaid/issue-brief/section-1115-medicaid-demonstration-waivers-the-current-landscape-of-approved-and-pending-waivers (accessed January 10, 2019).

NASEM (National Academies of Sciences, Engineering, and Medicine). 2015. *Mental disorders and disabilities among low-income children.* Washington, DC: The National Academies Press.

NASEM. 2016. *Parenting matters: Supporting parents of children ages 0–8.* Washington, DC: The National Academies Press.

NASEM. 2017. *Communities in action: Pathways to health equity.* Washington, DC: The National Academies Press.

NASEM. 2018. *Opportunities for improving programs and services for children with disabilities.* Washington, DC: The National Academies Press.

NASEM. 2019. *The promise of adolescence: Realizing opportunity for all youth.* Washington, DC: The National Academies Press.

Nath, J. B., S. Costigan, and R. Y. Hsia. 2016. Changes in demographics of patients seen at federally qualified health centers, 2005–2014. *JAMA Internal Medicine* 176(5):712–714.

NCDHHS (North Carolina Department of Health and Human Services). n.d. *Early childhood action plan.* https://www.ncdhhs.gov/about/department-initiatives/early-childhood/early-childhood-action-plan (accessed May 9, 2019).

NCQA (National Committee for Quality Assurance). 2018. *Prenatal and postpartum care (PPC).* https://www.ncqa.org/hedis/measures/prenatal-and-postpartum-care-ppc (accessed February 6, 2019).

NCQA. n.d. *Accounting for socioeconomic status in HEDIS measures.* https://www.ncqa.org/hedis/reports-and-research/hedis-and-the-impact-act (accessed June 20, 2019).

Newacheck, P. W., P. P. Budetti, and N. Halfon. 1986. Trends in activity-limiting chronic conditions among children. *American Journal of Public Health* 76(2):178–184.

NICHQ (National Institute for Children's Health Quality). 2016. *Promoting young children's (ages 0–3) socioemotional development in primary care.* Boston, MA: National Institute for Children's Health Quality.

NICHQ. n.d. *Monitoring, data, & evaluation.* https://www.healthystartepic.org/healthy-start-implementation/monitoring-data-and-evaluation (accessed July 19, 2019).

NIH (National Institutes of Health). 1989. *Caring for our future: The content of prenatal care. A report of the Public Health Service Expert Panel on the Content of Prenatal Care.* Bethesda, MD: National Institutes of Health.

NQF (National Quality Forum). 2016. *Perinatal and reproductive health 2015–2016. Final report.* Washington, DC: National Quality Forum.

NY (New York) Department of Health. 2017. *Value-based payment for children: Report to the NYS Medicaid VBP Workgroup.* New York: New York Department of Health.

Olson, C. A., S. D. McSwain, A. L. Curfman, and J. Chuo. 2018. The current pediatric telehealth landscape. *Pediatrics* 141(3):e20172334.

O'Malley, J., M. O'Keeffe-Rossetti, R. Lowe, H. Angier, R. Gold, M. Marino, B. Hatch, M. Hoopes, S. Bailey, J. Heintzman, C. Gallia, and J. DeVoe. 2016. Health care utilization rates after Oregon's 2008 Medicaid expansion: Within-group and between-group differences over time among new, returning, and continuously insured enrollees. *Medical Care Research and Review* 54(11):984–991.

Opray, N., R. M. Grivell, A. R. Deussen, and J. M. Dodd. 2015. Directed preconception health programs and interventions for improving pregnancy outcomes for women who are overweight or obese. *Cochrane Database of Systematic Reviews* 7:CD010932.

Oregon Health Authority. 2018. *CCO 2.0 Recommendations of the Oregon Health Policy Board.* Portland, OR: Oregon Health Authority Health Policy and Analytics Division.

Osterman, M. J. K., and J. A. Martin. 2018. Timing and adequacy of prenatal care in the United States, 2016. *National Vital Statistics Reports* 67(3):1–14.

Padarthy, S., K. Knudson, and S. Vattikuti. 2019. *The social determinants of health: Applying AI and machine learning to achieve whole person care.* Teaneck, NJ: Cognizant Digital Business.

Pai, N., S. Kandasamy, E. Uleryk, and J. L. Maguire. 2016. Social risk screening for pediatric inpatients. *Clinical Pediatrics* 55(14):1289–1294.

Palmer, L., A. Cook, and B. Courtot. 2010. Comparing models of maternity care serving women at risk of poor birth outcomes in Washington, DC. *Alternative Therapies in Health and Medicine* 16(5):48–56.

Park, E. H. M., and G. Dimigen. 1995. A cross-cultural comparison: Postnatal depression in Korean and Scottish mothers. *Psychologia* 38(3):199–207.

Pastor, P. N., C. A. Reuben, and C. R. Duran. 2015. *Reported child health status, Hispanic ethnicity, and language of interview: United States, 2011–2012. National health statistics reports; No. 82.* Hyattsville, MD: National Center for Health Statistics.

Patient-Centered Primary Care Collaborative. n.d. *Defining the medical home.* https://www.pcpcc.org/about/medical-home (accessed June 5, 2019).

Perrin, J. M. 2012. How can quality improvement enhance the lives of children with disabilities? *The Future of Children* 22(1):149–168.

Perrin, J. M., and T. G. Dewitt. 2011. Future of academic general pediatrics—areas of opportunity. *Academic Pediatrics* 11(3):181–188.

Perrin, J. M., M. W. Shayne, and S. R. Bloom. 1993. *Home and community care for chronically ill children.* New York: Oxford University Press.

Perrin, J. M., L. E. Anderson, and J. Van Cleave. 2014. The rise in chronic conditions among infants, children, and youth can be met with continued health system innovations. *Health Affairs* 33(12):2099–2105.

Perrin, J. M., E. Zimmerman, A. Hertz, T. Johnson, T. Merrill, and D. Smith. 2017. Pediatric accountable care organizations: Insight from early adopters. *Pediatrics* 139(2):e20161840.

Perrin, J. M., J. R. Asarnow, T. Stancin, S. P. Melek, and G. K. Fritz. 2019. Mental health conditions and health care payments for children with chronic medical conditions. *Academic Pediatrics* 19(1):44–50.

Picklesimer, A. H., D. Billings, N. Hale, D. Blackhurst, and S. Covington-Kolb. 2012. The effect of CenteringPregnancy group prenatal care on preterm birth in a low-income population. *American Journal of Obstetrics and Gynecology* 206(5):415.e411–415.e417.

Pillsbury, B. L. 1978. Doing the month: Confinement and convalescence of Chinese women after childbirth. *Social Science and Medicine* 12(1B):11–22.

Piper, J. M., E. F. Mitchel, Jr., and W. A. Ray. 1994. Presumptive eligibility for pregnant Medicaid enrollees: Its effects on prenatal care and perinatal outcome. *American Journal of Public Health* 84(10):1626–1630.

Poels, M., M. P. Koster, H. R. Boeije, A. Franx, and H. F. van Stel. 2016. Why do women not use preconception care? A systematic review on barriers and facilitators. *Obstetrical & Gynecological Survey* 71(10):603–612.

Radcliffe, J., D. Schwarz, and H. Zhao. 2013. The MOM Program: Home visiting in partnership with pediatric care. *Pediatrics* 132(Suppl 2):S153–S159.

Robbins, C., S. L. Boulet, I. Morgan, D. V. D'Angelo, L. B. Zapata, B. Morrow, A. Sharma, and C. D. Kroelinger. 2018. Disparities in preconception health indicators—Behavioral Risk Factor Surveillance System, 2013–2015, and Pregnancy Risk Assessment Monitoring System, 2013–2014. *Morbidity and Mortality Weekly Report Surveillance Summaries* 67(1):1–16.

Ross, L., and R. Solinger. 2017. *Reproductive justice: An introduction.* Vol. 1. Oakland, CA: University of California Press.

Rossin-Slater, M., and L. Uniat. 2019. *Paid family leave policies and population health.* Health policy brief. Bethesda, MD: Health Affairs.

Rudowitz, R., M. Musumeci, and C. Hall. 2019. *February state data for Medicaid work requirements in Arkansas.* Washington, DC: Kaiser Family Foundation.

Rushton, F. E., W. W. Byrne, P. M. Darden, and J. McLeigh. 2015. Enhancing child safety and well-being through pediatric group well-child care and home visitation: The Well Baby Plus Program. *Child Abuse and Neglect* 41:182–189.

Saha, S., M. C. Beach, and L. A. Cooper. 2008. Patient centeredness, cultural competence and healthcare quality. *JAMA* 100(11):1275–1285.

Sandel, M., M. Hansen, R. Kahn, E. Lawton, E. Paul, V. Parker, S. Morton, and B. Zuckerman. 2010. Medical-legal partnerships: Transforming primary care by addressing the legal needs of vulnerable populations. *Health Affairs* 29(9):1697–1705.

Sarvet, B., J. Gold, J. Q. Bostic, B. J. Masek, J. B. Prince, M. Jeffers-Terry, C. F. Moore, B. Molbert, and J. H. Straus. 2010. Improving access to mental health care for children: The Massachusetts Child Psychiatry Access Project. *Pediatrics* 126(6):1191–1200.

Schwarz, E. B., S. M. Parisi, S. M. Handler, G. Koren, G. Shevchik, and G. S. Fischer. 2013. Counseling about medication-induced birth defects with clinical decision support in primary care. *Journal of Women's Health* 22(10):817–824.

Sege, R. D., and L. Amaya-Jackson. 2017. Clinical considerations related to the behavioral manifestations of child maltreatment. *Pediatrics* 139(4):e2017010.

Sege, R., G. Preer, S. J. Morton, H. Cabral, O. Morakinyo, V. Lee, C. Abreu, E. De Vos, and M. Kaplan-Sanoff. 2015. Medical-legal strategies to improve infant health care: A randomized trial. *Pediatrics* 136(1):97–106.

Shekarchi, A., L. Gantz, and A. Schickedanz. 2018. Social determinant of health screening in a safety net pediatric primary care clinic. *Pediatrics* 142(1 Meeting Abstract):748.

Silva, R., M. Thomas, R. Caetano, and C. Aragaki. 2006. Preventing low birth weight in Illinois: Outcomes of the family case management program. *Maternal and Child Health Journal* 10(6):481–488.

Silverstein, M., C. Mack, N. Reavis, T. D. Koepsell, G. S. Gross, and D. C. Grossman. 2004. Effect of a clinic-based referral system to Head Start: A randomized controlled trial. *JAMA* 292(8):968–971.

Skogen, J. C., and S. Overland. 2012. The fetal origins of adult disease: A narrative review of the epidemiological literature. *Journal of the Royal Medical Society Short Reports* 3(8):59.

Smith, A. J. B., and A. T. Chien. 2019. Adult-oriented health reform and children's insurance and access to care: Evidence from Massachusetts health reform. *Maternal and Child Health Journal* 23(8):1008–1024.

Smith, R., S. Dobbins, A. Evans, K. Balhotra, and R. A. Dicker. 2013. Hospital-based violence intervention: Risk reduction resources that are essential for success. *Journal of Trauma and Acute Care Surgery* 74(4):976–980; discussion 980–982.

Solotaroff, R., J. Devoe, B. J. Wright, J. Smith, J. Boone, T. Edlund, and M. J. Carlson. 2005. Medicaid programme changes and the chronically ill: Early results from a prospective cohort study of the Oregon Health Plan. *Chronic Illness* 1(3):191–205.

Sommers, B. D., S. K. Long, and K. Baicker. 2015. Changes in mortality after Massachusetts health care reform. *Annals of Internal Medicine* 162(9):668–669.

Sommers, B. D., R. J. Blendon, E. J. Orav, and A. M. Epstein. 2016. Changes in utilization and health among low-income adults after Medicaid expansion or expanded private insurance. *JAMA Internal Medicine* 176(10):1501–1509.

Sommers, B. D., A. A. Gawande, and K. Baicker. 2017a. Health insurance coverage and health—what the recent evidence tells us. *New England Journal of Medicine* 377(6):586–593.

Sommers, B. D., B. Maylone, R. J. Blendon, E. J. Orav, and A. M. Epstein. 2017b. Three-year impacts of the Affordable Care Act: Improved medical care and health among low-income adults. *Health Affairs* 36(6):1119–1128.

Sommers, B. D., A. L. Goldman, R. J. Blendon, E. J. Orav, and A. M. Epstein. 2019. Medicaid work requirements—Results from the first year in Arkansas. Special report, June 19. *New England Journal of Medicine.* https://www.nejm.org/doi/full/10.1056/NEJMsr1901772 (accessed July 19, 2019).

Sonfield, A. 2017. Why protecting Medicaid means protecting sexual and reproductive health. In *Guttmacher Policy Review*, Vol. 20. Washington, DC: Guttmacher Institute.

Stancin, T., and E. C. Perrin. 2014. Psychologists and pediatricians: Opportunities for collaboration in primary care. *American Psychologist* 69(4):332–343.

Stecker, E. C. 2013. The Oregon ACO experiment—bold design, challenging execution. *New England Journal of Medicine* 368(11):982–985.

Stern, A. M. 2005. *Eugenic nation: Faults and frontiers of better breeding in modern America*, 1st ed. Berkeley, CA; Los Angeles, CA; London, UK: University of California Press.

Steuerle, C. E., and J. B. Isaacs. 2014. The scheduled squeeze on children's programs: Tracking the implications of projected federal spending patterns. *Health Affairs* 33(12):2214–2221.

Stille, C., R. M. Turchi, R. Antonelli, M. D. Cabana, T. L. Cheng, D. Laraque, J. Perrin, and Academic Pediatric Association Task Force on Family-Centered Medical Home. 2010. The family-centered medical home: Specific considerations for child health research and policy. *Academic Pediatrics* 10(4):211–217.

Stockwell, M. S., E. O. Kharbanda, R. A. Martinez, C. Y. Vargas, D. K. Vawdrey, and S. Camargo. 2012. Effect of a text messaging intervention on influenza vaccination in an urban, low-income pediatric and adolescent population: A randomized controlled trial. *JAMA* 307(16):1702–1708.

Straus, J. H., and B. Sarvet. 2014. Behavioral health care for children: The Massachusetts Child Psychiatry Access Project. *Health Affairs* 33(12):2153–2161.

Stuebe, A., J. E. Moore, P. Mittal, L. Reddy, L. K. Low, and H. Brown. 2019. Extending Medicaid coverage for postpartum moms. *Health Affairs Blog*, https://www.healthaffairs.org/do/10.1377/hblog20190501.254675/full (accessed June 12, 2019).

Suglia, S. F., K. C. Koenen, R. Boynton-Jarrett, P. S. Chan, C. J. Clark, A. Danese, M. S. Faith, B. I. Goldstein, L. L. Hayman, C. R. Isasi, C. A. Pratt, N. Slopen, J. A. Sumner, A. Turer, C. B. Turer, and J. P. Zachariah. 2018. Childhood and adolescent adversity and cardiometabolic outcomes: A scientific statement from the American Heart Association. *Circulation* 137(5):e15–e28.

Szilagyi, M., B. D. Kerker, A. Storfer-Isser, R. E. Stein, A. Garner, K. G. O'Connor, K. E. Hoagwood, and S. McCue Horwitz. 2016. Factors associated with whether pediatricians inquire about parents' adverse childhood experiences. *Academic Pediatrics* 16(7):668–675.

Taffel, S. 1978. *Prenatal care, United States, 1969–1975. DHEW Publication No. (PHS) 78-1911.* Hyattsville, MD: U.S. Department of Health, Education, and Welfare, Public Health Service, National Center for Health Statistics.

Tanner-Smith, E. E., K. T. Steinka-Fry, and M. W. Lipsey. 2014. The effects of CenteringPregnancy group prenatal care on gestational age, birth weight, and fetal demise. *Maternal and Child Health Journal* 18(4):801–809.

Team Up for Children. n.d. *Team Up for Children.* www.teamupforchildren.org (accessed April 16, 2019).

The Lancet. 2018. Campaigning for preconception health. *The Lancet* 391(10132):1749.

Thich, C. B. N. 2016. Doula support as a means to improve birth outcomes for minority women. *Master's Projects and Capstones 477.* https://repository.usfca.edu/capstone/477 (accessed April 12, 2019).

Thiel de Bocanegra, H., M. Braughton, M. Bradsberry, M. Howell, J. Logan, and E. B. Schwarz. 2017. Racial and ethnic disparities in postpartum care and contraception in California's Medicaid program. *American Journal of Obstetrics & Gynecology* 217(1):47. e41–47.e47.

Thielen, K. 2012. Exploring the group prenatal care model: A critical review of the literature. *The Journal of Perinatal Education* 21(4):209–218.

Tieu, J., E. Shepherd, P. Middleton, and C. A. Crowther. 2017a. Interconception care for women with a history of gestational diabetes for improving maternal and infant outcomes. *Cochrane Database of Systematic Reviews* 8:CD010211.

Tieu, J., P. Middleton, C. A. Crowther, and E. Shepherd. 2017b. Preconception care for diabetic women for improving maternal and infant health. *Cochrane Database of Systematic Reviews* 8:CD007776.

Too, G., T. Wen, A. K. Boehme, E. C. Miller, L. R. Leffert, F. J. Attenello, W. J. Mack, M. E. D'Alton, and A. M. Friedman. 2018. Timing and risk factors of postpartum stroke. *Obstetrics & Gynecology* 131(1):70–78.

Torpy, S. J. 2000. Native American women and coerced sterilization: On the Trail of Tears in the 1970s. *American Indian Culture and Research Journal* 24(2):1–22.

Trivette, C. M., and C. J. Dunst. 2014. *Community-based parent support programs.* http://www.child-encyclopedia.com/parenting-skills/according-experts/community-based-parent-support-programs (accessed January 30, 2019).

Tumin, D., R. Miller, V. T. Raman, J. C. Uffman, and J. D. Tobias. 2019. Patterns of health insurance discontinuity and children's access to health care. *Maternal and Child Health Journal* 23(5):667–677.

Turner Lee, N. 2018. Detecting racial bias in algorithms and machine learning. *Journal of Information, Communication and Ethics in Society* 16(3):252–260.

United Hospital Fund. 2018. *UHF and New York State partner to benefit youngest children.* https://uhfnyc.org/news/article/uhf-and-new-york-state-partner-to-benefit-youngest-children (accessed May 9, 2019).

U.S. Census Bureau. 2017. *CPS table creator [data tool].* https://www.census.gov/cps/data/cpstablecreator.html (accessed July 16, 2019).

Van Buren, R. 2018. *State approaches to financing social interventions through Medicaid.* https://www.macpac.gov/wp-content/uploads/2018/04/State-Approaches-to-Financing-Social-Interventions-through-Medicaid.pdf (accessed June 25, 2019).

Van Cleave, J., A. A. Boudreau, J. McAllister, W. C. Cooley, A. Maxwell, and K. Kuhlthau. 2015. Care coordination over time in medical homes for children with special health care needs. *Pediatrics* 135(6):1018–1026.

Vedam, S., K. Stoll, M. MacDorman, E. Declercq, R. Cramer, M. Cheyney, T. Fisher, E. Butt, Y. T. Yang, and H. Powell Kennedy. 2018. Mapping integration of midwives across the United States: Impact on access, equity, and outcomes. *PLoS ONE* 13(2):e0192523.

Verbiest, S., E. McClain, and S. Woodward. 2016. Advancing preconception health in the United States: Strategies for change. *Upsala Journal of Medical Sciences* 121(4):222–226.

Veugelers, P. J., and A. M. Yip. 2003. Socioeconomic disparities in health care use: Does universal coverage reduce inequalities in health? *Journal of Epidemiology and Community Health* 57(6):424–428.

Vonderheid, S. C., K. F. Norr, and A. S. Handler. 2007. Prenatal health promotion content and health behaviors. *Western Journal of Nursing Research* 29(3):258–276, discussion 277–283.

Waggoner, M. R. 2013. Motherhood preconceived: The emergence of the Preconception Health and Health Care Initiative. *Journal of Health Politics, Policy and Law* 38(2):345–371.

Wallace, J., and B. Sommers. 2016. Health insurance effects on preventive care and health: A methodological review. *American Journal of Preventive Medicine* 50(5 Suppl 1):S27–S33.

Weinick, R. M., and N. A. Krauss. 2000. Racial/ethnic differences in children's access to care. *American Journal of Public Health* 90(11):1771–1774.

Wherry, L., G. Kenney, and B. Sommers. 2016. The role of public health insurance in reducing child poverty. *Academic Pediatrics* 16(Suppl 3):S98–S104.

Whitworth, M., and T. Dowswell. 2009. Routine pre-pregnancy health promotion for improving pregnancy outcomes. *Cochrane Database of Systematic Reviews* 4:CD007536.

WHO (World Health Organization). n.d. *Chronic diseases and health promotion.* https://www.who.int/chp/chronic_disease_report/part2_ch2/en (accessed July 19, 2019).

Williams, S. G., C. M. Brown, K. H. Falter, C. J. Alverson, C. Gotway-Crawford, D. Homa, D. S. Jones, E. K. Adams, and S. C. Redd. 2006. Does a multifaceted environmental intervention alter the impact of asthma on inner-city children? *JAMA* 98(2):249–260.

Women's Preventive Services Initiative. n.d. *Well-woman preventive visits.* https://www.womenspreventivehealth.org/recommendations/well-woman-preventive-visits (accessed January 10, 2019).

Wong, C. A., J. M. Perrin, and M. McClellan. 2018. Making the case for value-based payment reform in children's health care. *JAMA Pediatrics* 172(6):513–514.

Woolf, S. H. 2019. Necessary but not sufficient: Why health care alone cannot improve population health and reduce health inequities. *Annals of Family Medicine* 17(3):196–199.

Yamauchi, M., M. J. Carlson, B. J. Wright, H. Angier, and J. E. DeVoe. 2013. Does health insurance continuity among low-income adults impact their children's insurance coverage? *Maternal and Child Health Journal* 17(2):248–255.

Yogman, M., and C. F. Garfield. 2016. Fathers' roles in the care and development of their children: The role of pediatricians. *Pediatrics* 138(1):e20161128.

Zero to Three. 2017. *HealthySteps evidence summary.* Washington, DC: Zero to Three.

Zero to Three. n.d.-a. *Become a site.* https://www.healthysteps.org/become-a-site (accessed July 18, 2019).

Zero to Three. n.d.-b. *National and site-level evaluations.* https://www.healthysteps.org/article/national-and-site-level-evaluations-9 (accessed May 8, 2019).

6

Creating Healthy Living Conditions
for Early Development

MEETING FUNDAMENTAL NEEDS TO SUPPORT
PRENATAL AND EARLY CHILDHOOD DEVELOPMENT

I am trying to get gainful employment. . . . We all have that same thing in common of trying to do better for ourselves, trying to turn things around and do the right thing. But it's hard, it's hard because the resources that are available to us—we don't know about them, we are not aware of them, we don't know how to connect to the resources that are available to us. —Parent on caregiver panel[1]

As described in earlier chapters, a child's most proximal influence in early development is the family unit, specifically the primary caregiver. Chapter 4 provides an overview of what children need from caregiver relationships and the critical role those relationships play for children to have the opportunity to flourish and thrive. However, these relationships do not exist in a vacuum, and neither do families—they are shaped by the social determinants of health (SDOH), as laid out in Chapter 3 (see also Figure 1-9). Families exist within the context of their communities, and all children need safe and healthy communities that promote optimal development. Healthy communities continuously create and improve physical and social environments and expand community resources that enable people to mutually support each other in daily life and in developing

---

[1] This quote is from a public meeting of the committee, held on October 1, 2018. The meeting webcast is available at www.nationalacademies.org/earlydevelopment (accessed July 29, 2019).

BOX 6-1
Chapter in Brief: Creating Healthy Living Conditions

Addressing the fundamental needs of families and children (i.e., economic stability, food security, and a safe and healthy living environment) is critical to achieving health and well-being during the prenatal through early childhood periods. This chapter identifies programs, policies, and systems changes that the committee concluded have the most evidence and promise for improving health and well-being outcomes for children and their caregivers, in addition to reducing disparities.
Chapter conclusions in brief:

- Increasing the economic resources families have available to meet basic needs when children are young (including prenatally) will improve children's health.
- Public programs that provide economic resources to families in the form of cash, tax credits, or in-kind benefits improve child health and development outcomes, which have long-lasting effects on health and educational outcomes.
- Income-support programs that are contingent on employment status or based on earned income have positive benefits for families yet may also have unintended consequences for child health and development outcomes through negative effects on attachment, breastfeeding, and caregiver stress. Thus, it is important to supplement work-support programs with basic support for families with young children that is not tied to employment.
- Given the importance of good nutrition for brain growth and development, providing resources to ensure families have access to sufficient and healthy foods can improve birth outcomes and child health outcomes.
- Child lead poisoning continues to be a pervasive problem in the United States. There are many effective programs and policies that, if implemented and funded, would prevent, or mitigate the impact of, lead poisoning prenatally and in early childhood.
- Healthy early development cannot occur without safe and stable housing. Lack of affordable housing and environmental hazards in housing disrupt healthy childhood development and parent/caregiver well-being.

to their maximum potential (CDC, 2009). Chapter 4 also makes the case that it is essential to mitigate caregiver stress so that caregivers have the capacity and supports to care for their children and to serve as buffers against adversities. (See Box 6-1 for an overview of this chapter. See Chapter 2 for a brief discussion of the biological mechanisms of buffering and Chapter 3 for discussion of the importance of stable and nurturing relationships.)

This chapter addresses the fundamental needs of families and children that are critical to achieving health and well-being. In the report conceptual framework (see Figure 1-9), these are the "healthy living conditions" situated in the second outermost circle, along with health systems and services (see Chapter 5) and early care and education (ECE) (see Chapter 7). Healthy living conditions are made up of the SDOH, or

- Lack of housing affordability and quality is an acute problem that dispro-portionately impacts people of color and contributes to health disparities among children.
- Current federal housing programs are not adequately funded, and there are not enough safe, affordable housing units in high-opportunity areas.
- Not all households experience the same level of risk of exposure to harmful environmental toxicants or pollutants. Poverty, substandard and/or unstable housing, race and ethnicity, and proximity to known sources of pollutants heighten pregnant women and children's risk of exposure and poor health and developmental outcomes.

Chapter recommendations in brief:

- Implement paid parental leave.
- Reduce barriers to participation to Special Supplemental Nutrition Program for Women, Infants, and Children and Supplemental Nutrition Assistance Program (SNAP) benefits; do not tie these benefits to parent employment for families with young children or for pregnant women.
- Increase the supply of high-quality, affordable housing that is available to families.
- Develop a comprehensive plan to ensure access to stable, affordable, and safe housing in the prenatal through early childhood periods.
- Test new Medicaid payment models that engage providers and other com-munity organizations in addressing housing safety concerns, especially those focused on young children.
- Address the critical gaps between family resources and family needs through a combination of benefits that have the best evidence of advancing health equity, such as a combination of increased SNAP benefits, increased housing assistance, and a basic allowance for young children.
- Support and enforce efforts to prevent and mitigate the impact of environmental toxicants during the preconception through early childhood periods.

more specifically, the social, economic, environmental, and cultural drivers of health and well-being. These determinants are interdependent, and together, they create conditions that influence child health and the ability of a caregiver to fulfill a child's basic needs for healthy development.

Based on the core scientific findings in this report, this chapter seeks to address the challenges—for example, the barriers highlighted in the quote that opened this chapter—caregivers face with respect to securing economic stability and a safe and healthy living environment during the prenatal through early childhood periods. The committee reviewed promising community-level models and policy opportunities that focus on key neurobiological and socio-behavioral mechanisms needed for healthy development that yield the greatest impact to both mitigate and forestall the impacts of early life adversities on health.

Systems changes are needed to target multiple SDOH that shape early development and well-being. Systems that children interact with are most effective when they take into account developmental science and evidence when they are created, thereby meeting children's developmental needs. There are changes that could be made based on this science to existing policies that would make them more responsive to the needs of children. The recommendations in this chapter aim to provide predictability and security in the lives of children and their families through ensuring economic stability and a healthy and safe living environment. While the chapter takes a social determinants approach to addressing early living conditions, it should be noted that there are some important contextual factors that are not discussed here. For example, research shows that factors such as public transit, access to parks and green space, and mass incarceration all shape inequities for children and families (see, for example, NASEM, 2017; Wildeman and Wang, 2017); however, these areas of programs, policies, and systems are not the focus of the solutions discussed in this report. The primary focus here is on the programs, policies, and systems changes that the committee has identified as having the most evidence and promise for improving health and well-being outcomes for children and their caregivers, in addition to reducing disparities. The chapter includes discussions of the existing evidence and committee recommendations for solutions to address economic stability and security, food security and nutrition, housing, neighborhood conditions, and environmental exposures and exposure to toxicants.

ECONOMIC STABILITY AND SECURITY

Children's well-being and future health outcomes are strongly related to family income, and as the review in Chapter 3 shows, poverty is associated with significant detrimental effects on children's health, development, and well-being. A systematic review of the literature concluded that the evidence supports the conclusion that the link between income and child outcomes is causal; that is, "money makes a difference in children's outcomes" (Cooper and Stewart, 2013). The study also finds evidence that money in early childhood is important, particularly for cognitive outcomes. Thus, reductions in childhood experiences of poverty, and increasing the resources available to families to meet their basic needs, would be expected to improve children's health and developmental outcomes.

Given the substantial evidence that money matters, an important factor in reducing health disparities in early childhood is to ensure that families with young children have sufficient resources. As the Council of Economic Advisers points out, current policies and public programs provide much less support for families when children are young compared to when they are school age, despite the needs and lower financial wherewithal, on average, of families with younger children (CEA, 2014). In this section, the committee reviews the evidence about U.S. safety net programs that are intended to increase financial resources of families with children through cash transfers or tax credits. In the following paragraphs, the committee assesses programs that provide targeted benefits to address food or housing shortfalls and programs to address neighborhood conditions. To retain a reasonable scope, the focus is on the largest safety net programs run by federal and state governments that are offered to families with young children or pregnant women, while acknowledging that local governments, nonprofit organizations, and religious organizations also provide resources to help families in need.

Furthermore, the committee acknowledges the importance of providing parents and other caregivers with pathways to sustained economic security, such as educational opportunities and workforce development training. Chapter 3, for example, highlights the salience of parental educational attainment and household income as determinants of child health, well-being, and educational outcomes. Thus, an approach that enhances educational and economic opportunities and ultimately financial sustainability for caregivers would benefit children and families. Community-based programs that promote economic well-being for families are one promising avenue for advancing economic security. One such example is the Dudley Street Neighborhood Initiative's Fair Chance for Family Success—funded by the Boston Promise Initiative in partnership with the Family Independence Initiative. This is a peer-to-peer financial literacy and learning program, which reports improved outcomes for participating families in terms of amount of money in savings accounts, checking accounts, total assets, and subsidy income (NASEM, 2017). Similarly, programs that enable workforce participation or retention could also help families get on a path to economic security. WorkAdvance is one program that allows employers to place individuals with moderate job skills into training programs for specific sectors that have high demand for local workers (NASEM, 2019). Evaluation data for this program suggested large increases in workforce participation, training completion, and credential acquisition at a 2-year follow-up (Hendra et al., 2016). While these types of programs are relevant to promoting healthy early development, the committee's approach in this report was to limit its scope to program, practice, and policy changes that had the strongest evidence for direct impacts on children and their well-being. Therefore, the committee did not include in-depth discussion of these types of economic and workforce support programs for caregivers in this chapter.

Policies and programs aimed at reducing the impact of poverty on children's health and well-being may provide cash benefits (directly, or indirectly through tax credits) or noncash or "in-kind" benefits, such as vouchers to buy food or housing. Alternatively, some programs directly provide food, housing, or education. This section first describes antipoverty programs designed to increase the level of (cash) resources families have, focusing on the two largest direct cash grant programs, Temporary Assistance for Needy Families (TANF) and Supplemental Security Income (SSI), and then on tax credits, focusing on the Earned Income Tax Credit (EITC) and the Child Tax Credits (CTCs). Next, paid parental leave is discussed as another option for supporting families' needs when children are young. The committee examined the evidence on the extent to which these programs (1) increase cash resources and thereby reduce poverty, (2) are associated with improved child health and development, including prenatal and birth outcomes, and (3) are associated with longer-term health,

---

BOX 6-2
Relevant Conclusions from *A Roadmap to Reducing Child Poverty* (2019)[a]

1. Poverty alleviation can promote children's development, both because of the goods and services that parents can buy for their children and because it may promote a more responsive, less stressful environment in which more positive parent–child interactions can take place.
2. Some children are resilient to a number of the adverse impacts of poverty, but many studies show significant associations between poverty and child maltreatment, adverse childhood experiences (ACEs), increased material hardship, worse physical health, low birth weight (LBW), structural changes in brain development, mental health problems, decreased educational attainment, and increased risky behaviors, delinquency, and criminal behavior in adolescence and adulthood. As for the timing and severity of poverty, the literature documents that poverty in early childhood, prolonged poverty, and deep poverty are all associated with worse child and adult outcomes.
3. Periodic increases in the generosity of the Earned Income Tax Credit (EITC) program have improved children's educational and health outcomes.
4. Supplemental Nutrition Assistance Program (SNAP) has been shown to improve birth outcomes and many important child and adult health outcomes.
5. The weight of the causal evidence indicates that income poverty itself causes negative child outcomes, especially when it begins in early childhood and/or persists throughout a large share of a child's life. Many programs that alleviate poverty either directly, by providing income transfers, or indirectly, by providing food, housing, or medical care, have been shown to improve child well-being.
6. Government tax and transfer programs modestly reduced the child poverty rate, defined by the Supplemental Poverty Measure (SPM), between 1967 and 1993 but became increasingly important after 1993 because of increases in government benefits targeted at poor and nearly poor. Between 1993 and 2016, SPM poverty fell by 12.3 percentage points, from 27.9 to 15.6 percent, more than twice as much as market-income-based poverty.
7. A number of other program and policy options lead to substantial reductions in poverty and deep poverty. Two involve existing programs—SNAP and housing vouchers. The option of a 40 percent increase in EITC benefits would also reduce child poverty substantially.

educational, and economic outcomes. Throughout this section, the committee explores concerns about the strength of the evidence and the possibility of unintended consequences of these programs (which might directly or indirectly impact children's health). The committee's conclusions and recommendations build off those made in the National Academies report *A Roadmap to Reducing Child Poverty* (NASEM, 2019), which provides a thorough analysis of the evidence for approaches to alleviate child poverty. Box 6-2 contains the conclusions from that report that are relevant to and informed this committee's conclusions and recommendations.

8. The 20 program and policy options [that the committee considered] generate disparate impacts across population subgroups in our simulations[a] Although virtually all of them would reduce poverty across all the subgroups we considered, disproportionately large decreases in child poverty occur only for black children and children of mothers with low levels of education. Hispanic children and immigrant children would benefit relatively less.

9. Two program and policy packages developed by the [Poverty Roadmap] committee met its mandated 50 percent reduction in both child poverty (defined as 100 percent of SPM) and deep poverty (defined as 50 percent of SPM). The first of these packages combines work-oriented policy expansions with increases in benefit levels in the housing voucher and SNAP. The second package combines work-oriented expansions with a child allowance, a child support assurance program, and elimination of immigrant restrictions on benefits built into the 1996 welfare reforms. Both packages increase work and earnings, and both are estimated to cost between $90 and $111 billion per year.

10. The committee was unable to formulate an evidence-based employment-oriented package that would come close to meeting its mandate of reducing child poverty by 50 percent. The best package it could design combines expansions of the EITC, the Child and Dependent Care Tax Credit, a minimum-wage increase, and a promising career development program. Although this package is estimated to add more than a million workers to the labor force, generate $18 billion in additional earnings, and cost the government only $8.6–$9.3 billion annually, its estimated reductions in child poverty are less than half of what is needed to meet the goal.

11. There is insufficient evidence to identify mandatory work policies that would reliably reduce child poverty, and it appears that work requirements are at least as likely to increase as to decrease poverty. The dearth of evidence also reflects underinvestment over the past two decades in methodologically strong evaluations of the impacts of alternative work programs.

---

[a] The charge of the National Academies committee that wrote the *A Roadmap to Reducing Child Poverty* report was to identify policies and programs that have the potential to reduce child poverty and deep poverty in the United States by half within 10 years. The committee examined 10 program and policy options. Four of them are tied to work, three of them modify existing safety net programs, two come from other countries, and the final one modifies existing provisions relating to immigrants. The committee then formulated two variations for each of the 10 options, yielding 20 scenarios in all.
SOURCE: NASEM, 2019.

Cash Assistance Programs (TANF, SSI)

TANF provides cash assistance and sometimes other supports, such as job search support or child care subsidies, for eligible families with dependent children. Because TANF is a block grant, each state establishes its own eligibility rules, determines the type and amount of assistance to be provided, and sets other requirements and services (within broad federal guidelines). TANF participation is time limited and is intended to promote economic self-sufficiency, work, and marriage (HHS, 2012). In fiscal year 2018, 1.2 million families and nearly 2.4 million children received TANF assistance on average each month (ACF Office of Family Assistance, 2019). TANF has been a shrinking component of the nation's social safety net for children since the passage in 1996 of the Personal Responsibility and Work Opportunity Reconciliation Act, when Aid to Families with Dependent Children (AFDC) was replaced by TANF. In 1996, 68 percent of low-income families with children received cash assistance through AFDC. In contrast, only 23 percent received TANF cash assistance in 2016 (CBPP, 2018a). In addition to reaching fewer low-income families, the size of grants has fallen in inflation-adjusted terms in most states. TANF benefits for a family of three in the median state were $447 per month in 2018 and have fallen by 20 percent in inflation-adjusted terms since 1996 (CBPP, 2018a). Overall, TANF is much less effective at reducing the severity of poverty than was the AFDC program: 18 percent compared to 56 percent of children moved out of deep poverty after receiving TANF versus AFDC grants (CBPP, 2018a).

Additional sources of direct cash support for families include the SSI for children and U.S. Social Security Administration (SSA) programs. Children "with physical or mental condition(s) that very seriously limit his or her activities" and that last for more than 1 year may qualify for SSI payments, which families can use to pay for basic needs, such as food and housing or medical care. To qualify, children need to meet the program's definition of eligibility and the family needs to have limited income and resources. In May 2019, about 1.1 million children under age 18 received an average monthly SSI payment of $674 (SSA, 2019). Nearly half (45 percent) of low-income families with an SSI recipient were lifted out of poverty by receiving SSI, according to a 2015 National Academies report (NASEM, 2015). Another 4 million children receive benefits through the Social Security program as children of deceased workers (survivor benefits), children of workers with disabilities (through Disability Insurance), or children of retired workers. Summing across these groups, about $3.6 billion flowed to children through SSI and SSA programs (SSA, 2019). It is likely that the bulk of these monies goes to older children rather than those under age eight; nonetheless, for the families receiving these payments, the increase in income helps them to meet basic needs.

These programs (TANF, SSI, and SSA) all have the potential to improve children's health by raising family incomes; however, eligibility is limited, and the size of the assistance provided, especially for TANF, has not kept pace with rising costs of basic needs, particularly of housing. In terms of federal expenditures, the $12 billion of TANF spending on children and $12 billion in SSI for children with disabilities are only a small portion of federal spending on children in low-income families (Hoynes and Schanzenbach, 2018; Isaacs et al., 2017b). See Figure 6-1 for a breakdown of government spending on children by program from 1990 to 2015. The 2019 National Academies report *A Roadmap to Reducing Child Poverty* estimated that reductions in child poverty based on the current TANF program are small because of the low proportion of low-income children receiving TANF and the level of benefits. That report did not include expansion of TANF in the main strategies proposed to reduce

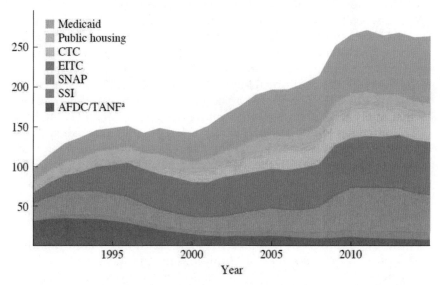

FIGURE 6-1 Government spending on children by program, 1990–2015.
NOTE: AFDC = Aid to Families with Dependent Children; CTC = Child Tax Credit; EITC = Earned Income Tax Credit; SNAP = Supplemental Nutrition Assistance Program; SSI = Supplemental Security Income; TANF = Temporary Assistance for Needy Families.
 [a] AFDC became TANF after the 1996 welfare reform. Dollars reported in billions of 2015 dollars.
SOURCE: Hoynes and Schanzenbach, 2018.

child poverty, primarily due to the lack of evidence and the difficulties of assessing the effects of block grants on child outcomes when states have considerable flexibility in how the money is spent (NASEM, 2019). In contrast, they estimated that the child poverty rate (based on the supplemental poverty measure) would be 1.8 and 2.3 percentage points higher without SSI and SSA benefits, respectively (NASEM, 2019). While these programs (TANF, SSI, and SSA) provide some income support for young children, much more of the spending on children is through tax credits and in-kind assistance for food and housing, which we examine next.

Supporting Children Through Tax Credits

In contrast to cash assistance received on a monthly basis, tax credits represent an alternative financing mechanism for income support. When a family receives a tax credit, the taxes they owe to the government are reduced, and when the tax credit is "refundable," the family receives a payment if the credit exceeds the tax owed. In theory, a tax credit can provide the same amount of income assistance to a family as a direct cash transfer, although in practice, the amount and timing of the payments differ between the two types of mechanisms. Economists generally regard tax credits as having advantages over direct cash transfers in terms of the ease of administering the program (less bureaucracy) and lesser stigma from participation (Nichols and Rothstein, 2016). However, the extra income from a tax credit or refund is typically available only once per year and only if the family files a tax return. The two primary tax credits that apply to U.S. families with young children are the EITC and the CTC, sometimes jointly referred to as working family tax credits. While this section's focus is the federal level, many states offer similar tax credits to working families. In theory, working family tax credits avoid the potential work disincentives of cash transfer programs, and research has demonstrated large increases in labor force participation, particularly for single mothers with children, as a result of the EITC (Nichols and Rothstein, 2016).

The EITC provides a refundable tax credit to eligible families based on earnings, number of children, and marital status. Initially implemented in 1975, the EITC has seen its level and coverage expanded with bipartisan support several times over the past 45 years. The Internal Revenue Service and the U.S. Census Bureau estimate that nationally, between 77 and 80 percent of eligible families claimed the EITC in 2015 (IRS, 2019). Although the take-up rate is high, outreach campaigns and use of tax preparation services or software can help increase the proportion of eligible families who receive the tax credit (Goldin, 2018). In 2016, the average EITC received by families with children was close to \$3,200, which lifted an estimated 3 million children out of poverty and reduced the severity of poverty for nearly 7 million more children (CBPP, 2018c).

The CTC[2] is structured similarly to the EITC as a tax credit that is (partially) refundable. Low- and moderate-income families can claim a tax credit for each of their children up to age 16. The Tax Cuts and Jobs Act of 2018 increased the CTC from \$1,000 to \$2,000 per child, with a maximum of \$1,400 that is refundable. More than 90 percent of American families with children receive the CTC, and the average amount received in 2018 was \$2,420 (per family) (TPC, n.d.). The average credit and share of families receiving the CTC is lower for families in the lowest income quintile because some of these families will not have enough earnings to qualify and the CTC is not fully refundable. Nonetheless, the estimated effect of the CTC on poverty is notable: the Center on Budget and Policy Priorities estimates that the CTC lifted about 1.6 million children out of poverty and reduced the severity of poverty for 6.7 million children in 2017 (CBPP, 2018b). Most families in the second, third, and fourth income quintiles receive the CTC, while those in the lowest bracket benefit less (TPC, n.d.). The boost of \$1,000–\$2,000 in the CTC is due to expire in 2025 (TPC, n.d.).

There is extensive research on the effects of the EITC on labor force participation (particularly of single mothers) and on health and educational outcomes for children in the United States. Less research has been conducted on the effects of the CTC, mostly because it was relatively small until recently. Given the similar structure of the CTC and EITC, many of the effects are expected to be the same, with the important exception that the CTC is available to most moderate-income families, unlike the EITC, which is targeted at families with low incomes.

As noted above, the EITC and the CTC together are effective in reducing child poverty: nearly 5 million children lived in families whose incomes were brought above the poverty level after including working family tax credits, and more than 7 million additional children experienced less severe poverty (CBPP, 2018c).[3] The poverty rate for children under 18 falls about 6 percentage points with the tax credits (16.4 percent compared to 22.8 percent without them) (Nichols and Rothstein, 2016). The reductions in child poverty are larger for these tax credits than other means-tested programs in the United States (Nichols and Rothstein, 2016). Given the well-established link between family income and health outcomes, by

---

[2] The refundable portion of the CTC is called the Additional Child Tax Credit (ACTC); here, both the ACTC and the CTC are included when referring to the CTC.

[3] Note that these estimates are based on data using the U.S. Census Bureau's Supplemental Poverty Measure.

increasing family incomes, these tax credits are likely to lead to improved child health. One advantage of studying the link between the EITC and outcomes is that researchers can use exogenous policy changes that increase families' income, avoiding the problem of endogenous income in studies of income–health links (Boyd-Swan et al., 2013).

While most studies have focused on the impacts of the EITC on labor force participation or reductions in poverty, a small but growing number of studies have examined the impacts of the EITC on health and education outcomes of children, both short and long term. Several studies found the EITC associated with higher birth weights and/or a reduction in the incidence of low birth weight (LBW) (Baker, 2008; Hoynes et al., 2012; Komro et al., 2019; Strully et al., 2010). Using quasi-experimental methods, Hoynes et al. (2012) estimated a decline of 2–3 percent in LBW occurrence for a $1,000 increase in the EITC, with larger effects for black than white women (among single women with a high school education or less). This study and one by Strully et al. (2010) also link EITC receipt with reduced rates of maternal smoking. In contrast, Baughman and Duchovny (2016) found that EITC receipt was not associated with improvements in parent-reported health status of children age birth to 5, although there were improvements for older children (age 6 to 14). Evidence linking the EITC to child cognitive or child development outcomes is limited (particularly for younger children). One study by Hamad and Rehkopf (2016) used an instrumental variable approach to estimate the impact of the EITC on child development. They found "modest but meaningful improvements" in child behavior and home environments. The article notes that one mechanism through which the EITC impacts child development is through improved mental health of mothers (Evans and Garthwaite, 2010) and that it may lead to reductions in maltreatment (Berger et al., 2017). Studies focused on older children also find positive associations with EITC receipt on test scores (Chetty et al., 2011; Dahl and Lochner, 2012) and college attendance (Manoli and Turner, 2018).

It is important to note that effects of the EITC on health outcomes may be a result of the increase in family income; however, the EITC also strongly impacts work incentives, and impacts on child health and development may be due to changes in parent employment. Increases in maternal employment may increase the family's income but also reduce the amount of time mothers spend with their children. How these changes impact children's health and development likely depends on the quality of nonparental child care used and the stress experienced by parents, in addition to income changes (Hoynes and Schanzenbach, 2018).

Unlike the working family tax credits, minimum-wage policies are not targeted specifically at low-income families with children.

Nonetheless, some economists argue that minimum-wage policies play an important and complementary role in reducing child poverty along with the EITC (Nichols and Rothstein, 2016). Research summarized by Nichols and Rothstein (2016) has demonstrated that the EITC provides a strong incentive for single mothers to work and has been a major factor underlying the rise in labor force participation of single mothers over the past two decades. An increase in the supply of labor, holding all else equal, could put downward pressure on wages, and the minimum wage provides a floor to keep wages from declining (Nichols and Rothstein, 2016). Parents who earn low wages benefit from a higher minimum wage in every paycheck along with receiving the tax credit when they file a tax return (CBPP, 2018c). A small number of studies also link increases in the minimum wage with health outcomes, though few examine children's health or birth outcomes. Two studies find small improvements in birth weight outcomes related to minimum-wage increases across states over time using quasi-experimental methods (Komro et al., 2016; Wehby et al., 2016). One study also found reductions in child maltreatment associated with higher minimum wages (Raissian and Bullinger, 2017). Given the evidence linking improved child health to higher family incomes, more research on the health effects of minimum-wage increases is needed to inform the policy debate.

Child Allowances

Many wealthy countries provide support to families through a child allowance or child benefit, which may be a cash grant or through the tax code. In the current U.S. tax code, the CTC and dependent child exemption act in many ways like a child allowance. The taxable income of families with dependent children is reduced, resulting in greater disposable income to meet the costs of raising children. A child allowance, distributed monthly, has two main advantages over the tax code approach. First, it helps families with short-term needs for cash to meet expenses, compared to a once-per-year distribution through the tax system. Second, the lowest-income families often cannot take full advantage of tax credits and exemptions if their income is so low that they do not owe income tax. A child allowance paid to families on a monthly basis and not tied to earnings or employment would provide support for many of the lowest-income children in the United States whose parents do not work or have unstable and insufficient earnings.

A number of child allowance proposals have been proposed in recent years (NASEM, 2019; Shaefer et al., 2018). Schaefer et al. (2018) proposed a universal child allowance of $250 per child per month, possibly offering $300 for children under age 6 and slightly less for each additional child. Schaefer et al. (2018) noted that while this amount would not come close to covering the full cost of raising a child, based on their review of the research, it is large enough to have a meaningful impact on families and children and is comparable to child allowances in other countries. The National Academies report *A Roadmap to Reducing Child Poverty* considered two options for a child allowance: about $2,000 and $3,000 per year. The reductions in child poverty are larger for these two policies than any of the other individual policy changes considered by the report (although the costs are also higher).

A few key principles are important when considering the parameters of a child allowance that is intended to improve health outcomes for young children. First, targeting payments to families with the youngest children acknowledges that families with younger children have lower incomes on average than families with older children (see Schaefer et al., 2018). In addition, some costs (particularly child care) are higher for younger than for older children. The nation provides sizable public resources to children starting at about age 5 when they enter the public K–12 education system. A child allowance targeted at children under age 5 would help to balance public investments in different age groups.

A universal program—in which all families with young children receive a child allowance—would reduce the stigma of participation relative to a means-tested program and may enhance social inclusion (NASEM, 2019, p. 148). While the costs of a universal program may exceed those of a targeted one, treating the allowance as taxable income would reduce the overall cost to the government. Alternatively, the child allowance could be phased out at 300 percent of the federal poverty level. Replacement of the current child tax credits with a monthly child allowance could provide families with a more regular source of cash income to support their children's needs (NASEM, 2019). Determining the specifics of a child allowance policy and funding mechanism requires additional research and modeling to compare the potential impacts on child health and health equity. In sum, based on the committee's review of the evidence and in accordance with the report *A Roadmap to Reducing Child Poverty*, there is strong evidence that programs that provide direct income transfers or basic necessities such as food and housing lead to improvements in child health and well-being (NASEM, 2019, p. 89). At the end of the chapter, the committee recommends expanding resources to support families with young children, with a child allowance as one important option to consider.

Paid Parental Leave

Maternal and paternal leave policies are generally intended to support mothers in recovering from childbirth and mothers and fathers in taking time off work to care for new infants. The United States remains one of the very few countries without a national paid guaranteed maternity leave policy. Across Organisation for Economic Co-operation and Development (OECD) countries, on average, mothers are entitled to 18 weeks of paid maternity leave (OECD, 2017). Although the United States is the only OECD country without a national-level policy of paid leave, California, New Jersey, New York, Rhode Island, Washington, Washington, DC, and, most recently, Massachusetts have passed legislation to implement paid leave at the state and local levels (Mass.gov, 2019; Raub et al., 2018). See Box 6-3 for more information on California as an example of a state that has implemented a paid leave policy. A number of studies of paid maternity leave have found positive health effects, particularly lower infant and child mortality (Heymann et al., 2011; Nandi et al., 2018). Stearns (2015) estimated that paid maternity leave through temporary disability insurance in the United States reduced LBW by 3.2 percent and early births by 6.6 percent, with larger effects for certain subgroups, including black and unmarried mothers (Stearns, 2015). While improved maternal and child outcomes have been associated with paid leave policies in other countries, a review by Almond et al. (2018) showed mixed findings on child health impacts across studies, depending in part on the length of the leave. They concluded that "facilitating short maternity leaves is highly beneficial, but extended maternity leaves do not have a positive effect" on child outcomes (Almond et al., 2018, p. 1406). Rossin-Slater (2011) estimated that the Family and Medical Leave Act (FMLA), which allows for 12 weeks of unpaid maternity leave, resulted in lower infant mortality and slightly higher birth weight outcomes for college-educated women. Overall, however, based on her review of the literature, Rossin-Slater stated that "while extensions in existing paid leave policies have had little impact on children's well-being, the evidence suggests that the introduction of short paid and unpaid leave programs can improve children's short- and long-term outcomes" (Rossin-Slater, 2011, p. 17).

Maternity leave policies have also been associated with higher rates of breastfeeding. As discussed in Chapter 3, breastfeeding provides important nutrition for developing infant brains and bodies; however, rates of exclusive breastfeeding for 6 months (as recommended by the World Health Organization and the American Academy of Pediatrics [AAP]) are low in the United States, especially among black women. Furthermore, the majority of mothers in the United States are not breastfeeding as long as they had planned (Mirkovic et al., 2014; Office of the Surgeon

BOX 6-3
Paid Family Leave in California

California was the first U.S. state to implement a comprehensive Paid Family Leave (PFL) program in 2004, authorized by Senate Bill 1661 (Chapter 901, Statutes of 2002). The PFL program provides eligible employees up to 6 weeks of wage replacement leave (55 percent of regular weekly earnings) when they take leave from work to bond with a new child or to care for a seriously ill family member. The program is funded by a payroll tax levied on employees, so employers do not bear any direct costs. PFL benefit levels are indexed to inflation. California built the PFL program on the existing State Disability Insurance system, so it is structured as an insurance benefit. California PFL was implemented as a virtually universal program—that is, almost all employees, excluding some self-employed persons, are eligible, regardless of the size of their employer.

The California Senate Office of Research reports that from 2004 to 2013, PFL applications increased overall, with almost a two-fold increase in claims filed by men. This increase among men was reported to be driven almost exclusively by the number of men filing claims for caring for a new child. Applications for PFL for the purpose of caring for a new child make up about 88 percent of all PFL claims. Data from 2013 indicate that on average, women took 5.5 weeks of leave to care for a new child, while men took 4.5 weeks. One analysis used a differences-in-differences approach to examine how the PFL program affected leave-taking from 1999 to 2010. The authors found that the program doubled the use of maternity leave in California, with notable increases among non-college-educated mothers with infants (from 2.4 to 7.7 percent), unmarried mothers (from 1.9 to 9.3 percent), and African American mothers (from 2.0 to 13.7 percent) (Rossin-Slater et al., 2011). Other research has studied the California PFL program in relation to child and family outcomes. For example, the passage of the PFL program has been found to be associated with increased rates of breastfeeding (Huang and Yang, 2015).

SOURCES: Applebaum and Milkman, 2011; California Senate Office of Research, 2014; Huang and Yang, 2015; Rossin-Slater et al., 2011.

General et al., 2011). While the Patient Protection and Affordable Care Act (ACA) has some protections for mothers who need to express milk while at work[4] (a critical component of successful breastfeeding for working mothers), many mothers are not given the time, appropriate space, and support needed to do so when in low-paying jobs (Murtagh and

---

[4] For example, the ACA updated the Fair Labor Standards Act to require U.S. firms with 50 or more employees to provide breastfeeding mothers with reasonable break time and space to express milk (DOL, 2018).

Moulton, 2011; Office of the Surgeon General et al., 2011). In a survey conducted by Declercq et al. (2013), 58 percent of women reported breast-feeding to be a challenge once they returned to work.

Paid leave "facilitates the initiation and continuation of breastfeed-ing" (Heymann et al., 2013). For example, a rigorous quasi-experimental study in California found that access to paid leave was associated with increased rates of exclusive and overall breastfeeding during the first 3, 6, and 9 months after birth (Huang and Yang, 2015). Studies (in both the United States and other developed countries) have found associations between maternity leave lasting at least 8 weeks and a higher probability of establishing breastfeeding (Guendelman et al., 2009; Ogbuanu et al., 2011; Skafida, 2012). Paid parental leave is hypothesized to increase mother–child attachment and give new mothers increased time to gain the skills and social support needed to maintain breastfeeding before returning to work.

The AEI-Brookings Working Group on Paid Family Leave published two reports in 2017 and 2018 that focused on paid parental leave and paid family care and medical leave, respectively. Based on the extant literature on paid parental leave and its impact on family outcomes, the 2017 report puts forth a federal paid parental leave proposal. In addition to physical health and cognitive outcomes for children, the report cites improved labor force participation as a positive outcome associated with paid leave. For example, California and New Jersey's paid leave policies saw increases in labor force attachment among women in the months surrounding child-birth (Byker, 2016). This is important because continued workforce par-ticipation can help sustain household income and individual income, as well as other economic indicators that have been linked to health and well-being (see, for example, NASEM, 2017; Woolf et al., 2015). The key elements of the AEI-Brookings federal paid leave proposal are mak-ing benefits available to both mothers and fathers, wage replacement of 70 percent up to a maximum limit of $600 per week for 8 weeks, and job protection for the individuals who take leave. The authors also suggest that such a federal paid leave program could be financed by a payroll tax levied on employees and/or savings in other areas of the budget (e.g., reduced tax expenditures in areas such as unemployment insurance or Social Security and disability programs) (AEI-Brookings Working Group on Paid Family Leave, 2017).

Summary and Conclusions

There is considerable evidence that "income matters" for health out-comes, especially in early childhood. The report *A Roadmap to Reducing Child Poverty* concludes that "the weight of the causal evidence does indeed indicate that income poverty itself causes negative child outcomes, especially when poverty occurs in early childhood or persists throughout a large portion of childhood" (NASEM, 2019, p. 2). There is also strong evidence that the reverse is true: increasing family resources to meet basic needs supports the health and development of young children. Given the high rate of child poverty in this country compared to other wealthy nations, as well as large disparities across racial and ethnic groups in poverty rates, reducing childhood poverty is a critical, foundational step in reducing health disparities in early childhood.

> *Conclusion 6-1: Increasing the economic resources families have available to meet basic needs when children are young (including prenatally) will improve children's health and has the potential to reduce health and developmental disparities in early childhood.*

One way to increase the resources families have for basic needs is through social insurance and safety net programs that provide cash or tax credits to families. Studies demonstrate improved health outcomes when families receive assistance through government programs, such as the EITC and SSI. These programs are associated with improved birth, health, and educational outcomes for young children, which will set them on a better trajectory for lifelong health and well-being.

> *Conclusion 6-2: Public programs that provide economic resources to families in the form of cash, tax credits, or in-kind benefits improve child health and development outcomes, which have long-lasting effects on health and educational outcomes.*

Much of the support provided to families with children in the United States is in the form of "work supports," where eligibility and the level of benefits are closely tied to employment and earnings. These policies help to reduce poverty by both increasing resources and encouraging employment (which also can lead to higher family income in the future). However, the report *A Roadmap to Reducing Child Poverty* determined that a work-oriented package of programs and policies would be the least effective of the four packages they considered in reducing the number of children in poverty (see Table 6-1 for a summary of the components of each of the four packages). That report also concluded that mandatory "work requirements are at least as likely to increase as decrease poverty" (NASEM, 2019) (see Box 6-2).

In addition to a limited impact on reducing child poverty, further expansions of the work-oriented safety net programs may have unintended negative consequences for child health if parent employment results in

TABLE 6-1 Components of the Four Packages and Their Estimated Costs and Impact on Poverty Reduction and Employment Change from *A Roadmap to Reducing Child Poverty*

		1. Work-oriented package	2. Work-based and universal support package	3. Means-tested supports and work package	4. Universal supports and work package
Work-oriented programs and policy	Expand EITC	X	X	X	X
	Expand Child Care Tax Credit	X	X	X	X
	Increase the minimum wage	X			X
	Roll out WorkAdvance	X			
Income support-oriented programs and policies	Expand housing voucher program			X	
	Expand SNAP benefits			X	
	Begin a child allowance		X		X
	Begin child support assurance				X
	Eliminate 1996 immigration eligibility restrictions				X
	Percent reduction in the number of poor children	−18.8%	−35.6%	−50.7%	−52.3%
	Percent reduction in the number of children in deep poverty	−19.3%	−41.3%	−51.7%	−55.1%
	Change in number of low-income workers	+1,003,000	+568,000	+404,000	+611,000
	Annual cost, in billions	$8.7	$44.5	$90.7	$108.8

SOURCE: NASEM, 2019.

lower rates of breastfeeding or disruptions to the attachment between infant and caregiver. Evidence of the importance of attachment and breast-feeding is discussed in Chapters 3 and 4. Work-oriented programs, such as the EITC, that increase families' incomes and increase employment are an important component of the social safety net. However, additional support for families with young children through paid parental leave or a child allowance that is not tied to parent employment would recognize the special needs of the earliest years in which parent time and attention are critically important for children's health and development. Both paid parental leave and income support, such as a child allowance not tied to employment, may provide parents with greater opportunity to take time out of the labor force to attend to their children's needs.

> *Conclusion 6-3: Income-support programs that are contingent on employment status or based on earned income have positive benefits for families yet may also have unintended consequences for child health and development outcomes through negative effects on attachment, breastfeeding, and caregiver stress. Thus, it is important to supplement work-support programs with basic support for families with young children that is not tied to employment.*

As noted above, additional income support for families with young children through paid parental leave would recognize the special needs of infants and their caregivers. Unpaid parental leave through FMLA does not cover all employees, and many families with low incomes are unable to afford to take an unpaid leave. Paid parental leave grants parents greater opportunity to take time out of the labor force to attend to their children's needs. Short, paid parental leave programs have been associated with positive health outcomes and higher rates of breastfeeding.

> **Recommendation 6-1: Federal, state, local, tribal, and territorial policy makers should implement paid parental leave. In partnership with researchers, policy makers should model variations in the level of benefits, length of leave, and funding mechanisms to determine alternatives that will have the largest impacts on improving child health outcomes and reducing health disparities.**

As of 2019, six states and Washington, DC, have paid leave programs, and the programs are financed through employee payroll taxes (AEI-Brookings Working Group on Paid Family Leave, 2017). Some proposals for paid family leave (PFL) follow a social insurance model in which employees contribute through payroll taxes to a government-administered social insurance fund. Other financing options include an employer mandate, tax credits to encourage employers, or general funds (Isaacs et al., 2017a). Because there are a variety of options to implement, structure, and administer a paid leave policy, cost estimates for this program vary widely. In its 2018 report, the AEI-Brookings Working Group on Paid Family Leave offered three methods for assessing the cost of a hypothetical 8-week paid family medical leave program[5] had it been operational in 2016. The three methods use (1) national-level data, assuming uptake would be similar to private-sector participation under FMLA; (2) state paid leave data, assuming participation would mirror the rates of the states with operational programs; and (3) a simulation model to combine national- and state-level data. Because these methods differ with respect to data sources and assumptions on program use, the cost estimates vary widely and drawing comparisons can be difficult. Based on their analyses, the authors estimate that the program could be expected to cost from 0.10 percent of total wages or $7.65 million total benefits paid (based on New Jersey's state paid leave program) to 0.61 percent of total wages or $46.3 million total benefits paid (based on the FMLA national survey).

The committee did not study in depth other income-enhancement strategies to boost family resources that are not targeted particularly to health outcomes or early childhood, but these may be important for supporting the health and well-being of families and children. The National Academies report *A Roadmap to Reducing Child Poverty* details a number of additional strategies to reduce child poverty through, for example, increases in the minimum wage, job training programs, child care subsidies, and child support assurance, in addition to the policies discussed in this section. There is limited evidence of the impacts of these on child health, with the exception of the minimum wage (discussed earlier). The National Academies report *A Roadmap to Reducing Child Poverty* provides a careful assessment of a set of feasible strategies that could be used to reduce child poverty by half within 10 years (see Table 6-1). As discussed in Chapter 2, the scientific evidence amassed since *From Neurons to Neighborhoods* has established that access to basic resources prenatally and in early childhood impact the developing child's brain and nervous system, immune function, and other organs (NRC and IOM, 2000). The toxic stress response of children living in poverty directly impacts behavioral and psychological well-being and substantially increases later-life risk for poor health and educational outcomes. Thus, reducing child poverty is a critically important, foundational strategy for improving child health outcomes and reducing health disparities in early childhood. Expansion of income-support programs that are not tied directly to parent earnings is likely to help those who need it most: children in deep poverty and the youngest children. Determining the specifics of a child allowance policy and funding mechanism requires additional

---

[5] The hypothetical program provides universal access to up to 8 weeks of family and medical leave, including parental leave, with benefits paid at 70 percent of usual weekly wages up to a cap of $600 per week.

research and modeling to compare the potential impacts on child health and health equity. At the end of the chapter, the committee recommends expanding programs to increase economic resources to support families with young children, with a child allowance as one important option to consider.

Policies that build family assets and wealth also deserve consideration in developing a national strategy to ensure that all children have an equal opportunity to reach their full health and developmental potential. Individual Development Accounts and child savings accounts, for example, are typically targeted toward building savings for home ownership or postsecondary education. These strategies may have longer-term impacts on child and family well-being. Increasing education levels, particularly of mothers, also would likely lead to improved economic security for families. These policies support the broader goal of human capital development and long-term economic growth.

FOOD SECURITY AND NUTRITION

As described in Chapter 3, adequate and nutritious food is critically important for health outcomes during the preconception, prenatal, and early childhood periods. At times, adequacy of specific nutrients is crucial, such as folic acid during pregnancy. In each of these developmental periods, the overall adequacy and healthiness of food intake influence current health and development and have effects lasting into adulthood. Furthermore, food insecurity may affect both children and parents through changes in eating habits and stress related to uncertainty and inadequacy of food availability. The neurobiological (and other) mechanisms underlying these effects were described in Chapters 2 and 3. In this section, we look at the programs and policies in the United States aimed at reducing food insecurity and improving nutrition and healthy eating, with a focus on the prenatal and early childhood periods.

Current Programs and Policies

Two major federal programs in the United States target the adequacy of food and nutrition for children living in households with limited resources: the Supplemental Nutrition Assistance Program (SNAP), formerly known as the Food Stamp Program, and the Special Supplemental Nutrition Program for Women, Infants, and Children (WIC). In this section we examine the evidence on the effects of these two programs on children's health and development. Note that programs that operate primarily in schools and early education settings, such as the National School Lunch and Breakfast Program, are discussed in Chapter 7.

SNAP

SNAP provides assistance to eligible individuals and families to purchase food. Participants use an Electronic Benefit Transfer (EBT) card that functions like a debit card to purchase food from authorized retailers, which include supermarkets, grocery and convenience stores, and farmers' markets (CBPP, n.d.). Many participants enroll in SNAP for a short time— from 2009 to 2012, approximately 48 percent of participants received benefits for 24 months or less (Irving and Loveless, 2015; RWJF, 2018).

Participants need to meet requirements regarding income (gross[6] and net[7] monthly income), resources (such as cash, money in checking and savings accounts, and vehicles), and nonfinancial standards to be eligible to receive SNAP benefits (Cronquist and Lauffer, 2019). Undocumented noncitizens of the United States are not eligible for SNAP, but noncitizens who have lived in the United States for at least 5 years, receive disability-related assistance, or are less than 18 years of age are eligible (if they also meet the aforementioned income, resource, and nonfinancial eligibility requirements) (USDA, 2018b). The program expects that participating households will spend about 30 percent of their own financial resources purchasing food; thus, the amount in SNAP benefits received by each participating household is calculated by multiplying the household's net monthly income by 0.3 and subtracting the result from the maximum monthly allotment[8] for the household size.

Each month of fiscal year 2017, SNAP served 42.1 million individuals in 20.8 million households. Children were 44 percent of SNAP participants and received 43 percent of SNAP benefits. On average, the program provided assistance to 8.6 million households with children (42 percent of all households served by SNAP) each month. Of the total number of SNAP participants, 8 percent were children with U.S. citizen status living with noncitizen adults (Cronquist and Lauffer, 2019).

While SNAP benefits can be spent only on eligible food items, these benefits add to the total resources the family has to spend on all necessities. The average monthly benefit of $255 per household "represents a sizable income transfer to participants, and is expected to change the amount or quality of food purchased" (Hoynes and Schanzenbach, 2018, p. 13). A recent Urban Institute report estimates that the SNAP program reduced the number of children living in poverty by more than

---

[6] Includes a household's total, nonexcluded income before any deductions have been made (USDA, 2018b).

[7] Gross income minus allowable deductions (USDA, 2018b).

[8] Maximum monthly allotments by household size are available at https://www.fns.usda.gov/snap/eligibility (accessed March 28, 2019).

one-quarter and the number in deep poverty by nearly half (Wheaton and Tran, 2018). The report also found that SNAP reduced the poverty gap (defined as the additional income needed to lift all low-income families out of poverty) by 37 percent for families with children. Given the evidence on the links between health outcomes and income, one would expect these sizable reductions in poverty to lead to improved health outcomes. A growing body of evidence shows that SNAP improves birth outcomes (Almond et al., 2011; East, 2018), although, as discussed below, relatively few studies focus on the effects of SNAP on the health outcomes of young children.

A review of studies prior to 2003 concluded that SNAP participation increased household food expenditures (USDA, 2004), which suggests that SNAP would reduce food insecurity among recipient households. Because families experiencing greater hardship are more likely to participate in SNAP, however, some studies of SNAP's effect on food insecurity have found mixed and null results (Gibson-Davis and Foster, 2006; Gundersen and Oliveira, 2001; Huffman and Jensen, 2008; Wilde, 2007; Wilde and Nord, 2005). Gregory et al. (2016) illustrate how estimates of the relationship between SNAP participation and food insecurity vary depending on statistical methods, demonstrating positive and negative estimates along with ones that were not significantly different from zero. They did conclude, however, that food insecurity was reduced by SNAP in a dose–response type model. Furthermore, according to an Urban Institute report, "controlling for selection into SNAP is important for disentangling the effect of SNAP receipt on food insecurity" (Ratcliffe and McKernan, 2010, p. 14). The authors found that the relationship between SNAP participation and food insecurity changed direction when they controlled for selection into SNAP using an instrumental variables approach. They concluded that SNAP participation reduced food insecurity by 16 percentage points (results for children not reported separately). Using methods to account for both selection and measurement error in reporting SNAP participation, Kreider et al. (2012) found a reduction of at least 8 percentage points in food insecurity for children, depending on the model assumptions. Deb and Gregory (2018) found that the effects of SNAP on food insecurity vary across the population; while it may have no effect for some, for those starting with low food security, it resulted in a much lower likelihood of food insecurity.

While SNAP increases household resources and reduces food insecurity for (at least) some families, studies of the impact of receiving food assistance on children's health outcomes are relatively rare. One study found that the introduction of the Food Stamp Program in California was associated with a reduction in infant birth weight, particularly among first-time teen mothers for whom birth rates increased overall

(Currie and Moretti, 2008). Potential mechanisms for this association could be related to fertility changes or the increased survival of LBW babies. The study findings also showed a small reduction in infant mortality for white babies in Los Angeles County. There is more recent evidence of a positive connection between receiving SNAP benefits (or food stamps) and improved birth outcomes. Almond et al. (2011) and East (2018) both found positive associations between food assistance during pregnancy and improved birth outcomes, using quasi-experimental methods. Almond et al. (2011) found larger improvements in birth weight outcomes for African American mothers and those living in high-poverty areas. They noted that these results occurred despite the fact that the Food Stamp Program was not designed to target pregnant women. See Figure 6-2 for data on the impact of in-utero exposures to food stamps on likelihood of birth weight below selected cut-offs.

With respect to other health outcomes for children, there is limited causal evidence. Kreider et al. (2012) reported improvements in child health outcomes (along with reductions in child food insecurity); however, the range of possible effect sizes is large. They accounted for both selection and underreporting of SNAP participation but did not specifically focus on young children. Most studies focus on adult health outcomes and found mixed results for adults (Kreider et al., 2012; see, for example,

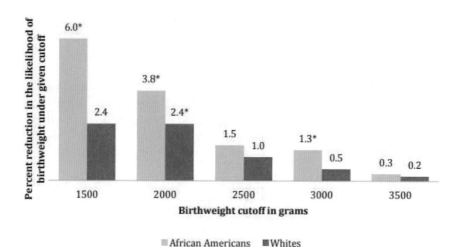

FIGURE 6-2 The impact of in-utero exposure to food stamps on likelihood of birth weight under selected cut-offs.
NOTES: * Denotes estimate statistically significantly different from zero. Data from Almond et al., 2011.
SOURCE: Hoynes and Schanzenbach, 2016.

Gregory and Deb, 2015; Yen et al., 2012). Overall, there is limited evidence on the causal effects of SNAP on children's health because there have been few opportunities for random assignment[9] or limited variation in policies over time or in different places to exploit with experimental or quasi-experimental methods (East, 2018).

While studies of direct or contemporaneous effects on children's health are limited, one recent study demonstrated a link between receipt of SNAP in childhood and adult health outcomes. Hoynes et al. (2016) found that adult health measured by the metabolic syndrome index was significantly better for those whose childhood families had access to food stamps, particularly in early childhood (before age 5). Long-term positive health effects of SNAP—that is, adult health outcomes for those receiving SNAP as children—are consistent with short-term health improvements during childhood. Similarly, East (2018) found positive effects of SNAP participation before age 5 on health outcomes when children were age 6–16, using quasi-experimental methods for a sample of children born in the United States to immigrant parents. While conclusions about the immediate impacts of SNAP on young children's health are provisional given the methodological challenges of estimating causality (Carlson and Keith-Jennings, 2018), the evidence of SNAP impacts on reduced food insecurity and later health outcomes suggests that children benefit in both the short and long run.

One of the concerns about the SNAP program has been the potential linkage between SNAP benefits and obesity, in both adults and children. Earlier studies that did not adequately control for selection into SNAP found positive correlations between SNAP and obesity, while other studies found reductions in obesity or no effects (Fan and Jin, 2015; Kreider et al., 2012). Myerhoefer and Yang concluded "the balance of evidence points to a small positive impact of SNAP participation on obesity for women" but that the results for "childhood obesity are less consistent" (Meyerhoefer and Yang, 2011, p. 313). For children, Kreider et al. (2012) concluded that the obesity rate was 5.3 percentage points lower due to SNAP.

In addition to reducing hunger and food insecurity, a second key objective of the nation's food assistance programs is to improve the healthfulness of American food consumption and provide nutrition education. Studies have examined the effect of SNAP on the quality or healthfulness of a family's food consumption as a possible mechanism through which SNAP might affect obesity (and other health) outcomes.

---

[9] Random assignment demonstration projects have been conducted recently and are under way in several sites as part of the Demonstration Projects to End Childhood Hunger project and the Healthy Incentives Pilot (Olsho et al., 2017; USDA, 2018a).

Most studies have focused on adult food intake, but Yen (2010) found no effect of the SNAP program on young children's nutrient intake. A number of demonstration projects have been conducted to evaluate ways to incentivize or influence consumption of healthful foods through SNAP. The Healthy Incentives Pilot (HIP) project provided a 30 percent rebate on purchases of a specified set of fruits and vegetables using SNAP benefits. Households receiving SNAP were randomly assigned to receive the rebate or not. The HIP evaluation reported that households receiving the rebates increased consumption of targeted fruits and vegetables by 26 percent, although some reported confusion and misunderstanding about how the rebate program worked and which vegetables and fruits were included (Olsho et al., 2017). The Summer EBT for Children pilot also was a random assignment design, but rather than targeting specific purchases, participants were provided with (an extra) $60 per month per school-age child. The evaluation study found modest improvements in several child nutritional outcomes and null effects for others (Collins and Klerman, 2017) even though this program did not specifically target or incentivize healthful food purchases. While SNAP benefits can be used to purchase almost any food item from participating retailers, recent pilot projects found that increased benefits and incentives for purchasing specific healthful foods can modestly impact some health-related and dietary outcomes. Proposals to restrict SNAP purchases to prohibit less healthful foods, such as sugary beverages, or to incentivize purchases of fruits and vegetables are highly controversial (Schwartz, 2017).

In summary, as discussed throughout this section, food assistance provided through SNAP is a major component of the nation's social safety net and reduces poverty and food insecurity for millions of families and children (Carlson and Keith-Jennings, 2018). While the evidence of SNAP's direct impact on children's health is limited, Hoynes et al. (2016) found that adults who received SNAP as children experienced a reduction of 5 percent in heart disease and 16 percent reduction in obesity. Improvements in adult health outcomes related to receipt of SNAP in early childhood suggest that children are benefiting as well. Based on Hoynes and Schanzenbach's (2018) summary of the literature examining links between SNAP participation and health outcomes, the National Academies (2019) report on reducing child poverty concluded that "many (but not all) of the methodologically strongest studies show SNAP benefits having positive impacts on health" (NASEM, 2019, p. 83). The report cites evidence that increasing SNAP benefits would substantially reduce child poverty and that current benefit levels do not account for food preparation time or geographic variation in food costs (Ziliak, 2016). Based on the evidence demonstrating the links between child health and family income or resources, increasing SNAP benefits would likely lead to improved child health and reduced health disparities.

Special Supplemental Nutrition Program for Women, Infants, and Children

WIC provides assistance through breastfeeding support and education, healthy foods, nutrition education and counseling, screening referrals to other services, and vouchers to purchase fruits and vegetables from authorized farmers' markets (USDA, 2015). WIC services are provided in many locations, including county health departments, hospitals, mobile clinics, community centers, schools, public housing sites, migrant health centers and camps, and Indian Health Service facilities (USDA, n.d.).

To be eligible to receive benefits, WIC participants need to meet all four categories of requirements: categorical, residential, income, and nutrition risk (USDA, 2018c). Infants younger than 1 year; children younger than 5 years; and women who are pregnant, postpartum (up to 6 months), or breastfeeding meet the WIC categorical requirement. To meet the residential requirement, participants need to reside in the state or local service area in which they apply but are not required to have lived in that area for a minimum amount of time. Participants also have to earn incomes at or below income standards that are set by state agencies, and fall within 100 and 185 percent of the federal poverty guidelines issued annually by the U.S. Department of Health and Human Services (HHS). Lastly, participants need to be determined by a health professional to have at least one medical (e.g., anemia, underweight) or dietary (e.g., poor diet) condition from a list of conditions indicating nutrition risk that is set by states (USDA, 2018c).

In fiscal year 2018, WIC served approximately 6.9 million people and cost the federal government about $5.3 billion (USDA, 2019). In 2016, it was estimated that 64 percent of individuals eligible to receive WIC benefits were children ages 1–4, 21 percent were pregnant and postpartum women, and 16 percent were infants for a total of 13.9 million individuals. Of these, 7.6 million (55 percent) received WIC benefits, with 86 percent of eligible infants receiving benefits but only 44 percent of children ages 1–4 receiving them (Trippe et al., 2019).

Numerous studies using varied methods have found evidence of improved birth outcomes for women participating in the WIC program (see, for example, Figlio et al., 2009; Fingar et al., 2017; Foster et al., 2010; Hoynes et al., 2011). These studies find reductions in the likelihood of LBW (Figlio et al., 2009; Hoynes et al., 2011) and reductions in infant mortality (Khanani et al., 2010). Figlio et al. (2009) studied the effect of WIC in Florida between 1997 and 2001 by matching infant birth records with school records for older siblings to identify those who were marginally eligible and marginally ineligible in order to form groups for comparison. They estimated a significant reduction in the likelihood of LBW among WIC participants, although there was no significant effect on average birth weight or gestational age. Studies generally have found that the effects of WIC on birth outcomes are stronger for women with lower education levels, those living in areas of high poverty, and African Americans (Hoynes et al., 2011; Khanani et al., 2010). Fingar et al. (2017) accounted for gestational age, which might bias estimates in other studies, and reported a significantly reduced risk of preterm birth, LBW, and prenatal death.

One of the potential channels through which WIC impacts birth outcomes is through changes in dietary quality and access to nutritional information and support for healthy behaviors, such as quitting smoking, for pregnant women. Participants can use their WIC vouchers only for specific foods, and changes in the approved foods after 2008 reflect dietary recommendations from AAP and the Institute of Medicine. The U.S. Department of Agriculture published a final rule in 2014 that provides for more purchases of fruits and vegetables, whole-grain options, yogurt and soy options in place of milk, and more flexibility to tailor food packages to individuals (Carlson and Neuberger, 2018). While there has been concern about the possibility that providing infant formula to new mothers reduces breastfeeding, the changes to food packages and incentives after 2014 have encouraged breastfeeding (NASEM, 2016). The rate of breastfeeding among WIC participants has risen 45 percent over 12 years, reducing the difference between all women and WIC participants (Carlson and Neuberger, 2018).

There is solid evidence linking the WIC program to improved nutrient intake and eating more healthful food, although many of the studies report household-level consumption and do not focus specifically on children. The introduction of the improved food packages in WIC led to noticeable improvements in the percentage of families reporting that they eat more whole grains, drink lower-fat milk, and consume more fruits and vegetables (Andreyeva and Luedicke, 2013; Chiasson et al., 2013; Whaley et al., 2012). Thus, the additional resources to purchase specific food items provided by the WIC program is associated with changes in the types of food consumed by households (Whaley et al., 2012). In the case of the HIP, these changes may have been due in part to "promotional effects," whereby the incentive for certain foods provides information to participants about which foods are healthier (Olsho et al., 2017).

By providing access to healthier foods and nutrition information, WIC would be expected to improve the health and developmental outcomes of young children. WIC may also reduce food insecurity. One study found that WIC participation reduced the number of children experiencing food insecurity by 20 percent (Kreider et al., 2016). There is also some evidence about the impact of WIC on young children's cognitive and socio-emotional development. Jackson (2015) used matching and fixed effects estimation methods and found improvements in cognitive development at age 2 and reading and math scores at age 11 for children whose mothers participated in WIC prenatally. In contrast, Arons et al. (2016) found no significant improvement in socio-emotional development among young children receiving WIC; however, their sample size was small. Based on the current literature, the extent to which WIC supports cognitive and noncognitive development in young children is still uncertain.

Overall, the evidence is solid that WIC leads to improved birth outcomes and improved dietary intake for participants, although there is less evidence that it directly improves children's health and development in the early years. Revisions to the food package and incentives for purchasing specific fruits and vegetables have led to improvements in dietary quality. Evidence of savings on health costs, particularly postpartum, from the mid-1990s suggested that (back then) the cost savings far exceeded program costs (GAO, cited in Carlson and Neuberger, 2018, p. 24). Nearly two-thirds of all infants and half of pregnant and postpartum women are eligible for WIC.[10] The broad reach of the WIC program has been viewed as a positive attribute, but some feel that it indicates that the program is not sufficiently targeted and resources could be spent more efficiently (Besharov and Call, 2009). However, many eligible families do not receive WIC benefits. In 2014, only half of eligible pregnant women participated, while 80 percent of eligible infants did (Johnson et al., 2017). While the WIC program is largely successful in supporting the health and nutrition of its recipients, investigating the barriers to participation and further studying heterogeneous effects on different subgroups are necessary to further understand its potential to reduce health disparities in early childhood. Furthermore, better coordination between the WIC program, ECE systems, and prenatal, postpartum, and pediatric care would allow for a more integrated systems approach to addressing children's nutrition and developmental needs. (See Chapter 8 for more on applying a systems approach to promoting equitable healthy development.) Box 6-4 describes Healthy Mothers on the Move as an example of a promising model to improve nutrition and healthy lifestyles.

Summary

Both the SNAP and WIC programs have been studied extensively, and a large body of literature points to strong associations between program participation and positive outcomes, including less food insecurity,

---

[10] See https://www.fns.usda.gov/wic/wic-eligibility-and-coverage-rates (accessed July 14, 2019).

BOX 6-4
Healthy Mothers on the Move (Healthy MOMs)/Madres
Saludables en Movimiento (Madres Saludables):
A Promising Model[a]

Healthy Mothers on the Move (Healthy MOMs)/Madres Saludables en Movimiento (Madres Saludables) was a culturally tailored intervention that encouraged healthy lifestyle practices for Latina and African American women in southwest and eastside Detroit. Informed by community-based participatory research that identified the needs of pregnant and postpartum women in the community, the program aimed to decrease excessive weight gain during pregnancy and excessive postpartum weight retention in order to reduce risk factors for obesity, gestational diabetes, and type 2 diabetes (Detroit URC, n.d.; University of Michigan Prevention Research Center, n.d.).

The program consisted of a "healthy lifestyle intervention" and a "healthy pregnancy intervention" that served as a control group. The former consisted of culturally tailored programs, including curriculum-based education and home visiting, designed to equip participants with knowledge on pregnancy, childbirth, postpartum, and maternal and infant development as well as skills and supports to develop healthy lifestyles and manage stress. The programs were conducted in English and Spanish by community health workers. The control intervention provided a culturally tailored education on the same topics in English and Spanish (Detroit URC, n.d.).

The efficacy of the intervention was demonstrated through positive findings from longitudinal comparisons of the two interventions (Detroit URC, n.d.; Kieffer et al., 2014; Thornton et al., 2006). Participants were found to have decreased fat and sugar consumption, increased vegetable and fiber consumption, and decreased risk of depression (REACH Detroit, 2018).

The program's multisector partners included the Community Health and Social Services Center, a community-based nonprofit providing primary health care and support services to underserved residents of Detroit; the Detroit Department of Health and Wellness Promotion; Friends of Parkside, a community-based nonprofit; Harper-Gratiot Neighborhood Service Organization, a health and human services agency; Latino Family Services; the Michigan Department of Community Health; Southwest Solutions; St. John Health System; and the University of Michigan Schools of Social Work, Public Health, and Nursing. The program was funded by the National Institute of Diabetes and Digestive and Kidney Diseases from 2002 to 2008.

---

[a] The committee used selection criteria to identify examples of promising models highlighted in this report (see Appendix A for a list of the criteria). These examples all apply developmental science and aim to advance health equity during the preconception through early childhood periods.

---

reductions in poverty, and greater consumption of healthy foods. The evidence is convincing that WIC, which is targeted to pregnant and postpartum women, infants, and young children, improves birth and postpartum outcomes. There is also strong evidence that SNAP improves birth outcomes and child health. In evaluating the impacts of both programs, however, confounding factors are important to consider: participants may be more disadvantaged than nonparticipants but also may self-select into the programs, and either factor may bias study estimates. A small but increasing number of studies use experimental and quasi-experimental methods to estimate causal effects, although few focus specifically on health outcomes for young children. In addition to providing additional resources to the family to meet their basic needs, both SNAP and WIC can increase the consumption of healthful foods through nutritional education and incentives.

Conclusion 6-4: Given the importance of good nutrition for brain growth and development (during the preconception, prenatal, and early childhood periods), providing resources to ensure families have access to sufficient and healthy foods can improve birth outcomes and child health outcomes.

Because safety net programs, such as WIC and SNAP, have been shown to improve birth outcomes and to reduce food insecurity for young children, the committee recommends:

Recommendation 6-2: Federal, state, local, territorial, and tribal agencies should reduce barriers to participation in the Special Supplemental Nutrition Program for Women, Infants, and Children (WIC) program and Supplemental Nutrition Assistance Program (SNAP) benefits. Receipt of WIC and SNAP benefits should not be tied to parent employment for families with young children or for pregnant women, as work requirements are likely to reduce participation rates.

As noted earlier, the National Academies report *A Roadmap to Reducing Child Poverty* concludes that the current level of SNAP benefits is inadequate. That report considers two options for increasing benefit levels: a 20 or 30 percent increase (along with a higher benefit amount for households with teenagers and a boost in summer benefits). The report also notes that SNAP has a larger effect on reducing deep poverty than other government assistance programs do. Given the strong evidence linking improved child food security and SNAP, along with evidence of longer-term positive outcomes, increases in SNAP benefit amounts are likely to reduce health disparities. This committee had insufficient evidence to compare the effects on health disparities of alternative means of increasing family resources, such as increasing SNAP benefits or providing a monthly child allowance. For the most part, a dollar increase in SNAP benefits will have the same effect as a cash dollar, although some families might increase food expenditures more with an increase in SNAP. Increasing family resources is a critical, foundational step to reduce child health disparities (see Conclusion 6-1). Careful study and modeling is needed to determine the most cost-effective way to do so, with particular attention to the potential impacts on child and caregiver health and well-being and maternal employment, attachment, and breastfeeding. At the end of the housing section in this chapter, the committee recommends expanding resources to support families with young children, with an increase in SNAP benefit levels as one important option to consider.

HOUSING

Housing Affordability and Child Health and Equity

Access to affordable housing is considered an "upstream" determinant of child development, as it has implications for housing quality (Evans et al., 2000), instability (Garboden et al., 2017; Jelleyman and Spencer, 2008), and loss of housing (Sandel et al., 2018)—all of which are well-established determinants of child health (Leventhal and Newman, 2010). Unaffordable housing, or "high housing cost burden"—typically defined as housing costs above 30 percent of household income—is a critical social issue (Desmond, 2018) that has worsened during the past several decades (Joint Center for Housing Studies at Harvard University, 2017). In 2016, 47 percent of all renters and more than three-quarters of families earning less than $30,000 had unaffordable housing (Joint Center for Housing Studies at Harvard University, 2017). At the extreme, nearly 110,000 children are estimated to be homeless on any given night in the United States, and more than half of families who used shelters in 2016 identified as African American or black (U.S. Interagency Council on Homelessness, 2018).

The evidence discussed in Chapter 3 suggests that lack of affordable and quality housing, housing instability, and overcrowding have significantly detrimental effects on the health, well-being, and development of infants, children, and families. For more information on the evidence supporting the role of affordable housing in promoting positive outcomes for child health and development, see Chapter 3.

Improving Housing Affordability and Quality

Federal housing assistance is provided through a number of programs, including the Housing Choice Voucher Program, public housing, and the Low Income Housing Tax Credit. The Housing Choice Voucher Program is the largest federal housing assistance program for people with low incomes. Administered by the U.S. Department of Housing and Urban Development (HUD), this program provides funds to local public housing agencies (PHAs). PHAs have latitude in how the program is administered and what populations are prioritized. Eligibility is based on average median income in the geographic area and stratified by extremely low income, very low income, and low income. A PHA has to provide 75 percent of its vouchers to people with extremely low incomes (Eligibility.com, 2019). Although HUD provides housing assistance through the Housing Choice Voucher Program to more than 2 million families per year (CBPP, 2019)—which ensures that participating households contribute no more than 30 percent of their income to rent (CBPP, 2017)—only one-quarter of all income-eligible households receive housing assistance (CBPP, 2017), and the average family will spend 26 months waiting for assistance (HUD, 2016). One analysis found that the percentage of families with children receiving rental assistance decreased by 13 percent since 2004, while "the number of families that paid more than half their income for rent or lived in severely substandard housing rose by 53 percent between 2003 and 2013, to nearly 3 million" (Mazzara et al., 2016).

HUD housing assistance can help families obtain improved housing quality and residential stability (social factors that are associated with child development and disparities) (Fischer, 2015; HUD, 2014, 2015). There is some evidence to suggest that housing assistance has a beneficial impact on child health (Slopen et al., 2018), although this is an underexplored area of research. Only a small number of studies have rigorously controlled for selection bias, thereby limiting interpretation of the results for many of the existing studies (Ahrens et al., 2016; Fenelon et al., 2018; Fertig, 2007; Jacob et al., 2015; Kimbro et al., 2011; Leech, 2012; Newman and Holupka, 2017; Slopen et al., 2018). According to an analysis by Chetty et al. (2016) of the Moving to Opportunity demonstration, the benefits of the voucher program may be greater for children who move when they are young (less than 13 years of age) and may "reduce the intergenerational persistence of poverty and ultimately save the government money" (Chetty et al., 2016, p. 860). (See the section on Improving Neighborhood Conditions for more on the Moving to Opportunity study.)

Although this program is designed to provide families with choices about residential location, new evidence suggests that the program falls short on multiple neighborhood characteristics for families with children (Mazzara and Knudsen, 2019). A 2019 study by the Center on Budget and Policy Priorities using HUD administrative data and Census survey data revealed that in the 50 largest metropolitan areas in the United States, voucher-assisted families with children are disproportionately clustered into high-poverty, low-opportunity, or minority-concentrated areas relative to the distribution of voucher-affordable housing across the metropolitan area. For example, 33 percent of families with children using vouchers reside in high-poverty neighborhoods (Census-tract poverty rate at or above 30 percent) even though only 22 percent of voucher units are in high-poverty neighborhoods. Similarly, 61 percent of voucher-assisted families of color with children reside in "minority-concentrated" areas (Census-tract percent of people of color is at least 20 percentage points greater than the proportion in the entire metropolitan area), although only 32 percent of voucher units are allocated to minority-concentrated areas (Mazzara and Knudsen, 2019). Some programs, such as the Baltimore Mobility Program, include intensive counseling and require the use of vouchers in low-poverty areas for at least 1 year (Darrah and DeLuca, 2014). However, lack of affordable units in higher-opportunity neighborhoods remains a barrier (Misra, 2016). Other barriers include inflexible limits on search periods for families to find units and landlord resistance to voucher clients (Sard et al., 2018).

A Roadmap to Reducing Child Poverty modeled "expansions of voucher availability rather than other modifications, such as an increase in the level of housing subsidies, primarily because most experts agree that limited availability is currently the primary barrier preventing subsidized housing programs from having a larger impact on poverty reduction" (NASEM, 2019, p. 146). That committee also noted that "there is as yet no consensus among researchers as to whether existing housing subsidy levels set by the government are sufficiently aligned with true market rents faced by low-income families" (NASEM, 2019, p. 146).

As discussed in Chapter 3, housing quality is also a contributor to child health and development. A systematic review found strong evidence of effectiveness for home interventions focused on addressing asthma triggers, including multifaceted, in-home, tailored interventions (including mattress and pillow covers, high-efficiency particulate air vacuums and air filters, and cleaning), cockroach control through integrated pest management (including e-strategies, reducing access points, and using low-toxicity gel-bait pesticides), and combined elimination of leaks and removal of moldy items (Krieger et al., 2010). Several of the reviewed studies focused on children. A systematic review conducted by Crocker et al. (2011) found that home-based, multitrigger, multicomponent interventions reduced asthma symptoms and school absenteeism, as well as asthma acute symptoms, among children and adolescents. These assessments and interventions are often performed by home visitors or community health workers and have been found to be effective in both urban and rural areas (Chew et al., 2003; Crain et al., 2002; Levy et al., 2006; Morgan et al., 2004). The actions taken as a result of these assessments and interventions have been found to reduce disparities in asthma-related outcomes based on race/ethnicity and income (Postma et al., 2009).

Similarly, a comprehensive review by the Health Impact Project found residential remediation to be an effective primary prevention strategy to reduce childhood lead exposure (Health Impact Project, 2017). This remediation can range from complete removal or permanent containment of lead paint to scraping and painting over existing paint and covering contaminated soil. Secondary prevention through screening by pediatricians and other health care providers of young children and treatment for those with elevated blood lead levels (BLLs) is also critical for mitigating potential long-term harm.

Several states, including Maryland and New York, have undertaken state- and municipality-level lead prevention and mitigation efforts that have led to significant decreases in childhood lead exposure and poisoning. In New York, the City of Rochester implemented a Lead-Based Paint Poisoning Prevention Ordinance in 2006, which requires inspections for lead paint as part of existing inspections of most rental properties built before 1978. In addition, New York requires that all children undergo BLL testing at ages 1 and 2, which is overseen by the state's health department. The health department also provides educational and environmental interventions for children who are found to have elevated BLLs (City of Rochester NY, n.d.).

Enacted in 1994 and modified in 2012, Maryland's Reduction of Lead Risk in Housing Act has helped to make housing units safer for children by requiring owners of rental properties built before 1978 to ensure their properties comply with a lead paint risk reduction standard. The state has also invested in strong public enforcement of the Act, which is coordinated by the Maryland Department of the Environment's Lead Poisoning Prevention Program.[11] Through partnerships with nonprofits that provide legal services, such as the Green & Healthy Homes Initiative,[12] the state has also increased compliance with the law via private enforcement (Trust for America's Health, n.d.). As of 2016, Maryland requires all children born in or after 2015 to undergo blood lead testing at ages 1 and 2 (Maryland Department of Health, 2016). The Maryland Department of Health and Mental Hygiene oversees the state's BLL testing efforts and other services, including case management follow-up for children found to have elevated BLLs and community education for parents, tenants, rental property owners, homeowners, and health care providers (Trust for America's Health, n.d.). As a result of these initiatives, from 1993 to 2015, the number of Maryland children under 6 years old whose BLLs were

---

[11] For more information, see https://mde.maryland.gov/programs/Land/LeadPoisoning Prevention/Pages/index.aspx (accessed March 21, 2019).

[12] For more information, see https://www.greenandhealthyhomes.org (accessed March 21, 2019).

10 µg/dl or higher decreased from 23.9 percent (14,564 of 60,912 children tested) to 0.3 percent (377 of 110,217 children tested). In addition, from 2013 to 2014 alone, the number of rental properties that were treated and received certification for compliance with the lead paint risk reduction standard increased from 28,000 to 57,603.

While the United States has reduced the number of children at risk of lead poisoning, it has not completely eliminated lead hazards, and those most at risk for lead exposure are low-income and minority children.

Conclusion 6-5: Child lead poisoning continues to be a pervasive problem in the United States. There are many effective programs and policies that, if implemented and funded, would prevent, or mitigate the impact of, lead poisoning prenatally and in early childhood. Concerted efforts are needed to continue to ensure progress—through both policy and regulatory actions—on this preventable but serious problem.

Many high-quality reviews of lead poisoning prevention have been completed and contain important recommendations for remediation and prevention. For example, a report by the Health Impact Project (2017) includes the following recommendations and findings:

- **Reduce lead in drinking water in homes built before 1986 and other places children frequent.** Removing leaded drinking water service lines from the homes of children born in 2018 would protect more than 350,000 children and yield $2.7 billion in future benefits, or about $1.33 per dollar invested.
- **Remove lead paint hazards from low-income housing built before 1960 and other places children spend time.** Eradicating lead paint hazards from older homes of children from low-income families would provide $3.5 billion in future benefits, or approximately $1.39 per dollar invested, and protect more than 311,000 children.
- **Increase enforcement of the federal renovation, repair, and painting rule.** Ensuring that contractors comply with the U.S. Environmental Protection Agency (EPA) rule that requires lead-safe renovation, repair, and painting practices would protect about 211,000 children born in 2018 and provide future benefits of $4.5 billion, or about $3.10 per dollar spent.
- **Reduce air lead emissions.** Eliminating lead from airplane fuel would protect more than 226,000 children born in 2018 who live near airports, generate $262 million in future benefits, and remove roughly 450 tons of lead from the environment every year.

BOX 6-5
Cincinnati Child Health-Law Partnership
(Child HeLP): A Promising Model[a]

Cincinnati Child Health-Law Partnership (Child HeLP), which began in 2008, is a medical–legal partnership between Cincinnati Children's Hospital and the Legal Aid Society of Greater Cincinnati. Child HeLP aims to support families experiencing legal and social issues that may be having detrimental effects on the health and well-being of their children. Physicians at Cincinnati Children's primary care clinics and social workers screen patient families for issues that may be affecting their children's health, such as food insecurity, inadequate housing, adverse childhood experiences, and poor-quality education. Physicians receive training to better identify legal and social issues, which has been shown to successfully increase their comfort level with and knowledge of the social determinants of health (SDOH) as well as their familiarity with available community resources (Klein et al., 2011). Families identified as experiencing such issues are referred to Child HeLP to receive legal advice and assistance from the Legal Aid Society, which transmits information back to the family's provider to maintain open communication between the family's medical and legal teams (Cincinnati Children's, n.d.).

Child HeLP is a part of a more comprehensive, multisector approach to improving child health and well-being called the All Children Thrive Learning Network. The network includes a number of partners from the medical, public health, social services, legal, and education sectors as well as local agencies and community and faith-based organizations. Partnerships among these myriad stakeholders focus on four specific areas to improve child health and well-being: providing community-connected primary care and behavioral health services, decreasing preterm birth and infant mortality, strengthening neighborhood social influences, and improving access and quality of education to improve 3rd grade reading level outcomes (Cincinnati Children's, n.d.). Since 2008, there have been 6,600 referrals

---

- Clean up contaminated soil.
- Improve blood lead testing among children at high risk of exposure, and find and remediate the sources of their exposure.
- Ensure access to developmental and neuropsychological assessments and appropriate high-quality programs for children with elevated BLLs.

Medical–Legal Partnerships

Medical–legal partnerships (MLPs) are multisector approaches to addressing legal issues, many of which are contributors to poor child health outcomes and disparities. Typically, a health care provider (or providers) partners with a legal aid entity to resolve a person or family's legal issues, including those related to housing, benefits, debt, or education. As discussed in more detail in *Communities in Action*, MLPs "play an

to the program, with 12,000 children and 6,100 adults helped.[b] One of Child HeLP's innovations is its practice of merging data sources and using geographic information system mapping to identify housing units with medium to high rates of housing code violations and high rates of pediatric asthma (Beck et al., 2014). Outreach to landlords and legal action have resulted in mitigation of asthma triggers (Beck et al., 2012).

Child HeLP has helped families improve the health and well-being of their children by addressing many issues related to the SDOH (Klein et al., 2013; Murphy et al., 2015; Sandel et al., 2010; Tyler, 2012). Families have received assistance in obtaining Supplemental Nutrition Assistance Program and Special Supplemental Nutrition Program for Women, Infants, and Children benefits, health insurance coverage, transportation to jobs, day care for young children, enrollment in school and special education services, and adequate housing to prevent homelessness. The program has also helped to prevent child maltreatment by resolving child custody disputes and obtaining relief for parents experiencing domestic violence (Cincinnati Children's, n.d.).

Dr. Kahn from Cincinnati Children's Hospital was quoted in a *New York Times* opinion piece as saying, "So much of child health is the result of poor social and physical living conditions for kids—food on the table, shelter, quality education. So much of what we do in pediatrics is driven by these broader well-being issues for the family. We do much better when we partner with groups that have that as a mission" (Rosenberg, 2014).

---

[a] The committee used selection criteria to identify examples of promising models highlighted in this report (see Appendix A for a list of the criteria). These examples all apply developmental science and aim to advance health equity during the preconception through early childhood periods.

[b] Robert S. Kahn, co-director of the Cincinnati Child-Health Law Partnership, presented to the committee at its public information gathering session in August 2018. Presentation slides are available at www.nationalacademies.org/earlydevelopment (accessed April 17, 2019).

important role in addressing the SDOH and are a relevant community-based solution for advancing health equity" (NASEM, 2017, p. 427).

A systematic review conducted by Martinez et al. found that "researchers have established more findings regarding the capacity of MLPs to address legal outcomes than their capacity to address health outcomes" (Martinez et al., 2017, p. 267); however, longer periods of study are likely needed to see improved health outcomes. Additional research is needed to identify child-specific health outcomes associated with MLPs.

MLPs represent a promising practice that has emerged over the past 10–15 years, and according to the National Center for Medical-Legal Partnerships,[13] there are now 333 MLPs in 46 states. See Box 6-5 for an example of a promising MLP between the Cincinnati Children's Hospital and the Legal Aid Society of Greater Cincinnati.

---

[13] See https://medical-legalpartnership.org (accessed July 19, 2019).

Promising Tools

The following section describes tools that are available to communities and show promise in addressing poor child health outcomes and disparities through solutions to improve the affordability, quality, and stability of housing.

ChangeLab Solutions and Abt Associates have created a comprehensive and detailed toolkit that describes policies and programs to help preserve, protect, and expand the number of affordable rental units in neighborhoods where demand for housing is rising (Allbee et al., 2015). The authors state that "to ensure that people of all incomes, races, and ethnicities can continue to afford housing in neighborhoods experiencing rising rents, most communities will require a multifaceted strategy," one that includes a combination of the policies and programs described. Grouped into six areas of focus, these policies and programs are summarized in Table 6-2.

Another promising tool is the National Healthy Housing Standard,[14] which "provides health-based provisions to fill gaps where no property maintenance policy exists" and is "a complement to the International Property Maintenance Code and other policies already in use by local and state governments and federal agencies for the upkeep of existing homes" (National Center for Healthy Housing, 2014). The resource details minimum standards for healthy and safe homes, with information on each provision's public health rationale and further references and resources. Since the resource's release, the National Center for Healthy Housing also developed an implementation tool to aid in the adoption of the standard (National Center for Healthy Housing, 2017).[15]

Summary

Based on the evidence discussed in this chapter and presented in Chapter 3 on the effects of housing affordability and quality on health and developmental outcomes, the committee has reached the following conclusions about housing needs.

Conclusion 6-6: Healthy early development cannot occur without safe and stable housing. Lack of affordable housing and environmental hazards in housing disrupt healthy childhood development and

---

[14] The National Healthy Housing Standard is available at https://nchh.org/resource/national-healthy-housing-standard-full-document (accessed March 21, 2019).

[15] The National Healthy Housing Standard implementation tool is available at https://nchh.org/resource/national-healthy-housing-standard-implementation-tool (accessed March 21, 2019).

TABLE 6-2 A Toolkit of Policies and Programs to Preserve, Protect, and Expand Affordable Housing

Area of Focus	Purpose	Policies and Programs
Preservation	Preserve the affordability of housing where low- and moderate-income renters already live	• Right of first refusal • Property tax incentives • Moving properties into subsidy programs • Preserving public housing through RAD*
Protection	Protect residents from the effects of rising rents or condo conversions by helping to reduce the risk of displacement or by helping them relocate to new units if necessary	• Good cause conviction policies • Condominium conversion protections • Rent stabilization
Inclusion	Ensure a share of new development is affordable to low- and moderate-income households	• Mandatory inclusionary zoning • Density bonuses and other voluntary inclusionary policies
Revenue Generation	Generate funding for affordable housing in neighborhoods experiencing rising rents and home prices by leveraging the development activity and economic growth associated with new development or redevelopment	• Tax increment financing • Linkage fees • Housing trust funds
Incentives	Offer a range of incentives to stimulate development of affordable housing in targeted areas	• Targeting of federal, state, and local housing resources • Local and state tax incentives • Parking incentives • Expedited permitting • Impact fees • Transfers of development rights
Property Acquisition	Gain control of desirable sites for development or redevelopment at affordable prices	• Using publicly owned land • Property acquisition funds

* Rental Assistance Demonstration (RAD) is a federal program that "converts public housing subsidies into a form that can be used as the basis for securing private financing and can be combined more easily with other subsidies" (Allbee et al., 2015, p. 23).
SOURCE: Allbee et al., 2015.

parent/caregiver well-being. Children require affordable, quality, and stable living conditions to ensure that they can develop to their full potential.

Conclusion 6-7: Housing affordability and quality is an acute problem that disproportionately impacts people of color and contributes to health disparities among children. Over half of black and Hispanic renters live in unaffordable housing, and health issues related to poor-quality housing, such as elevated blood lead levels and asthma, are more prevalent among these renters.

Conclusion 6-8: Current federal housing programs are not adequately funded, and there are not enough safe, affordable housing units in high-opportunity areas. Additional funding for programs such as housing vouchers can move families out of poverty and allow families to reallocate money for other basic needs that support child health and development. Incentives and/or regulations, along with enhanced programming, can increase the supply of affordable housing.

Given the evidence on the impact of housing for health and healthy child development, the committee recommends:

Recommendation 6-3: The U.S. Department of Housing and Urban Development, states, and local, territorial, and tribal public housing authorities should increase the supply of high-quality affordable housing that is available to families, especially those with young children.

Increasing the supply of high-quality affordable housing will likely require additional federal funding to HUD and commitment from state and other local governments, as well as additional incentives or regulations to promote the development of new housing units.

Recommendation 6-4: The Secretary of the U.S. Department of Health and Human Services, in collaboration with the U.S. Department of Housing and Urban Development and other relevant agencies, should lead the development of a comprehensive plan to ensure access to stable, affordable, and safe housing in the prenatal through early childhood period. This strategy should particularly focus on priority populations who are disproportionately impacted by housing challenges and experience poor health outcomes.

Additional collaborators for this project include the agencies and organizations that are part of the United States Interagency Council on Homelessness.[16] The plan could include cross-sectoral initiatives that draw on resources from the health sector, such as a joint voucher program between HUD and HHS, MLPs to address housing problems within the clinical setting, and local investments in civil legal services and eviction prevention programs to help families stay in their homes during a short-term economic crisis.

> **Recommendation 6-5: The Center for Medicare & Medicaid Innovation should partner with states to test new Medicaid payment models that engage providers and other community organizations in addressing housing safety concerns, especially focused on young children. These demonstrations should evaluate impact on health, health disparities, and total cost of care.**

Recognizing that reducing child poverty is a critically important, foundational strategy for improving child health outcomes and reducing health inequity, the committee recommends three key ways to ensure that families have the resources needed to meet children's basic needs. Founded in the review of the evidence of health impacts and the committee's expertise, the recommendation is based on increased resources for access to food and stable housing and income support in the form of a child allowance:

> **Recommendation 6-6: Federal, state, tribal, and territorial policy makers should address the critical gaps between family resources and family needs through a combination of benefits that have the best evidence of advancing health equity, such as increased Supplemental Nutrition Assistance Program benefits, increased housing assistance, and a basic income allowance for young children.**

The costs of providing more resources to families with young children by increasing SNAP benefits, housing assistance, or a child allowance depend on many parameters, including the size of the benefit per family

---

[16] The collaborators in this council are the Corporation for National and Community Service, General Services Administration, HHS, HUD, Office of Management and Budget, SSA, U.S. Department of Agriculture, U.S. Department of Commerce, U.S. Department of Defense, U.S. Department of Education, U.S. Department of Energy, U.S. Department of Homeland Security, U.S. Department of Justice, U.S. Department of Labor, U.S. Department of the Interior, U.S. Department of Transportation, U.S. Department of Veterans Affairs, U.S. Postal Service, and the White House Faith and Opportunity Initiative. See https://www.usich.gov (accessed June 15, 2019) for more information.

and how many families are eligible and take up the benefit. Changes in these benefits may induce changes in parent employment, earnings, and receipt of other public benefits, affecting the total cost to the government. Full-scale analysis of the cost and behavioral changes of these proposals was beyond this committee's scope; however, the work of the National Academies' Committee on Building an Agenda to Reduce the Number of Children in Poverty by Half in 10 Years in the report *A Roadmap to Reducing Child Poverty* does provide some illustrative examples of cost estimates. Using the Urban Institute's TRIM3 simulation model, the total change in annual government spending was estimated for a range of policy options (see the full report for the policy details and model assumptions). The change in government spending of increasing SNAP benefits by 20 percent was estimated at $26,414 million, including employment and earnings adjustments (NASEM, 2019, p. 533). The cost of increasing housing vouchers by 50 percent was similar ($24,134 million) (NASEM, 2019, p. 537). In contrast, the estimate for a child allowance of $2,000 per year for families with children ages 0–16 was $32,904 million (NASEM, 2019, p. 549).[17] A child allowance for families with children under age 6 would be considerably less costly. The actual costs of expanding SNAP or housing programs or creating a child allowance will depend on the size and scope of the program. Future research is needed to investigate how to implement these programs cost effectively and so that they will yield the greatest health benefits.

Increasing resources available for families with young children to meet their basic needs is of utmost urgency given the science-based connections between health and income for healthy development of young children and their later health and educational outcomes. While the National Academies' Committee on Building an Agenda to Reduce the Number of Children in Poverty by Half in 10 Years recommended other important strategies, such as expanding the EITC or the Child and Dependent Care Tax Credit and increasing minimum wage, this committee's recommendation focuses on strategies that are likely to have particularly important impacts on health outcomes for young children. These include a child allowance targeted at families with young children not yet in K–12 school and increasing SNAP benefit levels and housing assistance. A child allowance would fill in some of the gaps in the current safety net and particularly benefit the lowest-income children and those most at risk of poor health outcomes. The key advantage of a child allowance (over, for example, tax credits) is that funds are available to

---

[17] It is important to note that these estimates are net costs to the government, and they are not suitable for comparison to other cost estimates cited in this chapter.

families on an ongoing, monthly basis rather than once per year. In addition, under the current structure of the child and working family tax credits, the lowest-income families receive few benefits. Children whose parents are in unstable employment or not employed suffer the short- and long-term health consequences of living in poverty. Reducing health disparities requires reaching these children during their earliest years, regardless of parental employment. Increased SNAP benefits and housing allowances would address current inadequacies in both of these programs and provide targeted support for the critical food and housing needs of young children. Paid parental leave would also recognize and support the special needs of the earliest years, in which parental time and attention are critically important for children's health and development.

Another way to increase resources to families with young children would be to provide more funding to subsidize child care. For example, the National Academies' Committee on Building an Agenda to Reduce the Number of Children in Poverty by Half in 10 Years included the expansion of child care subsidies as one of their options for reducing childhood poverty, and guaranteeing access to subsidies for families below 150 percent of the federal poverty level would significantly increase resources available to low-income, working families. As noted in Chapter 3, only 15 percent of eligible families received Child Care and Development Block Grant subsidies in 2012 (Walker and Matthews, 2017). However, these subsidies would flow only to families who meet the work requirements and use an eligible care provider, so these resources would be less likely to help families in deep poverty or those with intermittent employment. While child care subsidies are an important work support for low-income families, the committee focused on programs with more evidence of positive effects on children's health and those not dependent on parental employment. As noted earlier in this chapter, expansions of the work-oriented safety net programs may have unintended negative consequences for child health if parent employment results in lower rates of breastfeeding or disruptions to the attachment between infant and caregiver. In order to provide supports for all children, it is important to supplement work-support programs with basic support for families with young children that is not tied to employment.

In addition to material resources to meet their basic needs, children need a nurturing and healthy environment, responsive and sensitive caregiving free of maltreatment, and opportunities to develop the socio-emotional and cognitive skills to be healthy and resilient. Families with adequate resources may be better able to provide these important determinants of health, yet income alone may not be sufficient to ensure positive health outcomes. Thus, while addressing families' basic material needs is a critically important strategy for improving health outcomes of young children, strategies that focus only on reducing child poverty are unlikely to be sufficient to eliminate poor health outcomes and health disparities in early childhood. Specific recommendations with regard to the child's environment and the importance of relationships are discussed in other chapters of this report. The importance of confronting and eliminating structural racism in order to eliminate health disparities is discussed in Chapters 3 and 8.

NEIGHBORHOOD CONDITIONS

Neighborhoods play a critical role in the health, well-being, and development of children. Those that provide families with access to high-quality education, employment opportunities, safety, high-quality health care, and other essential services are essential to supporting children's healthy development. Persistent and increasing economic inequality, however, has contributed to neighborhoods facing increased economic segregation and concentrated poverty whose conditions and lack of resources can negatively affect healthy development and limit opportunities for children to flourish.

Neighborhood conditions can be defined broadly as the overall community context that is shaped by the natural and built environment (e.g., housing structures and conditions, availability of sidewalks and open/green space, presence of vacant lots, environmental exposures) and the availability or lack of health-promoting goods and services (e.g., access to healthy foods, affordable and safe transportation), in addition to the social environment (e.g., community cohesion, residential segregation, violence). This section addresses neighborhood conditions broadly; other sections in this chapter discuss the evidence related to specific neighborhood-level factors, such as housing, environmental exposures, food security, and economic security.

Concentrated Disadvantage

Residential segregation persists in the United States and has contributed to neighborhoods experiencing concentrated disadvantage where intergenerational cycles of poverty and adversity can derail children's healthy development. Data from the 2010–2014 American Community Survey show that residential segregation by race and ethnicity has begun to decline slightly (Frey, 2015); however, economic residential segregation has increased (Rusk, 2017; Taylor and Fry, 2012).

Residential segregation, by race and ethnicity and by socioeconomic status and income, increases racial health disparities and has pronounced effects on children's health outcomes. Its effects include socioeconomic disadvantages, such as limited opportunities for high-quality education and employment; increased exposure to crime, violence, and environmental toxicants; and limited access to transportation options, healthy food options, and health care services, which in turn leads to disparities in the quality of services and treatment (Acevedo-Garcia et al., 2008). For children in particular, segregation limits their access to high-quality schools and after-school programs and to neighborhoods in which they can play and exercise safely (Acevedo-Garcia et al., 2007, 2008).

Although policies that promote and increase segregation (including Jim Crow laws, redlining, and discriminatory banking and foreclosure practices) no longer exist overtly, their effects have persisted and remain widespread in communities experiencing intergenerational poverty and trauma. Segregation limits socioeconomic resources available to those living in concentrated poverty and has resulted in disparities in rates of disease, availability of high-quality health care providers, and opportunities to engage in health-promoting behaviors. Its effects have also included access to a higher density of alcohol, tobacco, and fast food outlets, increased risk of exposure to environmental hazards and toxicants, and higher risk of exposure to violence. For more information on the historical and contemporary effects of segregation policies, see Chapter 3 of NASEM (2017), or Reskin (2012).

Exposure to Violence

Exposure to neighborhood crime and violence can significantly affect children's cognitive (Burdick-Will, 2018; Sharkey, 2010), emotional and behavioral (Kim et al., 2014; McCoy et al., 2016; Sharkey et al., 2012), and health outcomes. Improving neighborhood conditions to diminish exposure to crime and violence plays an important role in reducing children's biological stress and improving their health outcomes. For more on exposure to violence as an adverse childhood experience, see Chapter 3.

In addition to adversity faced at the individual level, repeated exposure to crime and violence can contribute to community trauma. A report by the Prevention Institute describes that "community trauma is not just the aggregate of individuals in a neighborhood who have experienced trauma from exposures to violence"; rather, symptoms of community trauma "are present in the closed-cultural environment, the physical/built environment, and the economic environment" (Pinderhughes et al., 2015). The report describes several community strategies to implement within each of these three environments to mitigate the negative effects of community trauma, build more resilient communities, and improve health and well-being outcomes (see Figure 6-3). The authors note that across all environments, approaches that are most effective will "build on indigenous knowledge, expertise, and leadership to produce strategies that are culturally relevant and appropriate" (Pinderhughes et al., 2015, p. 5).

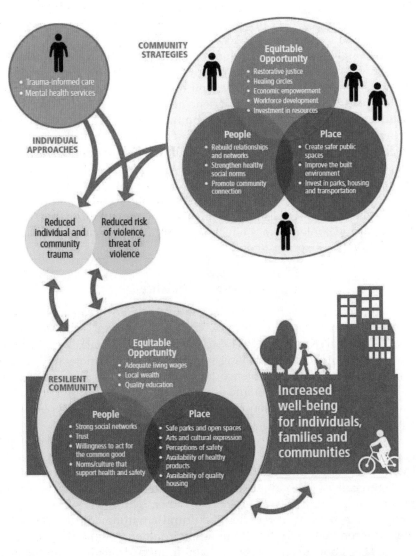

FIGURE 6-3 Promoting community resilience: from trauma to well-being.
SOURCES: Pinderhughes et al., 2015; figure provided by Prevention Institute, www.preventioninstitute.org.

Improving Neighborhood Conditions

HUD's Moving to Opportunity (MTO) study provides clear evidence that better neighborhood conditions are strongly associated with improved health and development outcomes (Kling et al., 2007; Ludwig et al., 2013). MTO randomized assistance designed to help low-income families move to less impoverished neighborhoods; after 10–15 years, adults chosen to receive that assistance had lower prevalence of obesity and diabetes and better subjective health outcomes than adults who were selected not to receive it (Ludwig et al., 2011). Despite these positive findings, the MTO experiment has also yielded mixed results. Early MTO studies resulted in findings that ran counter to the hypothesized outcomes; for example, Sanbonmatsu et al. (2006) found no evidence of improvement in academic outcomes for any age group 4–7 years after randomization. As noted previously in the chapter, Chetty et al. (2016) found strong evidence to suggest that children who moved to lower-poverty neighborhoods when they were young (i.e., under 13 years of age) were more likely to experience positive outcomes later in life, such as attending college and earning higher incomes. However, the study also showed contrary outcomes for those who moved when they were older. Other research indicates that while girls in the MTO experiment exhibited positive mental health outcomes (e.g., decreased rates of major depression and conduct disorder), boys experienced the opposite (e.g., increased rates of posttraumatic stress disorder, major depression, and conduct disorder) (Kessler et al., 2014). In terms of long-term outcomes (i.e., 10–15 years), Ludwig et al. (2013) concluded that moving to lower-poverty neighborhoods during childhood leads to improvements in adult physical and mental health, but not economic self-sufficiency.

MTO established that places matter for health but not what it is about them that matters most: it was not designed to tease apart which aspects of places drove those health improvements, nor did it specifically address prenatal or birth outcomes. Other studies have attempted to further illuminate which aspects of a neighborhood—for example, better economic environments, built environment features that promote healthy lifestyles, or improved social cohesion—might represent the most important levers for improving health and birth outcomes. Other than MTO, however, randomized studies on place and its impacts on health are extraordinarily rare, so the evidence is almost entirely limited to observational studies.

The Washington Center for Equitable Growth describes two approaches to addressing segregation within neighborhoods: (1) invest in neighborhoods to make the consequences of segregation less severe, and (2) reduce the level of segregation in neighborhoods directly (Sharkley, 2016).

Approaches to increase and shift investments to low-income communities include

1. Providing work supports (including supplemental wages and guaranteed public service jobs, as in the New Hope program, and services to residents of public housing developments and rent incentives to encourage work, as in the Job Plus program) for individuals and families in high-poverty communities;
2. Investing in evidence-based programs for young people, such as those that include tutoring or mentoring, sports activities, cognitive behavioral therapy, and summer jobs, which randomized trials have shown lead to increases in academic achievement and decreases in involvement in crime and violence;
3. Identifying and/or establishing a single institution in every low-income neighborhood "that takes ownership over the community and takes responsibility for all the residents within it, . . . so that everyone within that neighborhood knows that there is going to be an institution serving them for the long haul and will have resources sufficient to bring about long-term change" (Sharkley, 2016).

Addressing the lack of affordable housing is crucial to reducing segregation in neighborhoods directly (Sharkley, 2016). To improve housing affordability, the Washington Center for Economic Growth provides the following approaches:

1. Expanding the supply of housing vouchers. (See the following section on Housing Affordability for more on housing vouchers.)
2. Providing support to allow families to access opportunity neighborhoods.
3. Providing incentives and regulations to preserve and expand affordable housing in exclusive markets.
4. Establishing a long-range mobility bank (Sharkley, 2016).

In developing approaches to enable families to access opportunity neighborhoods, an important consideration is ensuring that adequate supports are available to families to buffer the negative effects of stress associated with moving to other communities. For an example of a promising initiative that aims to support and strengthen families by providing community-based supportive services, see Box 6-6.

ENVIRONMENTAL EXPOSURES AND EXPOSURE TO TOXICANTS

Each year, Americans are exposed to chemicals in the environment at increasingly greater levels. EPA tracks new chemical substances in its Toxic Substances Control Act (TSCA) Chemical Substance Inventory,

---

BOX 6-6
SHIELDS for Families: A Promising Model[a]

SHIELDS, started in 1991, provides multipronged community-based services and operates 34 different programs. SHIELDS' goals are to promote family reunification and support families remaining intact in the community, strengthen families by providing comprehensive and collaborative services, improve the general well-being of families through comprehensive health programs and preventive social services, and encourage self-sufficiency and economic independence by assisting individuals with obtaining employment and advancing education (SHIELDS for Families, 2011). SHIELDS consists of five divisions: child welfare, children and youth, mental health, substance abuse, and supportive services.

SHIELDS supports high-risk families in South Los Angeles, California, with several programs specifically for pregnant and parenting women and their children ages 0–5. SHIELDS' wraparound programs address employment, health services, housing, income and wealth, public safety, the social environment, and transportation. SHIELDS engages multiple sectors and is funded by private foundations, Los Angeles County, and federal grants. For wraparound support programs, SHIELDS has partnered with private hospitals, the Los Angeles Department of Children and Family Services, the Los Angeles Department of Probation, the Los Angeles Homeless Services Authority, Special Services for Groups, California's Post-Release Community Supervision jurisdiction, the California Department of Justice, training and vocational schools, and many more organizations and agencies.[b]

SHIELDS reports that 4,308 families were linked to more than 15,000 services through their family resource center; 362 families received mental health treatment; 78 percent of families successfully completed treatment; and 69 percent of families reunited with children (SHIELDS for Families, 2011).

---

[a] The committee used selection criteria to identify examples of promising models highlighted in this report (see Appendix A for a list of the criteria). These examples all apply developmental science and aim to advance health equity during the preconception through early childhood periods. Caregivers and representatives from SHIELDS for Families presented to the Committee at its public information gathering session in October 2018.

[b] For more information, see https://www.shieldsforfamilies.org (accessed April 17, 2019).

---

which is updated every 6 months (EPA, n.d.-c). Currently, more than 85,000 chemical substances are listed in the TSCA inventory, with companies introducing about 700 new substances each year (EPA, n.d.-a; Tollefson, 2016). As described in Chapter 3, many of these substances are related to poor health outcomes for mothers, infants, and children. In its review of the literature, the committee found that children (from fetal development through early childhood) are at greater risk than adults from adverse health effects of environmental exposures due to their smaller size and proportionally large intake of food, air, and water to body weight and are subject to rapid developmental processes that may be influenced and disrupted by chemicals and toxicants. Parents' exposures to environmental toxicants in the preconception phase also present a risk to early child development. Furthermore, as a result of exposure to toxicants, children are more likely than adults to suffer from developmental problems, chronic conditions, and death. The committee also concludes that

Conclusion 6-9: Not all households experience the same level of risk of exposure to harmful environmental toxicants or pollutants. Poverty, substandard and/or unstable housing, race and ethnicity, and proximity to known sources of pollutants heighten pregnant women and children's risk of exposure and poor health and developmental outcomes.

The following section provides a review of the limited research currently available that specifically examines policies and practices to reduce the risk of environmental exposures among preconception, prenatal, and postnatal populations.

Reducing the Risk of Environmental Exposures in the Home and in Child Care Settings

The Center for Medicaid and CHIP Services (CMCS) serves millions of pregnant women, children, and families by providing health care access to low-income families and families who would not otherwise qualify for health insurance. CMCS also establishes reimbursement criteria for these health services, including environmental exposure screening, testing, and case management. How these criteria are implemented varies by state, though some aspects of coverage are mandatory. For example, blood lead screening is mandated for Medicaid recipients at 12 and 24 months of age. However, states vary in how this mandate is implemented (CMS, n.d.). Some states provide these screenings only to Medicaid-enrolled children, while others offer universal screenings; one state, Arizona, has chosen to implement a targeted screening approach (Arizona Department of Health Services, 2017; CMS, 2016), while still others do not currently have a lead screening program (Dickman, 2017; NASHP, 2018). Moreover, some states require reporting the results to state health departments or the state lead registry, which may result in follow-up care or case management. Other states do not have a registry or other tracking system, and still others do not provide any form of follow-up to children with elevated BLLs.

Medicaid can cover home investigations of lead exposures, case management for exposed children, and support to states to implement education, screening, and outreach efforts to areas at high risk of lead exposure (CMS, 2017), though it is unclear how these programs are applied at local levels. In addition, greater collaboration with tribal nations is needed to improve state screening and registry efforts (PTFCEH, 2018), though some federally funded research studies have led to tribal law and policy updates to improve lead screening among children (Petersen et al., 2007). No other screening programs aimed at environmental exposures receive Medicaid support; lead exposure is an exception because of the estimated magnitude, frequency, and duration of exposure, the significance of the health impacts, and the potential for prevention (NASHP, 2017). However, several states have asserted regulatory authority over other environmental toxicants, including bisphenol A (BPA), cleaning agents in schools, and flame retardants (NCSL, 2017).

Child care settings represent another source of potential environmental exposures for children. With more than 13 million preschoolers in child care every day, including 6 million infants and toddlers (Amoah et al., 2016) (see Chapter 3 for more information on the number of children enrolled in various ECE programs), addressing potential environmental exposures in child care settings could reduce the risk of related health issues for a large proportion of children under age 6. Taking steps to address potential exposures can present challenges, as child care facilities may be located within individual homes, community centers, and office buildings, which may not be consistently assessed or regulated to reduce the risk of environmental exposures. Moreover, licensing guidelines vary, with limited requirements addressing child care provider training on mitigation of early childhood exposures. Reviewing existing state policies on the regulation of environmental exposures in child care facilities offers policy makers an opportunity to compare policy approaches and consider nonregulatory approaches to effect change (Environmental Law Institute, 2015).

In addition to reviewing existing policies, evaluating the effectiveness of training programs can also inform decision making around environmental exposure risk reduction. In a study of 60 child care centers in Washington, DC, an environmental risk assessment training was developed and tested that covered the following areas: (1) air quality, (2) arsenic, (3) asbestos, (4) built environment, (5) chemicals in art supplies, (6) lead, (7) mercury, (8) mold, (9) noise pollution, (10) pesticides and integrated pesticide management, (11) physical education and nutrition, (12) plastics, (13) radon, and (14) safe cleaning alternatives (Amoah et al., 2016). More than 580 child care workers received the training and pre-/post-assessments, and knowledge scores increased by about 20 percent, on average, between the two assessments. Nearly 70 percent of participating child care centers reduced their environmental risk assessment scores. This training is an important approach to reducing the environmental risk for children receiving child care outside the home.

Educational approaches are also effective at the level of the individual household. In a meta-analysis of seven community health worker–delivered interventions focused on reducing asthma symptoms, most of these significantly decreased asthma symptoms, lessened daytime activity limitations, and reduced emergency and urgent care use (Postma et al., 2009). Programs that included higher intensity and frequency of home visiting reported the most positive health outcomes. Similarly, in a systematic review of 20 studies focused on reducing the risk of asthma morbidity among children, most of them were effective in significantly reducing the number of days with asthma symptoms, school days missed, and asthma acute care visits (Crocker et al., 2011). The review examined studies expressly focused on informing multitrigger, multicomponent, home-based environmental interventions, which address the complex nature of reducing asthma risk within the home due to the many potential sources of risk. A randomized controlled trial aimed at educating pregnant women on reducing exposure to hazardous air pollutants resulted in a significant increase in preventive behaviors (Marzieh et al., 2017), demonstrating that interventions aimed at parents can also be effective in reducing the risk of toxic exposures for infants and children.

Reducing the Risk of Environmental Exposures in the Community

In a 2018 study, researchers linked 2011 National Emissions Inventory data with block groups from the 2009–2013 American Community Survey data (Mikati et al., 2018). For particulate matter of 2.5 micrometers or less in diameter ($PM_{2.5}$), those living in poverty and people of color experienced significantly higher levels of exposure compared to white individuals. Racial disparities, particularly for black Americans, were greater than for those living in poverty alone (Mikati et al., 2018). In a subsequent 2019 study, researchers found that, on average, non-Hispanic whites experience a "pollution advantage" (Tessum et al., 2019). In other words, they experience 17 percent less air pollution exposure, comparing the amount to which they are exposed and the amount that they are responsible for due to their consumption levels. In comparison, black and Hispanic Americans, on average, experience 56 percent and 63 percent excess exposure, respectively, relative to the exposure caused by their consumption (Tessum et al., 2019). While $PM_{2.5}$ exposure for all groups fell about 50 percent between 2002 and 2015 due to increased regulation and population density reductions near polluted areas, the inequities remain above and beyond this reduction. Scientists suggest addressing these inequities will likely require multilevel approaches, including reducing consumption levels, improving manufacturing and other processes to minimize pollution, and implementing more comprehensive measures, such as evaluating plans for construction and urban development with the purpose of reducing dependence on automobile transportation to manage and lessen current inequities, along with meaningfully involving communities in assessment processes to effect broader policy change (Schulz et al., 2016).

For example, researchers collaborated with the Rural Empower-
ment Association for Community Help in North Carolina to train middle
schoolers to assess asthma indicators, lung function, and air pollution
(Guidry et al., 2014). School administrators and students reported positive perspectives on the project, which offers an example for community-
based research aimed at improving air pollution in rural settings (Guidry
et al., 2014). In another example, the Community Action to Fight Asthma
Initiative in California used an environmental justice approach to reduce
risk factors for asthma in school-aged children. Statewide coalitions,
which included local residents and technical assistance experts, supported
policies to reduce children's exposures to environmental triggers. Technical assistance, community involvement, and multilevel strategies led
to policy change that addressed reduction of environmental inequities
(Kreger et al., 2011).

The BREATHE Project based in Barcelona, Spain, which aimed to
assess traffic-related air pollutant exposure among schoolchildren, is a
promising example of using complex measures and modeling to reduce
pollutant exposure (Rivas et al., 2018). Using advanced measurement
and statistical techniques, researchers identified eight factors/sources of
pollutants, including minerals, traffic, road dust, secondary sulfate and
organics, secondary nitrate, sea spray, heavy oil combustion, metallurgy,
and organic/textile/chalk, and were able to characterize the air quality
within and near 39 urban schools. This novel approach allows for detailed
mapping of exposure risk, which supports positive policy change through
data-driven decision making.

Community Infrastructure

Sustainable infrastructure is defined as

> systems that have the capacity to endure over a long period of time;
> enabling the human-built environment to thrive and providing an op-
> portunity for human society to improve its quality of life, without com-
> promising the integrity and availability of natural, economic, and social
> assets for future generations. (Hendricks et al., 2018, p. 2)

Properly managing infrastructure (i.e., replacing lead drinking water
pipes, mitigating flood zones to reduce damage to homes and schools,
and updating technology to ensure timely notification of emergent hazards) through the lens of assessing and maximizing sustainability therefore has important downstream implications for public health. This is
particularly the case with respect to ensuring that the necessary environment and resources are equitably available to support early childhood development and minimizing exposures to harms that arise from
poor infrastructure, lack of sustainable practices, and the concomitant
effects on the environment. Moreover, reducing these risks can lead to

cost savings. For example, the annual U.S. cost of environment-related pediatric disease in 2008 was estimated to be $76.6 billion, or 3.5 percent of total health care costs (Trasande and Liu, 2011). These costs are limited to pediatric diseases caused by environmental exposures. Including costs of pediatric diseases resulting from severe climate conditions' impact on aged or damaged infrastructure, such as heat-related deaths and illnesses and increased exposures to lead and other toxicants, mold and poor water quality from flooded and damaged dwellings, and poor air quality from increased forest fire smoke and smog, could support prioritization and decision making to best address failing infrastructure.

The United States currently faces a critical infrastructure crisis (Maxwell et al., 2018) as a result of decades of deferrals at every governmental level and lack of effective accountability on the side of private institutions to ensure essential infrastructure received necessary upgrades, including improvements that would minimize negative environmental impacts and ensure long-term sustainability (ASCE, 2017). Using strategies such as the framework put forth by Koehler et al. (2018) for improving community health through better environment decision making could provide important approaches to mitigate future harms and reduce costs. In addition, existing models do not specifically examine risks to early childhood development and ensuing costs. Additional research and environmental assessments are needed to ensure harms are minimized, especially for populations who are disproportionately impacted by harmful environmental exposures. Investing in the rebuilding of the nation's infrastructure at every level—waste and water management, walkable streets and parks, cleanup of toxic waste sites, and so on—along with strengthening capacity for community engagement and civil rights actions around environmental justice can provide a cross-sector approach that strengthens infrastructure in the United States, reducing potential harms to infants and children and ensuring lower medical costs for pediatric injury and disease associated with severe climate effects.

The Role of Civil Rights

Civil rights strategies are an important yet underused tool to promote clean and healthy communities for developing children. This was acknowledged as a community-driven solution to promote health equity in the 2017 National Academies report *Communities in Action: Pathways to Health Equity*. The report asserts that "civil rights, health, and environmental justice laws and policies provide a framework to promote equal access to publicly funded resources and prohibit discrimination based on race, color, national origin, income, gender, disability, and other factors" (NASEM, 2017, p. 351). Federal laws and civil rights legislation have historically been a codified source of rights to protect individuals and groups from harmful environmental exposures (see, for example, Title VI of the Civil Rights Act of 1964,[18] the National Environmental Policy Act,[19] and the Clean Water Act[20]). In 1994, an executive order was issued on Federal Actions to Address Environmental Justice in Minority Populations and Low-Income Populations.[21] Civil rights laws and their enforcement not only aim to protect populations in at-risk contexts—thereby reducing disparities—but also allow for a crosscutting approach that can apply to many of the determinants of health and development discussed in this report (e.g., housing, environmental exposures, education). (See Hahn et al. [2018] for a brief summary of civil rights history and discussion on the relationship between civil rights laws and the determinants of health.) Specifically, civil rights strategies can be used to mitigate discriminatory burdens, lower or remove barriers to community participation in decision making, and improve access to health and environmental benefits that are foundational to safe and healthy communities (NASEM, 2017; USDA, 2012).

At the state level, California's EPA operates an Environmental Justice Task Force, which develops initiatives in communities where compliance and enforcement can help mitigate or stop the harmful effects of exposure to pollution. At the community level, there are tools that can be employed to ensure that these rights are protected to engender equitable outcomes for children and families. For example, public health, civil rights, and environmental justice practitioners use a five-step planning framework by which to assess proposed or current environmental policies or practices for their potential to harm or benefit communities (Environmental Justice Leadership Forum on Climate Change, 2016; NASEM, 2017; The City Project, 2016)[22]:

1. Describe what is planned in terms that are understandable to the community;
2. Analyze the benefits and burdens on all people;
3. Analyze alternatives to what is being considered;

---

[18] Title VI of the Civil Rights Act of 1964 (42 U.S.C. § 2000d to 2000d-7): "No person in the United States shall, on the ground of race, color, or national origin, be excluded from participation in, be denied the benefits of, or be subjected to discrimination under any program or activity receiving Federal financial assistance" (DOL, n.d.).

[19] 42 U.S.C. § 4321 et seq.

[20] 33 U.S.C. § 1251 et seq.

[21] E.O. 12898. 59 FR 7629; February 16, 1994.

[22] This planning framework is based on Title VI, Executive Order 12898, case law, and best practices by federal agencies (NASEM, 2017).

4. Include people of color, low-income people, and other stakeholders in every step in the decision-making process; and
5. Develop an implementation plan to distribute benefits and burdens fairly and avoid discrimination.

(See NASEM [2017] for a more in-depth discussion about the planning
process, in addition to a few examples of communities that have successfully applied the process.)

The *Communities in Action: Pathways to Health Equity* report
(NASEM, 2017) also outlines some guidance for civil rights attorneys,
public health professionals, community groups, public agencies, recipients of public funding, foundations, and other stakeholders to advance
equity using civil rights tools (see Box 6-7 for a listing of these guiding
strategies).

Finally, based on the committee's expertise and its review of civil
rights legislation, literature, and past action to address equitable access
to the health-promoting social determinants, the authoring committee of

---

BOX 6-7
Guidance for Communities to Advance
Equity Using Civil Rights Tools

- Communities and other stakeholders can work together on compliance and
equity plans for programs or activities by recipients of public funding that use
the civil rights framework by describing what is to be done, analyzing the impact
on all communities, analyzing alternatives, including full and fair participation
by diverse communities, and promoting health equity.
- Compliance and equity plans can be used to guard against unjustified and un-
necessary discriminatory impacts, as well as against intentional discrimination,
in health and wellness programs and activities.
- Communities, when appropriate, can work with civil rights attorneys to use
problem-solving strategies, including coalition building, planning, data collection and analysis, media, negotiation, policy and legal advocacy out of court,
and access to justice through the courts.
- Communities can work with attorneys and public health experts together to
promote a better understanding of the civil rights dimension of the challenge
of health disparities and to show how to address these civil rights concerns
for their communities to ensure that civil rights laws against discrimination in
health and other publicly funded programs and activities are strengthened and
not rolled back.

SOURCE: Excerpted from NASEM, 2017.

Communities in Action: Pathways to Health Equity reached the following conclusions in its report:

> Civil rights approaches have helped mitigate the negative impacts of many forms of social and health discrimination. Continuing this work is needed to overcome discrimination and the structural barriers that affect health.
>
> Using civil rights approaches in devising and implementing community solutions to promote health equity can guard against unjustified and unnecessary discriminatory impacts, as well as against intentional discrimination in programs that affect health. For example, those implementing community solutions can employ methods and data in ways that include full and fair participation by diverse communities. (NASEM, 2017, p. 362)

Given the critical role of civil rights strategies in advancing health equity in communities, the report also included a recommendation to foundations and other funders to expand their community support beyond their traditional roles by supporting education, compliance, and enforcement related to civil rights law and other areas (see Recommendation 7-1 in NASEM [2017] for the full recommendation). The report acknowledges the barriers associated with federal tax laws that may preclude foundations from supporting such activities, but it also suggests the use of general operating funds as opposed to program-specific funds (NASEM, 2017). The alignment between this report and *Communities in Action* with respect to health equity and the applicability of civil rights strategies for addressing environmental exposures in communities warrants serious consideration of these findings and the abovementioned recommendation for promoting healthy and equitable early development.

Leveraging Clinical Settings to Reduce Environmental Exposure Risk

Recent evidence confirms that preconception and prenatal exposures can adversely impact fetal development, which may result in long-lasting health effects (Grandjean et al., 2015). Training tools for health practitioners offer a potentially promising prevention approach to reduce harmful environmental exposures and the risk of future adverse health effects for prenatal and preconception patients (Sathyanarayana et al., 2012). In a national online survey of more than 2,500 obstetricians, nearly 80 percent agreed that they can reduce patient exposures to environmental health hazards by counseling patients. However, half of respondents reported that they rarely take an environmental health history course, and less than 20 percent reported routinely asking about environmental exposures commonly found for pregnant women in the United States. Moreover, only 1

in 15 reported having any training on how to assess environmental exposures among patients (Stotland et al., 2014), demonstrating the need for
additional supports for providers, particularly given the complexity of
the assessment process. There are several online tools for providers to
use to triangulate exposure risk, yet the sheer number of possible chemical exposures, the relatively limited data available on possible risks, and
the expertise and time commitment needed to complete an assessment
may pose significant challenges for primary care or specialty providers
(Koehrn et al., 2017).

Medical Education on Environmental Health

Education on the effects of preconception and prenatal exposure to
environmental toxicants is largely insufficient in medical education and
curricula (Gehle et al., 2011; Tinney et al., 2015). Pediatric practice, which
has historically recognized the influence of environmental health exposures (Tinney et al., 2015), is an important setting to screen for exposure
to environmental toxicants. However, there are also earlier opportunities
to identify and ensure timely treatment for harmful exposures during the
preconception and prenatal periods (Tinney et al., 2015). Many professional organizations have emphasized the urgency and importance of
addressing exposure to environmental toxicants. In a joint committee
opinion from the American College of Obstetricians and Gynecologists
(ACOG) Committee on Health Care for Underserved Women and the
American Society for Reproductive Medicine (ASRM) Practice Committee, ACOG and ASRM call for "timely action to identify and reduce
exposure to toxic environmental agents while addressing the consequences of such exposure" (ACOG, 2013). The International Federation
of Gynaecology and Obstetrics, a professional organization of obstetrical
and gynecological associations from 125 countries that includes ACOG,
states that "obstetricians, gynecologists, midwives, women's health nurse
practitioners, nurses, and other health professionals should . . . make
environment health part of health care" and that "exposure to toxic environmental chemicals during pregnancy and breastfeeding is ubiquitous
and is a threat to healthy human reproduction" (Di Renzo et al., 2015).
However, despite broad consensus on the importance of addressing exposure to environmental toxicants, studies show that many obstetricians
and gynecologists do not screen their patients for harmful environmental
exposures (Grindler et al., 2018; Stotland et al., 2014).

While qualitative data suggest that pediatricians express an interest
and need for more training on environmental medicine topics (e.g., environmental history) (Kilpatrick et al., 2002; Trasande et al., 2006), this type
of education is not routinely included in pediatric curricula (Roberts and
Gitterman, 2003). The National Environmental Education and Training

Foundation and the Children's Environmental Health Network formed two working groups with expertise in medical and nursing education to explore opportunities to incorporate environmental health into pediatric education (McCurdy et al., 2004). After reviewing the transition from undergraduate student to professional status, the medical education working group recommended improving education about children's environmental health in medical school curricula, residence, training, and continuing medical education in addition to expanding fellowship training in children's environmental health. The nursing working group similarly recommended enhancing content on children's environmental health at the undergraduate, graduate, and continuing nursing education levels. Both working groups identified leverage points (i.e., key organizations and stakeholders) that could facilitate these changes.

There are several existing resources and strategies to accelerate the integration of environmental health into existing medical education and curricula. A work group of faculty members and residents[23] formed at a meeting convened by the Mid-Atlantic Center for Children's Health and the Environment and The George Washington University's Department of Obstetrics and Gynecology identified several approaches to better incorporate environmental health into medical education, including

1. Integrating environmental health into basic science courses and the organ systems approach (Gehle et al., 2011) into medical school and residency curricula;[24]
2. Implementing clinical training programs on environmental health, such as the model established by the University of California, San Francisco, Program on Reproductive Health and the Environment;[25]
3. Adding questions on environmental health to resident training and board-certifying exams[26] to ensure that programs will include environmental health in their curricula;

---

[23] Faculty members and residents who participated in the meeting represented 16 academic obstetrics-gynecology programs from 5 states (Delaware, Maryland, Pennsylvania, Virginia, and West Virginia) and Washington, DC.

[24] The George Washington University's Department of Obstetrics and Gynecology has a medical school and residency curriculum on environmental health specifically for obstetricians and gynecologists (Tinney et al., 2015).

[25] PHRE includes rotations programs for obstetrics-gynecology clinical trainees and maternal-fetal medicine fellows, as well as resources such as educational materials for patients and environmental health history forms for clinical practice for reproductive health professionals (Tinney et al., 2015).

[26] Such as those administered by the Council on Residency Education in Obstetrics and Gynecology, American Board of Obstetrics and Gynecology, and American Osteopathic Board of Obstetrics and Gynecology (Tinney et al., 2015).

4. Training leaders in medical education and faculty members on reproductive environmental health through the Association of Professors of Gynecology and Obstetrics; and

5. Requiring continuing education in environmental health[27] to ensure that practicing obstetricians and gynecologists receive introductory education to environmental health (Tinney et al., 2015).

There are also resources to support providers in offering their patients counseling and health education on environmental exposures. Located across the United States and Canada, Pediatric Environmental Health Specialty Units are a national network of experts in reproductive and children's environmental health who are located at academic medical centers and provide medical information and advice and respond to requests for information on the prevention, diagnosis, management, and treatment of the effects of environmental exposures on children and adults of child-bearing age (PEHSU, n.d.). AAP publishes a guide for pediatricians, *Pediatric Environmental Health*, which is meant to help identify, prevent, and treat pediatric environmental health problems (AAP Council on Environmental Health, 2012).

Similarly, the Organization of Teratology Information Specialists provides an online service known as MotherToBaby that provides evidence-based information on the safety of medications and other exposures during pregnancy and while breastfeeding to health care professionals and the general public (MotherToBaby, n.d.). Lastly, a collaborative initiative[28] known as SafetyNEST provides health care professionals and the general public with "accurate, evidence-based, and personalized information about the effects of toxic chemicals on prenatal and early childhood health" through an educational online platform (SafetyNEST, 2018).

Research, Monitoring, and Testing of Environmental Exposures

Existing conceptual frameworks fail to encapsulate the complexities inherent in early childhood development. The Public Health Eposome Conceptual Model attempts to capture the changing nature of these exposures, along with the life course considerations needed to accurately assess risk (Tulve, 2016). In particular, children may experience chemical

[27] The Agency for Toxic Substances and Disease Registry has created online resources on environmental health, including case studies on environmental medicine, for health professionals completing continuing education (Gehle et al., 2011; Tinney et al., 2015).

[28] Partners include the University of California, San Francisco, Program on Reproductive Health and the Environment; Icahn School of Medicine at Mount Sinai, American Medical Women's Association, and Universidade Federal do Paraná in Brazil (SafetyNEST, 2018).

exposures from their environments at every life stage throughout the life course. Children are exposed to chemicals in foods, water, air, and surfaces they touch, such as chemical residues on surfaces or in dust and soil. Revising existing conceptual models aims to improve evaluation and assessment of environmental exposures to improve accuracy, enhance the overall fit of statistical modeling, and ensure improved predictive power in research studies examining environmental exposures and effects on early childhood development.

In another approach, a conceptual framework relying on a holistic approach to maternal and child health research includes both psychosocial stressors and environmental hazards to better explain factors that influence poor health outcomes for populations that experience higher risks of environmental exposure. This approach makes it possible to include chronic stressors and environmental hazard exposures to better understand health inequities evident across income levels and racial and ethnic groups in the United States (Morello-Frosch and Shenassa, 2006).

Given the effect that environmental exposures have on some child mental health problems, researchers suggest "broadening outcomes to include dimensional measures of autism spectrum disorders (ASDs), attention-deficit hyperactivity disorder (ADHD), and child learning capacity, as well as direct assessment of brain function" (Rauh and Margolis, 2016, p. 1). Longitudinal studies examining these outcomes may inform how key exposures result in child mental health problems, which may better address or prevent these issues (Rauh and Margolis, 2016).

Existing Regulatory Approaches

The federal government plays an essential role in enhancing the resources and technical assistance available to states, tribes, and local agencies through programs, policy development, and implementation by the Centers for Disease Control and Prevention (CDC), EPA, U.S. Food and Drug Administration (FDA), U.S. Consumer Product Safety Commission (CPSC), and other relevant rule- and policy-making entities focusing on environmental exposures and children's health. In addition, many of these agencies collaborate on joint initiatives to address environmental exposures among American children and families. For example, CDC monitors environmental chemicals in children's blood, reports on trends over time, and establishes key recommendations for safe levels among children (CDC, 2019a). CDC also provides training and other resources to state, local, and tribal governments to support environmental health services, including tools focused on ensuring food safety and safe water (CDC, 2019b).

EPA also provides critical resources and supports to state, local, and tribal governments to reduce the risk of environmental exposures among children and to mitigate, if necessary, environments with high levels of contaminants. For example, through the *America's Children and the Environment* report, EPA reports on environmental health data, specifically concerning children, and establishes indicators to minimize potential adverse health outcomes related to environmental exposures. Areas of focus include criteria for air pollutants, drinking water contaminants, lead, mercury, cotinine, perfluorochemicals, phthalates, BPA, perchlorate, and certain health outcomes, such as respiratory diseases, childhood cancer, and neurodevelopmental disorders (EPA, n.d.-b). However, as EPA has noted, several scientific challenges exist with regard to children's environmental health, including (1) the dispersion of data and information across systems that are difficult to access, (2) the need to assess environmental health from a systems perspective, (3) the need for new and more complex methods and models to evaluate risks specific to the early life stage of development and how exposures could result in health outcomes in later life stages, and (4) the need for translational research to better support community action and decision making (EPA, 2015). FDA regulates products and ensures the safety of food, including infant formula, the levels of BPA in food, and ingredients in cosmetics. For example, in 2014, the FDA BPA Joint Emerging Science Working Group reviewed the scientific literature on BPA effects on humans and found existing margins of safety to be adequate for exposure to BPA due to food contact (e.g., BPA exposures from coatings used in food containers) (FDA, 2014). Similarly, CPSC regulates products that are manufactured for children and that may be used by children. For example, CPSC limits the levels of phthalates in toys (GPO, 2017).

In addition to federal regulations, state environmental and public health agencies engage in efforts to prevent environmental exposures and to translate existing data and research findings into actionable policies and practices. For example, Washington State has enacted the Washington Children's Safe Products Act to limit levels of lead, cadmium, phthalates, and certain flame retardants in children's products (Department of Ecology, 2008). California (DTSC, n.d.) and Oregon (Oregon Health Authority, 2017) have implemented similar efforts to reduce the levels of toxic chemicals in consumer products. In all, there are at least 72 laws in 25 states addressing BPA, green chemistry, decabromodiphenyl ether, biomonitoring, and chemical safety (NCSL, 2014). However, the development and implementation of state regulations vary widely from state to state.

Frank R. Lautenberg Chemical Safety for the 21st Century Act

The Frank R. Lautenberg Chemical Safety for the 21st Century Act was enacted in 2016, with overwhelming bipartisan support, and gives EPA the authority to regulate or ban new and existing chemicals that pose a risk to human health or health of the environment. Prior to this law, which amended the Toxic Substances Control Act, EPA bore the burden of proof to demonstrate that a chemical posed an "unreasonable risk" to public health or the environment. In addition, the law also required EPA to choose the "least burdensome" regulation with consideration of both public health and impact on the manufacturer (Gerlach, 2016). The law included new requirements for premarket testing of new chemicals ("EPA has to make an affirmative finding on the safety of a new chemical or significant new use of an existing chemical before it is allowed into the marketplace" [Camacho-Ramos, 2016]); ongoing risk evaluation of the toxicity of chemicals already in commerce ("EPA must develop a screening process for all existing chemicals that ranks them according to their level of risk, then develop a risk management strategy for chemicals that raise concerns" [Gerlach, 2016], and it is no longer required to select the "least burdensome" option); and a user fee (up to $25 million) charged to companies to cover the costs of risk evaluation. Importantly, for the first time, the law required EPA to specifically assess health threats to children, pregnant women, and other vulnerable populations (EDF, 2016). As of June 25, 2019, 60 new chemical reviews had been completed in May 2019. More than 2,300 new chemical reviews have been completed since enactment (EPA, 2019).

The President's Task Force on Environmental Health Risks and Safety Risks to Children

The President's Task Force on Environmental Health Risks and Safety Risks to Children was established by Executive Order 13045 in 1997.[29] The Task Force was created with multidisciplinary and cross-sector membership, including representation from the U.S. Departments of Agriculture, Education, Energy, Housing and Urban Development, Justice, Labor, and Transportation. According to the executive order, the mission of the Task Force is to

> Recommend to the president federal strategies for children's environmental health and safety, within the limits of the administration's budget, to include the following elements:
>
> a. statements of principles, general policy, and targeted annual priorities to guide the federal approach to achieving the goals of this order;
> b. a coordinated research agenda for the federal government, including steps to implement the review of research databases described in Section 4 of the executive order;

[29] For more information, see https://ptfceh.niehs.nih.gov (accessed April 8, 2019).

   c.   recommendations for appropriate partnerships among federal, state, local, and tribal governments and the private, academic, and non-profit sectors;

   d.   proposals to enhance public outreach and communication to assist families in evaluating risks to children and in making informed consumer choices;

   e.   an identification of high-priority initiatives that the federal government has undertaken or will undertake in advancing protection of children's environmental health and safety; and

   f.   a statement regarding the desirability of new legislation to fulfill or promote the purposes of this order (Executive Order 13045, 1997).

Over the years, the Task Force has developed and published guidance on federal strategies to protect children from environmental health and safety risks. These publications include information on strategies and programs to address topics such as childhood asthma (PTFCEH, n.d.), healthy housing (Federal Healthy Homes Work Group, 2013), and lead exposures (PTFCEH, 2016a). The Task Force's 2016 work plan identifies three areas of priority: (1) reducing lead exposures by addressing sources of lead (e.g., paint, drinking water, and consumer products), (2) protecting health in a changing climate by preparing families and communities to understand and mitigate the effects of climate change on children's health, and (3) reducing the burden of environment-related illnesses by addressing the environmental origins of diseases to promote health and reduce health disparities (PTFCEH, 2016b). The work plan also delineates short- and long-term strategies for making progress on these three priority areas. The strategies offer a multipronged approach by identifying opportunities for communication and engagement, educational innovation, regulation and policy, and research.

National Research Approaches to Establish the Effects of
Environmental Exposure

Fifteen years ago, spending on federal maternal and child health programs neared $57.5 billion. Most spending fell within HHS, but it also included several HHS agencies, as well as the U.S. Departments of Agriculture, Defense, Education, and HUD and EPA. A 2012 study examining these spending trends noted that supporting a continued focus on data sharing and integration of funding streams could yield synergistic effects and economies of scale. With a goal of realizing a coordinated, integrative maternal and child health (MCH) system, researchers recommended that federal, state, and local partners eliminate existing silos and increase community and consumer involvement (Kenney et al., 2012). It is unclear whether the federal government has attained these goals, and more research would support a re-evaluation of whether the implementation of federal MCH funding has resulted in improvements in outcomes, data sharing, or improved community participation. In particular, it is unclear how federal spending furthers goals related to the elimination or mitigation of environmental exposures from preconception through age 8. Additional research examining federal funding linked to environmental exposures for these populations could support decision making at multiple levels and across agencies charged with regulation of environmental exposures.

In 2016, the National Institutes of Health introduced the Environmental influences on Child Health Outcomes (ECHO) Program, a group of more than 70 cohort studies aimed at understanding the relationship between environmental exposures and five main domains: upper and lower airways; obesity; pre-, peri-, and postnatal outcomes; neurodevelopment; and positive health outcomes (ECHO, 2019a,b). ECHO has enrolled a combined sample of more than 50,000 children (ECHO, 2019a,b). Exposures are measured from before birth to 5 years of age, and outcome data are collected through adolescence (Forrest et al., 2018). Nearly 150 cohort-focused articles have been published in the first 3 years of the project. In February 2019, the project received single institutional review board approval to begin the ECHO-wide cohort data collection protocol (ECHO, 2019a). While the multiple measures over time on the same participants in longitudinal research provide important information on possible cause and effect relationships, pooled cohort studies offer the advantage of being able to include a variety of different population groups and multiple variables at the same time.

National survey data also continue to play a vital role in our understanding of environmental exposures among children. Biomonitoring data in the National Health and Nutrition Examination Survey (NHANES) among preschool-aged children are limited (Calafat et al., 2017) but offer an important key to establishing exposure trends among children as young as 3 years old, using both parental report and analysis of biomarkers within urine samples. With these methods, researchers detected more than 37 chemicals in children aged 3–5 years, including plasticizers, combustion products, personal care–product chemicals, and pesticides (Calafat et al., 2017). NHANES data also offer the opportunity to establish benchmarks for environmental exposures among children, which enables programs and community-based efforts to improve interventions to reduce the risk of environmental exposures. For example, in a recent study of farmworkers, researchers measured a significant reduction in the levels of pesticide metabolites among parents and children who received an educational intervention on steps to reduce transmission of pesticides in the home (Griffith et al., 2018). Moreover, NHANES data were key in establishing that children exposed to higher levels of one chemical were also exposed to higher levels of other chemicals (Hendryx and Luo, 2018), which may place them at higher risk for poor health outcomes.

Conclusions and Recommendations to Reduce Exposure to Environmental Toxins

Given the importance of safe early learning environments, as discussed above, the committee recommends:

Recommendation 6-7: The Administration for Children and Families, Maternal and Child Health Bureau, and federal and state regulators should strengthen environmental protection in early care and education settings through expanded workforce training, program monitoring, and regulations.

Training professionals who regularly interact with children and their families on how to prevent and mitigate exposure to environmental toxicants during early development is an important opportunity to advance health equity; therefore, the committee recommends:

Recommendation 6-8: Professional societies, training programs, and accrediting bodies should support expanded or innovative models for training of prenatal and childhood health care providers on screening, counseling, and interventions to prevent or mitigate toxic environmental exposures.

Given the need to continually monitor, prevent, and mitigate the impact of environmental toxicants in the preconception through early childhood period, it is critical that federal, state, local, tribal, and territorial governments continue their efforts in this area.

Recommendation 6-9: Federal, state, local, tribal, and territorial governments should support and enforce efforts to prevent and mitigate the impact of environmental toxicants during the preconception through early childhood period. This strategy should particularly focus on priority populations who are disproportionately impacted by harmful environmental exposures. This includes

- **Environmental Protection Agency (EPA) fully exercising the authorities provided by Congress to safeguard children's environmental health under the Toxic Substances Control Act as amended by the Frank R. Lautenberg Chemical Safety for the 21st Century Act.**

- Continued allocation of resources and technical assistance from the federal government through the Centers
  for Disease Control and Prevention (CDC), EPA, U.S. Food
  and Drug Administration (FDA), and the U.S. Consumer
  Product Safety Commission to translate existing data and
  research findings into actionable policies and practices.
- Ongoing review and updating of environmental exposure
  levels by federal agencies to reflect health and safety standards specific to the unique vulnerability of children (from
  fetal development through early development).

Other ongoing governmental activities that should be continued include regularly examining children and adolescents in NHANES and other national surveys for conditions related to environmental exposures, to track and monitor national and regional trends; development of policies and regulations requiring the remediation of persistent environmental exposure risks, including but not limited to children's exposures to lead, mercury, arsenic, and chemicals and by-products of manufacturing, and the continuation of environmental evaluations; and case management of children with demonstrated risk of environmental exposures, particularly within communities experiencing higher risk levels, such as those with disproportionate poverty rates, substandard housing, higher concentrations of air pollutants, and other risky exposures.

In summary, while the approaches discussed in this chapter offer a few promising practices or approaches, several unknowns continue to pose challenges to a comprehensive exposure reduction effort. For example, more research and monitoring is needed to assess the effects of multiple long-term chemical exposures, paternal exposure burden and effects, and potential interactions between chemical exposures and gene expression. Evaluation of new, systemic approaches to policy development and implementation with demonstrable effects of reducing or mitigating chemical exposures remains key (Wang et al., 2016). One possible example is genetic studies examining gene variations that may increase susceptibility to environmental exposures. Combining these data with prospective, longitudinal studies could expand our knowledge of the role of critical developmental stages in the etiology of childhood diseases related to chemical exposures and human development (Wright and Christiani, 2010) and lead to novel approaches to further reduce environmental exposure risk.

CONCLUSION

Creating healthy living conditions to promote optimal development requires a multipronged approach to support caregivers and families so that they may meet the fundamental needs of their children. This chapter builds on the evidence presented in Chapter 3 on early life influences and discusses the evidence on programs, policies, and systems changes to ensure that all children have access to healthy living conditions. Among the critical needs discussed in this chapter are access to nutrition, safe and stable housing, protection from environmental exposures, and importantly, economic resources to ensure these basic needs are met.

Based on its review of the extent literature and committee expertise, the committee offers program and policy recommendations to support families in promoting optimal development from the prenatal through early childhood periods. The conclusions and recommendations in this chapter emphasize the importance of public programs to provide access to economic resources, healthy foods, and stable housing. Furthermore, the recommendations highlight the many roles of government at all levels in shaping healthy early living conditions (e.g., removing barriers to accessing public nutrition programs, creating a comprehensive plan for healthy housing, passing legislation to authorize and fund paid parental leave, strengthening environmental protections in ECE settings). Implementation of the program and policy solutions in this chapter would enable families and caregivers to care for young children in healthy communities.

This chapter takes a systems perspective by delving into the multiple, interactive systems that shape the social, economic, and environmental determinants of health for children (see Chapter 8 for more on a systems approach to promote health equity during the prenatal through early childhood periods). The following chapter focuses on the ECE system and the various programs and policies that can be leveraged to promote health equity among children.

REFERENCES

AAP (American Academy of Pediatrics) Council on Environmental Health. 2012. *Pediatric environmental health*, 3rd ed., edited by R. A. Etzel. Elk Grove Village, IL: American Academy of Pediatrics.

Acevedo-Garcia, D., N. McArdle, T. L. Osypuk, B. Lefkowitz, and B. K. Krimgold. 2007. *Children left behind: How metropolitan areas are failing America's children*. Boston, MA: Harvard School of Public Health and the Center for the Advancement of Health.

Acevedo-Garcia, D., T. L. Osypuk, N. McArdle, and D. R. Williams. 2008. Toward a policy-relevant analysis of geographic and racial/ethnic disparities in child health. *Health Affairs* 27(2):321–333.

ACF (Administration for Children and Families) Office of Family Assistance. 2019. *TANF caseload data 2018*. https://www.acf.hhs.gov/ofa/resource/tanf-caseload-data-2018 (accessed May 2, 2019).

ACOG (American College of Obstetricians and Gynecologists). 2013. Committee opinion no. 575: Exposure to toxic environmental agents. *Obstetrics & Gynecology* 122(4):931–935.

AEI (American Enterprise Institute)-Brookings Working Group on Paid Family Leave. 2017. *Paid family and medical leave: An issue whose time has come*. Washington, DC: The Brookings Institution.

Ahrens, K. A., B. A. Haley, L. M. Rossen, P. C. Lloyd, and Y. Aoki. 2016. Housing assistance and blood lead levels: Children in the United States. *American Journal of Public Health* 106(11):2049–2056.

Allbee, A., R. Johnson, and J. Lubell. 2015. *Preserving, protecting, and expanding affordable housing: A policy toolkit for public health.* Oakland, CA: ChangeLab Solutions and Abt Associates.

Almond, D., H. W. Hoynes, and D. W. Schanzenback. 2011. Inside the war on poverty: The impact of food stamps on birth outcomes. *Review of Economics and Statistics* 93(2):387–403.

Almond, D., J. Currie, and V. Duque. 2018. Childhood circumstances and adult outcomes: Act II. *Journal of Economic Literature* 56(4):1360–1446.

Amoah, A. O., N. O. Witherspoon, J. Perodin, and J. A. Paulson. 2016. Findings from a pilot environmental health intervention at early childhood centers in the District of Columbia. *Journal of Public Health (Oxford)* 38(3):e209–e217.

Andreyeva, T., and J. Luedicke. 2013. Federal food package revisions: Effects on purchases of whole-grain products. *American Journal of Preventative Medicine* 45(4):422–429.

Applebaum, E., and R. Milkman. 2011. *Leaves that pay: Employer and worker experiences with paid family leave in California.* Washington, DC: Center for Economic and Policy Research.

Arizona Department of Health Services. 2017. *2018 Arizona targeted lead screening plan.* Phoenix, AZ: Arizona Department of Health Services.

Arons, A., C. Bolbocean, N. R. Bush, F. A. Tylavsky, and K. Z. LeWinn. 2016. Participation in the Special Supplemental Nutrition Program for Women, Infants, and Children is not associated with early childhood socioemotional development: Results from a longitudinal cohort study. *Preventive Medicine Reports* 4:507–511.

ASCE (American Society of Civil Engineers). 2017. *Infrastructure report card: A comprehensive assessment of America's infrastructure.* Reston, VA: ASCE.

Baker, K. 2008. *Do cash transfer programs improve infant health: Evidence from the 1993 expansion of the Earned Income Tax Credit.* Notre Dame, IN: University of Notre Dame.

Baughman, R., and N. Duchovny. 2016. State earned income tax credits and the production of child health: Insurance coverage, utilization, and health status. *National Tax Journal* 69(1):103–132.

Beck, A. F., M. D. Klein, J. K. Schaffzin, V. Tallent, M. Gillam, and R. S. Kahn. 2012. Identifying and treating a substandard housing cluster using a medical-legal partnership. *Pediatrics* 130(5):831–838.

Beck, A. F., B. Huang, R. Chundur, and R. S. Kahn. 2014. Housing code violation density associated with emergency department and hospital use by children with asthma. *Health Affairs* 33(11):1993–2002.

Berger, L. M., S. A. Font, K. S. Slack, and J. Waldfogel. 2017. Income and child maltreatment in unmarried families: Evidence from the Earned Income Tax Credit. *Review of Economics of the Household* 15(4):1345–1372.

Besharov, D. J., and D. M. Call. 2009. *The expansion of WIC eligibility and enrollment: Good intentions, uncontrolled local discretion, and compliant federal officials.* Washington, DC: American Enterprise Institute for Public Policy Research & University of Maryland Welfare Reform Academy.

Boyd-Swan, C., C. M. Herbst, J. Ifcher, and H. Zarghamee. 2013. *The Earned Income Tax Credit, health, and happiness. IZA DP No. 7261.* Bonn, Germany: The Institute for the Study of Labor.

Burdick-Will, J. 2018. Neighborhood violence, peer effects, and academic achievement in Chicago. *Sociology of Education* 91(3):205–223.

Byker, T. S. 2016. Paid parental leave laws in the United States: Does short-duration leave affect women's labor-force attachment? *American Economic Review* 106(5):242–246.

Calafat, A. M., X. Ye, L. Valentin-Blasini, Z. Li, M. E. Mortensen, and L.-Y. Wong. 2017. Co-exposure to non-persistent organic chemicals among American pre-school aged children: A pilot study. *International Journal of Hygiene and Environmental Health* 220(2):55–63.

California Senate Office of Research. 2014. *California's paid family leave program: Ten years after the program's implementation, who has benefited and what has been learned?* https://sor.senate.ca.gov/sites/sor.senate.ca.gov/files/Californias%20Paid%20Family%20Leave%20Program.pdf (accessed April 7, 2019).

Camacho-Ramos, I. A. 2016. *U.S. EPA/OPPT regulatory perspective on acute inhalation toxicity testing.* https://www.piscltd.org.uk/wp-content/uploads/2016/09/Camacho-presentation_acute-inhalation-tox-workshop_092206_v3_FINAL.pdf (accessed July 9, 2019).

Carlson, S., and B. Keith-Jennings. 2018. *SNAP is linked with improved nutritional outcomes and lower health care cost.* Washington, DC: Center on Budget and Policy Priorities.

Carlson, S., and Z. Neuberger. 2018. *WIC works: Addressing the nutrition and health needs of low-income families for 40 years.* Washington, DC: Center on Budget and Policy Priorities.

CBPP (Center on Budget and Policy Priorities). 2017. *Policy basics: Federal rental assistance.* Washington, DC. https://www.cbpp.org/research/housing/policy-basics-federal-rental-assistance (accessed June 25, 2019).

CBPP. 2018a. *Chart book: Temporary assistance for needy families.* Washington, DC: Center on Budget and Policy Priorities.

CBPP. 2018b. *Policy basics: The child tax credit.* https://www.cbpp.org/research/federal-tax/policy-basics-the-child-tax-credit (accessed May 1, 2019).

CBPP. 2018c. *Policy basics: The Earned Income Tax Credit.* https://www.cbpp.org/research/federal-tax/policy-basics-the-earned-income-tax-credit (accessed May 1, 2019).

CBPP. 2019. *National and state housing fact sheets & data.* https://www.cbpp.org/research/housing/national-and-state-housing-fact-sheets-data (accessed July 15, 2019).

CBPP. n.d. *SNAP retailers database.* https://www.cbpp.org/snap-retailers-database (accessed June 25, 2019).

CDC (Centers for Disease Control and Prevention). 2009. *Healthy places terminology.* https://www.cdc.gov/healthyplaces/terminology.htm (accessed April 18, 2019).

CDC. 2019a. *Fourth national report on human exposure to environmental chemicals.* 2019. https://www.cdc.gov/exposurereport/pdf/FourthReport_UpdatedTables_Volume1_Jan2019-508.pdf (accessed June 25, 2019).

CDC. 2019b. *Environmental health services.* https://www.cdc.gov/nceh/ehs (accessed June 25, 2019).

CEA (Council of Economic Advisers). 2014. *The economics of early childhood investments.* Washington, DC: Executive Office of the President.

Chetty, R., J. N. Friedman, and J. Rockoff. 2011. *New evidence on the long-term impacts of tax credits.* Paper read at Annual Conference on Taxation and Minutes of the Annual Meeting of the National Tax Association.

Chetty, R., N. Hendren, and L. F. Katz. 2016. The effects of exposure to better neighborhoods on children: New evidence from the moving to opportunity experiment. *American Economic Review* 106(4):855–902.

Chew, G. L., M. S. Perzanowski, R. L. Miller, J. C. Correa, L. A. Hoepner, C. M. Jusino, M. G. Becker, and P. L. Kinney. 2003. Distribution and determinants of mouse allergen exposure in low-income New York City apartments. *Environmental Health Perspectives* 111(10):1348–1351.

Chiasson, M. A., S. Findley, J. Sekhobo, R. Scheinmann, L. S. Edmunds, A. Faly, N. McLeod, and D. Gregg. 2013. Changing WIC changes what children eat. *Obesity* 21(7):1423–1429.

Cincinnati Children's. n.d. *Cincinnati child health-law partnership (child HeLP).* https://www.cincinnatichildrens.org/service/g/gen-pediatrics/services/child-help (accessed April 17, 2019).

City of Rochester NY (New York). n.d. *Lead paint—get prepared.* https://www.cityofrochester.gov/article.aspx?id=8589936091 (accessed March 20, 2019).

CMS (Centers for Medicare & Medicaid Services). 2016. *CMCS informational bulletin: Coverage of blood lead testing for children involved in Medicaid and the Children's Health Insurance Program.* https://www.medicaid.gov/federal-policy-guidance/downloads/cib113016.pdf (accessed July 15, 2019).

CMS. 2017. *Frequently asked questions (FAQs) health services initiatives.* https://www.medicaid.gov/federal-policy-guidance/downloads/faq11217.pdf (accessed June 25, 2019).

CMS. n.d. 2019. *Lead screening.* https://www.medicaid.gov/medicaid/benefits/epsdt/lead-screening/index.html (accessed June 25, 2019).

Collins, A. M., and J. A. Klerman. 2017. Improving nutrition by increasing Supplemental Nutrition Assistance Program benefits. *American Journal of Preventive Medicine* 52(2 Suppl 2):S179–S185.

Cooper, K., and K. Stewart. 2013. *Does money affect children's outcomes? A systematic review.* York, UK: Joseph Rowntree Foundation.

Crain, E. F., M. Walter, G. T. O'Connor, H. Mitchell, R. S. Gruchalla, M. Kattan, G. S. Malindzak, P. Enright, R. Evans, 3rd, W. Morgan, and J. W. Stout. 2002. Home and allergic characteristics of children with asthma in seven U.S. urban communities and design of an environmental intervention: The Inner-city Asthma Study. *Environmental Health Perspectives* 110(9):939–945.

Crocker, D. D., S. Kinyota, G. G. Dumitru, C. B. Ligon, E. J. Herman, J. M. Ferdinands, D. P. Hopkins, B. M. Lawrence, and T. A. Sipe. 2011. Effectiveness of home-based, multi-trigger, multicomponent interventions with an environmental focus for reducing asthma morbidity: A community guide systematic review. *American Journal of Preventive Medicine* 41(2):S5–S32.

Cronquist, K., and S. Lauffer. 2019. *Characteristics of Supplemental Nutrition Assistance Program households: Fiscal year 2017.* Alexandria, VA: U.S. Department of Agriculture, Food and Nutrition Service, Office of Policy Support.

Currie, J., and E. Moretti. 2008. Did the introduction of food stamps affect birth outcomes in California. In *Making Americans healthier: Social and economic policy as health policy*, edited by R. F. Schoeni, J. S. House, G. A. Kaplan, and H. Pollack. New York: Russell Sage Foundation. Pp. 122–144.

Dahl, G., and L. Lochner. 2012. The impact of family income on child achievement: Evidence from the Earned Income Tax Credit. *American Economic Review* 102:1927–1956.

Darrah, J., and S. DeLuca. 2014. "Living here has changed my whole perspective": How escaping inner-city poverty shapes neighborhood and housing choice. *Journal of Policy Analysis and Management* 33(2):350–384.

Deb, P., and C. A. Gregory. 2018. Heterogeneous impacts of SNAP on food insecurity. *Economic Letters* 173(C):55–60.

Declercq, E., C. Sakala, M. Corry, S. Applebaum, and A. Herrlich. 2013. *Listening to Mothers III: New mothers speak out.* Report of the National Survey of Women's Childbearing Experiences conducted October–December 2012 and January–April 2013. New York: Childbirth Connection.

Department of Ecology, Washington State. 2008. *Children's Safe Products Act.* https://ecology.wa.gov/Waste-Toxics/Reducing-toxic-chemicals/Childrens-Safe-Products-Act (accessed June 25, 2019).

Desmond, M. 2018. Heavy is the house: Rent burden among the American urban poor. *International Journal Urban and Regional Research* 42(1):160–170.

Detroit URC (Urban Research Center). n.d. *Healthy Mothers on the Move/Madres Saludables en Movimiento (Healthy MOMS).* http://www.detroiturc.org/index.php?option=com_content&view=article&id=15&Itemid=28 (accessed April 17, 2019).

Di Renzo, G. C., J. A. Conry, J. Blake, M. S. DeFrancesco, N. DeNicola, J. N. Martin, Jr., K. A. McCue, D. Richmond, A. Shah, P. Sutton, T. J. Woodruff, S. Z. van der Poel, and L. C. Giudice. 2015. International Federation of Gynecology and Obstetrics opinion on reproductive health impacts of exposure to toxic environmental chemicals. *International Journal of Gynecology & Obstetrics* 131(3):219–225.

Dickman, J. 2017. *Children at risk: Gaps in state lead screening policies.* https://saferchemicals.org/sc/wp-content/uploads/2017/01/saferchemicals.org_children-at-risk-report.pdf (accessed June 8, 2019).

DOL (U.S. Department of Labor). 2018. *Wage and Hour Division (WHD)*. https://www.dol.gov/whd/regs/compliance/whdfs73.htm (accessed July 9, 2019).

DOL. n.d. *Title VI, Civil Rights Act of 1964*. https://www.dol.gov/agencies/oasam/regulatory/statutes/title-vi-civil-rights-act-of-1964 (accessed October 1, 2019).

DTSC (Department of Toxic Substances Control, State of California). n.d. *Safer consumer products*. https://dtsc.ca.gov/scp (accessed January 29, 2019).

East, C. N. 2018. The effect of food stamps on children's health: Evidence from immigrants' changing eligibility. *The Journal of Human Resources* 0916-8197R2.

ECHO (Environmental influences on Child Health Outcomes). 2019a. *ECHO program activates first sites under the ECHO-wide cohort data collection protocol*. https://echochildren.org/echo-program-activates-first-sites-under-the-echo-wide-cohort-data-collection-protocol (accessed July 15, 2019).

ECHO. 2019b. *ECHO program receives green light to begin expansive child health research*. https://echochildren.org/echo-program-receives-green-light-to-begin-expansive-child-health-research (accessed July 15, 2019).

EDF (Environmental Defense Fund). 2016. *A new chemical safety law: The Lautenberg Act*. https://www.edf.org/health/new-chemical-safety-law-lautenberg-act (accessed July 15, 2019).

Eligibility.com. 2019. *Section 8 housing*. https://eligibility.com/section-8 (accessed March 26, 2019).

Environmental Justice Leadership Forum on Climate Change. 2016. *Environmental justice state guidance: How to incorporate equity and justice into your state clean power planning approach*. http://www.eesi.org/files/EJ-State-Guidance-Final-v5-jan-15-2016.pdf (accessed June 8, 2019).

Environmental Law Institute. 2015. *Reducing environmental exposures in child care facilities: A review of state policy*. https://www.eli.org/buildings/reducing-environmental-exposures-child-care-facilities (accessed June 25, 2019).

EPA (U.S. Environmental Protection Agency). 2015. *Children's environmental health: Research roadmap*. Washington, DC: U.S. Environmental Protection Agency, Office of Research and Development.

EPA. 2019. *Reviewing new chemicals under the Toxic Substances Control Act (TSCA)*. https://www.epa.gov/reviewing-new-chemicals-under-toxic-substances-control-act-tsca (accessed July 15, 2019).

EPA. n.d.-a. *About the TSCA Chemical Substance Inventory*. https://www.epa.gov/tsca-inventory/about-tsca-chemical-substance-inventory (accessed July 15, 2019).

EPA. n.d.-b. *Basic information about ACE*. https://www.epa.gov/ace/basic-information-about-ace (accessed July 12, 2019).

EPA. n.d.-c. *TSCA chemical substance inventory*. https://www.epa.gov/tsca-inventory (accessed July 12, 2019).

Evans, W., and C. Garthwaite. 2010. *Giving mom a break: The impact of higher EITC payments on maternal health. NBER Working paper 16296*. NBER Working Paper Series. Cambridge, MA: National Bureau of Economic Research.

Evans, G. W., N. M. Wells, H. Y. Chan, and H. Saltzman. 2000. Housing quality and mental health. *Journal of Consulting and Clinical Psychology* 68(3):526–530.

Executive Order 13045. 1997. Protection of children from environmental health risks and safety risks. *Federal Register* 62(78):19885–19888.

Fan, M., and Y. Jin. 2015. The Supplemental Nutrition Assistance Program and childhood obesity in the United States: Evidence from the National Longitudinal Survey of Youth 1997. *American Journal of Health Economics* 1(4):432–460.

FDA (U.S. Food and Drug Administration). 2014. *Bisphenol A (BPA): Use in food contact application*. https://www.fda.gov/food/food-additives-petitions/bisphenol-bpa-use-food-contact-application (accessed July 12, 2019).

Federal Healthy Homes Work Group. 2013. *Advancing healthy housing: A strategy for action.* https://www.hud.gov/sites/documents/STRATPLAN_FINAL_11_13.PDF (accessed June 25, 2019).

Fenelon, A., N. Slopen, M. Boudreaux, and S. J. Newman. 2018. The impact of housing assistance on the mental health of children in the United States. *Journal of Health and Social Behavior* 59(3):447–463.

Fertig, A. R. 2007. Public housing, health, and health behaviors: Is there a connection? *Journal of Policy Analysis and Management* 26(4):831–860.

Figlio, D., S. Hamersma, and J. Roth. 2009. Does prenatal WIC participation improve birth outcomes? New evidence from Florida. *Journal of Public Economics* 93(1–2):235–245.

Fingar, K. R., S. H. Lob, M. S. Dove, P. Gradziel, and M. P. Curtis. 2017. Reassessing the association between WIC and birth outcomes using a fetuses-at-risk approach. *Maternal and Child Health Journal* 21(4):825–835.

Fischer, W. 2015. *Research shows housing vouchers reduce hardship and provide platform for long-term gains among children.* Washington, DC: Center on Budget and Policy Priorities.

Forrest, C. B., C. K. Blackwell, and C. A. Camargo, Jr. 2018. Advancing the science of children's positive health in the National Institutes of Health Environmental influences on Child Health Outcomes (ECHO) Research Program. *The Journal of Pediatrics* 196:298–300.

Foster, E. M., M. Jiang, and C. M. Gibson-Davis. 2010. The effect of the WIC program on the health of newborns. *Health Services Research* 45(4):1083–1104.

Frey, W. H. 2015. *Census shows modest declines in black-white segregation.* https://www.brookings.edu/blog/the-avenue/2015/12/08/census-shows-modest-declines-in-black-white-segregation (accessed January 29, 2019).

Garboden, P. M., T. Leventhal, and S. Newman. 2017. Estimating the effects of residential mobility: A methodological note. *Journal of Social Service Research* 43(2):246–261.

Gehle, K. S., J. L. Crawford, and M. T. Hatcher. 2011. Integrating environmental health into medical education. *American Journal of Preventive Medicine* 41(4 Suppl 3):S296–S301.

Gerlach, C. 2016. *New Toxic Substances Control Act: An end to the Wild West for chemical safety?* http://sitn.hms.harvard.edu/flash/2016/new-toxic-substances-control-act-end-wild-west-chemical-safety (accessed March 21, 2019).

Gibson-Davis, C., and E. M. Foster. 2006. A cautionary tale: Using propensity scores to estimate the effect of food stamps on food insecurity. *Social Service Review* 80(1):93–126.

Goldin, J. 2018. *Tax benefit complexity and take-up: Lessons from the Earned Income Tax Credit.* Stanford law and economics Olin working paper 514. https://ssrn.com/abstract=3101160 (accessed May 2, 2019).

GPO (U.S. Government Publishing Office). 2017. Prohibition of children's toys and child care articles containing specified phthalates. *Federal Register* 82(207):49938–49982. https://www.govinfo.gov/content/pkg/FR-2017-10-27/pdf/2017-23267.pdf (accessed July 12, 2019).

Grandjean, P., R. Barouki, D. C. Bellinger, L. Casteleyn, L. H. Chadwick, S. Cordier, R. A. Etzel, K. A. Gray, E.-H. Ha, C. Junien, M. Karagas, T. Kawamoto, B. Paige Lawrence, F. P. Perera, G. S. Prins, A. Puga, C. S. Rosenfeld, D. H. Sherr, P. D. Sly, W. Suk, Q. Sun, J. Toppari, P. van Den Hazel, C. L. Walker, and J. J. Heindel. 2015. Life-long implications of developmental exposure to environmental stressors: New perspectives. *Endocrinology* 156(10):3408.

Gregory, C., and P. Deb. 2015. Does SNAP improve your health? *Food Policy* 50:11–19.

Gregory, C., M. P. Rabbitt, and D. C. Ribar. 2016. The Supplemental Nutrition Assistance Program and food insecurity. In *SNAP matters: How food stamps affect health and well-being,* edited by J. Bartfeld, C. Gundersen, T. M. Smeeding, and J. P. Ziliak. Stanford, CA: Stanford University Press. Pp. 74–106.

Griffith, W. C., E. M. Vigoren, M. N. Smith, T. Workman, B. Thompson, G. D. Coronado, and E. M. Faustman. 2018. Application of improved approach to evaluate a community intervention to reduce exposure of young children living in farmworker households to organophosphate pesticides. *Journal of Exposure Science & Environmental Epidemiology* 29(3):358–365.

Grindler, N. M., A. A. Allshouse, E. Jungheim, T. L. Powell, T. Jansson, and A. J. Polotsky. 2018. OB-GYN screening for environmental exposures: A call for action. *PLoS ONE* 13(5):e0195375.

Guendelman, S., J. L. Kosa, M. Pearl, S. Graham, J. Goodman, and M. Kharrazi. 2009. Juggling work and breastfeeding: Effects of maternity leave and occupational characteristics. *Pediatrics* 123(1):e38–e46.

Guidry, V. T., A. Lowman, D. Hall, D. Baron, and S. Wing. 2014. Challenges and benefits of conducting environmental justice research in a school setting. *NEW SOLUTIONS: A Journal of Environmental and Occupational Health Policy* 24(2):153–170.

Gundersen, C., and V. Oliveira. 2001. The food stamp program and food insufficiency. *American Journal of Agricultural Economics* 83(4):875–887.

Hahn, R. A., B. I. Truman, and D. R. Williams. 2018. Civil rights as determinants of public health and racial and ethnic health equity: Health care, education, employment, and housing in the United States. *SSM—Population Health* 4:17–24.

Hamad, R., and D. H. Rehkopf. 2016. Poverty and child development: A longitudinal study of the impact of the Earned Income Tax Credit. *American Journal of Epidemiology* 183(9):775–784.

Health Impact Project. 2017. *10 policies to prevent and respond to childhood lead exposure.* Washington, DC: The Pew Charitable Trusts and Robert Wood Johnson Foundation.

Hendra, R., D. H. Greenberg, G. Hamilton, A. Oppenheim, A. Pennington, K. Schaberg, and B. L. Tessler. 2016. *Encouraging evidence on a sector-focused advancement strategy: Two-year impacts from the WorkAdvance demonstration.* New York: MDRC.

Hendricks, M., M. Meyer, N. G. Gharaibeh, S. Van Zandt, J. Masterson, J. Cooper, Jr., J. Horney, and P. Berke. 2018. The development of a participatory assessment technique for infrastructure: Neighborhood-level monitoring towards sustainable infrastructure systems. *Sustainable Cities and Society* 38:265–274.

Hendryx, M., and J. Luo. 2018. Children's environmental chemical exposures in the USA, NHANES 2003–2012. *Environmental Science and Pollution Research* 25(6):5336–5343.

Heymann, J., A. Raub, and A. Earle. 2011. Creating and using new data sources to analyze the relationship between social policy and global health. *Public Health Reports* 126:127–134.

Heymann, J., A. Earle, and K. McNeill. 2013. The impact of labor policies on the health of young children in the context of economic globalization. *Annual Review of Public Health* 34(1):355–372.

HHS (U.S. Department of Health and Human Services). 2012. *What is TANF?* https://www.hhs.gov/answers/programs-for-families-and-children/what-is-tanf/index.html (accessed May 2, 2019).

Hoynes, H. W., and D. W. Schanzenbach. 2018. *Safety net investments in children.* Working paper 24594. NBER Working Paper Series. Cambridge, MA: National Bureau of Economic Research.

Hoynes, H., M. Page, and A. H. Stevens. 2011. Can targeted transfers improve birth outcomes?: Evidence from the introduction of the WIC program. *Journal of Public Economics* 95(7–8):813–827.

Hoynes, H., D. Miller, and D. Simon. 2012. Income, the Earned Income Tax Credit, and infant health. *American Economic Journal: Economic Policy* 7(1):172–211.

Hoynes, H., D. W. Schanzenbach, and D. Almond. 2016. Long-run impacts of childhood access to the safety net. *American Economic Review* 106(4):903–934.

Huang, R., and M. Yang. 2015. Paid maternity leave and breastfeeding practice before and after California's implementation of the nation's first paid family leave program. *Economics & Human Biology* 16:45–59.

HUD (U.S. Department of Housing and Urban Development). 2014. *Housing's and neighborhoods' role in shaping children's future.* https://www.huduser.gov/portal/periodicals/em/fall14/highlight1.html (accessed June 4, 2019).

HUD. 2015. *HUD reports continued high levels of "worst case housing needs."* https://archives.hud.gov/news/2015/pr15-014.cfm (accessed June 4, 2019).

HUD. 2016. *Picture of subsidized households.* https://www.huduser.gov/portal/datasets/assthsg.html (accessed June 4, 2019).

Huffman, S. K., and H. H. Jensen. 2008. Food assistance programs and outcomes in the context of welfare reform. *Social Science Quarterly* 89(1):95–115.

IRS (Internal Revenue Service). 2019. *EITC participation rate by states.* https://www.eitc.irs.gov/eitc-central/participation-rate/eitc-participation-rate-by-states (accessed May 1, 2019).

Irving, S. K., and T. A. Loveless. 2015. *Dynamics of economic well-being: Participation in government programs, 2009–2012: Who gets assistance?* Washington, DC: U.S. Department of Commerce, Economic and Statistics Administration, U.S. Census Bureau.

Isaacs, J., O. Healy, and H. E. Peters. 2017a. *Paid family leave in the United States: Time for a new national policy.* Washington, DC: The Urban Institute.

Isaacs, J. B., C. Lou, H. Hahn, J. Ovalle, and C. E. Steurle. 2017b. *Kids' share 2017: Report on federal expenditures on children through 2016 and future projections.* Washington, DC: The Urban Institute.

Jackson, M. I. 2015. Early childhood WIC participation, cognitive development and academic achievement. *Social Science & Medicine* 126:145–153.

Jacob, B. A., M. Kapustin, and J. Ludwig. 2015. The impact of housing assistance on child outcomes: Evidence from a randomized housing lottery. *Quarterly Journal of Economics* 130(1):465–506.

Jelleyman, T., and N. Spencer. 2008. Residential mobility in childhood and health outcomes: A systematic review. *Journal of Epidemiology and Community Health* 62(7):584–592.

Johnson, P., D. Betson, L. Blatt, and L. Giannarelli. 2017. *National- and state-level estimates of Special Supplemental Nutrition Program for Women, Infants, and Children (WIC) eligibles and program reach in 2014, and updated estimates for 2005–2013.* Special Nutrition Programs Report No. WIC-17-ELIG. Washington, DC: U.S. Department of Agriculture, Food and Nutrition Service, Office of Policy Support.

Joint Center for Housing Studies of Harvard University. 2017. *America's rental housing 2017.* Cambridge, MA: Harvard University.

Kenney, M. K., M. D. Kogan, S. Toomer, and P. C. van Dyck. 2012. Federal expenditures on maternal and child health in the United States. *Maternal and Child Health Journal* 16(2):271.

Kessler, R. C., G. J. Duncan, L. A. Gennetian, L. F. Katz, J. R. Kling, N. A. Sampson, L. Sanbonmatsu, A. M. Zaslavsky, and J. Ludwig. 2014. Associations of housing mobility interventions for children in high-poverty neighborhoods with subsequent mental disorders during adolescence. *JAMA* 311(9):937–947.

Khanani, I., J. Elam, R. Hearn, C. Jones, and N. Maseru. 2010. The impact of prenatal WIC participation on infant mortality and racial disparities. *American Journal of Public Health* 100(Suppl 1):S204–S209.

Kieffer, E. C., D. B. Welmerink, B. R. Sinco, K. B. Welch, E. M. Rees Clayton, C. Y. Schumann, and V. E. Uhley. 2014. Dietary outcomes in a Spanish-language randomized controlled diabetes prevention trial with pregnant Latinas. *American Journal of Public Health* 104(3):526–533.

Kilpatrick, N., H. Frumkin, J. Trowbridge, C. Escoffery, R. Geller, L. Rubin, G. Teague, and J. Nodvin. 2002. The environmental history in pediatric practice: A study of pediatricians' attitudes, beliefs, and practices. *Environmental Health Perspectives* 110(8):823–827.

Kim, S., J. Mazza, J. Zwanziger, and D. Henry. 2014. School and behavioral outcomes among inner city children: Five-year follow-up. *Urban Education* 49(7):835–856.

Kimbro, R. T., J. Brooks-Gunn, and S. McLanahan. 2011. Young children in urban areas: Links among neighborhood characteristics, weight status, outdoor play, and television watching. *Social Science and Medicine* 72(5):668–676.

Klein, M. D., R. S. Kahn, R. C. Baker, E. E. Fink, D. S. Parrish, and D. C. White. 2011. Training in social determinants of health in primary care: Does it change resident behavior? *Academic Pediatrics* 11(5):387–393.

Klein, M. D., A. F. Beck, A. W. Henize, D. S. Parrish, E. E. Fink, and R. S. Kahn. 2013. Doctors and lawyers collaborating to help children—outcomes from a successful partnership between professions. *Journal of Health Care for the Poor and Underserved* 24(3):1063–1073.

Kling, J. R., J. B. Liebman, and L. F. Katz. 2007. Experimental analysis of neighborhood effects. *Econometrica* 75(1):83–119.

Koehler, K., M. Latshaw, T. Matte, D. Kass, H. Frumkin, M. Fox, B. F. Hobbs, M. Wills-Karp, and T. A. Burke. 2018. Building healthy community environments: A public health approach. *Public Health Reports* 133(Suppl 1):S35–S43.

Koehrn, K., J. Hospital, A. Woolf, and J. Lowry. 2017. Pediatric environmental health: Using data on toxic chemical emissions in practice. *Current Problems in Pediatric and Adolescent Health Care* 47(11):281–302.

Komro, K. A., M. D. Livingston, S. Markowitz, and A. C. Wagenaar. 2016. The effect of an increased minimum wage on infant mortality and birth weight. *American Journal of Public Health* 106(8):1514–1516.

Komro, K. A., S. Markowitz, M. D. Livingston, and A. C. Wagenaar. 2019. Effects of state-level earned income tax credit laws on birth outcomes by race and ethnicity. *Health Equity* 3(1):61–67.

Kreger, M., K. Sargent, A. Arons, M. Standish, and C. D. Brindis. 2011. Creating an environmental justice framework for policy change in childhood asthma: A grassroots to treetops approach. *American Journal of Public Health* 101(Suppl 1):S208.

Kreider, B., J. Pepper, C. Gundersen, and D. Jolliffe. 2012. Identifying the effects of SNAP (food stamps) on child health outcomes when participation is endogenous and misreported. *Journal of the American Statistical Association* 107(499):958–975.

Kreider, B., J. V. Pepper, and M. Roy. 2016. Identifying the effects of WIC on food insecurity among infants and children. *Southern Economic Journal* 82(4):1106–1122.

Krieger, J., D. E. Jacobs, P. J. Ashley, A. Baeder, G. L. Chew, D. Dearborn, H. P. Hynes, J. D. Miller, R. Morley, F. Rabito, and D. C. Zeldin. 2010. Housing interventions and control of asthma-related indoor biologic agents: A review of the evidence. *Journal of Public Health Management and Practice* 16(Suppl 5):S11–S20.

Leech, T. G. 2012. Subsidized housing, public housing, and adolescent violence and substance use. *Youth & Society* 44(2):217–235.

Leventhal, T., and S. Newman. 2010. Housing and child development. *Children and Youth Services Review* 32(9):1165–1174.

Levy, J. I., D. Brugge, J. L. Peters, J. E. Clougherty, and S. S. Saddler. 2006. A community-based participatory research study of multifaceted in-home environmental interventions for pediatric asthmatics in public housing. *Social Science & Medicine* 63(8):2191–2203.

Ludwig, J., L. Sanbonmatsu, L. Gennetian, E. Adam, G. J. Duncan, L. F. Katz, R. C. Kessler, J. R. Kling, S. T. Lindau, R. C. Whitaker, and T. W. McDade. 2011. Neighborhoods, obesity, and diabetes—a randomized social experiment. *New England Journal of Medicine* 365(16):1509–1519.

Ludwig, J., G. J. Duncan, L. A. Gennetian, L. F. Katz, R. C. Kessler, J. R. Kling, and L. Sanbonmatsu. 2013. Long-term neighborhood effects on low-income families: Evidence from Moving to Opportunity. *American Economic Review Papers and Proceedings* 103(3):226–231.

Manoli, D., and N. Turner. 2018. Cash-on-hand and college enrollment: Evidence from population tax data and the Earned Income Tax Credit. *American Economic Review: Economic Policy* 10(2):242–271.

Martinez, O., J. Boles, M. Muñoz-Laboy, E. C. Levine, C. Ayamele, R. Eisenberg, J. Manusov, and J. Draine. 2017. Bridging health disparity gaps through the use of medical legal partnerships in patient care: A systematic review. *Journal of Law, Medicine & Ethics* 45(2):260–273.

Maryland Department of Health. 2016. *Lead poisoning prevention in Maryland: What's new?* https://phpa.health.maryland.gov/OEHFP/EH/Pages/LeadTesting.aspx (accessed March 21, 2019).

Marzieh, A., T. Sedigheh Sadat, Z. Saeed Motesaddi, H. Ali Reza, B. Andrea, and M. Ali. 2017. A behavioral strategy to minimize air pollution exposure in pregnant women: A randomized controlled trial. *Environmental Health and Preventive Medicine* 22(1):1–8.

Mass.gov. 2019. *Department of Family and Medical Leave (DFML).* https://www.mass.gov/orgs/department-of-family-and-medical-leave (accessed July 15, 2019).

Maxwell, K., S. Julius, A. Grambsch, A. Kosmal, L. Larson, and N. Sonti. 2018. Built environment, urban systems, and cities. In *Impacts, risks, and adaptation in the United States: Fourth national climate assessment*, Vol. 2, edited by D. R. Reidmiller, C. W. Avery, D. R. Easterling, K. E. Kunkel, K. L. M. Lewis, T. K. Maycock, and B. C. Stewart. Washington, DC: U.S. Global Change Research Program. Pp. 438–478.

Mazzara, A., and B. Knudsen. 2019. *Where families with children use housing vouchers: A comparative look at the 50 largest metropolitan areas.* Washington, DC: Poverty & Race Research Action Council.

Mazzara, A., B. Sard, and D. Rice. 2016. *Rental assistance to families with children at lowest point in decade.* Washington, DC: Center on Budget and Policy Priorities.

McCoy, D. C., A. L. Roy, and C. C. Raver. 2016. Neighborhood crime as a predictor of individual differences in emotional processing and regulation. *Developmental Science* 19(1):164–174.

McCurdy, L. E., J. Roberts, B. Rogers, R. Love, R. Etzel, J. Paulson, N. O. Witherspoon, and A. Dearry. 2004. Incorporating environmental health into pediatric medical and nursing education. *Environmental Health Perspectives* 112(17):1755–1760.

Meyerhoefer, C. D., and M. Yang. 2011. The relationship between food assistance and health: A review of the literature and empirical strategies for identifying program effects. *Applied Economic Perspectives and Policy* 33(3):304–344.

Mikati, I., A. F. Benson, T. J. Luben, J. D. Sacks, and J. Richmond-Bryant. 2018. Disparities in distribution of particulate matter emission sources by race and poverty status. *American Journal of Public Health* 108(4):480–485.

Mirkovic, K. R., C. G. Perrine, K. S. Scanlon, and L. M. Grummer-Strawn. 2014. Maternity leave duration and full-time/part-time work status are associated with US mothers' ability to meet breastfeeding intentions. *Journal of Human Lactation: Official Journal of International Lactation Consultant Association* 30(4):416–419.

Misra, T. 2016. Baltimore's housing voucher program almost gets it right. *CityLab.* https://www.citylab.com/equity/2016/01/baltimore-affordable-housing-voucher-opportunity/421722 (accessed March 26, 2019).

Morello-Frosch, R., and E. D. Shenassa. 2006. The environmental "riskscape" and social inequality: Implications for explaining maternal and child health disparities. *Environmental Health Perspectives* 114(8):1150–1153.

Morgan, W. J., E. F. Crain, R. S. Gruchalla, G. T. O'Connor, M. Kattan, R. Evans, 3rd, J. Stout, G. Malindzak, E. Smartt, M. Plaut, M. Walter, B. Vaughn, and H. Mitchell. 2004. Results of a home-based environmental intervention among urban children with asthma. *New England Journal of Medicine* 351(11):1068–1080.

MotherToBaby. n.d. *About us.* https://mothertobaby.org/about-us (accessed April 5, 2019).

Murphy, J. S., E. M. Lawton, and M. Sandel. 2015. Legal care as part of health care: The benefits of medical-legal partnership. *Pediatric Clinics* 62(5):1263–1271.

Murtagh, L., and A. D. Moulton. 2011. Working mothers, breastfeeding, and the law. *American Journal of Public Health* 101(2):217–223.

Nandi, A., D. Jahagirdar, M. C. Dimitris, J. A. Labrecque, E. C. Strumpf, J. S. Kaufman, I. Vincent, E. Atabay, S. Harper, A. Earle, and S. J. Heymann. 2018. The impact of parental and medical leave policies on socioeconomic and health outcomes in OECD countries: A systematic review of the empirical literature. *The Milbank Quarterly* 96(3):434–471.

NASEM (National Academies of Sciences, Engineering, and Medicine). 2015. *Mental disorders and disabilities among low-income children*. Washington, DC: The National Academies Press.

NASEM. 2016. *Review of WIC food packages: Proposed framework for revisions: Interim report*. Washington, DC: The National Academies Press.

NASEM. 2017. *Communities in action: Pathways to health equity*. Washington, DC: The National Academies Press.

NASEM. 2019. *A roadmap to reducing child poverty*. Washington, DC: The National Academies Press.

NASHP (National Academy for State Health Policy). 2017. *Lead screening and treatment in Medicaid and CHIP*. https://nashp.org/wp-content/uploads/2017/02/Lead-Screening.pdf (accessed June 25, 2019).

NASHP. 2018. *State health care delivery policies promoting lead screening and treatment for children and pregnant women (5.21.18)*. https://nashp.org/wp-content/uploads/2018/05/NASHP-Lead-Policy-Scan-5-21-18_updated.pdf (accessed June 25, 2019).

National Center for Healthy Housing. 2014. *National healthy housing standard (full document, 2018 update)*. Columbia, MD: National Center for Healthy Housing.

National Center for Healthy Housing. 2017. *National healthy housing standard—implementation tool*. https://nchh.org/resource/national-healthy-housing-standard-implementation-tool (accessed March 21, 2019).

NCSL (National Conference of State Legislators). 2014. *Toxic Substances Control Act reform*. http://www.ncsl.org/research/environment-and-natural-resources/state-chemical-statutes.aspx#statelaws (accessed July 12, 2019).

NCSL. 2017. *NCSL policy update: State statutes on chemical safety*. http://www.ncsl.org/research/environment-and-natural-resources/ncsl-policy-update-state-statutes-on-chemical-safety.aspx (accessed June 25, 2019).

Newman, S., and C. S. Holupka. 2017. The effects of assisted housing on child well-being. *American Journal of Community Psychology* 60(1–2):66–78.

Nichols, A., and J. Rothstein. 2016. The Earned Income Tax Credit. In *Economics of means-tested transfer program in the United States*, Vol. 1, edited by R. A. Moffitt. Chicago, IL: University of Chicago Press. Pp. 137–218.

NRC and IOM (National Research Council and Institute of Medicine). 2000. *From neurons to neighborhoods: The science of early childhood development*. Washington, DC: National Academy Press.

OECD (Organisation for Economic Co-operation and Development). 2017. PF2.1: *Key characteristics of parental leave systems*. https://www.oecd.org/els/soc/PF2_1_Parental_leave_systems.pdf (accessed July 15, 2019).

Office of the Surgeon General, CDC (Centers for Disease Control and Prevention), and Office on Women's Health. 2011. *The Surgeon General's call to action to support breastfeeding*. Rockville, MD: Office of the U.S. Surgeon General.

Ogbuanu, C., S. Glover, J. Probst, J. Liu, and J. M. Hussey. 2011. The effect of maternity leave length and time of return to work on breastfeeding. *Pediatrics* 127(6):e1414–e1427.

Olsho, L. E. W., J. A. Klerman, S. H. Bartlett, and C. W. Logan. 2017. Rebates to incentivize healthy nutrition choices in the Supplemental Nutrition Assistance Program. *American Journal of Preventative Medicine* 52(2 Suppl 2):S161–S170.

Oregon

Oregon Health Authority. 2017. *Toxic-free kids: A report to the governor and the 79th Oregon legislative assembly.* Portland, OR: Oregon Health Authority, Public Health Division.

PEHSU (Pediatric Environmental Health Specialty Units). n.d. *About the PEHSU program.* https://www.pehsu.net/About_PEHSU.html (accessed April 5, 2019).

Petersen, D. M., M. Minkler, V. B. Vasquez, M. C. Kegler, L. H. Malcoe, and S. Whitecrow. 2007. Using community-based participatory research to shape policy and prevent lead exposure among Native American children. *Progress in Community Health Partnerships: Research, Education, and Action* 1(3):249–256.

Pinderhughes, H., R. A. Davis, and M. Williams. 2015. *Adverse community experiences and resilience: A framework for addressing and preventing community trauma.* Oakland, CA: Prevention Institute.

Postma, J., C. Karr, and G. Kieckhefer. 2009. Community health workers and environmental interventions for children with asthma: A systematic review. *Journal of Asthma* 46(6):564–576.

PTFCEH (President's Task Force on Environmental Health Risks and Safety Risks to Children). 2016a. *Key federal programs to reduce childhood lead exposures and eliminate associated health impacts.* https://ptfceh.niehs.nih.gov/features/assets/files/key_federal_programs_to_reduce_childhood_lead_exposures_and_eliminate_associated_health_impactspresidents_508.pdf (accessed June 25, 2019).

PTFCEH. 2016b. *President's task force on environmental health risks and safety risks to children work plan.* https://ptfceh.niehs.nih.gov/activities/assets/files/presidents_task_force_work_plan_508.pdf (accessed April 17, 2019).

PTFCEH. 2018. *Federal action plan to reduce childhood lead exposures and associated health impacts.* Washington, DC: President's Task Force on Environmental Health Risks and Safety Risks to Children.

PTFCEH. n.d. *Asthma and the environment: A strategy to protect children.* https://ptfceh.niehs.nih.gov/activities/assets/files/asthma_and_the_environment_a_strategy_to_protect_children.pdf (accessed June 25, 2019).

Raissian, K. M., and L. R. Bullinger. 2017. Money matters: Does the minimum wage affect child maltreatment rates? *Children and Youth Services Review* 72:60–70.

Ratcliffe, C., and S. McKernan. 2010. *How much does SNAP reduce food insecurity?* Washington, DC: Urban Institute.

Raub, A., A. Nandi, A. Earle, N. D. G. Chorny, E. Wong, P. Chung, P. Batra, A. Schickedanz, B. Bose, J. Jou, D. Franken, and J. Heymann. 2018. *Paid parental leave: A detailed look at approaches across OECD countries.* Los Angeles, CA: World Policy Analysis Center.

Rauh, V. A., and A. E. Margolis. 2016. Research review: Environmental exposures, neurodevelopment, and child mental health—new paradigms for the study of brain and behavioral effects. *Journal of Child Psychology and Psychiatry* 57(7):775–793.

REACH (Racial and Ethnic Approaches to Community Health) Detroit. 2018. *Healthy Mothers on the Move (Healthy MOMS)/Madres Saludables en Movimiento (Madres Saludables).* http://www.reachdetroit.org/about/HealthyMoms (accessed April 17, 2019).

Reskin, B. 2012. The race discrimination system. *Annual Review of Sociology* 38:17–24.

Rivas, I., X. Querol, J. Wright, and J. Sunyer. 2018. How to protect school children from the neurodevelopmental harms of air pollution by interventions in the school environment in the urban context. *Environment International* 121:199–206.

Roberts, J. R., and B. A. Gitterman. 2003. Pediatric environmental health education: A survey of U.S. Pediatric residency programs. *Ambulatory Pediatrics* 3(1):57–59.

Rosenberg, T. 2014. When poverty makes you sick, a lawyer can be the cure. *The New York Times,* July 17.

Rossin-Slater, M. 2011. The effects of maternity leave on children's birth and infant health outcomes in the United States. *Journal of Health Economics* 30(2):221–239.

Rossin-Slater, M., C. J. Ruhm, and J. Waldfogel. 2011. *Effects of California's paid family leave program on mothers' leave-taking and subsequent labor market outcomes.* Cambridge, MA: National Bureau of Economic Research.

Rusk, D. 2017. *Economic segregation is replacing racial segregation in large U.S. metro areas.* https://www.dcpolicycenter.org/publications/economic-polarization (accessed January 29, 2019).

RWJF (Robert Wood Johnson Foundation). 2018. *SNAP supports children and families.* Princeton, NJ: Robert Wood Johnson Foundation.

SafetyNEST. 2018. *SafetyNEST science.* https://uploads.strikinglycdn.com/files/3770c2fa-680a-4eb7-b1e0-116bdf601a64/SafetyNEST_Summary_2018.pdf (accessed April 5, 2019).

Sanbonmatsu, L., J. R. Kling, G. J. Duncan, and J. Brooks-Gunn. 2006. *Neighborhoods and academic achievement: Results from the Moving to Opportunity experiment.* NBER Working paper 11909. NBER Working Paper Series. Cambridge, MA: National Bureau of Economic Research.

Sandel, M., M. Hansen, R. Kahn, E. Lawton, E. Paul, V. Parker, S. Morton, and B. Zuckerman. 2010. Medical-legal partnerships: Transforming primary care by addressing the legal needs of vulnerable populations. *Health Affairs* 29(9):1697–1705.

Sandel, M., R. Sheward, S. Ettinger de Cuba, S. M. Coleman, D. A. Frank, M. Chilton, M. Black, T. Heeren, J. Pasquariello, P. Casey, E. Ochoa, and D. Cutts. 2018. Unstable housing and caregiver and child health in renter families. *Pediatrics* 141(2):e20172199.

Sard, B., D. Rice, A. Bell, and A. Mazzara. 2018. *Federal policy changes can help more families with housing vouchers live in higher-opportunity areas.* https://www.cbpp.org/research/housing/federal-policy-changes-can-help-more-families-with-housing-vouchers-live-in-higher (accessed June 25, 2019).

Sathyanarayana, S., J. Focareta, T. Dailey, and S. Buchanan. 2012. Environmental exposures: How to counsel preconception and prenatal patients in the clinical setting. *American Journal of Obstetrics and Gynecology* 207(6):463–470.

Schulz, A., G. Mentz, N. Sampson, M. Ward, R. Anderson, R. de Majo, B. Israel, T. Lewis, and D. Wilkins. 2016. Race and the distribution of social and physical environmental risk. *Du Bois Review* 13(2):285–304.

Schwartz, M. B. 2017. Moving beyond the debate over restricting sugary drinks in the Supplemental Nutrition Assistance Program. *American Journal of Preventive Medicine* 52(2):S199–S205.

Shaefer, L., S. Collyer, G. Duncan, K. Edin, I. Garfinkel, D. Harris, T. M. Smeeding, J. Waldfogel, C. Wimer, and H. Yoshikawa. 2018. A universal child allowance: A plan to reduce poverty and income instability among children in the United States. *The Russell Sage Foundation Journal of the Social Sciences* 4(2):22–42.

Sharkey, P. 2010. The acute effect of local homicides on children's cognitive performance. *Proceedings of the National Academy of Sciences of the United States of America* 107(26):11733–11738.

Sharkey, P. T., N. Tirado-Strayer, A. V. Papachristos, and C. C. Raver. 2012. The effect of local violence on children's attention and impulse control. *American Journal of Public Health* 102(12):2287–2293.

Sharkley, P. 2016. *Confronting neighborhood segregation.* https://equitablegrowth.org/confronting-neighborhood-segregation (accessed January 11, 2019).

SHIELDS for Families. 2011. *Annual report.* https://www.shieldsforfamilies.org/download/annual-reports/SHIELDS_ANNUAL_10-11.pdf (accessed April 17, 2019).

Skafida, V. 2012. Juggling work and motherhood: The impact of employment and maternity leave on breastfeeding duration: A survival analysis on growing up in Scotland data. *Maternal and Child Health Journal* 16(2):519–527.

Slopen, N., A. Fenelon, S. Newman, and M. Boudreaux. 2018. Housing assistance and child health: A systematic review. *Pediatrics* 141(6):e20172742.

SSA (U.S. Social Security Administration). 2019. *Monthly statistical snapshot, May 2019.* https://www.ssa.gov/policy/docs/quickfacts/stat_snapshot (accessed July 15, 2019).

Stearns, J. 2015. The effects of paid maternity leave: Evidence from temporary disability insurance. *Journal of Health Economics* 43:85–102.

Stotland, N. E., P. Sutton, J. Trowbridge, D. S. Atchley, J. Conry, L. Trasande, B. Gerbert, A. Charlesworth, and T. J. Woodruff. 2014. Counseling patients on preventing prenatal environmental exposures—a mixed-methods study of obstetricians. *PLoS ONE* 9(6):e98771.

Strully, K. W., D. H. Rehkopf, and Z. Xuan. 2010. Effects of prenatal poverty on infant health: State earned income tax credits and birth weight. *American Sociological Review* 75(4):534–562.

Taylor, P., and R. Fry. 2012. *The rise of residential segregation by income.* Washington, DC: Pew Research Center.

Tessum, C. W., J. S. Apte, A. L. Goodkind, N. Z. Muller, K. A. Mullins, D. A. Paolella, S. Polasky, N. P. Springer, S. K. Thakrar, J. D. Marshall, and J. D. Hill. 2019. Inequity in consumption of goods and services adds to racial–ethnic disparities in air pollution exposure. *Proceedings of the National Academy of Sciences of the United States of America* 116(13):6001.

The City Project. 2016. U.S. Civil Rights Commission civil rights and environmental justice and enforcement by EPA. *The City Project Blog.* http://www.cityprojectca.org/blog/archives/43798 (accessed June 3, 2019).

Thornton, P. L., E. C. Kieffer, Y. Salabarria-Pena, A. Odoms-Young, S. K. Willis, H. Kim, and M. A. Salinas. 2006. Weight, diet, and physical activity-related beliefs and practices among pregnant and postpartum Latino women: The role of social support. *Maternal and Child Health Journal* 10(1):95–104.

Tinney, V. A., J. A. Paulson, S. L. Bathgate, and J. W. Larsen. 2015. Medical education for obstetricians and gynecologists should incorporate environmental health. *American Journal of Obstetrics & Gynecology* 212(2):163–166.

Tollefson, J. 2016. US chemicals law set for overhaul. *Nature* 534. https://www.nature.com/news/polopoly_fs/1.19973!/menu/main/topColumns/topLeftColumn/pdf/nature.2016.19973.pdf?origin=ppub (accessed July 15, 2019).

TPC (Tax Policy Center). n.d. *What is the Child Tax Credit?* https://www.taxpolicycenter.org/briefing-book/what-child-tax-credit (accessed May 1, 2019).

Trasande, L., and Y. Liu. 2011. Reducing the staggering costs of environmental disease in children, estimated at $76.6 billion in 2008. *Health Affairs (Millwood)* 30(5):863–870.

Trasande, L., M. L. Schapiro, R. Falk, K. A. Haynes, A. Berhmann, M. Vohmann, E. D. Stremski, C. Eisenberg, C. Evenstad, H. A. Anderson, and P. J. Landrigan. 2006. Pediatrician attitudes, clinical activities and knowledge of environmental health in Wisconsin. *Wisconsin Medical Journal* 105(2):45–49.

Trippe, C., C. Tadler, P. Johnson, L. Giannarelli, and D. Betson. 2019. *National- and state-level estimates of WIC eligibility and WIC program reach in 2016.* Alexandria, VA: U.S. Department of Agriculture, Food and Nutrition Service, Office of Policy Support.

Trust for America's Health. n.d. *Maryland's efforts to prevent and respond to childhood lead exposure.* https://www.tfah.org/story/marylands-efforts-to-prevent-and-respond-to-childhood-lead-exposure (accessed March 20, 2019).

Tulve, N. 2016. Development of a conceptual framework depicting a child's total (built, natural, social) environment in order to optimize health and well-being. *Journal of Environment and Health Science* 2(2):1–8.

Tyler, E. T. 2012. Aligning public health, health care, law and policy: Medical-legal partnership as a multilevel response to the social determinants of health. *Journal of Health & Biomedical Law* 8:211–247.

University of Michigan Prevention Research Center. n.d. *Promoting healthy lifestyles among women.* http://prc.sph.umich.edu/projects/promoting-healthy-lifestyles-among-women (accessed April 17, 2019).

U.S. Interagency Council on Homelessness. 2018. *Homelessness in America: Focus on families with children.* Washington, DC: U.S. Interagency Council on Homelessness.

USDA (U.S. Department of Agriculture). 2004. *Effects of food assistance programs on nutrition and health.* Washington, DC: Economic Research Service.

USDA. 2012. *Environmental justice strategic plan: 2012–2014.* Washington, DC: U.S. Department of Agriculture.

USDA. 2015. *Women, infants and children (WIC): About WIC—WIC at a glance.* https://www.fns.usda.gov/wic/about-wic-wic-glance (accessed March 28, 2019).

USDA. 2018a. *Evaluation of demonstration projects to end childhood hunger: Interim evaluation report (summary).* Washington, DC: USDA Food and Nutrition Service.

USDA. 2018b. *Supplemental Nutrition Assistance Program (SNAP). Am I eligible for SNAP?* https://www.fns.usda.gov/snap/eligibility (accessed March 28, 2019).

USDA. 2018c. *Women, infants and children (WIC). WIC eligibility requirements.* https://www.fns.usda.gov/wic/wic-eligibility-requirements (accessed March 28, 2019).

USDA. 2019. *WIC program.* https://www.ers.usda.gov/topics/food-nutrition-assistance/wic-program (accessed April 1, 2019).

USDA. n.d. *Special Supplemental Nutrition Program for Women, Infants, and Children (WIC).* https://www.fns.usda.gov/wic (accessed July 15, 2019).

Walker, C., and H. Matthews. 2017. *CCDBG participation drops to historic low.* Washington, DC: Center for Law and Social Policy.

Wang, A., A. Padula, M. Sirota, and T. J. Woodruff. 2016. Environmental influences on reproductive health: The importance of chemical exposures. *Fertility and Sterility* 106(4):905–929.

Wehby, G., D. Dave, and R. Kaestner. 2016. *Effects of the minimum wage on infant health.* NBER working paper 22373. NBER Working Paper Series. Cambridge, MA: National Bureau of Economic Research.

Whaley, S. E., L. D. Ritchie, P. Spector, and J. Gomez. 2012. Revised WIC food package improves diets of WIC families. *Journal of Nutrition Education and Behavior* 44(3):204–209.

Wheaton, L., and V. Tran. 2018. *The antipoverty effects of the Supplemental Nutrition Assistance Program.* Washington, DC: The Urban Institute.

Wilde, P. 2007. Measuring the effect of food stamps on food insecurity and hunger: Research and policy considerations. *Journal of Nutrition* 137:307–310.

Wilde, P., and M. Nord. 2005. The effect of food stamps on food security: A panel data approach. *Review of Agricultural Economics* 27(3):425–432.

Wildeman, C., and E. A. Wang. 2017. Mass incarceration, public health, and widening inequality in the USA. *The Lancet* 389(10077):1464–1474.

Woolf, S. H., L. Aron, D. L, S. M. Simon, E. Zimmerman, and K. X. Luk. 2015. *How are income and wealth linked to health and longevity?* Washington, DC, and Richmond, VA: Urban Institute and Center on Society and Health.

Wright, R., and D. Christiani. 2010. Gene-environment interaction and children's health and development. *Current Opinion in Pediatrics* 22(2):197–201.

Yen, S. T. 2010. The effects of SNAP and WIC programs on nutrient intakes of children. *Food Policy* 35(6):576–583.

Yen, S. T., D. J. Bruce, and L. Jahs. 2012. Supplemental Nutrition Assistance Program participation and health; evidence from low-income individuals in Tennessee. *Contemporary Economic Policy* 30(1):1–12.

Ziliak, J. P. 2016. *Modernizing SNAP benefits. Policy proposal 2016-06, The Hamilton Project.* Washington, DC: The Brookings Institution.

7

Promoting Health Equity Through Early Care and Education

INTRODUCTION

Several important threads are evident throughout this report: the importance of intervening early, preferably before adversity occurs, but if not, soon after; the inextricable interplay between genes and the child's environment in producing health; the need to support caregivers of children—those who spend significant time with children and therefore have an important impact on children's growth and development; and the need to create healthy, supportive environments. Knowing that most young children participate in some type of nonparental care on a regular basis (formal or informal arrangements), the early care and education (ECE) platform is a significant opportunity for health promotion and advancing health equity (see the committee's conceptual model, Figure 1-9, in Chapter 1). ECE is defined here as nonparental care that occurs outside the child's home. ECE services may be delivered in center-based settings, school-based settings, or home-based settings (i.e., a setting other than a child's home) (NASEM, 2018); however, this chapter also discusses programs that support parents, such as home visiting. Education itself is incredibly important when it comes to health (García, 2015). Because educational attainment positively correlates with health outcomes, investments in ECE are critical to decreasing disparities to set the stage for future success (Barnett, 2013; NASEM, 2017a). In this chapter, the committee discusses how to apply the important learnings from early development to the ECE system, including the importance of a properly supported and trained ECE workforce, access to quality ECE, and

---

BOX 7-1
Chapter in Brief: Early Care and Education

This chapter discusses the role of early care and education (ECE) in ensuring that children are healthy and ready to learn, with a focus on incorporating health and health equity into a comprehensive approach to school readiness and success. The chapter examines the evidence linking ECE to health and health equity outcomes through leveraging such programs and systems as platforms to deliver health-related services, social-emotional and behavioral curricula, and interventions to support parents and the home environment as well as educators and other members of the ECE workforce. The chapter also emphasizes the importance of improving the quality, access, and affordability of ECE programs, especially for underserved populations.

Chapter conclusions in brief:

- For ECE programs to contribute significantly to a health promotion and equity strategy, there is a need to intentionally, cohesively, and simultaneously address adequate funding that supports comprehensive, evidence-based standards and practices that promote health equity in the ECE system, an adequately compensated and competent workforce, a connection to community resources and support, continuous quality improvement, and a systematic examination of effectiveness at multiple levels.
- Policies and systems that prepare and support early childhood educators and program leaders, including those in public schools, need to incorporate the latest evidence about how educators can better support children's school readiness and success by fostering their health and well-being. This would entail providing comprehensive supports and resources to degree

---

resources to support these needs. At the end of the chapter, the committee provides recommendations detailing the specific actions needed to ensure that ECE meets its potential to promote child health and well-being. See Box 7-1 for an overview of the chapter.

While ECE has primarily focused on whether it improves children's cognitive and social-emotional development, as well as academic readiness, there is some indication that ECE may influence child (and even adult) health outcomes, including physical, emotional, and mental health (Campbell et al., 2014; D'Onise et al., 2010; Muennig et al., 2011). What is also of critical importance is *how* ECE is related to children's cognitive development, social-emotional development, academic readiness and achievement, and health and well-being, as well as how it can lead to health equity. Hahn and colleagues (2016) postulate that ECE advances health equity through several interrelated systems (see Figure 7-1).

ECE programs increase children's cognitive, social, and health outcomes through enhancing children's motivation for school and readiness

granting institutions and preparation programs, including the development of curricula, textbooks, practicum experiences, toolkits, and fact sheets, with an emphasis on equitable practices that address the diverse experiences and needs of children and families.

- Maximizing the impact of ECE on positive childhood development and health and well-being at the community or population levels will require increasing public funds for ECE programs. Currently, eligibility for ECE programs is limited, and among eligible families, access is low due to lack of funding and availability of programs and services. Therefore, even if existing publicly funded programs have the resources to provide robust supports that improve young children's health and well-being, they will not reach most children, especially those who live in low-income households or experience adverse experiences and toxic stressors.

Chapter recommendations in brief:

- Develop a comprehensive approach to school readiness that explicitly incorporates health outcomes, standards, and practices and leverages ECE systems and programs, including home visiting.
- Develop and strengthen coursework, practicums, and ongoing professional learning opportunities that focus on competencies of educators, principals, and ECE program directors that are critical to children's health, school readiness, and life success.
- Develop and implement a strategic plan to (1) improve the quality of ECE programs by adopting health-promoting standards, and (2) expand access to comprehensive, high-quality, and affordable ECE programs across multiple settings.

to learn and identifying problems that impede learning. This, in turn, helps children improve their cognitive ability and social and emotional competence while increasing their use of preventive health care. There is also evidence that participation in a high-quality early learning program is associated with children's self-regulation; approaches to learning, such as their motivation and persistence; and executive function (EF) skills, which are domain-general skills that transfer to many areas of development, including learning to read, making friends, and dealing with new challenges (Holliday et al., 2014; Pianta et al., 2009; Yoshikawa et al., 2013). These short-term outcomes of ECE are then expected to lead to lower risk of dropping out of school, greater school engagement, and subsequently better educational attainment, which results in increased income and health care, decreased social and health risk, and improved health equity. Traditionally, ECE is thought of as being confined to a specific age range. For this report, the committee discusses ECE in the context of birth through 8–10 years of age. Another National Academies report,

476

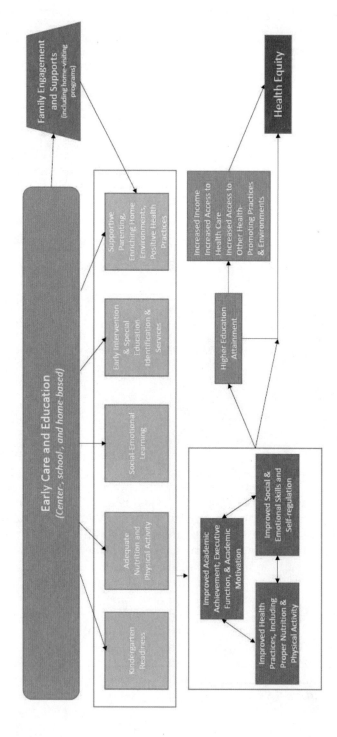

FIGURE 7-1 Conceptual framework: How ECE is linked to health promotion and health equity.
SOURCE: Informed by Hahn et al., 2016.

The Promise of Adolescence: Realizing Opportunity for All Youth, picks up from here, discussing health and development from the onset of puberty into adolescence and early adulthood (NASEM, 2019).

DIRECT LINKS BETWEEN ECE AND HEALTH EQUITY

Health, social-emotional, and other health-related behavioral outcomes are some of the most commonly reported from evaluations of ECE programs, aside from the often-cited cognitive outcomes (Cannon et al., 2017; Carney et al., 2015; Fisher et al., 2014; Rossin-Slater, 2015). ECE programs have been shown to reduce externalizing and internalizing behaviors (Carney et al., 2015), improve social-emotional skills (D'Onise et al., 2010; Hahn et al., 2016), reduce substance use (Cannon et al., 2017; Jones et al., 2015), and improve physical health or well-being (D'Onise et al., 2010; Rossin-Slater, 2015; Sabol and Hoyt, 2017). ECE can produce this range of results through different pathways. It can provide services to children and/or their parents directly that impact their health outcomes and related skills and behaviors; implement evidence-based curricula or interventions to improve children's social-emotional skills, which are associated with both short- and long-term health and cognitive effects; and support the training and well-being of early childhood educators.

While reviews of the research literature suggest that ECE programs can be a promising lever for improving health outcomes and equity, they also show instances where ECE programs have weak, nonexistent, or even negative impact on children's behavior and health (Cannon et al., 2017; D'Onise et al., 2010; Hahn et al., 2016; Herbst and Tekin, 2011; Rossin-Slater, 2015). These mixed and negative findings could reflect factors such as lack of program quality, poor fidelity to the program model, and limited program duration. The following section takes a deeper dive into specific ECE programs or interventions that have produced significant results on health and discusses their characteristics.

Links Between ECE and Health Outcomes

A number of studies and reviews of the literature have found positive relationships between participation in ECE programs and physical health indicators and outcomes (Hahn et al., 2016; Kay and Pennucci, 2014). Most of the associated benefits tend to be related to obesity, access to health care, and early screenings and detection. For example, low-income preschoolers enrolled in a center-based program are less likely to experience food insecurity than if they were cared for by parents exclusively or by an unrelated adult in a home setting (Gundersen and Ziliak, 2014). Using a quasi-experimental methodology on data from the Eunice Kennedy

Shriver National Institute of Child Health and Human Development's Study of Early Child Care and Youth Development (NICHD SECCYD), Sabol and Hoyt (2017) found that 4-year-olds who attended center-based ECE programs had lower blood pressure when they were 15 years old than those who were in a home-based environment, whether that was with a parent, a relative, or a nonrelative.

Hahn et al. (2016) sought to examine the impact of ECE on fostering the health equity outcomes of low-income and racial and ethnic minority children through a meta-analysis. They focused on state and district programs, the federal Head Start program, and foundational model programs, such as the HighScope Perry Preschool Project (PPP) and Carolina Abecedarian (ABC) program. They included studies that were for children aged 3 or 4 years; primarily focused on low-income or racial and ethnic minority populations; were not conducted only in the summer; were based on behavioral interventions; included assessment of effects on children's health and health-related or academic outcomes; and had a control or comparison population and provided enough data for analysts to calculate effect size and adjust for confounding. Findings were included for the following outcomes: standardized achievement (effect found across program types); high school graduation (effect found only for Head Start); grade retention (effect found across program types); assignment to special education (Head Start was not evaluated on this measure; effect found for all other programs); and crime (effect found across all program types) (see Table 7-1 for more information). Additional analyses examining the persistence of effect of programs on academic achievement and cognitive ability showed a rapid decrease of effects after the program ended, then a gradual decline over time. Higher program quality based on observational data and having teachers with a bachelor's degree or higher had greater effects on student standardized achievement. There were insufficient data to examine impact of class size, hours, duration, or benefits of additional components, such as family engagement or health access. In sum, there was consistent evidence that center-based ECE programs improved educational and health-related outcomes for low-income and ethnic minority preschool-age children, with some indication of long-term outcomes. Hahn et al. (2016) further note that the fade-out of center-based ECE effects for cognitive and achievement outcomes could likely be because many low-income and ethnic minority children are likely to attend low-resourced (i.e., lower-quality) elementary schools and have teachers with fewer credentials. Others, such as Duncan and Magnuson, have postulated that "preschool programs may affect something other than basic achievement and cognitive test scores, and perhaps these other program impacts, unlike achievement and cognitive impacts, persist over time" (Duncan and Magnuson, 2013, p. 120). That

TABLE 7-1 Effects of Center-Based Early Childhood Education Programs on Education, Social, and Health-Related Outcomes (data for all program types combined)

Outcome (number of studies; program types included)	Mean Age at Follow-Up, y	Standardized Mean Difference (95% CI)	Effect Meaningful?	Consistent Across Body of Evidence?
Test scores (27 studies; all types)	3.7	0.29 (0.23–0.34)	Yes	Yes
High school graduation (7 studies; all types)	20.0	0.20 (0.07–0.33)	Yes	Yes
Grade retention (12 studies; all types)	17.0	−0.23 (−0.43 to −0.02)	Yes	Yes
Assignment to special education (6 studies; state and district and model programs)	15.5	−0.28 (−0.49 to −0.08)	Yes	Yes
Crime (5 studies; all types)	25.0	−0.23 (−0.45 to 0.05)	Yes	No
Teen birth (3 studies; Head Start and model programs)	18.0	−0.46 (−0.92 to 0.0)	Yes	No
Self-regulation (5 studies; state and district and Head Start programs)	18.0	0.21 (0.14–0.28)	Yes	Yes
Emotional development (7 studies; state and district and Head Start programs)	4.0	0.04 (−0.05 to 0.12)	No	No

SOURCE: Hahn et al., 2016.

is, looking at discrete and constrained skills, such as letter naming, may not be good predictors, whereas focusing on unconstrained skills, such as self-regulation and expressive language, would be more appropriate. Thus, there is more to understand about the fade-out effect, or arguably the catch-up effect, especially in the changing landscape where more children are in out-of-home settings.

The research is equivocal, however, especially for health, social, and emotional outcomes. Herbst and Tekin (2011) found that 4-year-old children of single mothers who were enrolled in nonparental care through a child care subsidy were more likely to be obese or overweight when they were kindergartners than those who stayed home. As with a study by Hawkinson and colleagues (2013), this study also found an association between subsidy use and poor cognitive outcomes. A review of 37 studies found "generally null effects of preschool interventions across a range of health outcomes" (D'Onise et al., 2010, p. 1432), leading the authors to caution against relying on a "flimsy evidence base" to inform policy (D'Onise et al., 2010, p. 1432). However, the study did find "a general trend toward beneficial effects, with particularly beneficial effects for overweight and obesity, mental health, social competency, and crime prevention" (D'Onise et al., 2010, p. 1432). They also found that across the studies, half of the comparisons related to immunization and general health yielded positive impacts (and none produced adverse effects).

Foundational Research in ECE

The foundational studies of the HighScope PPP and Carolina ABC project provide the most robust findings regarding the link between ECE and health equity throughout the life course. As described below, these two programs—which occurred in two different states and were conducted by two different teams in two different decades—have similar short- and long-term outcomes. They also shared some common characteristics: they focused on children with the greatest needs and employed an educated and responsive teacher, low child–teacher ratio, active and language-rich learning opportunities, child assessment, and home visiting and family support activities.

Some caution, however, should be taken in generalizing these findings due to the limitations of these studies. They occurred more than 50 years ago, when most children in poverty did not have access to early education services and programs. The samples, primarily African American children, are not representative of the general population. They were also small and continued to decrease over time. Finally, these controlled programs have not been adequately replicated at a large scale. It is also critical to note that not all children in the treatment groups performed at the highest level and in the end, did not surpass their more economically advantaged peers. For example, in the PPP study almost one-third of children from the treatment groups were arrested five or more times by age 40, almost one-third did not graduate high school, and almost two-thirds of children from the treatment group required public assistance as adults (Gomby et al., 1995). Thus, these programs did not equalize the outcomes for children from low-income households in comparison to their higher-income peers.

While PPP and ABC provide a blueprint to build from to support children's school readiness, achievement, and health equity throughout the life course, policy makers and practitioners alike need to base their decisions on lessons beyond those from these studies, such as more contemporary ECE programs and interventions discussed in this chapter, to ensure that all children, especially children with the greatest needs, have the same opportunity to thrive and lead healthy lives.

HighScope Perry Preschool Project (PPP)

The HighScope PPP started in 1962 with a focus on serving 3- and 4-year-olds (it was 1–2 years long) with a home visiting component. The program aims to promote social and cognitive development in children who are at risk due to poverty. Schweinhart and Weikart (1997) showed that students enrolled in the program in 1986 had more positive behavior and attitudes than students in the control group (Schweinhart and Weikart, 1997). In addition, experimental evaluations of study participants in their teens and 20s showed that even years later, when study participants were in their teens and 20s, students formerly enrolled in the program "had higher academic grades and earnings, higher rates of high school graduation, fewer arrests and out-of-wedlock births, and lower levels of welfare receipt than their peers who were not in a preschool program" (Child Trends, 2012). Furthermore, children in the intervention group had higher rates of safety-belt use and engaged in fewer risky health behaviors, such as smoking and illicit substance use, in adulthood compared to those in the control group. At age 27, former PPP students were more likely to be employed and had higher earnings than students in the control group (Child Trends, 2012; Schweinhart et al., 2005). This continued into age 40, with former PPP students having higher earnings, committing fewer crimes, and being more likely to hold a job and to have graduated from high school than adults who did not participate in PPP. In 2019, Heckman and Karapakula presented findings from the HighScope PPP Age 55 Study (Heckman and Karapakula, 2019a). They indicated that the program kept parent engagement active longer, which resulted in more warmth and less authoritarian parenting. They also found that at age 55, the female participants in the early childhood intervention group had lower cortisol (39.01 versus 89.29 picograms per milligram) compared to the control group, and the male participants were less likely to have high cholesterol levels (mean differences in high cholesterol[1] were 0.71 in the treatment group versus 0.94 in the control group). Female participants

---

[1] High total cholesterol indicates whether total cholesterol concentration in milligrams per deciliter is 220 or higher.

in the intervention group were also less likely to be uninsured for a prolonged period compared to the control group (Heckman and Karapakula, 2019b). In addition, they reported intergenerational effects for children of intervention participants: completion of high school, good health status, stable employment, and a history of never having been suspended and arrested (Heckman and Karapakula, 2019a).

Carolina Abecedarian (ABC) Study

The Carolina ABC Study is a center-based intervention that enrolled families between 1972 and 1977 based on a high-risk index. During recruitment, 111 infants were matched on high-risk scores and then assigned to preschool treatment or control status. Fifty-seven infants were assigned to the experimental group and 54 to the control group (Campbell et al., 2012). The families in the study were mostly African American with young mothers, less than a high school education, unmarried, living in multigenerational homes, and reporting no earned income (Campbell et al., 2012). The service delivery model for the experimental group was a 5-year, full-day, year-round, center-based program with a comprehensive curriculum (LearningGames®) (Sparling and Lewis, 1979) focused on educational games addressing children's cognition, language, and adaptive behavior. The program also emphasized health care and family support programs. Activities were individualized for the child's needs, with more conceptual and group-oriented activities as children got older. Families in both the experimental and control groups received supportive social services. Findings showed that children in the 0–5 intervention group had better cognitive, academic, and emotional outcomes (Ramey and Ramey, 2004). This also had persistent effects when children were in their 20s, with children in the treatment group having better intellectual test performance and reading and mathematics test scores, more years of education, and a greater likelihood of being enrolled in college (Campbell et al., 2012; Frank Porter Graham Child Development Institute, 2012). By age 30, the treatment group was more likely to have completed a bachelor's degree, have consistent employment, not use public assistance, and have delayed parenthood. Regarding health outcomes, Campbell et al. (2014) found through biomedical data that children in the intervention group at age 35 had significantly lower risk factors for cardiovascular and metabolic disease, especially for male participants (i.e., mean systolic blood pressure for the control group was 143 versus 126 for boys in the intervention group). "One in four males in the control group was affected by metabolic syndrome, while none in the treatment group were" (Ramey, 2018, p. 539).

Looking across the body of research, Head Start appears to be particularly effective at promoting young children's physical health (see

Box 7-2 for more information on Head Start). The Head Start Impact Study showed that children enrolled in the program had better access to dental care while they were in the program and to health insurance when they were in kindergarten (Puma et al., 2012). Broader reviews of research on Head Start show positive impacts on obesity, immunization, screening for hearing and vision problems, and even child mortality (Belfield and Kelly, 2013; Rossin-Slater, 2015; Yoshikawa et al., 2013). In addition, in their review of Early Child Longitudinal Study-Birth Cohort (ECLS-B) data, Belfield and Kelly (2013) found that Head Start provided its participants "protective effects against . . . asthma, respiratory ailments, allergies, and being on medication" (Belfield and Kelly, 2013, p. 322). Lee et al. (2013) used data from ECLS-B to analyze low-income children's nutrition, weight, and health care receipt at kindergarten entry. They compared (a) Head Start participants and all nonparticipants, and (b) Head Start participants and children in pre-kindergarten (pre-K), other center-based care, other nonparental care, or only parental care using propensity score–weighted regressions. They found Head Start effects were larger compared to informal child care settings rather than center-based settings. Specifically, Head Start children had lower body mass index (BMI) scores and probability of being overweight compared to children in home-based settings; had better healthy eating habits than children in center- and home-based settings; and were also more likely to have dental care checkups compared to children in any other type of setting, including pre-K and center-based settings. Furthermore, dosage appears to matter. Frisvold and Lumeng (2011) analyzed administrative data from more than 1,500 children from Head Start programs in Michigan from 2001 to 2006 and found that children who participated in full-day Head Start were 25 percent less likely to be obese at the end of an academic year than those who enrolled in half-day programs. The effect seems to be more pronounced for boys and African American children.

One reason that Head Start stands out among ECE programs with respect to impact on physical health outcomes may be that the program design includes a robust health component (such as requiring programs to provide diverse nutrition and health services, helping families receive physical examinations by scheduling screening appointments or offering screenings directly onsite, assisting families in applying for age-appropriate health care services, providing health promotion activities directly onsite, and tracking each child's health progress) (Lee et al., 2013). In their review of the literature, Yoshikawa et al. (2013) concluded that "in contrast to the literature on Head Start and health outcomes, there are almost no studies of the effects of public prekindergarten on children's health" (Yoshikawa et al., 2013, p. 5) because pre-K programs typically do not provide health-related services.

BOX 7-2
About Head Start

Head Start is a program of the U.S. Department of Health and Human Services that provides comprehensive early childhood education, health, nutrition, and parent involvement services to low-income children and their families.

Program quality in Head Start and Early Head Start programs is defined by the Head Start Program Performance Standards (HSPPS), which include provisions related to teaching and the learning environment, curricula, child screenings and assessment, oral health practices, child nutrition, child mental health and social-emotional well-being, and family engagement. In addition, HSPPS includes standards of practice for special populations, including tribal communities, dual-language learners, children with disabilities, and pregnant women.

The federal government assesses the extent to which programs meet HSPPS through the Designation Renewal System. Programs are evaluated on a regular basis, and if deficiencies are found, programs are required to recompete for their federal grant. If the program does not achieve a high level of classroom and teacher-child interaction quality, as measured by the Classroom Assessment Scoring System (CLASS), it will need to recompete. Generally, Head Start programs score well on the Emotional Support and Classroom Organization domains of the CLASS assessment (about a 6 out of 7), but the average score for Instructional Support is only a 2.9. "In only two states (Kentucky and Vermont) were scores statistically significantly above 3 such that we can be confident the state average exceeds the threshold" (Barnett and Friedman-Krauss, 2016, p. 5).

Head Start's standards stand out among the major early care and education programs for its attention to the holistic needs of children and families (including health care) and value placed on engaging families as partners and leaders. Programs are required to help children and families access health services (including insurance), promote oral health, meet children's nutritional needs, and work with mental health consultants. Programs also need to develop strategies to communicate with parents; implement intake and assessment processes to identify families' strengths and needs; connect them to resources that support family well-being, including family safety, health, and economic stability (HHS, 2018); increase their capacity to support their children's learning and development; and include them in the governance of the program. Finally, Head Start programs have to establish relationships with other programs that serve families in their communities, such as health care providers, schools, child care, libraries and museums, housing agencies, and other social services agencies.

In 2016, the federal government released updated standards for Head Start (previously not updated since the authorization of the Improving Head Start for School Readiness Act of 2007) to reflect the latest research on child development and program quality. More research is needed to elucidate how these changes have affected program quality and outcomes.

SOURCES: HHS, 2017; Rose, 2010.

However, pre-K programs can incorporate such services and potentially achieve similar outcomes. A recent evaluation of the Universal Pre-K (UPK) program in New York City found that the expansion of the program "led to increases in rates of diagnosis of asthma and vision problems, to increased rates of screening for immunization or infectious disease, and to increased rates of treatment of hearing and vision problems" among Medicaid recipients who were eligible for UPK (Hong et al., 2017, p. 3). The researchers attribute some of these findings to UPK's program requirements, which include immunizations and developmental screenings for all enrolled students. In other words, by incorporating direct services[2] into their program design, Head Start and New York City's UPK initiative have become opportunities to effect broad improvements in young children's health outcomes.

Head Start and the UPK program in New York City are just two examples of large-scale, publicly funded ECE programs that have demonstrated generally positive results for preschool children. Others include state-funded pre-K programs in Georgia, New Jersey, North Carolina, and Oklahoma and district-run programs, like that of Boston. In a review of the body of research behind these and other large, publicly funded programs, Phillips et al. (2017) concluded that there is robust evidence of short-term benefits, especially in cognitive and academic skills. However, "the available evidence about the long-term effects of state pre-k programs offers some promising potential but is not yet sufficient to support confident overall and general conclusions about long-term effects" (Phillips et al., 2017, p. 10). For example, Lipsey et al. (2018) found that although children who participated in the Tennessee pre-K program demonstrated better cognitive skills than the control group, this advantage was lost or even reversed by 2nd or 3rd grade.

Still, the promising results from large-scale, publicly funded pre-K programs, in light of the impacts that Head Start and New York City's UPK program have on young children's health outcomes, suggest that ECE programs that serve significant proportions of young children can be a platform for interventions that promote health equity.

Home-Based Child Care Programs

Home-based child care is regulated family child care and family, friend, and neighbor care (Porter et al., 2010b). As mentioned earlier, it is a common arrangement for many young children in the United States,

---

[2] For example, immunization and a valid and reliable developmental screening tool to identify students with potential developmental delays and English Language Acquisition support needs.

particularly those from low-income families and families of color (Porter et al., 2010b). As Porter et al. note, "parents use these arrangements for a variety of reasons, including convenience, flexibility, trust, shared language and culture, and individual attention from the caregiver" (Porter et al., 2010a, p. 1). Home-based child care also serves as a primary non-parental care arrangement for infants and toddlers (Corcoran et al., 2019). (See Chapter 3 for statistics by race, ethnicity, and income.)

While most young children who are not yet enrolled in kindergarten participate in some kind of weekly center- or school-based early childhood program, 41 percent of them receive care weekly from a relative, and 22 percent participate in nonrelative care in a home environment (Corcoran et al., 2019). (Twelve percent of young children receive care in more than one of these settings on a weekly basis.) The number of children in center-based care increases as children get older. Furthermore, about 3.6 million of the approximately 3.7 million home-based providers are "unlisted": they are not registered with, licensed by, or regulated by a public agency. Together, these home-based providers serve more than 7 million young children (National Survey of Early Care and Education Project Team, 2016). Children of color are more likely to receive care from a relative, while white children are more likely to participate in nonrelative home-based care. Infants and toddlers are more likely to be cared for in a home setting—whether with a relative or nonrelative—while preschool-aged children are more likely to be enrolled in a center- or school-based program. Families with a household income of $75,000 or less are also more likely to put their young children in relative care (Corcoran et al., 2019). Thus, to the extent that regulations and policies related to safety and quality promote better care and child development, the youngest children, low-income children, and children of color could disproportionately lack access to ECE opportunities that are more equipped to support their cognitive, social-emotional, and healthy development.

The majority of evidence linking ECE to children's health, education, and well-being is primarily from center- and school-based programs. Some studies have shown a link between home-based programs and children's academic skills and social-emotional development. For example, Iruka and Forry (2018) found that children in home-based programs that were high quality and engaged frequently in enriching literacy and numeracy activities (e.g., learning names of letters, learning the conventions of print, using manipulatives, using a measuring instrument, learning about shapes and patterns) were likely to have stronger reading and math skills compared to children in home-based programs that were low quality and engaged in fewer enriching activities. This is consistent with prior work by Forry et al. (2013) using data from a multistate study of a professional development intervention showing that the quality of home-based programs, their child-centered beliefs (e.g., progressive beliefs that children should have autonomy and be allowed to express their ideas), and their perceptions of job demands were related to children's school readiness, emotional health (e.g., initiative, self-control, and attachment), and internalizing and externalizing problem behaviors.

However, mostly correlational data indicate that children in centers compared to family child care homes had higher cognitive, language, and school readiness scores but increased likelihood of contracting communicable illnesses and otitis media (ear infection), which is likely due to the large group size (Bradley and Vandell, 2007). While the data are mixed, there is indication that children in home-based programs have stronger social-emotional competence compared to children who attended center-based programs (Belsky et al., 2007). In their analyses examining multiple child care arrangement and children's academic and behavioral outcomes, Gordon et al. (2013) found that preschool children, on average, scored higher on reading and math assessments when they attended centers alone or centers in combination with home-based programs than home-based programs only or parental care. There were no differences in children's social-emotional development between families who used or did not use multiple care arrangements. The stronger benefits for children's cognitive and school readiness skills for center-based compared to home-based programs have also been seen for Latino children (Ansari and Winsler, 2012).

These better academic outcomes for center- versus home-based programs are likely due to higher teacher education and more training opportunities (Bradley and Vandell, 2007). However, the larger group size in center-based programs may preclude sensitive individual care and attending to children's social-emotional needs, which could exacerbate problem behaviors (Gordon et al., 2013). There is still a need for more rigorous examination of the differential impact based on program type and accounting for differences in teacher education and training, sociodemographics of children and families, and more robust health-related outcomes.

Quality Rating and Improvement Systems (QRISs)

Motivated in part by ECE research, states and localities have implemented QRISs to promote and enhance ECE program quality across various sectors and settings, including schools, community-based organizations (center- and home-based), and Head Start. State and local policy makers have used research linking high-quality early childhood education and children's outcomes in developing QRISs to ensure that children, especially disadvantaged children, are attending high-quality education programs during the early years. QRISs could serve as a unifying framework for defining quality across ECE programs and a defined pathway for achieving it. Moreover, without a strategy such as a QRIS, ECE programs could have inequitable resources for improvement, exacerbating the variance of quality among programs and leading to inequitable outcomes for children, families, and communities. When funded adequately and supported as a unifying strategy for ECE, QRISs can raise the overall quality of the ECE system and create more equity across communities.

Almost all QRISs measure staff training and education and assess the classroom or learning environment (Burchinal et al., 2015). Factors such as parent-involvement activities, business practices, child–staff ratios, and national accreditation status vary by state (Burchinal et al., 2015; Zellman and Perlman, 2008). QRISs serve multiple purposes, including providing a standardized method to rate program quality—based on a set of criteria—and to make the program rating information available to parents, as is done with restaurant ratings. The rating system is built on the primary assumption that parents often lack good information about program quality and that such information would inform their decisions on program selection (Burchinal et al., 2015). Consequently, providers who work with lower-quality programs would be incentivized to enhance the quality of their program or leave the market (Burchinal et al., 2015; Zellman and Perlman, 2008). In addition, QRISs represent a systematic approach to providing a range of technical assistance, resources, and incentives for programs to improve their quality (Burchinal et al., 2015). This could entail consultation on quality improvement, increased investments for professional development scholarships, microgrants for other targeted efforts, and increased subsidy payments for more highly rated programs (Burchinal et al., 2015). It has been noted that regarding QRIS,

> the goal of these efforts is to foster and support providers' efforts to improve the quality of care they provide. Thus, [QRISs] attempt to improve quality by affecting both the demand for high-quality care and the supply of such care. Of course, the success of such efforts rests on the ability of rating systems to accurately identify and measure key aspects of quality and the willingness of providers to participate in a rating system. (Burchinal et al., 2015, p. 255; see also Zellman and Perlman, 2008)

Validation of QRISs has yielded mixed findings. The Race to the Top—Early Learning Challenge Grant resulted in a proliferation of QRIS validation studies. Prior to this, most research on QRISs was descriptive and focused on issues of implementation. A recent synthesis of the validation studies by Tout et al. (2017) from 10 states found that while these ECE rating systems were valid (i.e., independent observations indicated meaningful differences across levels), most programs were, on average, providing a moderate level of quality and inconsistently associated with child outcomes, mostly for social-emotional development and EF outcomes.

There has been a limited focus on children's physical health. In their synthesis of states' QRIS validation studies, Tout et al. (2017) found that only two states focused on physical development, which included BMI and fine and gross motor skills. One state found a link between its QRIS and children's fine motor development, indicating that higher-rated programs were associated with improved fine motor development. Several states have included nutrition, physical activity, and screen time as part of their QRIS standards (Gabor and Mantinan, 2012). In their report to examine state efforts to address obesity prevention in QRISs, Gabor and Mantinan (2012) found specific standards, including a focus on nutrition (including standards), physical activity and screen time limits, professional development for staff and teachers, and sharing information about nutrition and physical activity with families.

The differences in system designs across states make it difficult to draw general conclusions from these validation studies about their links to various domains of children's development, especially health. The voluntary nature of QRISs in most states and the varying standards also make it difficult to establish a causal link between them and child outcomes. Even with these limitations, the QRIS is one *potential*, and perhaps underused, platform that could increase the use of evidence-based, health-promoting practices and standards in a mixed-delivery system by unifying leadership and governance, standards, financing, stakeholder engagement, improvement supports, accountability, and continuous quality improvement. As QRISs expand, mature, and become better funded, they could serve as the one point of entry that promotes high-quality programming across various settings (e.g., home, school, centers) and provides more children, especially children with the greatest needs, with access to beneficial ECE experiences that meet their comprehensive needs regardless of program funding.

Early Intervention for Children with Developmental Disabilities

Early Intervention[3] services support the early development of children with developmental delays or specific health conditions that could lead to delay (e.g., genetic disorder, birth defect, hearing loss). These services and programs intend to help children catch up and increase their chances for school and life success, though most of this work falls

---

[3] Early intervention refers to services for children ages 0–3. Early childhood special education refers to services for children ages 3–5.

to parents and families. Early intervention services are provided under the Individuals with Disabilities Education Act (IDEA). Eligible children are able to receive services free of charge (or at a reduced rate) through federal grants to states. Each state has its own definition of developmental delay and its own process for determining eligibility and identifying eligible children. Families with children under age 3 who qualify for early intervention receive an Individualized Family Service Plan that defines goals and the types of services that will support the family and child. Children older than age 3 who are eligible for special education services under IDEA meet with school professionals to develop an Individualized Education Program to support their educational goals.

Some of the specialists who work with children include speech-language pathologists, who help with communication speech and language delays; physical therapists, who strengthen children's movement, gross motor skills, and physical development; occupational therapists, who improve fine motor, cognitive, sensory processing, and communication skills; nurses, who support children's health status and address feeding and growth concerns; social workers, who assess and support children's social and emotional development; and developmental therapists, who design learning activities to promote children's learning and social interaction skills.

Early Intervention (Children Under 3 Years Old)

A substantial body of research supports the effectiveness of early intervention for children's functioning (Bruder, 2010; Guralnick, 2005). However, these studies suffer from methodological limitations, such as sample heterogeneity, lack of control groups, narrowly defined outcomes, and inappropriateness of standardized measures of intelligence (Bruder, 2010). Nevertheless, there is a body of research indicating that children who receive early intervention services (Part B or Part C) are less likely to see a decline in their functioning over time, with effect sizes of 0.5 to 0.75 of the standard deviation (Guralnick, 1998). This is supported by a foundational meta-analysis of 31 studies examining the effect of early intervention, which found that early intervention was "effective in promoting developmental progress in infants and toddlers with biologically based disabilities" (Shonkoff and Hauser-Cram, 1987, p. 650). The mean effects of early intervention services ranged from 0.43 for motor development to 1.17 for language development. In particular, they found that "programs that served a heterogeneous group of children, provided a structured curriculum, and targeted . . . parents and children together appeared to be the most effective" (Shonkoff and Hauser-Cram, 1987, p. 650).

In their study of community-based early intervention services for children who were in neonatal intensive care units (NICUs), Litt et al. (2018) analyzed retrospective data from the U.S. Department of Education's National Early Intervention Longitudinal Study and found that longer and more intensive services were associated with higher kindergarten skills ratings and the importance of following up after children left the NICU. These findings are consistent with those from McManus et al. (2012) in their longitudinal study of mother–infant dyads from three NICUs in southeastern Wisconsin. They matched pairs of dyads using propensity-score matching to reduce selection bias and estimate the effect of early intervention services on cognitive function trajectories. They found that service receipt was positively associated with children's cognitive functioning and trajectory and more maternal supports (e.g., mothers' report of emotional, informational, child care, financial, respite, and other support) was associated with better outcomes for families over time. Unfortunately, national data indicate that children who qualify for early intervention services are not likely to receive them, with this issue especially pronounced for black children (Boyd et al., 2018).

Most of the recent evidence about early intervention has primarily focused on children with autism spectrum disorder (ASD), which "is characterized by severe and sustained impairment in communication and social interaction and restricted patterns of ritualistic and stereotyped behaviors manifested [before] 3 years old" (APA, 2013). Children with ASD often qualify for early intervention services, usually because they are not developing in social, play, language, and cognitive domains at the expected pace (Landa, 2018). In her review of the efficacy of early interventions for young children with or at risk for ASD, Landa (2018) found that greater intervention intensity (hours and duration in months) and fidelity of implementation were associated with greater child gains. One of the applied behavior analysis approaches for children with ASD is called Early Intensive Behavioral Intervention (EIBI), which focuses on remediation of deficient language, imitation, pre-academics, self-help, and social interaction skills (Peters-Scheffer et al., 2011). In a meta-analysis examining the effectiveness of EIBI, Peters-Scheffer and colleagues (2011) found that the experimental groups outperformed the control groups on IQ, nonverbal IQ, expressive and receptive language, and adaptive behavior, with differences of 4.96–15.21 points on standardized tests. Reichow (2011) offered a similar conclusion in his overview of five meta-analyses of EIBI for young children with ASD, but he also stressed the importance of more information about child characteristics, additional knowledge on the characteristics of EIBI programs used in real-world settings, and guidelines focused on the intensity, duration, level of treatment fidelity, and therapist experience and/or training necessary to achieve optimal outcomes.

There are disparities in service access for economically disadvantaged and racial and ethnic minority families who have children with ASD (Boyd et al., 2018), and these children are also "at risk for poorer outcomes in comparison to their white and higher-income counterparts, including a more severe symptom presentation (e.g., more severe language and cognitive delays)" (Boyd et al., 2018, p. 20; CDC, 2014; Cuccaro et al., 2007; Fountain et al., 2012). One posited rationale for these poorer outcomes is lower-quality or fewer services (Boyd et al., 2018) and lower likelihood of being referred for services (Delgado and Scott, 2006).

Early Intervention/Special Education (Children 3 Years Old and Older)

Special education provides children with disabilities with specialized services designed to "prepare them for further education, employment, and independent living."[4] "Practitioners are responsible for providing specific services, instructional strategies or routines, and resources that mitigate the impact of the disability on a child's learning or behavior" (Morgan et al., 2010, p. 236). "Helping the child to benefit from the school's curriculum should in turn increase subsequent educational and societal opportunities" (ED, 2018; Morgan et al., 2010, p. 236).

The majority of students with disabilities performed in the "below basic" achievement level in all four areas of measurement (mathematics and reading, in 4th and 8th grade) in 2017. The gaps between students with disabilities and those without disabilities are substantial (Advocacy Institute, 2019). Youth with disabilities are also more likely to drop out of school, be delinquent, be unemployed, earn less, and be unsatisfied with their adult lives (Blackorby and Wagner, 1996; Horowitz et al., 2017; Thurlow et al., 2002). There is some evidence that at the end of the school year, youth placed in special education classrooms sometimes score lower on measures of reading, writing, and mathematics skills than they did at the start of the school year (Lane et al., 2005; Morgan et al., 2010).

Establishing rigorous evidence for special education services through randomized controlled trials (RCTs) is not possible because of the legal entitlement to these services for children meeting eligibility criteria, the small sample sizes, and the distinct categories and severities of disabilities (Hocutt, 1996). Thus, different quasi-experimental approaches (e.g., propensity matching) are used to gauge the impact of special education services on children's outcomes. In one study using propensity-score matching with data from the Early Childhood Longitudinal Study-Kindergarten Class (ECLS-K), 1998–1999, which is a large-scale, nationally representative sample of U.S. schoolchildren, Morgan et al. (2010) examined whether

---

[4] Individuals with Disabilities Education Improvement Act. P.L. 108-446.

children receiving special education services displayed (1) greater reading or mathematics skills, (2) positive learning-related behaviors, or (3) less frequent externalizing or internalizing problem behaviors than closely matched peers not receiving such services. The results indicated that special education services had either a negative or statistically non-significant impact on children's learning or behavior but a small positive effect on children's learning-related behaviors, such as their attention on task. Part of these findings may be due to the settings in which children are receiving services. For example, a review conducted by Ruijs and Peetsma (2009) examining the effects of inclusion on students with and without special education showed neutral to positive effects of inclusive education. Specifically, they found that students with special educational needs performed academically better in inclusive than noninclusive settings, possibly because they could learn from more able students or be more motivated to succeed because of the academic focus. Mixed results were found for social-emotional development, with some positive outcomes on social and emotional ratings and negative outcomes based on peer perceptions.

Other Issues in Special Education

Disproportionality in identification Skiba et al.'s (2005) analyses of cross-sectional state-level data indicated that black and Hispanic children were overrepresented in special education. They found this for multiple disability conditions, including intellectual disability, emotional disturbance, speech-language impairment, and learning disability. This supported prior work conducted by Oswald et al. (1999) using cross-sectional, nationally representative, and district-level data showing that minorities were overrepresented in special education, specifically in the mild mental retardation and serious emotional disturbance categories. Oswald et al. (1999) defined disproportionality as "the extent to which membership in a given ethnic group affects the probability of being placed in a specific special education disability category" (Oswald et al., 1999, p. 198), such as mild mental retardation. Morgan et al. (2015), using ECLS-K 1998 data, found minority students were underrepresented, which contradicts previous findings. Analyses of ECLS-K data of multiyear longitudinal observations and extensive covariate adjustment for potential child-, family-, and state-level confounds showed that minority children were consistently less likely than similar white, English-speaking children to be identified as having a disability and so to receive special education services. From kindergarten entry to the end of middle school, racial and ethnic minority children were less likely to be identified as having learning disabilities, speech or language impairments, intellectual disabilities, health impairments, or emotional disturbances. Language-minority children were less likely to be identified as having learning disabilities or speech or language impairment (Morgan et al., 2015). Many reasons likely account for the mixed findings, including cross-sectional versus longitudinal data, national compared to state or local data, child- versus school-level data, special education category, and trying to equate white and ethnic minority children when the latter are more likely to experience larger risk factors for developmental delay (e.g., poverty).

Nutrition Support Programs

For young students in elementary grades, schools are critical settings to support their health, such as in the area of nutrition. The National School Lunch Program (NSLP) was established under the National School Lunch Act, signed by President Harry Truman in 1946, to "safeguard the health and well-being of the Nation's children and to encourage the domestic consumption of nutritious agricultural commodities and other foods" (USDA, 2017). The largest of the five school- and center-based programs, NSLP fed about 30 million children each school day in 2014 and cost $12.7 billion (CBO, 2015). In 2014, 52 percent of school-aged children (ages 5–18) participated in NSLP, and 23 percent participated in the School Breakfast Program (SBP) (CBO, 2015). Almost half of all lunches served are provided free to students, with an additional 10 percent at reduced prices. Ethnic minority students participate in NSLP at slightly higher levels than white students, and students from low-income households participate at higher rates than those from higher-income households (Ralston et al., 2008). Ninety-four percent of schools, both public and private, choose to participate in the program (though they are not required to offer NSLP meals). NSLP accounts for 17 percent of the total federal expenditures for all food and nutrition assistance programs (Ralston et al., 2008). School meals are required to meet nutritional targets for calories, protein, calcium, iron, and vitamins. Recent changes in standards have made these meals healthier by reducing salt and saturated fat and increasing servings of fruits and vegetables. While such policies should theoretically lead to improvements in health and nutrition, there is emerging evidence that children may be less likely to consume healthier meals. Some schools have also stopped participating in NSLP because of the increased costs. To be sure, these findings are from only a few studies, and more research on the overall impact on higher nutrition standards is needed (Gundersen, 2015).

Under separate legislation, this program provides free, reduced-price, and full-price breakfasts to students. Other related programs include the Summer Food Service Program (also known as the Summer Meals Program), which extends the availability of free breakfasts and lunches into the summer months in low-income areas; the Special Milk Program, which provides subsidized milk to schools; and the After-School Snack Program, which "reimburses schools for healthy snacks given to students in educational after-school programs" (Ralston et al., 2008, p. 5). Food insecurity increases during the summer months, when children do not have access to NSLP, and the Summer Food Service Program could alleviate this problem. As of 2012, the Summer Food Service Program has a budget of under $400 million and serves a fraction of the children that NSLP serves (Gundersen, 2015). Alternatively, Supplemental Nutrition Assistance Program (SNAP) benefits can be increased during the summer months. Based on one demonstration project, it is estimated that an increase of about $2 billion in SNAP could minimize the spike in food insecurity during the summer (Gundersen and Ziliak, 2014).

Based on the report from Ralston et al. (2008), there is mixed evidence on the impact of NSLP on obesity and nutrition. For example, some studies show that children who participate in NSLP have higher intake of key nutrients and lower intake of sweets compared to nonparticipants. Other studies find high intakes of fat and sodium, which may be due to school programs not following the guidelines about fat and sodium levels. This mixed finding may be due to selection effect. For example, in their examination of NSLP on children's behavior, health, and academic outcomes, Dunifon and Kowaleski-Jones (2003) found that NSLP was associated with an increase in children's externalizing behavior and health limitation (i.e., limitation in being able to participate in regular activities) and a decrease in their math scores. However, once family-level factors associated with the selection of children's NSLP participation were adjusted, the effects attenuated. Even after addressing selection effects, there are still mixed findings about the impact of NSLP, with some studies finding participants likely to be overweight (e.g., Schanzenbach, 2009) and others (Gundersen, 2015; Hofferth and Curtin, 2005) finding no effect on obesity. Recent studies to address missing counterfactuals and systematic under-reporting of program participation (Gundersen et al., 2012) through causal analytical approaches found some indication of a positive link between NSLP and health outcomes. For example, Gunderson et al. (2012), using data from the 2001–2004 National Health and Nutrition Examination Survey study conducted by the National Center for Health Statistics and the Centers for Disease Control and Prevention, found that NSLP reduced the prevalence of food insecurity by at least 3.8 percent, the rate of poor health by at least 29 percent, and the rate of obesity by at least 17 percent.

While questions remain about the impact of NSLP on child outcomes, there is consistent evidence about the SBP. Whereas almost all schools participate in NSLP, about 75 percent are part of the SBP, serving 13.2 million children in 2013 (Gundersen and Ziliak, 2014). Frisvold (2015) used the National Assessment of Educational Progress (NAEP) and ECLS-K to determine the impact of SBP on school achievement. Using the NAEP data, he found that availability of SBP increases math by 9 percent of a standard deviation and reading achievement by 5–12 percent of a standard deviation. ECLS-K data show that SBP increases math achievement by 2.7 percent of a standard deviation, reading achievement by 2.0 percent of a standard deviation, and science achievement by 0.9 percent of a standard deviation each school year. Gleason and Dodd (2009) also found a positive effect of SBP but not NSLP on children's health. Specifically, they found that participation in the SBP is associated with lower BMI but saw no evidence for participation in NSLP and BMI. This association is strongest among white children and not significant for Hispanic children. The mechanism of the effect between SBP and learning is likely through improvement in nutrition, such as increased milk and fruit consumption and decreased soda consumption (Frisvold, 2015).

Beyond NSLP and SBP, there is a need to conduct in-depth examination of other food and nutrition programs. The Child and Adult Care Food Program (CACFP) reimburses child care programs (both centers and homes) and after-school programs for meals and snacks. Funded at about $3 billion and serving 3.3 million children in 2013, it is much smaller than NSLP and SBP. One study using the ECLS-B dataset found that participating in CACFP was not associated with any changes in the experience of food insecurity (Gundersen and Ziliak, 2014).

Summary

The PPP and ABC studies were seminal because they inspired research on *why* the early years are so important to cognitive and health outcomes. They also inspired the design and implementation of large-scale, publicly funded ECE programs that the field continues to evaluate, improve, and refine over time—many of which are discussed in this chapter. The evidence linking health equity to ECE programs and services, including Head Start, pre-K, early intervention, special education, and nutrition programs, is mixed. However, the totality of the research demonstrates effects that are generally positive, albeit with small effect sizes and nonfindings in some instances. This indicates that ECE can play an important role in improving health outcomes that could lead to health equity and there is value in continuing to ensure that children have high-quality early learning experiences from birth, though programs may differ in standards, practices, auspices, workforce, dosage, and timing. In order to maximize the impact of ECE, the field will have to better understand how the lessons of PPP and ABC apply (or not) in the current context, with a different counterfactual (i.e., more children with access to some ECE) and more diverse children and programs that operate under different funding systems and auspices. The field will also have to learn from contemporary large-scale, publicly funded programs and identify essential ingredients that lead to robust health outcomes and health equity. Only then can ECE be meaningfully part of a health promotion strategy that ensures children with the greatest needs are being served, that their needs are met early and consistently (e.g., through early intervention and nutrition), and in a diversity of settings (e.g., home- or center-based care) through a unifying system that provides high-quality access for all children.

LINKAGES BETWEEN ECE AND HEALTH EQUITY THROUGH SOCIAL-EMOTIONAL DEVELOPMENT

Social-Emotional/Behavioral Development

Social-emotional skills, including emotional processes, social/interpersonal skills, and cognitive regulation (Jones and Bouffard, 2012), in young children have been shown to predict later health outcomes and behaviors, such as substance use or abuse, mental health problems (e.g., depression), and teen pregnancy (Conti et al., 2010; Jones et al., 2015; Moffitt et al., 2011).[5] Conversely, externalizing behaviors are associated with later behavioral and academic problems, such as grade retention, school dropout, and lower school engagement (Schindler et al., 2015). Social-emotional skills are especially critical for children and families who experience trauma because of the ways in which such adverse events can impact brain development and affect children's cognitive and healthy development (see Chapter 2 for more details). For these children and families, those adults, professionals, and programs in both early childhood settings and public schools that provide nurturing and safe environments and bolster self-regulation and social-emotional skills can help mitigate the effects of and build resilience in the face of traumatic experiences (Bartlett et al., 2017). (See Box 7-3 for definitions of key terms.)

How effective are ECE programs in providing such environments? Some reviews of ECE programs have found adverse effects on children's social behaviors, especially externalizing behaviors (D'Onise et al., 2010). Analyses of data from the ECLS (Loeb et al., 2007; Magnuson et al., 2007) and the NICHD SECCYD (Belsky et al., 2007) found that participation in

---

[5] Jones and Bouffard define these core skills further: "Emotional processes include emotional knowledge and expression, emotional and behavioral regulation, and empathy and perspective-taking. Social/interpersonal skills include understanding social cues, interpreting others' behaviors, navigating social situations, interacting positively with peers and adults, and other prosocial behavior. Cognitive regulation includes attention control, inhibiting inappropriate responses, working memory, and cognitive flexibility or set shifting" (Jones and Bouffard, 2012, p. 4).

BOX 7-3
Key Terms Related to Social-Emotional Development

- **Executive function** (along with self-regulation skills) is made up of the mental processes that enable someone to plan, focus attention, remember instructions, and juggle multiple tasks successfully. The brain needs this skill set to filter distractions, prioritize tasks, set and achieve goals, and control impulses (Center on the Developing Child at Harvard University, n.d.).
- **Social-emotional development** is the change over time in children's ability to react to and interact with their social environment. It is complex and includes many different areas of growth, such as temperament, attachment, social skills or social competence, and emotional regulation (The Urban Child Institute, 2019).
- **Social-emotional learning** is the process through which children and adults acquire and effectively apply the knowledge, attitudes, and skills necessary to understand and manage emotions, set and achieve positive goals, feel and show empathy for others, establish and maintain positive relationships, and make responsible decisions (CASEL, n.d.).

ECE was associated with more reports of behavior problems, including increased externalizing behaviors and lower self-regulation, but also better cognitive outcomes, such as vocabulary and early reading and math skills. More time in ECE appears to be correlated with more pronounced behavioral issues, and the relationship sometimes persisted beyond kindergarten. See Figure 7-2 for an organizing framework for promoting social-emotional outcomes.

However, studies that examined different kinds of ECE or specific interventions in these programs reveal that ECE and public education can be vehicles for cultivating social-emotional skills and reducing bullying behaviors for older children through effective professional development, coaching, and use of evidence-based curricula. For example, an evaluation of the Chicago School Readiness Program shows that the combination of training in classroom management and job-embedded coaching helped Head Start teachers create more "emotionally and behaviorally supportive classroom environments" and reduced children's emotional and behavioral challenges and improved their EF skills (Raver, 2012, p. 683). Based on the broader body of research, the evaluators further suggested that results like these may lead to "biobehavioral benefits with health impact," such as lower cortisol in reaction to stress and lower risk of obesity (Raver, 2012, p. 684).

Another teacher training program implemented in Head Start programs, Incredible Years, produced "small but statistically significant improvements in children's knowledge of emotions, social problem-solving

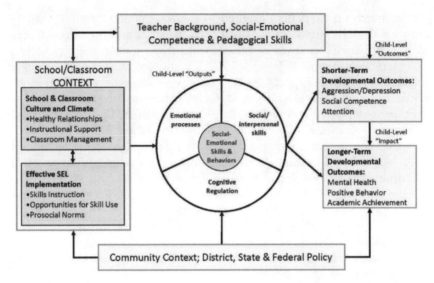

FIGURE 7-2 Organizing framework for social and emotional learning (SEL).
NOTE: Adapted from collaborative work conducted with Celene Domitrovich as part of the Preschool to Elementary School SEL Assessment Workgroup, Collaborative for Academic, Social and Emotional Learning.
SOURCE: Jones and Bouffard, 2012.

skills, and social behaviors" but no impact on children's problem behaviors or EFs (inhibition, working memory, cognitive flexibility), except among those who were exhibiting the most challenging behaviors at the beginning of the school year (Morris et al., 2014, p. 9 of the executive summary). The Good Behavior Game is a behavior management program for elementary schools, and evaluations show that children who participated in it were less likely to behave disruptively. As young adults, they were also less likely to receive diagnoses of conduct or personality disorders or use mental health services than a control group (NASEM, 2016b).

Other trainings for educators offer more direct support inside the classroom. The Early Childhood Consultation Partnership provides mental health consultation to ECE programs that serve children from birth through age 5 in Connecticut. Consultants work with early childhood educators for 8 weeks, at 4–6 hours per week, to improve the social-emotional environment of the classroom, behavior management strategies, and interactions and support for specific children with social-behavioral challenges. An evaluation using randomized assignment showed that preschoolers whose teachers participated in the intervention were rated as exhibiting less externalizing behaviors, such as hyperactivity, restlessness, and impulsivity (Gilliam et al., 2016a).

Research on curricula designed to improve young children's social-emotional skills yields generally positive but sometimes mixed findings. For instance, a study of Head Start programs that were randomly assigned to implement Preschool PATHS showed that it had "small to moderate positive impacts on . . . children's knowledge of emotions, social problem-solving skills, and social behaviors" but no impact on their problem behaviors or EF (Morris et al., 2014, p. 13 of the executive summary). Another RCT of the PATHS curriculum led to high levels of social competence, reduced aggression, and improved print knowledge but only for children who started the year with low levels of EF (Bierman et al., 2008). The researchers followed these children for 1 more year, examining 13 child outcomes at the end of kindergarten. In general, they found a sustained, small to moderate impact on social-emotional skills (as opposed to language and literacy), including enhanced learning engagement, improved social competence, and reduced aggression. The effects were especially strong among children who entered low-achieving schools (Bierman et al., 2014).

Another curriculum, Tools of the Mind, was designed to increase EF in young children—especially preschoolers and kindergarteners. The curriculum relies heavily on play-based learning, and teachers who use it with fidelity spend about 80 percent of each day promoting EF. In a study using randomized assignment, children who experienced the curriculum consistently outperformed those who did not on a variety of EF tasks (Diamond et al., 2007). Other studies showed that the curriculum has greater impact on children who may need more support, such as those who attend high-poverty schools (Blair and Raver, 2014) or have issues with hyperactivity or inattention (Solomon et al., 2017). However, Farran et al. (2015) found that children who participated in the Tools curriculum generally performed no better than those in the control group in EF tasks, and in some cases, the control group children performed better. Importantly, the researchers found that the teachers in the treatment group spent less than half of their class time on activities from the curriculum. In addition, while these teachers generally implemented the activities, *how* they interacted with children (e.g., time spent on content areas, listening versus talking, positive behavioral reinforcement, scaffolding) was not significantly different than their counterparts in the control group. These findings led the researchers to wonder whether a "reliance on a curriculum to affect child outcomes may be less important than changing interaction patterns in the classroom" (Farran et al., 2015, p. 83).

Looking at older, school-aged children, a meta-analysis of 213 school-based social-emotional learning (SEL) programs showed that "students demonstrated enhanced SEL skills, attitudes, and positive social behaviors following intervention, and also demonstrated fewer conduct problems and had lower levels of emotional distress" (Durlak et al., 2011, pp. 412–413). For example, Second Step is a violence prevention curriculum aimed at a wider range of children from ages 4 to 14. Through short (20–50-minute) lessons, classroom management support, and parent training, the program has been found to reduce aggressive behaviors (NASEM, 2016b, p. 198).

Across the above interventions, one key ingredient for success appears to be curricula that are intentionally designed to promote targeted skills and strong training and professional development (McClelland et al., 2017; Morris et al., 2014). In addition, when they are effective, they appear to have compensatory effects for those children who live or learn in more challenging or adverse environments. As described earlier, SEL can encompass a range of skills. Effective curricula or interventions are explicit about which specific skills are targeted and have intentionally designed activities or program components that target those skills. In their meta-analysis of 31 studies that focused on externalizing behaviors, Schindler et al. (2015) found that ECE programs that implemented "enhancements" or interventions that target specific social-emotional competencies were more effective at improving children's behaviors than those that relied on a "global" curriculum that addressed children's learning and developmental domains comprehensively. Durlak et al. (2011) suggest that effective programs use curricula that are "SAFE": sequenced (activities that are designed to connect and build on each other to strengthen social-emotional skills), active (instruction based on active learning strategies), focused (curricula designed to support SEL), and explicit (targeting specific social-emotional skills rather than general development in this domain).

Beyond the design of the intervention or curriculum, the support provided to early childhood educators who implement SEL programs also appears to matter. In their study of Head Start programs, Morris et al. (2014) attribute successful interventions to high-quality training followed by opportunities to practice new strategies in the classroom and ongoing support from coaches who provide feedback. Raver (2012) and Gilliam et al. (2016a) also emphasize this level of support for educators. However, Schindler et al. (2015) found that interventions that focused more on improving children's social-emotional skills directly (e.g., through specific activities or lessons in a curriculum) are more effective than training teachers to use more effective behavioral management strategies: while "the addition of a caregiver behavior management training program enhancement was not associated with significant reductions in externalizing behavior problems" (Schindler et al., 2015, p. 253), the "addition of a child social skills training enhancement . . . resulted in half of a standard deviation reduction in externalizing behavior problems . . . which is nearly twice as large as the effect found in a previous study for high-quality social and emotional learning programs implemented in primary and secondary schools" (Schindler et al., 2015, p. 257).

That said, as described above, research on early childhood mental health consultation programs may point to a promising way to improve teachers' performance in the classroom. In a qualitative analysis of six statewide or local early childhood mental health consultation programs, Duran et al. (2009) found that effective programs share three core components:

- A robust infrastructure for implementation, including strong leadership, clear program design, clear organizational structure, effective hiring, training, support and supervision of staff, strong partnerships, evaluation, and funding;
- Highly qualified consultants, defined as having a master's degree in a mental health field, demonstrating core knowledge and skills, and able to develop strong relationships with colleagues, providers, and families; and
- High-quality and comprehensive services that are child centered and targeted to both classrooms and homes, including referral to services that providers and families may need beyond consultation.

In addition, interventions at the classroom or teacher level are more likely to be effective if they are supported by the leadership and broader culture of the school or ECE program. Effective educators are more able to demonstrate their competencies if they work under supportive leadership and policies (IOM and NRC, 2015). Similarly, in its review of the research on antibullying efforts, which focuses mostly on school-aged children, the National Academies' Committee on the Biological and Psychosocial Effects of Peer Victimization: Lessons for Bullying Prevention emphasized the importance of implementing interventions across all school contexts (not just the classroom) and involving all school staff (NASEM, 2016b). For example, the playground or the lunch room can be a "hotspot" for aggressive behaviors as well as an opportunity to promote prosocial interactions. (See Box 3-4 in Chapter 3 for this committee's findings on the effects of bullying in early childhood.)

Finally, it is unclear how critical it is for SEL interventions—whether through a curriculum or consultation—to include a parent education or engagement component. Many programs do so to ensure that the strategies implemented in the classroom are reinforced at home (Duran et al., 2009; McClelland et al., 2017). For example, Fast Track is an intervention for students in grades 1 through 10 that is designed to improve children's social, cognitive, and problem-solving skills by addressing the "interactions of influences" across the school, the home, and the individual

(NASEM, 2016b, p. 201). Longitudinal RCTs of the program found that participants showed lower incidence of diagnoses of psychiatric or behavioral disorders through high school and "reduced adult psychopathology at age 25 among high-risk early-starting conduct-problem children" (NASEM, 2016b, p. 201). Unfortunately, the evaluation was not able to disaggregate the impact of the parent engagement component.

Other research had ambiguous findings. In one small, quasi-experimental study of the Incredible Years program, Williford and Shelton (2008) found that parents in the intervention group were more likely to report the use of effective parenting skills, but they did not observe a significantly lower or different level of disruptive behavior when compared with those in the control group. The two groups also did not differ in their experience of stress. The researchers posited that more robust and targeted interventions may be needed for families, as opposed to relying on a supplement to a classroom-based or teacher-focused intervention. In their qualitative review, Duran et al. (2009) also found that "engaging parents/caregivers can be difficult because they believe the services are unwarranted, unfamiliar, or stigmatizing, or because various factors impede their ability to actively participate in consultation activities (e.g., transportation, time constraints)" (p. 8 of the executive summary).

Perhaps a better approach to strengthening social-emotional development through ECE is to consider the comprehensive array of cross-sector strategies that meet the needs of children and families. The evidence described above suggests that early childhood educators are more effective at promoting social-emotional development when they have access to effective training and consultation and evidence-based curricula. But even with those supports, ECE programs and educators may lack the capacity to fully provide what children and families need, especially recipients who have experienced trauma, chronic stress, or adverse experiences. ECE programs and teachers may need to partner with other community agencies that provide services, such as screening, referrals, and enrollment in programs outside the ECE sector (e.g., mental health, legal, child welfare) (Caringi et al., 2015). Such an approach would be aligned with the way the National Child Traumatic Stress Network conceives of a "trauma-informed child- and family-services system" (Bartlett et al., 2017, p. 8) (see Box 7-8 in this chapter for more).

An example of such a cross-sector strategy to support the multiple domains of children's development, especially the environments of school-aged children, is through implementation of full-service schools (Zigler and Finn-Stevenson, 2007). Full-service community schools (FSCSs) focus on "integrat[ing] academic, health, and social supports with youth and community development strategies," (Biag and Castrechini, 2016, pp. 157–158), which is especially critical for children and families experiencing multiple challenges. "The goal is to more efficiently use resources to bolster students' learning, strengthen families, and promote healthy communities" (Biag and Castrechini, 2016, pp. 157–158; Blank et al., 2003). By coordinating services at school (by colocating or other mechanisms), community schools try to address service fragmentation and encourage more communication and collaboration among providers and educators (Biag and Castrechini, 2016). There is mixed evidence relating FSCSs with student outcomes. Using longitudinal data from six high-poverty majority-Latino community schools, Biag and Castrechini (2016) examined how participation in a FSCS influenced students' educational outcomes. The results indicated that participating in a FSCS that included family engagement opportunities and extended learning programs was associated with modest gains in students' attendance and achievement in math. In another example of FSCS, Whitehurst and Croft (2010) found that the Harlem Children's Zone did not produce higher academic gains than some other charter schools not identified as FSCSs. These mixed findings are likely due to the variation in FSCSs and their communities (Sanders, 2016), thus indicating a need for more effectiveness studies. Unfortunately, many of the evaluations on FSCSs to date have focused on academic outcomes, which calls for an intentional focus on health and social-emotional outcomes. See Box 7-4 for an example of a promising model that was designed to close the achievement gap by providing wraparound services for families.

Other school and education reform efforts found to have an effect on children's learning and behavior are the Comer School Development Program (SDP) and the 21st Century Community Learning Centers (21st CCLC). The Comer SDP was developed by James Comer and the Child Study Center at Yale University in 1968 to improve the educational experiences of low-income ethnic minority children. This model includes three mechanisms (School Planning and Management Team, Student and Staff Support Team, and Parent/Family Team); three operations (Comprehensive School Plan, Staff Development Plan, and monitoring and assessment); and three guiding principles (collaboration, consensus decision making, and no-fault problem solving) (Lunenburg, 2011). SDP is implemented in 1,150 schools across the world. Studies of SDP schools show significant student gains in achievement, attendance, behavior, and overall adjustment (Lunenburg, 2011). It is theorized that the SDP model effect manifests through improvement in school climate, indicated by improved relationships among staff and students, collaboration among staff, and central focus on students (Lunenburg, 2011). Quasi-experimental design studies have shown that students in SDP schools in comparison to students in matched non-SDP schools showed significant gains in achievement, behavior, and overall school adjustment (Haynes

---

BOX 7-4
The Northside Achievement Zone: A Promising Model[a]

The Northside Achievement Zone's (NAZ's) goal is to permanently close the achievement gap and end generational poverty in North Minneapolis. Together with its partner organizations, NAZ works with low-income families as they put their children on a path to college. NAZ's wraparound framework effectively supports low-income children of color so that they will graduate from high school prepared for college—the programming begins in early childhood.

To end the achievement gap, NAZ offers family classes; early childhood education scholarships; general improvements to public, public charter, and parochial schools in the area to support academic excellence for all children; after-school and full-day summer tutoring programs; and health and wellness programs. The health and wellness focus is rooted in the knowledge that behavioral issues are often related to traumatic experiences or adverse childhood experiences and can result in removal or expulsion from schools and after-school programs. A licensed clinical social worker meets with families who have experienced trauma and/or children who present behavioral health issues and follows a diagnostic process to help support children and their families.

The target age group is young children (ages 0–11) and their families, with some other developing programs supporting adolescents and young adults through college. The program, which was first established in 2003, originally focused on reducing violence in North Minneapolis. In 2008, residents, community organizations, and NAZ joined forces to find solutions to "seemingly intractable" issues in their neighborhood. Together, they developed the model of wraparound services for North Minneapolis's low-income families to close the "achievement gap."

By providing wraparound services focused on education, career training and financial education, and housing stabilization for children and their families, NAZ addresses several social determinants of health, including education, employment, the social environment, housing, income and wealth, and public safety.

The program is a collaborative effort among a broad range of nonprofit direct service providers, nonprofit advocacy organizations, school systems (parochial, public charter, and public district), universities, county government agencies, and Minneapolis's Public Housing Authority. These partners provide critical components of best-practice supports from prenatal development through college.

As of early 2019, NAZ has proven to reach the families that are furthest behind and in greatest need—73 percent of NAZ families make less than $30,000 per year; 98 percent are families of color; and 79 percent are African American. Between the 2016–2017 and 2017–2018 school years, NAZ family and scholar participation increased by almost 15 percent. NAZ data also support two or more layered strategies for closing the achievement gap—NAZ scholars with two or more layers of educational support (coach, expanded learning opportunities, anchor school) are more than twice as likely to be proficient in both reading and math, compared to just one layer.

NOTE: Data provided by program results summary.
   [a] The committee used selection criteria to identify examples of promising models highlighted in this report (see Appendix A for a list of the criteria). These examples all apply developmental science and aim to advance health equity during the preconception through early childhood periods.
SOURCES: Northside Achievement Zone, 2019, n.d.

and Comer, 1990a,b). Studies have emphasized the importance of implementation of key components of the SDP to find evidence of effectiveness (Cook et al., 1999; Haynes et al., 1998).

The 21st CCLC program provides students in high-poverty communities across the nation with the opportunity to participate in academic enrichment and youth development programs designed to enhance their well-being (ED, 2010). Programs provide the following activities: academic enrichment learning programs; tutoring; supplemental educational services; homework help; mentoring; recreational activities; career or job training for youth; drug and violence prevention, counseling, and character education programs; expanded library service hours; community service or service-learning programs; and activities that promote youth leadership (ED, 2010). Studies of 21st CLCC have been mixed, with limited significant findings associated with gains in achievement scores and some gains in parental involvement in school and student commitment to work (Durlak and Weissberg, 2013). In their review of after-school programs beyond the 21st CLCC, Durlak and Weissberg (2013) found four evidence-based practices that formed the acronym SAFE: (S) step-by-step training approach, (A) emphasis on active forms of learning through practicing new skills, (F) focused specific time and attention on skill development, and (E) explicitness in defining the skills being promoted. Students who participated in SAFE programs had more positive social behaviors (effect size of 0.29 versus 0.06 for other programs), reduction in problem behaviors (effect size of 0.30 versus 0.08 for other programs), school grades (effect size of 0.22 versus 0.05 for other programs), self-perception (effect size of 0.37 versus 0.13 for other programs), and academic achievement (effect size of 0.20 versus 0.02 for other programs). Thus, there is a need to examine and incorporate these evidence-based approaches in all aspects of learning during the school day or extended day.

Social-Emotional Learning, Trauma-Informed Care, and Suspensions and Expulsions

Suspensions and expulsions in ECE or K–12 settings are often used as a deterrent for misbehavior, which could be due to many factors, including learning disabilities and social-emotional needs in response to trauma, chronic stress, and adverse experiences. "Suspension" is either out-of-school or in-school suspension, which often lasts from 1 to 10 days but varies across states and localities. "Expulsion" is the permanent removal of students from an ECE or school setting. The U.S. Department of Education's Office for Civil Rights (ED OCR, 2016) found that students with disabilities served by the IDEA (11 percent) are more than twice as likely to receive one or more out-of-school suspensions compared to students without disabilities (5 percent). More than 1 out of 5 American Indian or Alaska Native (22 percent), Native Hawaiian or other Pacific Islander (23 percent), black (23 percent), and multiracial (25 percent) boys with disabilities served by the IDEA received one or more out-of-school suspensions, compared to 1 out of 10 white (10 percent) boys with disabilities served by the IDEA. Black students are 2.3 times as likely to receive a referral to law enforcement or be subject to a school-related arrest as white students (ED OCR, 2016), emphasizing the need for trauma-informed approaches in schools.

Turning to children in general education, more than 250 preschoolers are suspended or expelled daily (Malik, 2017). Estimates show that as many as 8,710 3- and 4-year-old children may be expelled from or pushed out of their state-funded preschool or pre-K classrooms annually—a rate nearly three times that of students in kindergarten through 12th grade. In child care centers, expulsion rates are 13 times what they are in kindergarten through 12th grade. These rates are particularly pernicious for black children, who are suspended and expelled at much higher rates than their peers. Black preschoolers are 3.6 times more likely to receive one or more suspensions than white preschoolers (Meek and Gilliam, 2016). Black children represent only 19 percent of preschool enrollment but are 47 percent of children receiving one or more out-of-school suspensions; in comparison, white children are 41 percent of preschool enrollment but 28 percent of children receiving one or more out-of-school suspensions (Boyd et al., 2018; Meek and Gilliam, 2016).

Various scholars, and more recently, Gilliam et al. (2016b), suggested that teachers' implicit bias may be the underlying cause for this "push-out" of black children, especially boys, from these early learning settings as teachers view black children as older and more culpable (Goff et al., 2014). These biased views and attitudes about black children are likely to contribute to children's disengagement in school. In a meta-analytic study using 53 studies examining the link between suspension and student outcomes, Noltemeyer et al. (2015) found an inverse relationship between suspension and achievement and a positive relationship between suspension and school dropout. Effect sizes ranged from 0.10 for in-school suspension and 0.24 for out-of-school suspension to 0.32 for the effect of suspension on achievement tests. There was an effect size of 0.28 for the effect of suspension on school dropout. Noltemeyer et al. (2015) also found that the percentage of male ethnic minority students and family socioeconomic status (SES) moderated the relationship between suspension and achievement; this was also the case for school dropout. This indicates that the exclusionary practices are not beneficial for students' achievement and learning process and may heighten risk for children from ethnic and low-SES households. These practices are especially harmful when they contribute to pushing students of color into the school-to-prison pipeline (see Box 7-5 for more information).

In response to suspension and expulsion, there have been two general approaches for training professionals—trauma-informed care (TIC) and implicit bias training (see the section on supports for the ECE professional for an overview of both approaches to help address suspension and expulsion issues).

Social-Emotional Learning and Dual-Language Learners

Research suggests that children who are bilingual tend to have better self-regulation skills than their monolingual peers (Castro et al., 2013). They have enhanced ability to control their attention and greater EF skills, such as planning, working memory, and cognitive flexibility. Researchers

---

BOX 7-5
School-to-Prison Pipeline

The school-to-prison pipeline refers to "policies and practices that are directly and indirectly pushing students of color out of school and on a pathway to prison" (National Education Association, n.d.). These policies and practices "disproportionately [place] students of color, including those who identify as LGBTQ [lesbian, gay, bisexual, transgender, and queer], have disabilities, and/or are English language learners, into the criminal justice system for minor school infractions and disciplinary matters, subjecting them to harsher punishments than their white peers for the same behaviors" (National Education Association, n.d.).

Disproportionate rates of school discipline, such as suspensions and expulsions, in early care and education (ECE) are one means through which children of color are driven to the criminal justice and welfare systems. Based on U.S. Department of Education national civil rights data from the 2013–2014 school year, a Government Accountability Office analysis (2018) found that black students, boys, and students with disabilities experienced disproportionately high rates of suspension and expulsion (GAO, 2018). For detailed information on the welfare and criminal justice systems and their effects on adolescent health and well-being through a life course perspective, see the 2019 National Academies report *The Promise of Adolescence: Realizing Opportunity for All Youth*.

Addressing the school-to-prison pipeline and its deleterious effects on the health, well-being, and development of children of color (into adolescence and across the life course) requires attention from ECE providers, as the origins of the pipeline are often established in ECE settings through disproportionate rates of discipline to young children of color, particularly boys. ECE providers can help to dismantle the pipeline through the aforementioned strategies—specifically, countering unconscious biases and cultural stereotyping and fostering greater cultural competency through trainings on antiracism, implicit bias, and mindfulness.

attribute this advantage to bilingual children's experiences at paying attention to their environment and other contextual cues to understand when to use one language over another (Castro et al., 2013). A 2017 National Academies report concluded that dual-language learners (DLLs) "who have a strong base in their [home language] and acquire high levels of English proficiency will realize the cognitive, linguistic, social, and cultural benefits of becoming bilingual" (NASEM, 2017b, p. 175). Conversely, DLLs' loss of proficiency in their home language may also compromise their social-emotional development. For instance, "children who do not develop and maintain proficiency in their home language may lose their ability to communicate with parents and family members and risk becoming estranged from their cultural and linguistic heritage" (NASEM, 2017b, p. 175).

Thus, to strengthen DLLs' social-emotional health and self-regulation, it is important for ECE and elementary schools to foster their home language skills. Research also shows that when educators implement evidence-based practices that support bilingual development, DLLs' maintenance of their home language does not come at the cost of their proficiency in English (NASEM, 2017b).

LINKAGES BETWEEN ECE AND HEALTH EQUITY THROUGH PARENTING AND THE HOME ENVIRONMENT

Another crucial pathway through which ECE leads to health equity is the family and home environment (see Chapter 4 for the importance of family cohesion and support). As indicated in the pathway by Hahn et al. (2016), ECE programs support a positive, enriching, and stable home environment through parents' participation in educational, social, health, and job training opportunities. This pathway can lead to improvement in children's and families' cognitive, social, and health outcomes, which then impacts children's outcomes that lead to higher education attainment and health equity. This pathway is particularly supported by the National Academies report *Parenting Matters: Supporting Parents of Children Ages 0–8* (NASEM, 2016a), which emphasized the evidence about strengthening parental knowledge, attitudes, and practices to improve children's cognitive and social-emotional well-being. Specifically, it found that parental knowledge of child development is positively associated with parent behaviors. Parents with knowledge of evidence-based parenting practices, especially those related to promoting children's physical health and safety, such as vaccination and use of seat belts, are more likely to engage in those practices.

Ample evidence exists that parental knowledge of how to meet their children's basic physical (e.g., hunger) and emotional (e.g., wanting to be held or soothed) needs, as well as of how to read infants' cues and signals, ensures proper child growth and development (Bowlby, 2008; Chung-Park, 2012; Regalado and Halfon, 2001; Zarnowiecki et al., 2011). Parents' attitudes about specific practices, such as breastfeeding and engagement in children's education, were related to parents' behaviors and use of services. They found strong evidence that the following parenting practices are important to children's physical health and safety and emotional and behavioral, social, and cognitive competence: (a) contingent responsiveness ("serve and return")—adult behavior that occurs immediately after a child's behavior and is related to the child's focus of attention, such as a parent smiling back at a child; (b) warmth and sensitivity; (c) routines and reduced household chaos; (d) shared book reading and talking to children; (e) practices that promote children's health and safety—in particular, prenatal care, breastfeeding, vaccination, ensuring adequate nutrition and physical activity, monitoring, and household and vehicle safety; and (e) use of appropriate (less harsh) discipline (McClelland et al., 2017).

The pathway linking ECE to health equity through supporting responsive parenting and a quality home environment is generally supported by many programs, including the three foundational early childhood programs, each of which included a significant family engagement component—the HighScope PPP, focused on 3- and 4-year olds, the Carolina ABC Study, focused on children birth to age 3, and the Chicago Child-Parent Centers (CPCs) (see Box 7-6). While these studies are quite old, focused on particular populations (i.e., African Americans), and specific to local areas, in addition to being unable to disentangle the impact of teacher practices compared to family engagement practices, they provide long-term and intergenerational evidence of the importance of engaging with families while also providing high-quality learning experiences in classrooms. Other early childhood programs, including home visiting programs that serve mothers prenatally and last until the children are 3 years old and family engagement programs for preschool- and school-age children, provide additional support for the links between ECE and healthy equity through parenting.

Family Engagement Programs

The focus on family engagement has been bolstered by the recent federal funds for parent and family community engagement centers (U.S. Department of Education [ED] Statewide Family Engagement Center Program through the Consolidated Appropriations Act of 2018). As reviewed in the *Parenting Matters* report, some ECE programs "provide full- or part-time classroom-based services (center or family child care) for children

---

BOX 7-6
Chicago Child-Parent Centers (CPCs)

The Chicago CPC "began in the Chicago public schools in 1967 through federal funding from the Elementary and Secondary Education Act of 1965. . . . The 24 centers provide comprehensive services under the direction of the Head Teacher and in collaboration with the elementary school principal, as well as parent resource teachers, the school-community representative, bachelor's level classroom teachers, nurses, speech therapists, and school psychologists" (Temple and Reynolds, 2007, pp. 133–134). The CPC's comprehensive services included an intensive parent involvement component, outreach, and attention to health and nutrition. Participation in the CPC preschool intervention relative to the usual enrichment program was associated with significantly higher rates of school completion by age 24, significantly lower rates of juvenile arrest for both violent and nonviolent offenses, lower rates of school remedial services, stable employment, health insurance coverage, and lower likelihood of depressive symptoms (Temple and Reynolds, 2007). School-age intervention was associated with lower rates of school remedial services and receipt of public aid. Extended intervention for 4–6 years was linked to significantly lower rates of remedial education, juvenile arrests for violent offense, receipt of disability assistance, and private insurance coverage.

---

from birth to age five" that "often include parenting education and other services for families (sometimes starting prenatally)" (NASEM, 2016a, p. 159). To address the overall conditions of families, these programs are designed to improve parenting knowledge, attitudes, and practices with the goal of supporting children's cognitive and social-emotional development and success in school (Brooks-Gunn et al., 2000; Chase-Lansdale and Brooks-Gunn, 2014; Fantuzzo et al., 2013). These parent-focused programs have several different structures. For example, some include parent supports (and parent self-sufficiency support) as well as intensive classroom-based services for children that are multipronged. Others offer services that are primarily classroom-based with either some parenting education services or some parent self-sufficiency services (NASEM, 2016a).

In their examination of the impact of Head Start on child outcomes through parenting, Puma et al. (2012) did not find significant differences on parenting-related measures, included disciplinary practices, educational supports, parenting styles, parent participation in and communication with the school, and parent and child time together (NASEM, 2016a). With respect to Early Head Start, there was some evidence that programs that were mixed delivery (center and home) had favorable and consistent impact on parenting outcomes, including sensitive parenting and language-rich environments.

Other school-based parent engagement programs have been found to be effective for children's outcomes. For example, the Companion Curriculum uses Head Start teachers to encourage parents' participation in the classroom and provides workshops and activity spaces in the classroom that focus on training parents to engage in parent–child learning activities (Mendez, 2010; NASEM, 2016a). There were no benefits for parents, but there was significant improvement in children's vocabulary in a quasi-experimental study (Mendez, 2010). Another example is documented in the *Parenting Matters* report (NASEM, 2016a, p. 163):

> The Kids in Transition to School (KITS) Program is a short-term, targeted, evidence-based intervention aimed at increasing early literacy, social skills, and self-regulatory skills among children who are at high risk for school difficulties. This program provides a 24-session readiness group for children that promotes social-emotional skills and early literacy as well as a 12-session parent workshop focused on promoting parent involvement in early literacy and the use of positive parenting practices. In a pilot efficacy trial with 39 families, Pears and colleagues found that children in families who received the KITS intervention demonstrated early literacy and social skill improvements as compared with their peers who did not receive the intervention (Pears et al., 2014). In randomized controlled studies, foster children who received the intervention exhibited improvements in social competence, self-regulation skills, and early literacy skills. (Pears et al., 2007, 2012, 2013)

Two-generational model programs, such as Head Start, Project Redirection, New Chance demonstration, Ohio's Learning and Earning Program, Teen Parent Demonstration, and the Comprehensive Child Development Program from the 1980s and 1990s, offered mothers a wide range of services, including parenting classes, job training, mandatory schooling, and child care (Granger and Cytron, 1999; NASEM, 2016a; Polit, 1989). Many of these programs have not resulted in significant positive outcomes, at least based on older versions of the models (NASEM, 2016a). The new iterations of two-generation models focus

> on the education benefits to children of high-quality ECE programs and higher parental levels of education and labor force motivation. Parenting knowledge, attitudes, and practices may be improved, but the improvement comes indirectly through higher parental job skills and education and reduced household stress rather than explicit programming directed at parenting skills. (NASEM, 2016a, p. 166)

Examples of these new iterations that have evaluations planned or under way are the CareerAdvance Community Action Project of Tulsa, Oklahoma; The Annie E. Casey Foundation Atlanta Partnership; and the Housing Opportunity and Services Together project (NASEM, 2016a; see Chase-Lansdale and Brooks-Gunn, 2014, for others).

There are also other family-focused interventions for school-age children. In one example, the ParentCorps program, parent groups (see Box 7-7; also documented in NASEM, 2016a)—"co-facilitated by teachers and mental health professionals with expertise in behavior management— are used to help parents establish structure and routines for children, teach positive parenting practices (e.g., positive reinforcement and consistent consequences), and provide opportunities for facilitator-observed parent– child interactions" (NASEM, 2016a, p. 171). In addition to reduced behavior problems among children in the treatment group, parents displayed more effective parenting practices than in the control group. Parents in the treatment group reported using more effective disciplinary practices and receiving higher scores on tests of knowledge of effective behavior management strategies; in addition, higher-quality parenting was observed for parent–child interactions by the research team (Brotman et al., 2011).

As documented in the *Parenting Matters* report (NASEM, 2016a), Getting Ready is an evidence-supported intervention that targets parents' decision-making role at school (Sheridan et al., 2010). The program includes parent–teacher conferences, monthly family socialization, and teacher home visits with parents using structured interactions. The goal is to actively engage parents in learning and behavior goal setting and decision making. "Together, teachers and parents identify learning opportunities at home and school and plan how educators and parents can complement each other's efforts to promote learning and track children's growth. Priorities include affirming parents' competence, increasing their access to information on child development, and reinforcing positive parenting practices" (Knoche et al., 2012; NASEM, 2016a, pp. 171–172). Knoche et al. (2012) identified treatment effects for parental warmth and sensitivity, learning support, and autonomy support. Sheridan et al. (2014) found that, relative to children in the control group, children in the Getting Ready intervention had a significantly greater decline in disruptive behaviors such as difficulty standing still and tendency to run around; however, no differences were seen for other learning-related behaviors. Children's language and literacy were also improved, and one study found some evidence that the program's effects on achievement were greatest for children at highest risk for underachievement (that is, those children whose parents have less than a high school education and those who did not speak English prior to treatment) (Sheridan et al., 2011). Thus, there is some evidence that schools' partnership and engagement with parents through specific and structured approaches are related to improved parenting and child academic and behavioral outcomes; unexpectedly, these outcomes seem stronger in older age groups. However, caution is warranted because these are not national studies and, in many instances, are localized and researcher controlled, unlike the Head Start and Early Head Start studies.

BOX 7-7
ParentCorps: A Promising Model[a]

ParentCorps is a universal school-based program for all children in pre-kindergarten (pre-K) or early childhood settings that aims to help students develop foundational skills for learning. The program takes a family-centered approach by building on the strengths of culturally diverse families and engaging parents as partners. ParentCorps is now offered as an "evidence-based enhancement" to Pre-K for All programs throughout New York City (NYU School of Medicine, 2019). ParentCorps includes three key components that are designed to strengthen home–school connections and provide high-quality (i.e., safe, predictable, and nurturing) environments for students based on the scientific evidence that this will help students to develop strong social, emotional, and behavioral regulation skills.

1. Program for pre-K students ("Friends School"): 14-week curriculum for students on social, emotional, and behavioral regulation skills (materials offered in English and Spanish).
2. Program for parents of pre-K students: 14-week program for parents to promote the use of evidence-based strategies for enhancing social, emotional, and behavioral regulatory skills (materials offered in English and Spanish).
3. Professional development for staff: group and individual learning opportunities for pre-K and kindergarten teachers and assistants, mental health professionals, parent support staff, and school leaders to promote the use of evidence-based strategies for enhancing home–school connections and to strengthen social, emotional, and behavioral regulation skills.

ParentCorps works to buffer the effects of early adversity, such as poverty, by engaging and supporting parents and early childhood professionals in the community. The program takes a multisector approach by engaging professionals in early care and education and health. The primary social determinants of health that it targets are education, the social environment, and health services. ParentCorps has been found to yield positive outcomes for children through age 8 in urban schools in areas of concentrated poverty. These include improvements in areas of academic achievement, behavioral outcomes, and obesity outcomes (Brotman et al., 2011, 2012, 2013, 2016; Dawson-McClure et al., 2015). In addition, a cost-effectiveness analysis estimated $4,387 in long-term cost savings per individual in health care, criminal justice, and productivity expenditures after factoring program costs and increased life expectancy by 0.27 quality-adjusted life years (Hajizadeh et al., 2017).

---

[a] The committee used selection criteria to identify examples of promising models highlighted in this report (see Appendix A for a list of the criteria). These examples all apply developmental science and aim to advance health equity during the preconception through early childhood periods.

Home Visiting Programs

One particular early childhood program focused on supporting parents and enhancing positive parenting and reducing/preventing child abuse and maltreatment is home visiting (see Chapter 4 for additional background on home visiting, including health impacts and a committee recommendation). Home visiting (which targets families with pregnant women and children from birth through age 5—though most attend until children are 3 years old) has been found to increase parental knowledge and practices and reduce parental stress and depression while also supporting child health and reducing maltreatment. The general short-term outcomes of home visiting programs include (1) decreasing parent stress, depression, and isolation; (2) increasing family self-sufficiency; (3) enhancing parenting knowledge of child development; (4) increasing self-efficacy in the parenting role; (5) healthier parent–child relationships and interactions; (6) increasing positive guidance and decreasing harsh punishment; and (7) supporting children's learning. The long-term outcome is to enhance children's well-being, social competence, and school readiness.

Based on strict criteria for what counted as evidence and a systematic review of that evidence (adapted in part from ED's What Works Clearinghouse),[6] the U.S. Department of Health and Human Services' (HHS's) Home Visiting Evidence of Effectiveness identified many effective models that impact various outcomes, including positive parenting practices, family economic self-sufficiency, child health, child development and school readiness, and reductions in child maltreatment. Regarding positive parent practices, the review shows that

> while many individual evaluations of home visiting programs have shown impacts on parenting practices tied to positive developmental outcomes, the average impacts of home visiting on parenting practices are not large. Nor is there a strong pattern of effects on parenting practices across evaluation studies and home visiting models. (NASEM, 2016a, p. 151)

None of the home visiting models were linked to reductions in juvenile delinquency, family violence, and crime. Healthy Families America, however, had one or more favorable impacts in each of the eight domains, and Nurse-Family Partnership had favorable impacts in seven domains, followed by Early Head Start—Home Visiting with favorable impacts in five domains. See the *Parenting Matters* report for synthesis of home visiting and various models, and the Home Visiting Evidence for Effectiveness website by HHS's Administration for Children and Families for

---

[6] For more information, see Institute of Education Sciences. n.d. *What Works Clearinghouse. Find What Works.* https://ies.ed.gov/ncee/wwc/FWW (accessed July 15, 2019).

a recent examination of all home visiting models.[7] These findings are consistent with the 2019 results from the Mother and Infant Home Visiting Program Evaluation (MIHOPE) and MIHOPE–Strong Start Studies of Evidence-Based Home Visiting, namely, that MIHOPE found positive effects on some family outcomes (e.g., home environment) but MIHOPE–Strong Start found little effect on birth outcomes and prenatal behaviors (Michalopoulos et al., 2019).

In summary, there is some evidence linking family engagement, including home visiting and support, to children's health and well-being. While it is challenging to disentangle family engagement and support from ECE classroom practices, there is indication that supporting family functioning and processes and providing resources and strategies will likely lead to better outcomes for parents themselves and their children, resulting in health equity. Current evidence indicates the importance of tailoring services and programs to meet the needs of individual families and ensuring that families and children with the greatest needs are engaged throughout the duration of the program/services. With new approaches to family engagement and support, such as the Two Gen 2.0 models, more actionable evidence is emerging about how best to support children and their families in the early years.

LINKAGES BETWEEN ECE AND HEALTH EQUITY THROUGH SUPPORTS FOR THE ECE PROFESSIONAL

The salutary effects that ECE can have on the physical, mental, and social-emotional health of children—whether through the inclusion of comprehensive services, evidence-based curriculum, high-quality professional development and supports, or effective family engagement—can be disrupted if the ECE professionals themselves are not trained or supported to implement best practices or navigate systems of services for children and families outside the ECE sector. Since the release of the National Academies report *Transforming the Workforce for Children Birth Through Age 8: A Unifying Foundation* (IOM and NRC, 2015), there has been increased interest from funders, policy makers, and advocates in overhauling the professional preparation and ongoing supports for early childhood educators so that these experiences—and the policies and funding that shape them—better reflect the science of early development.[8] For example, states

---

[7] For more information, see U.S. Department of Health and Human Services. n.d. *Home Visiting Evidence of Effectiveness*. See https://homvee.acf.hhs.gov (accessed June 14, 2019).

[8] See initiatives from national organizations, such as Power to the Profession, National Governors Association, and Council of Chief State School Officers, and state-led initiatives, such as in Colorado, Minnesota, and Nebraska.

and national organizations have developed statements of core professional competencies that inform the training of these educators. The report found that, in most cases, these statements need to be updated to follow recent developments in science and research. Some of these areas are especially relevant to promoting young children's health and well-being, such as knowledge and skills related to working effectively with children who have experienced chronic stress, trauma, and adversity; collaboration with professionals in ECE or the education sector; promotion of self-regulation and related EFs; and support for DLLs. Incorporating these issues into efforts to improve policies, systems, and programs that prepare and support early childhood educators is critical to maximizing the potential of ECE programs to improve health outcomes and equity. For example, teachers, especially those who work with students who experience trauma, can be more effective if they receive more training and education on mental health issues and skills to access relevant services from that sector (Hydon et al., 2015).

Training and supports for early childhood educators are needed to help them adjust their practice to acknowledge their own biases and their understanding that children's behavioral challenges and learning difficulties are often due to the toxic stress response and undiagnosed and untreated trauma (Matthews et al., 2018; Ramirez et al., 2012). It is important to note that these trainings are critical for supporting children's learning and healthy development beyond addressing suspension and expulsion. Whether or not children are suspended or expelled, many are exposed to traumatic experiences, including abuse and neglect, family and media violence, community or school violence, loss of a parent, parents dealing with substance abuse, and mental or other health challenges. In turn, children who experience trauma can exhibit behaviors in ECE programs and schools that may indicate social-emotional challenges. Box 7-8 describes a trauma-informed service system for children and families.

Trauma-Informed Care or Practices

TIC is defined as a "recognition of the pervasiveness of trauma and a commitment to identify and address it early . . . [and it] involves seeking to understand the connection between presenting symptoms and behaviors and the individual's past trauma history" (Hodas, 2006, p. 5) (see Box 7-9 for more information). TIC can be provided in multiple settings by trained, committed professionals who understand the principles of a TIC system, including

a. trauma and how it may impact children's identity, how they will view the world, and coping mechanisms;

b. children and their contexts, including their family and commu-
    nity contexts, and supporting children to be active in their healing
    process;
c. services that are strengths based and promote children's self-
    control and coping skills; and
d. the service relationship, which is based on relationships and trust
    that is earned over time.

BOX 7-8
Trauma-Informed Child- and Family-Service Systems

A trauma-informed child- and family-service system is one in which all parties recognize and respond to the impact of traumatic stress on those who have contact with the system, including children, caregivers, and service providers. Programs and agencies within such a system infuse and sustain trauma awareness, knowledge, and skills into their organizational cultures, practices, and policies. They act in collaboration with all of those who are involved with the child, using the best available science, to facilitate and support the recovery and resiliency of the child and family.

SOURCE: The National Child Traumatic Stress Network, n.d.

BOX 7-9
Trauma-Informed Care Strategies for Educators

The following trauma-informed care strategies for educators are adapted from The National Child Traumatic Stress Network child welfare trauma training toolkit.

1. Develop a crisis plan with resources.
2. Maximize the child's sense of safety.
3. Assist children in reducing overwhelming emotion.
4. Help children make new meaning of their trauma history and current experiences.
5. Address the impact of trauma and subsequent changes in the child's behavior, development, and relationships.
6. Coordinate services with other agencies.
7. Utilize comprehensive assessment of the child's trauma experiences and their impact on the child's development and behavior to guide services.
8. Support and promote positive and stable relationships in the life of the child.
9. Provide support and guidance to the child's family and caregivers.
10. Manage professional and personal stress.

SOURCE: Child Welfare Committee, The National Child Traumatic Stress Network, 2013.

There is emerging evidence about the impact of TIC and trauma-informed practices (TIPs) for children's outcomes and well-being. For example, Zakszeski et al. (2017) conducted a review to describe the implementation and evaluation of trauma-focused school practices. They found that most approaches used Cognitive Behavioral Intervention for Trauma in Schools, followed by drama instruction, eye movement desensitization and reprocessing training, coping/social skill instruction, and comprehensive, multitiered systems. Zakszeski et al. (2017) found that most of the studies reported positive treatment outcomes, especially reduction in symptoms of trauma and internalizing problems, but effect sizes were not included to determine magnitude. The limitation of the studies in this review was that most occurred with subpopulations of children rather than across the student population. There has been a call for more rigorous study and review of TIC and TIP beyond their implementation (Bryson et al., 2017). See Box 7-10 for an example of a promising model that employs a cognitive behavioral intervention to address trauma in schools.

Implicit Bias Training

Implicit biases are unconscious and involuntary attitudes that can influence one's affect, behavior, and cognitive processes (Boysen, 2010). It has been suggested that implicit bias is one reason for the disproportionality of suspension and expulsion rates for black children and children with special needs. That is, educators may see the normative behaviors of black children in particular as dangerous and aggressive, even when there is no evidence of misbehavior (Gilliam et al., 2016b). Implicit bias training may be a potential strategy to counter these unconscious biases. Evidence is emerging on the impact of implicit bias training, mostly from the public health and nursing sectors. One core feature of implicit bias training is cultural competence, which "is the process and ability of an individual or organization to function effectively within different cultural situations" (Betancourt et al., 2003; Cross et al., 1989; Gallagher and Polanin, 2015, p. 333); it "combines a set of congruent behaviors with attitudes and knowledge that facilitate an individual or a system to work successfully in various cultural contexts other than their own culture" (Gallagher and Polanin, 2015, p. 333). See Box 7-11 for more information on the importance of cultural competence and sensitivity in ECE.

Scholars caution about the focus on cultural competence without antiracist training. A literature review by Allen (2010) indicates that cultural competence training could be strengthened by antiracist training to adequately ensure that professionals are able to

> challenge discrimination experienced by minority cultural groups, such as ethnocentrism, cultural biases, and overt and covert discrimination

BOX 7-10
Cognitive Behavioral Intervention for Trauma
in Schools: A Promising Model[a]

Cognitive Behavioral Intervention for Trauma in Schools (CBITS) is a mental health intervention that was designed and first implemented in 2001 to target students from 5th through 12th grade who have witnessed or experienced traumatic life events (CBITS, n.d.-a). CBITS uses cognitive behavioral techniques, implemented in a school setting. The program includes 10 group sessions, 1–3 individual therapy sessions, 2 parent psychoeducational sessions, and 1 teacher education session.

CBITS works to address posttraumatic stress symptoms in students who are 10–18 years old. The program uses cognitive behavioral therapy techniques to address a growing issue: 20–50 percent of children in the United States are affected by violence, as victims or witnesses, and even more are exposed to natural disasters, accidents, and traumatic losses (Stein et al., 2011). These experiences, which disproportionately affect low-income and minority children, can cause posttraumatic stress symptoms, leading to behavioral problems, poorer school performance, more days of school absence, and depression and anxiety (Stein et al., 2011). CBITS addresses several social determinants of health (health systems and services, education, and the social environment) and engages multiple sectors (mental health providers, nonprofit community-based organizations, public schools, the Substance Abuse and Mental Health Services Administration and other federal agencies, state governments, and universities).

Evidence suggests that CBITS is effective, and it has been implemented widely across the United States and abroad (Stein et al., 2011). The Journey Mental Health Center in Dane County, Wisconsin, has successfully implemented CBITS in local public schools since 2004, and feedback consistently shows that it reduces symptoms, increases the potential for positive school performance, and creates a forum for open communication with students (CBITS, n.d.-b). The University of Maryland Center for Mental Health (CMH) has also used CBITS in Baltimore schools since 2004. CBITS was met with such enthusiasm from participants and providers that CMH has continued provide annual trainings for its clinicians and began conducting trainings for mental health practitioners at schools, many of whom are actively using CBITS at the request of the Maryland State Department of Education. When CBITS was implemented between 2008 and 2010 in more than 100 schools in the Los Angeles Unified School District, 81 percent of participants across grades 5–10 reported improvement in posttraumatic stress disorder symptoms, with 63 percent falling below the clinical range.

---

[a] The committee used selection criteria to identify examples of promising models highlighted in this report (see Appendix A for a list of the criteria). These examples all apply developmental science and aim to advance health equity during the preconception through early childhood periods.

due to racial difference . . . [and cultural competence training may limit] culture to a static entity and reduces understanding of peoples' behavior to prescribed cultural norms. This promotes cultural stereotyping with the risk of discrimination and it fails to account for individual and family differences within cultural groups. (Allen, 2010, p. 315)

BOX 7-11
Integrating Cultural Competence and Sensitivity into ECE

Beyond implicit bias training, it is important to broadly integrate cultural competency and sensitivity into early care and education (ECE) policies and practices to make progress on health equity. Chapter 4 discusses the role of culture as a contextual determinant of development. Based on this, ECE is an optimal platform to embrace and build from cultural practices of the populations being served. Integrating cultural competency can provide continuity between the home environment and the ECE setting, and is an opportunity to engage parents as co-teachers. Given the cultural differences that some children may experience, their understanding of specific behaviors and learning methods will inevitably differ based on their community of origin. For example, based on community values, a child may learn most effectively from child-directed interactions, observing other social actors, or observing third-party interactions in which they are not involved. An understanding of cultural norms for certain groups of children would best position ECE professionals to incorporate specific teaching practices that are consistent with what the child is experiencing at home.

One example of cultural competence training from the nursing literature is called "transcultural nursing," which "is concerned with comparing differences and similarities between cultures regarding caring values and life practices to predict the care needs of individuals and promote culturally [appropriate] care. In this approach, culture is defined as attitudes, values, beliefs, and life practices learned and shared by people in a particular social group, which are passed on down generations, affecting individuals' thinking and actions" (Allen, 2010, p. 315; Leininger and McFarland, 2002). This cultural competence training model and others similarly focus on meaningful, thoughtful, and humble interactions, and teaching individuals from different cultural backgrounds needs to be based on knowledge about specific cultural beliefs, attitudes, and practices. In a meta-analysis to examine the effect of educational interventions designed to enhance cultural competence in professional nurses and nursing students, Gallagher and Polanin (2015) found, in general, moderate to large positive effects. This is consistent with previous studies (e.g., Maina et al., 2018), including a meta-analysis conducted by Smith et al. (2006). These studies, however, were limited in their lack of an articulated definition of cultural competence, implementation, rigorous design, and self-rating measures, which calls for more rigorous, well-defined multimethod studies in this area.

SOURCES: Allen, 2010; Galindo et al., 2019; Gallagher and Polanin, 2015; Maina et al., 2018; Schneidman and Woodward, 2016; Silva et al., 2015; Smith et al., 2006; Sperry et al., 2018.

However, there is an absence of a validated antiracist training and intervention.

Other options to address unconscious bias are mindfulness training and prejudice habit breaking. It is theorized that mindfulness training could reduce implicit bias by (1) deactivating the "prejudice network," which involves the activation of the amygdala (or threat responses) and reduces the ventromedial prefrontal cortex (or the empathy and "humanizing" pathway) (Burgess et al., 2017); (2) meditating to increase one's ability to become aware of implicit biases, once they are activated, and to engage in self-regulatory processes to behave in less discriminatory and prejudicial ways; (3) reducing stress and internal sources of cognitive load that contribute to the activation and application of implicit biases; (4) activating empathy and compassion, which reduce the activation and application of implicit bias and promote willingness to engage with members of stigmatized groups; and (5) improving one's ability to communicate and focus on the other person's individual characteristics rather than their group membership. While Burgess et al. (2017) provide a strong rationale for mindfulness as a strategy to address implicit bias, there is a need for systematic implementation and examination in this area. It should also be noted that in order to maximize mindfulness, it is imperative for individuals to recognize their own implicit bias, any privilege that comes with their social status, and unintentional microaggressions (i.e., "brief and commonplace daily verbal, behavioral, or environmental indignities, whether intentional or unintentional, that communicate negative slights and insults") (Godsil et al., 2014; Sue et al., 2007).

Devine's prejudice habit-breaking framework argues that implicit biases are deeply entrenched habits developed through socialization experiences (Devine et al., 2012). "Breaking the habit" of implicit bias therefore requires learning about the contexts that activate the bias and how to replace the biased responses with responses that reflect one's nonprejudiced goals. Thus, when people who are opposed to prejudice believe they have acted with bias, they will seek out information to help them break this habit of prejudice or bias. That training includes (1) stereotype replacement (recognizing stereotypic responses within oneself and society), (2) counter-stereotypic imaging (imagining examples of outgroup members who counter popularly held stereotypes), (3) individuating (viewing others according to their personal rather than stereotypic characteristics), (4) perspective taking (adopting the perspective of a member of the stigmatized group), and (5) contact (increasing exposure to outgroup members). In an RCT, Devine et al. (2012) showed that participants in an 8-week habit-breaking training showed significant decrease in their explicit bias but also became more acutely aware of discrimination in society. This study was conducted with introductory graduate students who were likely biased in their willingness to participate. There is a need for more rigorous examination of this training approach with educational professionals and those caring for and teaching young children.

Supporting ECE Workforce Well-Being

In addition, even the most competent early childhood educators will not be effective if they are not physically, mentally, and social-emotionally healthy. Educators who have strong social-emotional awareness and skills are more likely to develop close, constructive relationships with children, implement SEL programs effectively, and be more able to create a positive classroom climate. Conversely, educators who are stressed, depressed, or have low social-emotional skills are more likely to be less sensitive and warm toward children and have more conflictual relationships with them. Since children who live in high-stress communities or with adverse conditions benefit the most from warm, enriching interactions with adults, it is critically important for them to be in ECE programs in which the educators are social-emotionally healthy and strong (Becker et al., 2017; IOM and NRC, 2015; Jones and Bouffard, 2012; Roberts et al., 2019; Whitaker et al., 2015). Indeed, McClelland et al. (2017) found that effective social-emotional interventions often include building teachers' own social-emotional skills, as well as children's.

Unfortunately, it has been well documented that compared to other fields, the ECE workforce experiences a high level of stress and depression; one reason is the stress of low compensation and benefits (see IOM and NRC, 2015). Most of them (53 percent) participate in at least one of four public support or health care programs for low-income individuals, compared to 21 percent of the U.S. workforce in general (Whitebook et al., 2018). On average, child care teachers earn less than $11 per hour, or about $22,000 per year—barely over the federal poverty guidelines for a family of three. There is also emerging evidence (Borntrager et al., 2012; Hydon et al., 2015) that when educators work with children who experience trauma and significant adverse experiences, whether in ECE programs or public schools, they can experience "secondary traumatic stress" (STS), or "the natural consequent behaviors and emotions resulting from *knowing* about a traumatizing event experienced by a significant other—the stress resulting from helping or wanting to help a traumatized or suffering person" (Hydon et al., 2015, p. 320).

Which supports or interventions can help educators manage or mitigate their general social-emotional health and their experience of stress, depression, or STS? For early childhood educators, an analysis of the National Survey of Early Care and Education found that "informal workforce supports" that help teachers feel that they are a part of a team and respected as professionals were related to lower stress. Studies of public school teachers by Borntrager et al. (2012) and Caringi et al. (2015) similarly found that working in schools that provided or encouraged peer support was associated with lower STS. In addition, stable classroom assignments were related to lower stress, as was (unsurprisingly) higher pay. Teachers with higher household incomes (more than $45,000 per year) experienced less stress than those earning less (Madill et al., 2018). In another analysis, Roberts et al. (2019) found that early childhood educators who had no health insurance, received high professional demands with few work-related resources, and had multiple jobs were more likely to have depressive symptoms. Interestingly, Madill et al. (2018) found that more formal professional supports, such as small group size and access to professional development or coaching, were not related to early childhood educators' experience of stress.

There is emerging evidence that professional support that is targeted to improve the mental and social-emotional well-being of educators could be helpful. In their small, qualitative study, Caringi et al. (2015) reported that teachers' practice of "self-care" techniques helped them manage their stress. In her small study of educators and caregivers in a residential program for AIDS-affected children and youth, Lucas (2007) found that training on "reframing" and realistic goal setting with children and parents led to a decrease in emotional exhaustion. (Reframing has teachers identify children's and families' strengths and assets rather than their faults, which helps teachers approach problems and obstacles collaboratively with those they serve rather than treating these as issues they need to "fix" on their own.)

Another promising type of intervention is to improve "dispositional mindfulness" (Becker et al., 2017; Hydon et al., 2015). Mindfulness is related to the ability to regulate one's emotions, thoughts, and attention. People who are mindful are more aware of their thoughts, feelings, and reactions to their surroundings and better able to refrain from judgment, which enables them to react more calmly to a given situation and to better understand others' perspectives and behaviors before responding. In one study based on a survey of 1,001 Head Start teachers, those who were more mindful had closer relationships with children and less conflict with them, partly because mindfulness is also associated with fewer depressive symptoms.

> A mindful disposition may help teachers view challenging interactions with more equanimity. Alternatively, mindful teachers may have fewer challenging interactions. Their attention and focus may help them to be proactive in their guidance of young children, structuring the classroom for successful interactions and diffusing potentially difficult situations before they begin. . . . Teachers who are more mindful may be better able

to disengage from depressive or ruminative thoughts, and experience fewer difficult exchanges with children. Additionally, a mindful disposition may help teachers appraise stressors differently, such that children's difficult behavior may not be perceived as a threat. Mindful teachers may be aware of situations that may elicit challenging behavior, and take action to engage in reappraisal to regulate their emotional response. (Becker et al., 2017, p. 48)

One program, called Cultivating Awareness and Resilience in Education (CARE), has demonstrated impact on teachers' mindfulness. CARE provides 30 hours of training in group-based settings and individual sessions with trainers. The program includes "emotion skills instruction, mindfulness practices, and compassion-building activities" (Becker et al., 2017, p. 49). RCTs with elementary teachers showed improvements in their mindfulness and emotional regulation. In one of those studies, researchers also observed improvements in teachers' emotional support for students (Becker et al., 2017).

This study also indicated that for programs of this nature to be viable and sustainable, school leaders' buy-in is necessary. Strong leadership is influential in early childhood educators' professional support systems (IOM and NRC, 2015). While local program administrators and leaders may not be able to improve educators' professional preparation programs, compensation levels, or benefit packages on their own, they are critical to establishing an organization and environment that supports their staff's mental health and minimizes stress—whether through opportunities for them to collaborate or appreciate each other's work, training on topics such as TIC, or self-care interventions, like mindfulness training.

ECE CONCLUSIONS AND RECOMMENDATIONS

Below, the committee provides conclusions and recommendations, based on the information reviewed in this chapter, to ensure adequate resources for ECE programs and educators, support and improve competencies for the ECE workforce, and improve access to ECE for eligible children. The goal of these recommendations is to advance the ECE system to promote health equity during the early childhood period to set the course for good health and well-being into adulthood.

Allocation of Adequate Resources to Support Health-Promoting ECE Programs and Educators

ECE programs, including systems that support and ensure standards for high quality (e.g., QRISs), can be comprehensive platforms for ensuring all children are healthy and prepared for school and life. That can only occur if these programs and systems adopt specific practices and processes that have been shown to have such impacts and set a threshold that ensures all participating programs are sufficiently high quality, as opposed to more general benchmarks related to quality (e.g., teacher education levels, class size, professional development). Furthermore, current funding levels for child care, pre-K, and Head Start generally are not based on systematic estimates of the cost of quality, including those elements that promote better health outcomes. It is also critical to consider the cost of funding programs to ensure that they reach all eligible children. Until that has been remedied, our nation will not maximize the potential of ECE programs to promote the health and school readiness of young children, especially those who tend to fall on the wrong side of the health equity equation (e.g., low-income children and children of color).

For ECE to be part of a system that ensures children are healthy and ready for school and life, these programs need

- Adequate resources to support the "whole child," including cognitive, emotional, social, and physical development, regardless of setting (e.g., home, center, or school). This includes adequately supporting programs' implementation of standards and content that are health promoting (e.g., high-quality nutrition and physical activity) for child, family, and staff outcomes, ensuring children's access to effective early intervention and special education services, and tailoring specific resources and supports for various settings and providers (e.g., home-based providers);
- The ability to implement the recommendation from the National Academies reports *Transforming the Workforce for Children Birth Through Age 8: A Unifying Foundation* (IOM and NRC, 2015) and *Transforming the Financing of Early Care and Education* (NASEM, 2018) addressing the level of compensation and access to basic benefits (such as health care and housing); ensuring work environments and conditions that respect the demands of the ECE profession, including adequate resources and opportunities for teamwork (e.g., planning time, substitutes); offering ongoing training to maintain educators' own emotional well-being; and developing school and program leaders' knowledge and competencies in creating an organizational culture that supports the social-emotional health and well-being of children, families, and educators;
- The capacity (funding, staffing, skill sets) to provide or make referrals (and follow-up) to various agencies or integrated

partnerships with professionals from various sectors or organizations (e.g., home visitors, social workers, health services) that meet the various needs of children and their families;

- An SEL component that has the following characteristics:
  - o Strong training and support (e.g., job-embedded coaching, early childhood mental health consultants) for educators on specific SEL skills;
  - o Curricula intentionally designed to build specific SEL skills through sequenced and active learning experiences;
  - o Promotion of a supportive organizational culture and climate by engaging the involvement of the leaders, paraprofessionals, and other staff of the school or ECE program; and
  - o Supports for the social-emotional health of parents and early childhood professionals and staff, including leaders.
- Educators who are well trained and well supported to develop critical professional competencies and support children's social, emotional, and physical health. Educators need to develop specialized skills that ensure children are healthy and prepared for school. In order for them to use these skills effectively, their own physical, emotional, and mental health needs to be supported; and
- Adequate resources and support to systematically identify factors that support or hinder integration at the federal, state, and local levels, as well as the impact of this effort for children, families, and communities.

Conclusion 7-1: For early care and education programs to contribute significantly to a health promotion and equity strategy, there is a need to intentionally, cohesively, and simultaneously address adequate funding that supports a comprehensive equity-promoting early care and education system, well-compensated and competent workforce, connection to community resources and support, continuous quality improvement, and systematic examination of effectiveness at multiple levels.

Recommendation 7-1: The committee recommends that early care and education (ECE) systems and programs, including home visiting, adopt a comprehensive approach to school readiness. This approach should explicitly incorporate health promotion and health equity as core goals. Implementing this approach would require the following actions:

- **Federal, state, local, tribal, and territorial governments and other public agencies (e.g., school districts, city governments,** public–private partnerships) that have decision-making power over ECE programs should establish program standards and accountability systems, such as a quality rating and improvement system, linked with better school readiness and health outcomes and provide adequate funding and resources to implement and sustain these standards effectively.

- The Office of Child Care and the Office of Head Start at the federal level, along with state, local, tribal, and territorial early care and other education agencies, should assess the full cost of implementing standards that promote health outcomes and equity as described above, including supporting educators' own health and well-being, and work with Congress to align funding levels of the major federal ECE programs—child care subsidy and Head Start—accordingly.
- Health and human service entities, the federal Early Learning Interagency Policy Board, state Early Childhood Advisory Councils, and federal, state, local, tribal, and territorial agencies that oversee home visiting and ECE programs should ensure greater programmatic coordination and policy alignment to ensure effective allocation of resources.
- The Office of Planning, Research & Evaluation in the Administration for Children and Families, along with the U.S. Department of Education, should examine the feasibility and seek resources to conduct (a) an implementation study to examine the design and implementation of this comprehensive ECE approach that incorporates health standards and (b) an outcomes study that examines the impact on children's school readiness and achievement, and health outcomes, with particular attention to eliminating disparities and gaps prior to school entry.

Health-Focused Competencies of the Workforce

The ECE workforce and other professionals are critical in implementing evidence-based practices in ECE settings that support children's well-being, leading to health equity. However, there is a need for systems and supports to strengthen their competencies and skills, as well as stability, in supporting health-promoting and health equity practices.

Conclusion 7-2: Policies and systems that prepare and support early childhood educators and program leaders, including those in public schools, need to incorporate the latest evidence about how to support children's school readiness and success by fostering the health and well-being of children. This would entail providing comprehensive supports and resources to degree granting institutions and preparation programs, including the development of curricula, textbooks, practicum experiences, toolkits, and fact sheets.

Recommendation 7-2: Building off the 2015 Institute of Medicine and the National Research Council report *Transforming the Workforce for Children Birth Through Age 8*, the committee recommends that degree granting institutions, professional preparation programs, and providers of ongoing professional learning opportunities develop or strengthen coursework or practicums that focus on competencies of educators, principals, and early care and education program directors that are critical to children's health, school readiness, and life success.

Specific areas include

- Strengthening professionals' understanding of and capacity to collaborate with professionals from other sectors, such as health and social work (interprofessional learnings);
- Implementing practices and policies based on the understanding of the link between biology and children's learning and development and impact on children's readiness for school and school success;
- Educating professionals about unconscious biases and practices that undermine the learning and social-emotional health of diverse children and their families;
- Training and coaching on effective antibias and culturally responsive practices that strengthen professionals' effectiveness in supporting the learning, social-emotional health, and well-being of diverse children and families (including DLLs); and
- Effectively implementing practices and policies informed by understanding of trauma, adverse childhood experiences, toxic stress, and racism.

Access and Affordability

Children who experience comprehensive high-quality ECE early in life and for multiple years are likely to show stronger cognitive, academic, and social-emotional outcomes over time. Unfortunately, many children who could benefit the most from ECE are less likely, for various reasons, to access these high-quality ECE environments early and for longer periods. To ensure health promotion and health equity in the early years, there is a need to ensure that these programs are available to and affordable for families as early as possible and as long as possible.

Conclusion 7-3: Maximizing the impact of early care and education (ECE) on positive childhood development, health, and well-being at the community or population level will require increasing public funds for ECE programs. Currently, eligibility for ECE programs is limited, and among eligible families, access is low due to lack of funding and availability of programs and services. Therefore, even if existing publicly funded programs have the resources to provide robust supports that improve young children's health and well-being, they will not reach most children, especially those who live in low-income households or experience adverse experiences and toxic stressors.

Recommendation 7-3: Federal, state, local, tribal, and territorial policy makers should work with the U.S. Department of Health and Human Services (HHS), the Office of Head Start, and Office of Child Care to develop and implement a plan to

a. **Improve the quality of early care and education (ECE) programs by adopting the health-promoting standards discussed in Recommendation 7-1, such as building on the performance standards of Early Head Start and Head Start, and**
b. **Within 10 years, expand access to such comprehensive, high-quality, and affordable ECE programs across multiple settings to all eligible children. Disproportionately underserved populations should be prioritized.**

The Secretary of HHS should conduct a process evaluation to inform the expansion effort, and, once implemented, conduct rigorous and comparative outcomes studies to ensure that the expansion is having the intended impacts on children and families, with particular attention on what group(s) may be benefiting.

The strategic plan should be modeled after and build on the relevant performance standards of Early Head Start and Head Start, which emphasize mixed settings, the whole child, family and community engagement, transition between home and school, and continuous quality improvement. It should also strengthen the program components discussed in this chapter that lead to stronger school readiness and health outcomes, including mitigating the impact of adverse experiences and toxic stress for children, families, teachers, and staff. Critical components include a comprehensive social-emotional strategy that encompasses both the classroom (curriculum, teacher training, and support) and program or school (leadership, culture, and climate) levels and educators who have the competencies described in Recommendation 7-2. The plan should identify strategies to bolster capacity and resources of new and existing programs to implement these more ambitious standards, including by incentivizing collaboration among Head Start, pre-K, and child care programs. Implementation of this plan will likely require funding from Congress.

A national evaluation led by the Office of Head Start, Office of Child Care, Office of the Assistant Secretary for Planning and Evaluation, and Office of Planning, Research & Evaluation in the Administration for Children and Families is needed to examine and inform the design, implementation, and effect of this expanded access and strengthening of Early Head Start and Head Start to enhance children's school readiness and achievement and health outcomes.

Heeding the findings from the Head Start Impact Study that program implementation and workforce challenges vary widely from site to site, which leads to variable outcomes (Phillips et al., 2017), the improvement and scale-up strategy described in this recommendation should include mechanisms that help new providers incorporate program features and conditions that are associated with stronger outcomes. For example, an evaluation can provide rapid-cycle feedback (see Chapter 8 for more) to ensure faithful implementation of the "upgraded" program model and fidelity and to inform ongoing midcourse corrections as needed to reach targeted health outcomes. This study will help to identify factors that supported or hindered expansion and access at the federal, state, and local levels, as well as the impact of this effort for children, families, and communities.

State policy makers (e.g., governors, legislators, agency leaders, pre-K administrators) should also consider how pre-K funding and policies can support the program and workforce characteristics discussed in this chapter that are associated with health outcomes. State pre-K programs are highly variable, and some will be better positioned to serve as a platform for promoting health equity than others. In the final analysis, the committee believes that among the major publicly funded ECE programs, Head Start's history, program design, quality standards, targeted populations, and evidence base make a useful platform from which to build expanded access to comprehensive high-quality ECE programs. Health promotion (including social-emotional health) and family engagement are already important goals of the program that can be strengthened based on evidence from this report. The program's historical focus on children furthest from opportunity can help address inequities among different racial and income groups. With an intentional effort to bolster its health-promoting strategies, provide adequate resources for educators and leaders to implement them effectively, and expand access to all eligible children, Head Start can be a critical element of our nation's cross-sector approach to improving child health and reducing inequities.

CONCLUSION

The ECE system is a critical setting to provide young children with a strong foundation for skill building and positive learning, as well as shaping social-emotional, cognitive, and physical health. This chapter delves into the evidence on ECE programs and childhood outcomes with respect to the many different service settings (e.g., home-, school-, and center-based care). In addition, the committee highlights salient issues and populations related to health equity throughout the chapter, such as early intervention for children with developmental disabilities, DLLs, and implicit bias training for educators. Based on its review of the evidence and committee expertise, the committee applies the evidence to provide recommendations in the areas of allocating adequate resources to support ECE programs and educators, supporting and training the workforce, and improving access to quality ECE for eligible children. By targeting these key areas that are instrumental to an effective and equitable system, the committee identifies a comprehensive approach to leveraging and enhancing the current ECE system to promote health equity. The following chapter integrates the crosscutting themes from the report and applies them to inform a systems approach to promote equitable prenatal and childhood development.

REFERENCES

Advocacy Institute. 2019. *National Assessment of Educational Progress (NAEP)*. http://www.advocacyinstitute.org/NAEP/NationPerformance2013-15-17.shtml (accessed April 2, 2019).

Allen, J. 2010. Improving cross-cultural care and antiracism in nursing education: A literature review. *Nurse Education Today* 30(4):314–320.

Ansari, A., and A. Winsler. 2012. School readiness among low-income, Latino children attending family childcare versus centre-based care. *Early Child Development and Care* 182(11):1465–1485.

APA (American Psychiatric Association). 2013. *Diagnostic and statistical manual*, 5th ed. Washington, DC: American Psychiatric Association.

Barnett, W. S. 2013. *Getting the facts right on pre-K and the president's pre-K proposal*. New Brunswick, NJ: National Institute for Early Education Research.

Barnett, W. S., and A. H. Friedman-Krauss. 2016. *State(s) of Head Start*. New Brunswick, NJ: National Institute for Early Education Research.

Bartlett, J. D., S. Smith, and E. Bringewatt. 2017. *Helping young children who have experienced trauma: Policies and strategies for early care and education.* Publication #2017-19. Bethesda, MD: Child Trends.

Becker, B. D., K. C. Gallagher, and R. C. Whitaker. 2017. Teachers' dispositional mindfulness and the quality of their relationships with children in Head Start classrooms. *Journal of School Psychology* 65:40–53.

Belfield, C. R., and I. R. Kelly. 2013. Early education and health outcomes of a 2001 U.S. birth cohort. *Economics & Human Biology* 11(3):310–325.

Belsky, J., D. L. Vandell, M. Burchinal, K. A. Clarke-Stewart, K. McCartney, and M. T. Owen. 2007. Are there long-term effects of early child care? *Child Development* 78(2):681–701.

Betancourt, J. R., A. R. Green, J. E. Carrillo, and O. Ananeh-Firempong, 2nd. 2003. Defining cultural competence: A practical framework for addressing racial/ethnic disparities in health and health care. *Public Health Reports* 118(4):293–302.

Biag, M., and S. Castrechini. 2016. Coordinated strategies to help the whole child: Examining the contributions of full-service community schools. *Journal of Education for Students Placed at Risk* 21(3):157–173.

Bierman, K. L., R. L. Nix, M. T. Greenberg, C. Blair, and C. E. Domitrovich. 2008. Executive functions and school readiness intervention: Impact, moderation, and mediation in the Head Start REDI program. *Development and Psychopathology* 20(3):821–843.

Bierman, K. L., R. L. Nix, B. S. Heinrichs, C. E. Domitrovich, S. D. Gest, J. A. Welsh, and S. Gill. 2014. Effects of Head Start REDI on children's outcomes 1 year later in different kindergarten contexts. *Child Development* 85(1):140–159.

Blackorby, J., and M. Wagner. 1996. Longitudinal postschool outcomes of youth with disabilities: Findings from the National Longitudinal Transition Study. *Exceptional Children* 62(5):399–413.

Blair, C., and C. C. Raver. 2014. Closing the achievement gap through modification of neurocognitive and neuroendocrine function: Results from a cluster randomized controlled trial of an innovative approach to the education of children in kindergarten. *PLoS ONE* 9(11):e112393.

Blank, M. J., A. Melaville, and B. P. Shah. 2003. *Making the difference: Research and practice in community schools.* Washington, DC: The Coalition for Community Schools.

Borntrager, C., J. C. Caringi, R. van den Pol, L. Crosby, K. O'Connell, A. Trautman, and M. McDonald. 2012. Secondary traumatic stress in school personnel. *Advances in School Mental Health Promotion* 5(1):38–50.

Bowlby, J. 2008. *A secure base: Parent-child attachment and healthy human development.* New York: Basic Books.

Boyd, B. A., I. U. Iruka, and N. P. Pierce. 2018. Strengthening service access for children of color with autism spectrum disorders: A proposed conceptual framework. *International Review of Research in Developmental Disabilities* 54:1–33.

Boysen, G. A. 2010. Integrating implicit bias into counselor education. *Counselor Education and Supervision* 49(4):210–227.

Bradley, R. H., and D. L. Vandell. 2007. Child care and the well-being of children. *Archives of Pediatrics and Adolescent Medicine* 161(7):669–676.

Brooks-Gunn, J., L. J. Berlin, and A. S. Fuligni. 2000. Early childhood intervention programs: What about the family? In *Handbook of early childhood intervention,* 2nd ed., edited by J. P. Shonkoff and S. J. Meisels. New York: Cambridge University Press. Pp. 549–588.

Brotman, L. M., E. Calzada, K. Y. Huang, S. Kingston, S. Dawson-McClure, D. Kamboukos, A. Rosenfelt, A. Schwab, and E. Petkova. 2011. Promoting effective parenting practices and preventing child behavior problems in school among ethnically diverse families from underserved, urban communities. *Child Development* 82(1):258–276.

Brotman, L. M., S. Dawson-McClure, K. Y. Huang, R. Theise, D. Kamboukos, J. Wang, E. Petkova, and G. Ogedegbe. 2012. Early childhood family intervention and long-term obesity prevention among high-risk minority youth. *Pediatrics* 129(3):e621–e628.

Brotman, L. M., S. Dawson-McClure, E. J. Calzada, K. Y. Huang, D. Kamboukos, J. J. Palamar, and E. Petkova. 2013. Cluster (school) RCT of ParentCorps: Impact on kindergarten academic achievement. *Pediatrics* 131(5):e1521–e1529.

Brotman, L. M., S. Dawson-McClure, D. Kamboukos, K. Y. Huang, E. J. Calzada, K. Goldfeld, and E. Petkova. 2016. Effects of ParentCorps in prekindergarten on child mental health and academic performance: Follow-up of a randomized clinical trial through 8 years of age. *JAMA Pediatrics* 170(12):1149–1155.

Bruder, M. B. 2010. Early childhood intervention. *Exceptional Children* 76(3):339–355.

Bryson, S. A., E. Gauvin, A. Jamieson, M. Rathgeber, L. Faulkner-Gibson, S. Bell, J. Davidson, J. Russel, and S. Burke. 2017. What are effective strategies for implementing trauma-informed care in youth inpatient psychiatric and residential treatment settings? A realist systematic review. *International Journal of Mental Health Systems* 11:36.

Burchinal, M., K. Magnuson, D. Powell, and S. S. Hong. 2015. Early childcare and education. In *Handbook of child psychology and developmental science: Ecological settings and processes*, Vol. 4, edited by M. H. Bornstein, T. Leventhal, and R. M. Lerner. Hoboken, NJ: John Wiley & Sons. Pp. 223–267.

Burgess, D. J., M. C. Beach, and S. Saha. 2017. Mindfulness practice: A promising approach to reducing the effects of clinician implicit bias on patients. *Patient Education and Counseling* 100(2):372–376.

Campbell, F. A., E. P. Pungello, M. Burchinal, K. Kainz, Y. Pan, B. H. Wasik, O. A. Barbarin, J. J. Sparling, and C. T. Ramey. 2012. Adult outcomes as a function of an early childhood educational program: An Abecedarian Project follow-up. *Developmental Psychology* 48(4):1033–1043.

Campbell, F., G. Conti, J. J. Heckman, S. H. Moon, R. Pinto, E. Pungello, and Y. Pan. 2014. Early childhood investments substantially boost adult health. *Science* 343(6178):1478–1485.

Cannon, J. S., M. R. Kilburn, L. A. Karoly, T. Mattox, A. N. Muchow, and M. Buenaventura. 2017. *Investing early: Taking stock of outcomes and economic returns from early childhood programs.* Santa Monica, CA: RAND Corporation.

Caringi, J. C., C. Stanick, A. Trautman, L. Crosby, M. Devlin, and S. Adams. 2015. Secondary traumatic stress in public school teachers: contributing and mitigating factors. *Advances in School Mental Health Promotion* 8(4):244–256.

Carney, R., B. Stratford, K. A. Moore, A. Rojas, and P. Daneri. 2015. *What works for reducing problem behaviors in early childhood: Lessons from experimental evaluations.* Bethesda, MD: Child Trends.

CASEL (Collaborative for Academic, Social, and Emotional Learning). n.d. *What is SEL?* https://casel.org/what-is-sel (accessed April 2, 2019).

Castro, D. C., E. E. García, and A. M. Markos. 2013. *Dual language learners: Research informing policy.* Chapel Hill, NC: The University of North Carolina, Frank Porter Graham Child Development Institute, Center for Early Care and Education—Dual Language Learners.

CBITS (Cognitive Behavioral Intervention for Trauma in Schools). n.d.-a. *Home.* http://cbitsprogram.org (accessed July 15, 2019).

CBITS. n.d.-b. *Cognitive behavioral intervention for trauma in schools: Success stories.* http://cbitsprogram.org/success-stories (accessed June 11, 2019).

CBO (Congressional Budget Office). 2015. *Child nutrition programs: Spending and policy options.* Washington, DC: Congressional Budget Office.

CDC (Centers for Disease Control and Prevention). 2014. Prevalence of autism spectrum disorder among children aged 8 years—Autism and Developmental Disabilities Monitoring Network, 11 sites, United States, 2010. *Morbidity and Mortality Weekly Report Surveillance Summaries* 63(2):1–21.

Center on the Developing Child at Harvard University. n.d. *Executive function & self-regulation.* https://developingchild.harvard.edu/science/key-concepts/executive-function (accessed April 2, 2019).

Chase-Lansdale, P. L., and J. Brooks-Gunn. 2014. Two-generation programs in the twenty-first century. *The Future of Children* 24(1):13–39.

Child Trends. 2012. *HighScope Perry Preschool.* https://highscope.org/perry-preschool-project (accessed July 9, 2019).

Child Welfare Committee, National Child Traumatic Stress Network. 2013. *Child welfare trauma training toolkit: Comprehensive guide*, 3rd ed. Los Angeles, CA, and Durham, NC: National Center for Child Traumatic Stress.

Chung-Park, M. S. 2012. Knowledge, opinions, and practices of infant sleep position among parents. *Military Medicine* 177(2):235–239.

Conti, G., J. Heckman, and S. Urzua. 2010. The education-health gradient. *American Economic Review* 100(2):234–238.

Cook, T. D., F.-N. Habib, M. Phillips, R. A. Settersten, S. C. Shagle, and S. M. Degirmencioglu. 1999. Comer's School Development Program in Prince George's County, Maryland: A theory-based evaluation. *American Educational Research Journal* 36(3):543–597.

Corcoran, L., K. Steinley, and S. Grady. 2019. *Early childhood program participation, results from the National Household Education Surveys Program of 2016.* Washington, DC: U.S. Department of Education, National Center for Education Statistics, Institute of Education Sciences.

Cross, T., B. Bazron, K. Dennis, and M. Isaacs. 1989. *Towards a culturally competent system of care: A monograph on effective services for minority children who are severely emotionally disturbed.* Washington, DC: Georgetown University Child Development Center.

Cuccaro, M. L., J. Brinkley, R. K. Abramson, A. Hall, H. H. Wright, J. P. Hussman, J. R. Gilbert, and M. A. Pericak-Vance. 2007. Autism in African American families: Clinical-phenotypic findings. *American Journal of Medical Genetics, Part B: Neuropsychiatric Genetics* 144b(8):1022–1026.

Dawson-McClure, S., E. Calzada, K. Y. Huang, D. Kamboukos, D. Rhule, B. Kolawole, E. Petkova, and L. M. Brotman. 2015. A population-level approach to promoting health child development and school success in low-income, urban neighborhoods: Impact on parenting and child conduct problems. *Prevention Science* 16(2):279–290.

Delgado, C. E. F., and K. G. Scott. 2006. Comparison of referral rates for preschool children at risk for disabilities using information obtained from birth certificate records. *The Journal of Special Education* 40(1):28–35.

Devine, P. G., P. S. Forscher, A. J. Austin, and W. T. Cox. 2012. Long-term reduction in implicit race bias: A prejudice habit-breaking intervention. *Journal of Experimental Social Psychology* 48(6):1267–1278.

Diamond, A., W. S. Barnett, J. Thomas, and S. Munro. 2007. Preschool program improves cognitive control. *Science* 318(5855):1387–1388.

D'Onise, K., J. W. Lynch, M. G. Sawyer, and R. A. McDermott. 2010. Can preschool improve child health outcomes? A systematic review. *Social Science & Medicine* 70(9):1423–1440.

Duncan, G. J., and K. Magnuson. 2013. Investing in preschool programs. *Journal of Economic Perspectives* 27(2):109–132.

Dunifon, R., and L. Kowaleski-Jones. 2003. The influences of participation in the National School Lunch Program and food insecurity on child well-being. *Social Service Review* 77(1):72–92.

Duran, F., K. Hepburn, M. Irvine, R. Kaufmann, B. Anthony, N. Horen, and D. Perry. 2009. *What works?: A study of effective early childhood mental health consultation programs.* Washington, DC: Georgetown University Center for Child and Human Development.

Durlak, J. A., and R. P. Weissberg. 2013. Afterschool programs that follow evidence-based practices to promote social and emotional development are effective. In *Expanding minds and opportunities: Leveraging the power of afterschool and summer learning for student success, section 3: Recent evidence of impact*, edited by T. K. Peterson. Washington, DC: Collaborative Communications Group. Pp. 24–28.

Durlak, J. A., R. P. Weissberg, A. B. Dymnicki, R. D. Taylor, and K. B. Schellinger. 2011. The impact of enhancing students' social and emotional learning: A meta-analysis of school-based universal interventions. *Child Development* 82(1):405–432.

ED (U.S. Department of Education). 2010. *21st Century Community Learning Centers (21st CCLC) analytic support for evaluation and program monitoring: An overview of the 21st CCLC performance data: 2008–09 (sixth report)*. Washington, DC: U.S. Department of Education.

ED. 2018. *40th annual report to Congress on the implementation of the Individuals with Disabilities Education Act, 2018*. Washington, DC: U.S. Department of Education, Office of Special Education and Rehabilitative Services, Office of Special Education Programs.

ED OCR (Office for Civil Rights). 2016. *2013-2014 Civil Rights Data Collection: A first look. Key data highlights on equity and opportunity gaps in our nation's public schools*. Washington, DC: U.S. Department of Education, Office for Civil Rights.

Fantuzzo, J., V. Gadsden, F. Li, F. Sproul, P. McDermott, D. Hightower, and A. Minney. 2013. Multiple dimensions of family engagement in early childhood education: Evidence for a short form of the Family Involvement Questionnaire. *Early Childhood Research Quarterly* 28(4):734–742.

Farran, D. C., S. J. Wilson, D. Meador, J. Norvell, and K. Nesbitt. 2015. *Experimental evaluation of the Tools of the Mind pre-K curriculum: Technical report. (Working paper)*. Nashville, TN: Peabody Research Institute, Vanderbilt University.

Fisher, B., A. Hanson, and T. Raden. 2014. *Start early to build a healthy future: The research linking early learning and health*. Chicago, IL: Ounce of Prevention Fund.

Forry, N., I. U. Iruka, K. Tout, J. Torquati, A. Susman-Stillman, D. Bryant, and M. P. Daneri. 2013. Predictors of quality and child outcomes in family child care settings. *Early Childhood Research Quarterly* 28(4):893–904.

Fountain, C., A. S. Winter, and P. S. Bearman. 2012. Six developmental trajectories characterize children with autism. *Pediatrics* 129(5):e1112–e1120.

Frank Porter Graham Child Development Institute. 2012. *The Abecedarian Project: High-quality early child care has long-lasting effects*. FPG Snapshot #66. https://fpg.unc.edu/sites/fpg.unc.edu/files/resources/snapshots/FPG_Snapshot66_2012.pdf (accessed July 9, 2019).

Frisvold, D. E. 2015. Nutrition and cognitive achievement: An evaluation of the School Breakfast Program. *Journal of Public Economics* 124:91–104.

Frisvold, D. E., and J. C. Lumeng. 2011. Expanding exposure: Can increasing the daily duration of Head Start reduce childhood obesity? *Journal of Human Resources* 46(2):373–402.

Gabor, V., and K. Mantinan. 2012. *State efforts to address obesity prevention in child care quality rating and improvement systems*. Ann Arbor, MI: Altarum Institute.

Galindo, C., S. Sonnenschein, and A. Montoya-Ávila. 2019. Latina mothers' engagement in children's math learning in the early school years: Conceptions of math and socialization practices. *Early Childhood Research Quarterly* 47:271–283.

Gallagher, R. W., and J. R. Polanin. 2015. A meta-analysis of educational interventions designed to enhance cultural competence in professional nurses and nursing students. *Nurse Education Today* 35(2):333–340.

GAO (U.S. Government Accountability Office). 2018. *K–12 education: Discipline disparities for black students, boys, and students with disabilities*. Washington, DC: U.S. Government Accountability Office.

García, E. 2015. *Inequalities at the starting gate: Cognitive and noncognitive skills gaps between 2010–2011 kindergarten classmates*. Washington, DC: Economic Policy Institute.

Gilliam, W. S., A. N. Maupin, and C. R. Reyes. 2016a. Early childhood mental health consultation: Results of a statewide random-controlled evaluation. *Journal of the American Academy of Child and Adolescent Psychiatry* 55(9):754–761.

Gilliam, W. S., A. N. Maupin, C. R. Reyes, M. Accavitti, and F. Shic. 2016b. *Do early educators' implicit biases regarding sex and race relate to behavior expectations and recommendations of preschool expulsions and suspensions? A research study brief.* New Haven, CT: Yale University Child Study Center.

Gleason, P. M., and A. H. Dodd. 2009. School breakfast program but not school lunch program participation is associated with lower body mass index. *Journal of the American Dietetic Association* 109(Suppl 2):S118–S128.

Godsil, R. D., L. R. Tropp, P. A. Goff, and J. A. Powell. 2014. *Addressing implicit bias, racial anxiety, and stereotype threat in education and health care.* Perception Institute.

Goff, P. A., M. C. Jackson, B. A. Di Leone, C. M. Culotta, and N. A. DiTomasso. 2014. The essence of innocence: Consequences of dehumanizing black children. *Journal of Personality and Social Psychology* 106(4):526–545.

Gomby, D. S., M. B. Larner, C. S. Stevenson, E. M. Lewit, and R. E. Behrman. 1995. Long-term outcomes of early childhood programs: Analysis and recommendations. *The Future of Children* 5(3):6–24.

Gordon, R. A., A. Colaner, M. L. Usdansky, and C. Melgar. 2013. Beyond an "either-or" approach to home- and center-based child care: Comparing children and families who combine care types with those who just use one. *Early Childhood Research Quarterly* 28(4):918–935.

Granger, R. C., and R. Cytron. 1999. Teenage parent programs a synthesis of the long-term effects of the new chance demonstration, Ohio's learning, earning, and parenting program, and the teenage parent demonstration. *Evaluation Review* 23(2):107–145.

Gundersen, C. 2015. Food assistance programs and child health. *The Future of Children* 25(1):91–109.

Gundersen, C., and J. P. Ziliak. 2014. *Childhood food insecurity in the U.S.: Trends, causes, and policy options.* Princeton, NJ: The Future of Children.

Gundersen, C., B. Kreider, and J. Pepper. 2012. The impact of the National School Lunch Program on child health: A nonparametric bounds analysis. *Journal of Econometrics* 166(1):79–91.

Guralnick, M. J. 1998. Effectiveness of early intervention for vulnerable children: A developmental perspective. *American Journal on Mental Retardation* 102(4):319–345.

Guralnick, M. J. 2005. Early intervention for children with intellectual disabilities: Current knowledge and future prospects. *Journal of Applied Research in Intellectual Disabilities* 18:313–324.

Hahn, R. A., W. S. Barnett, J. A. Knopf, B. I. Truman, R. L. Johnson, J. E. Fielding, C. Muntaner, C. P. Jones, M. T. Fullilove, and P. C. Hunt. 2016. Early childhood education to promote health equity: A community guide systematic review. *Journal of Public Health Management and Practice* 22(5):e1–e8.

Hajizadeh, N., E. R. Stevens, M. Applegate, K. Y. Huang, D. Kamboukos, R. S. Braithwaite, and L. M. Brotman. 2017. Potential return on investment of a family-centered early childhood intervention: A cost-effectiveness analysis. *BMC Public Health* 17(1):796.

Hawkinson, L. E., A. S. Griffen, N. Dong, and R. A. Maynard. 2013. The relationship between child care subsidies and children's cognitive development. *Early Childhood Research Quarterly* 28(2):388–404.

Haynes, N. M., and J. P. Comer. 1990a. Helping black children succeed: The significance of some social factors. In *Going to school: The African American experience,* edited by K. Lomotey. Albany, NY: State University of New York Press.

Haynes, N. M., and J. P. Comer. 1990b. The effects of a school development program on self-concept. *The Yale Journal of Biology and Medicine* 63(4):275–283.

Haynes, N. M., C. L. Emmons, and D. W. Woodruff. 1998. School Development Program effects: Linking implementation to outcomes. *Journal of Education for Students Placed at Risk* 3(1):71–85.

Heckman, J. J., and G. Karapakula. 2019a. *Intergenerational and intragenerational externalities of the Perry Preschool Project*. Working Paper 2019-033. Chicago, IL: Human Capital and Economic Opportunity Global Working Group, University of Chicago.

Heckman, J. J., and G. Karapakula. 2019b. *The Perry Preschoolers at late midlife: A study in design-specific inference*. NBER Working paper no. 25888. Cambridge, MA: National Bureau of Economic Research.

Herbst, C. M., and E. Tekin. 2011. Child care subsidies and childhood obesity. *Review of Economics of the Household* 9(3):349–378.

HHS (U.S. Department of Health and Human Services). 2017. *Head Start program facts: Fiscal year 2017*. https://eclkc.ohs.acf.hhs.gov/about-us/article/head-start-program-facts-fiscal-year-2017 (accessed April 18, 2019).

HHS. 2018. *Family well-being: Strategies to support family safety, health, and financial stability*. Washington, DC: U.S. Department of Health and Human Services, Administration for Children and Families, Office of Head Start, Office of Child Care; National Center on Parent, Family and Community Engagement.

Hocutt, A. M. 1996. Effectiveness of special education: Is placement the critical factor? *The Future of Children* 6(1):77–102.

Hodas, G. R. 2006. *Responding to childhood trauma: The promise and practice of trauma informed care*. Pennsylvania Office of Mental Health and Substance Abuse Services. http://www.childrescuebill.org/VictimsOfAbuse/RespondingHodas.pdf (accessed July 11, 2019).

Hofferth, S. L., and S. Curtin. 2005. Poverty, food programs, and childhood obesity. *Journal of Policy Analysis and Management* 24(4):703–726.

Holliday, M. R., A. Cimetta, C. Cutshaw, D. Yaden, and R. Marx. 2014. Protective factors for school readiness among children in poverty. *Journal of Education for Students Placed at Risk* 19:125–147.

Hong, K., K. Dragan, and S. Glied. 2017. *Seeing and hearing: The impacts of New York City's universal prekindergarten program on the health of low-income children*. Working Paper 23297. Cambridge, MA: National Bureau of Economic Research.

Horowitz, S. H., J. Rawe, and M. C. Whittaker. 2017. *The state of learning disabilities: Understanding the 1 in 5*. New York: National Center for Learning Disabilities.

Hydon, S., M. Wong, A. K. Langley, B. D. Stein, and S. H. Kataoka. 2015. Preventing secondary traumatic stress in educators. *Child and Adolescent Psychiatric Clinics of North America* 24(2):319–333.

IOM and NRC (Institute of Medicine and National Research Council). 2015. *Transforming the workforce for children birth through age 8: A unifying approach*. Washington, DC: The National Academies Press.

Iruka, I., and N. D. Forry. 2018. Links between patterns of quality in diverse settings and children's early outcomes. *Journal of Education* 198(1):95–112.

Jones, D. E., M. Greenberg, and M. Crowley. 2015. Early social-emotional functioning and public health: The relationship between kindergarten social competence and future wellness. *American Journal of Public Health* 105(11):2283–2290.

Jones, S. M., and S. M. Bouffard. 2012. Social and emotional learning in schools: From programs to strategies. *Social Policy Report* 26(4):1–33.

Kay, N., and A. Pennucci. 2014. *Early childhood education for low-income students: A review of the evidence and benefit-cost analysis*. Doc. No. 14-01-2201. Olympia, WA: Washington State Institute for Public Policy.

Knoche, L. L., S. M. Sheridan, B. L. Clarke, C. P. Edwards, C. A. Marvin, K. D. Cline, and K. A. Kupzyk. 2012. Getting Ready: Results of a randomized trial of a relationship-focused intervention on the parent–infant relationship in rural Early Head Start. *Infant Mental Health Journal* 33(5):439–458.

Landa, R. J. 2018. Efficacy of early interventions for infants and young children with, and at risk for, autism spectrum disorders. *International Review of Psychiatry* 30(1):25–39.

Lane, K. L., J. H. Wehby, M. A. Little, and C. Cooley. 2005. Students educated in self-contained classrooms and self-contained schools: Part II—how do they progress over time? *Behavioral Disorders* 30(4):363–374.

Lee, R., F. Zhai, W. Han, J. Brooks-Gunn, and J. Waldfogel. 2013. Head Start and children's nutrition, weight, and health care receipt. *Early Child Development and Care* 28(4):723–733.

Leininger, M., and M. McFarland. 2002. *Transcultural Nursing Concepts, Theories, Research and Practice*, 3rd ed. New York: McGraw-Hill.

Lipsey, M. W., D. C. Farran, and K. Durkin. 2018. Effects of the Tennessee Prekindergarten Program on children's achievement and behavior through third grade. *Early Childhood Research Quarterly* 45:155–176.

Litt, J. S., M. M. Glymour, P. Hauser-Cram, T. Hehir, and M. C. McCormick. 2018. Early intervention services improve school-age functional outcome among neonatal intensive care unit graduates. *Academic Pediatrics* 18(4):468–474.

Loeb, S., M. Bridges, D. Bassok, B. Fuller, and R. W. Rumberger. 2007. How much is too much? The influence of preschool centers on children's social and cognitive development. *Economics of Education Review* 26(1):52–66.

Lucas, L. 2007. The pain of attachment—"You have to put a little wedge in there": How vicarious trauma affects child/teacher attachment. *Childhood Education* 84(2):85–91.

Lunenburg, F. C. 2011. The Comer School Development Program: Improving education for low-income students. *National Forum of Multicultural Issues Journal* 8(1):1–14.

Madill, R., T. Halle, T. Gebhart, and E. Shuey. 2018. *Supporting the psychological well-being of the early care and education workforce: Findings from the National Survey of Early Care and Education*. OPRE Report 2018-49. Washington, DC: U.S. Department of Health and Human Services, Administration for Children and Families, Office of Planning, Research & Evaluation.

Magnuson, K. A., C. Ruhm, and J. Waldfogel. 2007. Does prekindergarten improve school preparation and performance? *Economics of Education Review* 26(1):33–51.

Maina, I. W., T. D. Belton, S. Ginzberg, A. Singh, and T. J. Johnson. 2018. A decade of studying implicit racial/ethnic bias in healthcare providers using the implicit association test. *Social Science & Medicine* 199:219–229.

Malik, R. 2017. New data reveals 250 preschoolers are suspended or expelled every day. *Center for American Progress*. https://www.americanprogress.org/issues/early-childhood/news/2017/11/06/442280/new-data-reveal-250-preschoolers-suspended-expelled-every-day (accessed June 14, 2019).

Matthews, H., R. Ullrich, and W. Cervantes. 2018. *Immigration policy's harmful impacts on early care and education*. Washington, DC: Center for Law and Social Policy.

McClelland, M. M., S. L. Tominey, S. A. Schmitt, and R. Duncan. 2017. SEL interventions in early childhood. *The Future of Children* 21(1):33–47.

McManus, B. M., A. C. Carle, and J. Poehlmann. 2012. Effectiveness of Part C early intervention physical, occupational, and speech therapy services for preterm or low birth weight infants in Wisconsin, United States. *Academic Pediatrics* 12(2):96–103.

Meek, S. E., and W. S. Gilliam. 2016. Expulsion and suspension in early education as matters of social justice and health equity. *NAM Perspectives*. Discussion Paper, National Academy of Medicine, Washington, DC. doi: 10.31478/201610e.

Mendez, J. L. 2010. How can parents get involved in preschool? Barriers and engagement in education by ethnic minority parents of children attending Head Start. *Cultural Diversity and Ethnic Minority Psychology* 16(1):26–36.

Michalopoulos, C., S. S. Crowne, X. A. Portilla, H. Lee, J. H. Filene, A. Duggan, and V. Knox. 2019. *A summary of the results from the MIHOPE and MIHOPE—Strong Start studies of evidence-based home visiting.* OPRE Report 2019-09. Washington, DC: U.S. Department of Health and Human Services, Administration for Children and Families, Office of Planning, Research & Evaluation.

Moffitt, T. E., L. Arseneault, D. Belsky, N. Dickson, R. J. Hancox, H. Harrington, R. Houts, R. Poulton, B. W. Roberts, S. Ross, M. R. Sears, W. M. Thomson, and A. Caspi. 2011. A gradient of childhood self-control predicts health, wealth, and public safety. *Proceedings of the National Academy of Sciences of the United States of America* 108(7):2693–2698.

Morgan, P. L., M. Frisco, G. Farkas, and J. Hibel. 2010. A propensity score matching analysis of the effects of special education services. *The Journal of Special Education* 43(4):236–254.

Morgan, P. L., G. Farkas, M. M. Hillemeier, R. Mattison, S. Maczuga, H. Li, and M. Cook. 2015. Minorities are disproportionately underrepresented in special education: Longitudinal evidence across five disability conditions. *Educational Research* 44(5):278–292.

Morris, P., S. K. Mattera, N. Castells, M. Bangser, K. Bierman, and C. Raver. 2014. *Impact findings from the Head Start CARES demonstration: National evaluation of three approaches to improving preschoolers' social and emotional competence.* OPRE Report 2014-44. Washington, DC: U.S. Department of Health and Human Services, Administration for Children and Families, Office of Planning, Research & Evaluation.

Muennig, P., D. Robertson, G. Johnson, F. Campbell, E. P. Pungello, and M. Neidell. 2011. The effect of an early education program on adult health: The Carolina Abecedarian Project randomized controlled trial. *American Journal of Public Health* 101(3):512–516.

NASEM. 2016a. *Parenting matters: Supporting parents of children ages 0–8.* Washington, DC: The National Academies Press.

NASEM. 2016b. *Preventing bullying through science, policy, and practice.* Washington, DC: The National Academies Press.

NASEM. 2017a. *Communities in action: Pathways to health equity.* Washington, DC: The National Academies Press.

NASEM. 2017b. *Promoting the educational success of children and youth learning English: Promising futures.* Washington, DC: The National Academies Press.

NASEM. 2018. *Transforming the financing of early care and education.* Washington, DC: The National Academies Press.

NASEM. 2019. *The promise of adolescence: Realizing opportunity for all youth.* Washington, DC: The National Academies Press.

National Education Association. n.d. *Discipline and the school-to-prison pipeline (2016).* https://ra.nea.org/business-item/2016-pol-e01-2 (accessed June 14, 2019).

National Survey of Early Care and Education Project Team. 2016. *Characteristics of home-based early care and education providers: Initial findings from the National Survey of Early Care and Education.* OPRE Report 2016-13. Washington, DC: U.S. Department of Health and Human Services, Administration for Children and Families, Office of Planning, Research & Evaluation.

New, R. S., and M. Cochran. 2007. *Early childhood education (four volumes): An international encyclopedia,* Vol. 1–4. Westport, CT: Praeger Publishers. http://www.encyclopedias.biz/dw/Encyclopedia%20of%20Early%20Childhood%20Education.pdf (accessed July 10, 2019).

Noltemeyer, A. L., R. M. Ward, and C. McLoughlin. 2015. Relationship between school suspension and student outcomes: A meta-analysis. *School Psychology Review* 44(2):224–240.

Northside Achievement Zone. 2019. *NAZ results summary: An innovative approach that is working.* Minneapolis, MN: Northside Achievement Zone.

Northside Achievement Zone. n.d. *What is NAZ?* https://northsideachievement.org/who-we-are (accessed April 2, 2019).

NYU (New York University) School of Medicine. 2019. *ParentCorps Langone Health.* https://med.nyu.edu/departments-institutes/population-health/divisions-sections-centers/health-behavior/center-early-childhood-health-development/parentcorps (accessed July 11, 2019).

Oswald, D. P., M. J. Goutinho, A. M. Best, and N. Singh. 1999. Ethnic representation in special education: The influence of school-related economic and demographic variables. *The Journal of Special Education* 32(4):194–206.

Pears, K. C., P. A. Fisher, and K. D. Bronz. 2007. An intervention to promote social emotional school readiness in foster children: Preliminary outcomes from a pilot study. *School Psychology Review* 36(4):665–673.

Pears, K. C., H. K. Kim, and P. A. Fisher. 2012. Effects of a school readiness intervention for children in foster care on oppositional and aggressive behaviors in kindergarten. *Children and Youth Services Review* 34(12):2361–2366.

Pears, K. C., P. A. Fisher, H. K. Kim, J. Bruce, C. V. Healey, and K. Yoerger. 2013. Immediate effects of a school readiness intervention for children in foster care. *Early Education and Development* 24(6):771–791.

Pears, K. C., C. V. Healey, P. A. Fisher, D. Braun, C. Gill, H. M. Conte, J. Newman, and S. Ticer. 2014. Immediate effects of a program to promote school readiness in low-income children: Results of a pilot study. *Education and Treatment of Children* 37(3):431–460.

Peters-Scheffer, N., R. Didden, H. Korzilius, and P. Sturmey. 2011. A meta-analytic study on the effectiveness of comprehensive ABA-based early intervention programs for children with autism spectrum disorders. *Research in Autism Spectrum Disorders* 5(1):60–69.

Phillips, D. A., M. W. Lipsey, K. A. Dodge, R. Haskins, D. Bassok, M. R. Burchinal, G. J. Duncan, M. Dynarski, K. A. Magnuson, and C. Weiland. 2017. *Puzzling it out: The current state of scientific knowledge on pre-kindergarten effects. A consensus statement.* Washington, DC: The Brookings Institution.

Pianta, R. C., W. S. Barnett, M. Burchinal, and K. R. Thornburg. 2009. The effects of preschool education: What we know, how public policy is or is not aligned with the evidence base, and what we need to know. *Psychological Science in the Public Interest* 10(2):49–88.

Polit, D. F. 1989. Effects of a comprehensive program for teenage parents: Five years after project redirection. *Family Planning Perspectives* 21(4):164–187.

Porter, T., T. Nichols, P. Del Grosso, C. Begnoche, R. Hass, L. Vuong, and D. Paulsell. 2010a. *A compilation of initiatives to support home-based child care.* Washington, DC, and Princeton, NJ: Office of Planning, Research & Evaluation, Administration for Children and Families, and Mathematica Policy Research.

Porter, T., D. Paulsell, P. Del Grosso, S. Avellar, R. Hass, and L. Vuong. 2010b. *A review of the literature on home-based child care: Implications for future directions.* Washington, DC: Administration for Children and Families, Office of Planning, Research & Evaluation.

Puma, M., S. Bell, R. Cook, C. Heid, P. Broene, F. Jenkins, A. Mashburn, and J. Downer. 2012. *Third-grade follow-up to the Head Start Impact Study: Final report.* OPRE Report 2012-45. Washington, DC: U.S. Department of Health and Human Services, Administration for Children and Families, Office of Planning, Research & Evaluation.

Ralston, K., C. Newman, A. Clauson, J. Guthrie, and J. Buzby. 2008. *The National School Lunch Program: Background, trends, and issues.* Economic Research Report Number 61. Washington, DC: U.S. Department of Agriculture.

Ramey, C. T. 2018. The Abecedarian approach to social, educational, and health disparities. *Clinical Child and Family Psychology Review* 21(4):527–544.

Ramey, C. T., and S. L. Ramey. 2004. Early learning and school readiness: Can early intervention make a difference? *Merrill-Palmer Quarterly* 50(4):471–491.

Ramirez, M., Y. Wu, S. Kataoka, M. Wong, J. Yang, C. Peek-Asa, and B. Stein. 2012. Youth violence across multiple dimensions: A study of violence, absenteeism, and suspensions among middle school children. *The Journal of Pediatrics* 161(3):542–546.

Raver, C. C. 2012. Low-income children's self-regulation in the classroom: Scientific inquiry for social change. *American Psychologist* 67(8):681–689.

Regalado, M., and N. Halfon. 2001. Primary care services promoting optimal child development from birth to age 3 years: Review of the literature. *Archives of Pediatrics and Adolescent Medicine* 155(12):1311–1322.

Reichow, B. 2011. Overview of meta-analyses on early intensive behavioral intervention for young children with autism spectrum disorders. *Journal of Autism and Developmental Disorders* 42(4):512–520.

Roberts, A. M., K. C. Gallagher, A. M. Daro, I. U. Iruka, and S. L. Sarver. 2019. Workforce well-being: Personal and workplace contributions to early educators' depression across settings. *Journal of Applied Developmental Psychology* 61:4–12.

Rose, E. 2010. *The promise of preschool: From Head Start to universal pre-kindergarten.* New York: Oxford University Press.

Rossin-Slater, M. 2015. Promoting health in early childhood. *The Future of Children* 25(1):35–64.

Ruijs, N. M., and T. T. D. Peetsma. 2009. Effects of inclusion on students with and without special educational needs reviewed. *Educational Research Review* 4(2):67–79.

Sabol, T. J., and L. T. Hoyt. 2017. The long arm of childhood: Preschool associations with adolescent health. *Developmental Psychology* 53(4):752–763.

Sanders, M. 2016. Leadership, partnerships, and organizational development: Exploring components of effectiveness in three full-service community schools. *School Effectiveness and School Improvement* 27(2):157–177.

Schanzenbach, D. W. 2009. Do school lunches contribute to childhood obesity? *The Journal of Human Resources* 44(3):684–709.

Schindler, H. S., J. Kholoptseva, S. S. Oh, H. Yoshikawa, G. J. Duncan, K. A. Magnuson, and J. P. Shonkoff. 2015. Maximizing the potential of early childhood education to prevent externalizing behavior problems: A meta-analysis. *Journal of School Psychology* 53(3):243–263.

Schneidman, L., and A. L. Woodward. 2016. Are child-directed interactions the cradle of social learning? *Psychological Bulletin* 142(1):1–17.

Schweinhart, L. J., and D. P. Weikart. 1997. The High/Scope Preschool Curriculum Comparison Study through age 23. *Early Childhood Research Quarterly* 12(2):117–143.

Schweinhart, L. J., J. Montie, Z. Xiang, W. S. Barnett, C. R. Belfield, and M. Nores. 2005. *Lifetime effects: The High/Scope Perry Preschool study through age 40.* Ypsilanti, MI: High Scope Press.

Sheridan, S. M., L. L. Knoche, C. P. Edwards, J. A. Bovaird, and K. A. Kupzyk. 2010. Parent engagement and school readiness: Effects of the Getting Ready intervention on preschool children's social-emotional competencies. *Early Education and Development* 21(1):125–156.

Sheridan, S. M., L. L. Knoche, K. A. Kupzyk, C. P. Edwards, and C. A. Marvin. 2011. A randomized trial examining the effects of parent engagement on early language and literacy: The Getting Ready intervention. *Journal of School Psychology* 49(3):361–383.

Sheridan, S. M., L. L. Knoche, C. P. Edwards, K. A. Kupzyk, B. L. Clarke, and E. M. Kim. 2014. Efficacy of the Getting Ready intervention and the role of parental depression. *Early Education and Development* 25(5):746–769.

Shonkoff, J. P., and P. Hauser-Cram. 1987. Early intervention for disabled infants and their families: A quantitative analysis. *Pediatrics* 80(5):650–658.

Silva, K. G., P. M. Shimpi, and B. Rogoff. 2015. Young children's attention to what's going on: Cultural differences. *Advances in Child Development and Behavior* 49:207–227.

Skiba, R. J., L. Poloni-Staudinger, A. B. Simmons, and L. R. C. Feggins-Azziz. 2005. Unproven links: Can poverty explain ethnic disproportionality in special education? *The Journal of Special Education* 39(3):130–144.

Smith, T. B., M. G. Constantine, T. W. Dunn, J. M. Dinehart, and J. A. Montoya. 2006. Multi-cultural education in the mental health professions: A meta-analytic review. *Journal of Counseling Psychology* 53(1):132–145.

Solomon, T., A. Plamondon, A. O'Hara, H. Finch, G. Goco, P. Chaban, L. Huggins, B. Ferguson, and R. Tannock. 2017. A cluster randomized-controlled trial of the impact of the Tools of the Mind curriculum on self-regulation in Canadian preschoolers. *Frontiers in Psychology* 8:2366.

Sparling, J., and I. Lewis. 1979. *Learningames for the first three years: A guide to parent-child play.* New York: Walker and Company.

Sperry, D. E., L. L. Sperry, and P. J. Miller. 2018. Reexamining the verbal environments of children from different socioeconomic backgrounds. *Child Development* 90(4):1303–1318.

Stein, B. D., L. H. Jaycox, S. H. Kataoka, M. Wong, A. K. Langley, J. L. Avila, A. Bonilla, P. Castillo-Campos, J. B. Cohen, K. L. Dean, J. L. DuClos, M. N. Elliott, P. Escudero, A. Fink, S. Fuentes, K. L. Gegenheimer, K. Halsey, A. P. Mannarino, E. Nadeem, V. K. Ngo, V. P. O'Donoghue, M. Schonlau, M. M. Scott, P. Sharma, W. Wenli Tu, D. Walker, and C. Zaragoza. 2011. *Helping children cope with violence and trauma: A school-based program that works.* Santa Monica, CA: RAND Corporation.

Sue, D. W., C. M. Capodilupo, G. C. Torino, J. M. Bucceri, A. M. B. Holder, K. L. Nadal, and M. Esquilin. 2007. Racial microaggressions in everyday life: Implications for clinical practice. *American Psychologist* 62(4):271–286.

Temple, J. A., and A. J. Reynolds. 2007. Benefits and costs of investments in preschool education: Evidence from the Child–Parent Centers and related programs. *Economics of Education Review* 26(1):126–144.

The National Child Traumatic Stress Network. n.d. *Creating trauma-informed systems.* https://www.nctsn.org/trauma-informed-care/creating-trauma-informed-systems (accessed June 10, 2019).

The Urban Child Institute. 2019. *Social and emotional development in early childhood? The first years last a lifetime.* http://www.urbanchildinstitute.org/resources/publications/good-start/social-and-emotional-development (accessed June 14, 2019).

Thurlow, M., M. Sinclair, and D. Johnson. 2002. *Students with Disabilities who drop out of School—Implications for policy and practice. National Center on Secondary Education and Transition Issue Brief* 1(2). http://www.ncset.org/publications/viewdesc.asp?id=425 (accessed April 18, 2019).

Tout, K., K. Magnuson, S. Lipscomb, L. Karoly, R. Starr, H. Quick, and J. Wenner. 2017. *Validation of quality ratings used in quality rating and improvement systems (QRIS): A synthesis of state studies.* OPRE Report 2017-92. U.S. Department of Health and Human Services. https://www.acf.hhs.gov/opre/resource/validation-quality-ratings-used-quality-rating-improvement-systems-qris-a-synthesis-of-state-studies (accessed June 28, 2019).

USDA (U.S. Department of Agriculture). 2017. *PART 210—National School Lunch Program.* https://www.fns.usda.gov/part-210%E2%80%94national-school-lunch-program (accessed July 10, 2019).

Whitaker, R. C., T. Dearth-Wesley, and R. A. Gooze. 2015. Workplace stress and the quality of teacher–children relationships in Head Start. *Early Childhood Research Quarterly* 30:57–69.

Whitebook, M., C. McLean, L. J. E. Austin, and B. Edwards. 2018. *The Early Childhood Workforce Index—2018.* Berkeley, CA: Center for the Study of Child Care Employment, University of California, Berkeley.

Whitehurst, G. J., and M. Croft. 2010. *The Harlem Children's Zone, Promise Neighborhoods, and the broader, bolder approach to education.* Washington, DC: Brown Center on Education Policy at Brookings.

Williford, A. P., and T. L. Shelton. 2008. Using mental health consultation to decrease disruptive behaviors in preschoolers: Adapting an empirically-supported intervention. *Journal of Child Psychology and Psychiatry* 49(2):191–200.

Yoshikawa, H., C. Weiland, J. Brooks-Gunn, M. R. Burchinal, L. M. Espinosa, W. T. Gormley, J. Ludwig, K. A. Magnuson, D. Phillips, and M. J. Zaslow. 2013. *Investing in our future: The evidence base on preschool education.* Washington, DC, and New York: Society for Research in Development and Foundation for Child Development.

Zakszeski, B. N., N. E. Ventresco, and A. R. Jaffe. 2017. Promoting resilience through trauma-focused practices: A critical review of school-based implementation. *School Mental Health* 9(4):310–321.

Zarnowiecki, D., N. Sinn, J. Petkov, and J. Dollman. 2011. Parental nutrition knowledge and attitudes as predictors of 5–6-year-old children's healthy food knowledge. *Public Health Nutrition* 15(7):1284–1290.

Zellman, G. L., and M. Perlman. 2008. *Child-care quality rating and improvement systems in five pioneer states: Implementation issues and lessons learned.* Santa Monica, CA: RAND Corporation.

Zigler, E., and M. Finn-Stevenson. 2007. From research to policy practice: The school of the 21st century. *American Journal of Orthopsychiatry* 77(2):175–181.

8

A Systems Approach to Advance Early Development and Health Equity

INTRODUCTION

Advancing health equity in the preconception through early childhood periods cannot be achieved by any one sector alone. It will take action, collaboration, and alignment across all sectors that frequently interact with children and families and the professionals who serve them. Additionally, better alignment among systems will need to be accompanied by an increase in overall investment in early life: many of the systems best positioned to address early life drivers of health inequities are chronically underresourced, and improved collaboration may only be possible if resources are available to adopt, scale, and spread best practices within a redesigned and better aligned cross-sector ecosystem. There is likely no single, sweeping change that will create a new and better system of care that can address the variety of needs and challenges identified in this report; rather, steady progress integrating and connecting the efforts of the systems already in place, along with improved investments in those systems, will lead incrementally but steadily to improvements in health equity over time. Systems change is not an easy strategy; it seldom yields speedy returns, and it may not be sufficient without an investment of resources designed to take advantage of new and better aligned approaches. However, given that disparities are systematically generated, it is likely a necessary precursor to real and widespread advances in health equity. (See Box 8-1 for a brief overview of this chapter.)

As defined in Chapter 1, systems are collections of interacting, interdependent parts that function as a whole. For the purposes of this report,

---

BOX 8-1
Chapter in Brief: A Systems Approach

There are many opportunities to overcome key barriers to strengthen a systems approach to advance health equity in the preconception through early childhood periods. The crucial stakeholders who need to be involved and the alignment, measures, and research that are needed for systems change are discussed in this chapter based on the committee's assessment of the literature in Chapters 2–7 in this report. Recommendations in brief:

- Develop cross-sector initiatives that align strategies to address barriers to data sharing and integration, cross-sector financing, and other challenges to cross-sector collaboration.
- Enhance detection of early-life adversity and improve response systems.
- Develop adversity and trauma-informed systems.
- Build a diverse, culturally informed workforce in all relevant systems.
- Improve access to programs and policies across systems that provide parental or caregiver supports and help build or promote family attachments and functioning. For families with intensive support needs, develop programs or initiatives designed to provide comprehensive wraparound services.
- Integrate care and services across the health continuum, including the adoption of models that provide comprehensive support for the whole person by leveraging and connecting existing community resources.
- Support payment reform to allow for upstream investment.
- Support research that advances the state of the science in several critical ways to advance health equity, including exploring alternative methods to address complex causality and expanding research into individual differences in response to adversity and treatment.

---

most systems are social constructs and organized around a key functional area (e.g., education, health care, criminal justice). Systems have existing patterns and structures that define how people tend to move through them. This chapter summarizes the opportunities to overcome key barriers to strengthen a systems approach, the crucial stakeholders who need to be involved, and the necessary alignment, measures, and research based on the committee's assessment of the literature in Chapters 2–7 in this report. The committee identified eight crosscutting recommendation areas where multiple sectors need to take action.

Systems Characteristics That Impede Advancing Health Equity

There are many systems characteristics that act as barriers to spreading and scaling up evidence-based and promising programs and approaches to reduce health disparities and advance health equity.

Sometimes barriers are simply financial—scaling programs requires significant and sustained investments in a world with limited resources and many competing priorities. However, the barriers often stem from policy or structural arrangements that could be altered with sufficient political will or from knowledge gaps that could be addressed with appropriate research, well-targeted dissemination, and thoughtfully considered implementation assistance. Some of the key system barriers that prevent moving forward with what is known to work include the following.

Systems Are Designed to React, Not to Prevent

Many systems are designed in response to a challenge or crisis—people are sick or lack jobs—and operate with the primary goal of mitigating the negative impacts of those challenges. Few systems are set up to think ahead to the root causes of the problem and to address those causes, and as a result, resources are applied downstream. In fact, many systems are explicitly not allowed to spend resources upstream (on prevention, for example) because the upstream factors are seen as a different system's challenge to address, and that other system has its own budget and goals. Current programs and policies are operating in an interconnected world, where one system's cause is another system's effect, and the carefully partitioned systems each address only the portion of the problem that falls explicitly within their purview. From the perspective of a life course approach—where failing to invest early means missing critical windows to set positive health trajectories, and the later an intervention comes, the more difficult it is to change negative trajectories—this fractured approach is an impediment to reaching health equity in the preconception through early childhood periods and beyond.

Systems Are Structured to Take the Short-Term View

Currently, systems are poorly structured to incentivize long-term thinking and planning. The pressures of annual budget and performance cycles make investment in long-term gains challenging, and savings are often disincentivized by penalizing systems that reduce costs with a subsequent reduction in payment rates or budget allocations. Often, payments or budgets for systems are based on prior experiences that do not reflect transformed realities. For example, early efforts to integrate behavioral health into primary care faced formidable barriers because payment rates are based on prior experience that does not include many mental or behavioral health services, making transformation extraordinarily difficult to catalyze. From an economic and political standpoint, the benefits of early care and education (ECE) are generally not realized until after children enter school, and sometimes even later in life. Additionally, when the root causes of poor outcomes are interconnected across systems but the financial stakes are not, misaligned incentives emerge whereby each partner fears they may put in significant work and expense to change an outcome, only to see the savings realized primarily by someone else. As Teutsch and Berger noted, "If everyone is focused only on his own task, no one is responsible for ensuring that our nation's investments are well utilized, let alone best utilized, to improve health" (Teutsch and Berger, 2005, p. 486).

Systems Typically Have a Singular Focus

A multisystem approach to health equity is difficult when involved systems are primarily built to specialize in one aspect of the health continuum (and whose main goal might not even be health). Which system responds to risks that might generate poor health outcomes, how that work is organized, which system is allowed to address it, and the way funds flow to support a response are all built within highly specialized silos with distinct rules, regulations, strategies, and normative practices. There are relatively few system architectures ready-made to advance cross-sector work and few easy pathways to conceptualize, implement, or pay for it. In addition, those who work within systems might feel a strong sense of special expertise and ownership over their area of focus, which may cause a reluctance to invite others to share hard-earned professional "turf." Overcoming both the structural and cultural barriers to integrating systems will be no easy task, but structures that align the interests of different sectors—for example, by creating shared savings or other models that reward systems or actors within systems for contributing to one another's positive outcomes—may help overcome some of these inherent challenges.

Systems Take a Narrow View of the Biological and Social Context

Scientific and institutional systems tend to segment the biological and social; in the context of early life, they are often poorly set up to address the symbiotic relationship between biological development and social context. Even within settings that address health and development explicitly, such as pediatric clinics, there tends to be segmentation of biological risk (assessed by clinicians or pharmacists) from social risk (assessed by social workers or therapists), lacking clear processes for developing a plan for each that is informed by the other.

Systems Undervalue Community Expertise

Current systems tend to value formal knowledge attained through traditional, credentialed academic channels but often undervalue knowledge of culture, community, populations, or other context gained through lived experiences. Those making decisions about how to serve some communities, or even those providing the service, often do not reflect or live in the communities being served. When the experiences of those most impacted by inequities are not represented in strategies to address them, there is a risk of developing solutions that do not connect with, will not be used by, or do not meet the actual needs of the population for whom they are intended, which may ultimately exacerbate the very disparities that are intended to be addressed.

OPPORTUNITIES TO STRENGTHEN A SYSTEMS APPROACH

Throughout this report, the committee has explored key factors that help set the odds for long-term health and health equity outcomes and made recommendations suitable for actors within key systems and institutions to help improve those odds. While the actions taken by each system identified in this report are important components of improving health equity, one of the committee's important findings—that the forces driving health inequities are systemic and profoundly interconnected across those systems—suggests that a larger strategy is also needed to advance health equity in the long term. When outcomes are driven by forces that cut across multiple systems, even doing everything perfectly within one system is not enough. Multisector causality requires a multisector response.

Based on the committee's assessment of the needed changes in Chapters 2–7, the corresponding recommendations contained in each chapter, and its collective expertise, the committee identified eight cross-cutting recommendations that need to be adopted by all systems that frequently touch the lives of children and families and the professionals who serve them. These recommendations represent part of a comprehensive strategy for improving the overall system's ability to address the early-life drivers of health inequity. These strategies draw on the evidence presented in this report and reflect the key insights from the core principles presented in Chapter 1. These recommendations can optimize the impact of the strategies in this report and create a framework where what is known to work can be made to work for more people, under more circumstances, and with a greater overall impact on health equity.

Support Cross-Sector Initiatives Across the Health Continuum

Achieving health equity is a systems challenge. It will not be improved solely by developing and deploying programs aimed at individuals experiencing poor outcomes—until the root causes are addressed, negative health outcomes will persist. Young people experience adverse and positive exposures that cumulatively help shape their odds for good health over the life course, but within systems, those exposures occur at systematically different rates for different groups of people. They also intersect profoundly—the early-life exposures and experiences that shape health are multidimensional and fall under the purview of multiple social and cultural systems (see Chapters 2 and 3 for more information). These different exposures and experiences result in different cumulative odds for good health over the life course, odds that are ultimately expressed in the form of disparate outcomes between groups.

Early efforts to adopt cross-sector approaches were often impeded by the challenges of data sharing. The regulatory structure that governs data use and data privacy offers important protections for individual consumers, but it was also largely developed without considering the limitations it might place on cross-sector interventions by communities seeking to collectively address complex problems with roots in multiple systems. The distinct regulations for different sectors (e.g., Health Insurance Portability and Accountability Act of 1996 in health care and Family Educational Rights and Privacy Act of 1974 in education) have different criteria for data use, and while some allow data to be combined for the purposes of research or evaluation, there are few legal pathways available to make *operational* use of cross-sector data in ways that would help co-manage common populations or address common root causes with coordinated, cross-sector approaches. By providing a regulatory architecture to support data sharing between the key systems identified in this report, policy makers and systems leaders could dramatically improve communities' ability to adopt, scale, and spread cross-sector interventions.

A second key challenge of cross-sector work stems from how public dollars are organized. Resources tend to be allocated in a siloed manner: this money is for health care, that money is for education, and so on. In general, most systems have strict administrative rules on how their funding can be spent and limited ability to direct it at work that occurs outside of their system, even if that work is critical to that same system to achieve its desired outcomes. However, in reality, these issues are not confined to the convenient boundaries within which finances are organized, and if the problem that is creating poor outcomes for a system does not happen to fall within its boundaries, that system is left with only a limited ability to address it. Creating pathways for funds within a system to flow to activities outside the system, especially when there is strong evidence that those activities will result in improved outcomes, is critical to building effective cross-sector initiatives. A recent example of this is an effort under way by health care provider Kaiser Permanente—it plans to spend $200 million on fighting homelessness and building more low-cost housing in eight states, plus Washington, DC.[1]

---

[1] See https://about.kaiserpermanente.org/community-health/news/kaiser-permanente-announces-three-initiatives-to-improve-communi for more information (accessed April 16, 2019).

In addition to allowing for investments across sectors, it is important to consider how any *savings* generated by those investments might be shared. In the absence of shared savings models, a "wrong pocket" problem is often created, whereby system partners fear they may invest in the work only to see the outcomes or savings accrue to others. There are currently few validated methodologies for measuring shared savings— especially given the data-sharing challenges that have already been highlighted—or mechanisms for capturing those savings and distributing them among the participating partners. Making headway on shared savings models could help create powerful aligned incentives that help cross-sector initiatives create, sustain, and spread their work. One strategy to address this problem is to develop and test shared savings models that allow sectors whose work helps the outcomes in another sector "share the savings" generated by that work. This would help create aligned incentives that acknowledge intersectional causes and reward intersectional work.

Finally, licensure and certification requirements vary dramatically across fields; in many emerging fields, they are virtually nonexistent. However, services that impact health are sometimes also delivered by paraprofessionals, peers, or other workforces that either lack formal professional licensure standards or use standards that are not recognized by larger, more established systems that would pay for such services (IOM, 2001). Payment rules for many systems often require more traditional certification, so this barrier hinders using nontraditional workforces, which may be closer to the communities being served and could have similar lived experiences, to deliver services that help create health within the context of collaborative cross-sector work.

While there has been significant work around the key components necessary to establish successful cross-sector initiatives (see examples in Chapters 5, 6, and 7), a number of key barriers remain, including cultural, ideological, or normative barriers around perceived ownership of specific content areas that may limit cross-sector communication and cooperation that policy makers and leaders can help address.

Recommendation 8-1: Policy makers and leaders in the health care, public health, social service, criminal justice, early care and education/education, and other sectors should support and invest in cross-sector initiatives that align strategies and operate community programs and interventions that work across sectors to address the root causes of poor health outcomes. This includes addressing structural and policy barriers to data integration and cross-sector financing and other challenges to cross-sector collaboration.

These initiatives could include collective impact strategies, Accountable Communities for Health,[2] Health in All Policies[3] initiatives, or other models of aligned, cross-sector community action in service to shared health and health equity goals. (See Chapter 8 of the 2017 National Academies report *Communities in Action: Pathways to Health Equity* for more information on Health in All Policies and other collective impact strategies to foster multisector collaboration.)

Enhance Detection of Early-Life Adversity and Improve Response Systems

As discussed throughout this report, adversities in early life— including adverse childhood experiences and other adverse experiences or exposure to key social determinants of health (SDOH), such as housing instability or food insecurity—help set the odds for poor health outcomes later in life. Early-life adversity is especially important for a number of reasons: first, it occurs at points of high plasticity for key biological systems that shape health over the long term; second, it occurs during a period of critical development in the social, emotional, and cognitive domains of self; third, it increases the likelihood of additional exposures to adversity later in the life course; and fourth, it may impact future resilience to additional exposures (see Chapter 2 for more information). Early adversities make a negative health trajectory more likely; left unaltered, such trajectories will play out across decades and result in differences in health outcomes within and across generations. Early detection and rapid response are essential to help mitigate the long-term effects of exposure to adversity by adjusting the trajectories back toward positive health as early as possible.

Early detection and rapid response would require a number of steps across systems, such as developing and promoting screening tools and procedures that can be adopted, implemented, and scaled to improve monitoring and fast reaction. Screening approaches that can be adopted within

---

[2] "Accountable health initiatives, most commonly referred to as accountable communities for health (ACHs), have been implemented nationwide in response to or as a result of contributions from state innovation model grants and community transformation grants, through collaborations with state Medicaid programs, or through other policy and financial incentives" (Mongeon et al., 2017). They bring together partners from health, social service, and other sectors to improve population health and clinical-community linkages within a geographic area (Spencer and Bianca, 2016).

[3] "Health in All Policies is a collaborative approach to improving the health of all people by incorporating health considerations into decision-making across sectors and policy areas. The goal of Health in All Policies is to ensure that all decision-makers are informed about the health consequences of various policy options during the policy development process" (Rudolph et al., 2013, p. 6).

and connected across settings, such as the health care and early learning systems, and that make frequent contact with young families during the first years of a child's life are especially critical because they represent the best opportunities to detect early and act decisively in response.

Professionals who frequently interact with children and caregivers—clinicians, teachers, or personnel in social service or other agencies, for example—need training to understand the effects of early-life adversity and the associated toxic stress response on the physiological and psychosocial development of young people. These trainings need to move beyond awareness training to include how to respond effectively within the context of their field and how to refer across sectors when needed.[4] Dedicated staff are also needed to help professionals refer children and families to services outside of that system (e.g., social workers embedded within the relevant systems). These professionals need to know how their approach to treatment or service provision will vary based on the results of a child's adversity screen. (See below for more on transdisciplinary needs.)

It is also necessary to develop rapid response or referral systems that can bring a range of community resources to bear when early-life trauma and adversity is detected. These systems should include information and service pathways and the ability to "close the loop" back to the referring agency or partner so that responses are coordinated across the continuum of health. Accomplishing this will require changes to regulatory limitations on how data can be shared across sectors or between professionals with different qualifications and licensure systems.

> **Recommendation 8-2: Policy makers and leaders in the health care, public health, social service, criminal justice, early care and education/education, and other sectors should adopt and implement screening for trauma and adversities early in life to increase the likelihood of early detection. This should include creating rapid response and referral systems that can quickly bring protective resources to bear when early-life adversities are detected, through the coordination of cross-sector expertise, as covered in Recommendation 8-1.**

Rapid response and referral systems will require implementing and scaling screening across key settings, enhancing trauma response training, and ensuring support for these systems.

---

[4] For example, the Alberta Family Wellness Initiative in Canada has developed a "Brain Story Certification Course" that teaches the foundational science of brain development to help professionals in all fields who interact with families with children. See https://www.albertafamilywellness.org/training (accessed July 19, 2019) for more information.

Develop Adversity and Trauma-Informed Systems

Early-life trauma and adversity are key factors that help set the odds for poor health outcomes across the life course, but *how systems respond* to that trauma is nearly as important. Once adversity or trauma occurs, it cannot be erased. However, its effects also are not destiny: effective services can help mitigate the impact of adversity on health across the life course. Most systems are designed to capture discrete data elements about their service domain, but exposure to social adversity or trauma is often contextual, captured via narrative interactions with patients or clients. These are also sensitive personal data with additional layers of privacy protections. Because these data are not easily shared within or across systems, however, people seeking help at multiple points of service often have to tell the story of their trauma over and over again. Mechanisms that allow service providers to have the needed data and context about their clients at the point of care could ensure that their service options are appropriate to clients' financial, social, cultural, and personal situations. For example, when service options are presented that require resources a client cannot possibly access (e.g., financial cost-sharing, transportation), the client's status as an "outsider" is reinforced. When systems have mechanisms to meet clients where they are, clients will be more supported and understood and be more likely to adhere to recommendations, remain engaged with the system, and receive the help they need.

Many clients feel distress not just from past life events but from interactions with the system itself: they feel unwelcome or stigmatized when they seek services due to their race, poverty, sexual or gender identity, or other factors. It is critical to train service providers on discrimination and stigma to ensure all persons feel welcome receiving services in any setting, so that they will engage in and benefit from those important services. As noted in Chapter 7, trauma-informed care (TIC) and implicit bias training reflects the understanding that a child's or family's behavioral or health challenges are often due to experiences of toxic stress and undiagnosed and untreated trauma, and with implicit bias among those they interact with in the education or other systems. Furthermore, systems delivering services to people with traumatic histories are also at risk of retraumatizing clients if they do not act in a trauma-informed manner. There are strategies for TIC that can be used to prevent and mitigate the impact of implicit biases (see Chapter 7 for more strategies and Recommendation 8-8 for research needs on this topic). Furthermore, harmonizing eligibility criteria across programs and systems is needed so that when children or families experiencing trauma or adversity enter a system, professionals can take a holistic perspective and refer them to cross-sector services; children and families would also be more likely to be eligible for needed services in other systems.

Recommendation 8-3: Policy makers and leaders in the health care, public health, social service, criminal justice, early care and education/education, and other sectors should adopt best practices and implement training for trauma-informed care and service delivery. Sector leadership should implement trauma-informed systems that are structured to minimize implicit bias and stigma and prevent retraumatization. Standards for trauma-informed practice exist in a variety of service sectors, including health care and social services; those standards should be replicated and implemented across systems.

Build a Diverse, Culturally Informed Workforce

Building a high-quality health, early learning, or social services system will not improve outcomes if people do not engage with the system(s), and the populations where health inequities are most strongly expressed are often the least likely to engage in systems designed to serve them because they have not historically felt welcomed in those systems. Most systems are built to specifications that are responsive to dominant culture norms and practices, but there is no perfect system that works for everyone. Systems need to move beyond *what works* and address the question of *what works for whom, and under what circumstances*? Some communities may prefer to receive care and services via alternative modes; in a manner of their choosing; or from providers who look and speak like them or understand their unique cultural or community identity. Offering services to caregivers and children in culturally and linguistically appropriate ways is critical to ensuring that good systems exist and that the people who have historically had the poorest outcomes engage in these systems as partners in generating health.

System actions to offer culturally and linguistically appropriate services include training service providers to be attuned to and respect cultural and other identity differences and ensuring that systems have a range of appropriate linguistic services available for providers. Furthermore, systems that ensure that signage, forms, and data processes that clients use are available in multiple modes and languages facilitate participation in these systems. Another system action relates to the integration of workforces across sectors in the early-life period. Complementary disciplines can be drawn from to create teams that promote transdisciplinary service delivery. This might include traditional service providers and the expanded use of paraprofessionals, community health workers, peer support specialists, parent advisors, or others who bring expertise in, and lived experiences that are relevant to, the communities or populations being served. Bringing transdisciplinary providers together is just the first step; standards and workflows that allow these teams to collaborate effectively may need to be developed so that each functions at the top of its license to provide comprehensive wraparound support for families that need it.

Another system action is expanding the workforce in early-life-serving sectors to ensure that service providers reflect the diversity of their communities and that people of diverse racial, ethnic, cultural, sexual orientation, gender expression, or other identities have access to more service providers who look like them and reflect their experiences. This could be accomplished through mentoring programs, outreach into culturally specific communities when recruiting or hiring, or scholarship programs to "plant the seeds" to introduce more diverse communities into fields where some communities are underrepresented.

> **Recommendation 8-4: Policy makers and leaders in the health care, public health, social service, criminal justice, early care and education/education, and other sectors should develop a transdisciplinary and diverse workforce to implement culturally competent service delivery models. The workforce should reflect the diversity of populations who will engage in sector services.**

Align Across Systems to Enhance Early-Life Supports for Caregivers

Parental and caregiver supports are critical for promoting prosocial attachment, nurturing, and healthy family relationships that foster the healthy development of youth (see Chapter 4). Supporting caregivers should be an essential goal of multiple systems (e.g., caregivers who do not have to worry about access to health care have a better opportunity to remain healthy and maintain positive relationships with their children, caregivers with adequate housing may experience reduced strain and be better able to bond with their children, and caregivers whose children are receiving effective early-life education and developmental supports may feel better equipped as effective and engaged parents).

Better support for caregivers will increase the likelihood of positive nurturing relationships between caregivers and children, and improvements in the multiple systems that are touch points for children and families should explicitly address caregiver support. Such changes may include encouraging the development of programs and policies that provide support for the whole family unit, including parents, children, and other important members of the family's extended caregiving system. Strategies include moving away from segmented policies, such as those that consider eligibility for supports or services separately for parents and children (e.g., child-only health insurance versus a family plan), and instead consider programs that incorporate or leverage the extended family unit or other close social networks.

Another strategy is enacting policies and programs that provide assistance to families without requiring a separation between caregivers and children that might negatively impact attachments and family functioning, especially in early life. For example, programs could offer families with young children certain financial or other assistance that does not include extensive requirements to leave the home in order to work or perform other tasks, which reduces the opportunities for developing, maintaining, and supporting healthy family attachments and functioning. (See Chapter 6 for examples.)

Efforts could be promoted to create wraparound services for families with greater needs, offering multiple types of assistance designed to support caregivers along a variety of dimensions within a single program or setting, even or especially if those services come from traditionally segmented or siloed systems in the community. Bundled services require less time for caregivers to navigate the systems, allowing more time for them to focus on effective caregiving. (See Chapters 4, 5, and 7 for examples of integrated and wraparound care.)

> **Recommendation 8-5: Policy makers and leaders in the health care, public health, social service, criminal justice, early care and education/education, and other sectors should improve access to programs or policies that explicitly provide parental or caregiver supports and help build or promote family attachments and functioning by engaging with the families as a cohesive unit. For families with intensive support needs, develop programs or initiatives designed to provide comprehensive wraparound supports along a number of dimensions, such as health care, education, and social services, designed to address needs related to the social determinants of health that are integrated and community based.**

Support Integration of Care and Services Across All Dimensions of Health and Community

Integration refers to establishing standards by which services are delivered in ways that break down traditional silos and are informed by and responsive to the intersection of health and the key drivers of health. This might include social domains (such as social support, cultural identity, or community cohesion; see Chapter 4), clinical domains of health (such as physical, mental, behavioral, or dental health; see Chapter 5), economic domains (such as income, housing stability, or food security; see Chapter 6), and educational domains (such as access to high-quality ECE programs or others; see Chapter 7). Integrated service models cohesively connect and align along the health continuum, address health holistically, and often include both primary prevention designed to forestall health crises, and screening and response systems designed to act quickly when needs are identified.

A whole-family approach calls for integrating services at the point of care or intervention. Thus, the committee's vision for programs and services is that families have access to an array of clinical, early educational, family developmental, and psychosocial support and economic help in their communities. Rather than fragmented programs, the vision calls for easy and coordinated access across the breadth of needed services for households—viewed from a life course perspective and one that ensures equity in access and use. Achieving this integration takes substantial work and community leadership, with programs having only limited incentives to collaborate, share accountability, and pool resources across sectors. The 2017 National Academies report *Communities in Action: Pathways to Health Equity* provides principles and examples of integration at the community level (NASEM, 2017).

Integration and whole-family clinical care models are one example. This could include integrating the delivery of clinical care to include physical, mental, behavioral, and dental health services and connecting clinical care with other services for families (nutrition, early childhood programs, housing) either through a "one-stop" colocation strategy or a seamless and easy referral process with strong information sharing, "warm" handoffs between providers, and a "no wrong door" policy that helps people get whatever help they need easily through any entry point.

New models that integrate services to address the SDOH should follow this model. These include service delivery models that integrate supports across a range of SDOH, especially housing, transportation, food security, and social support, with a particular focus on family social supports and programs that integrate informal social networks into the health care, ECE, and services ecosystem (see Chapter 5 for recommendations on this for the clinical care system and its connections to other sectors). Another strategy is integration across settings and sectors, such as establishing community centers that include health care, nutrition, parent education, and resources to identify social needs and adversity and to help families find resources, or supporting church- or community-based programs, such as health care/community partnerships (see Chapter 5 of NASEM [2017], for in-depth examples of these types of partnerships), to extend the reach of health or social service programs into culturally specific or otherwise historically underserved communities.

Recommendation 8-6: Policy makers and leaders in the health care, public health, social service, criminal justice, early care and education/education, and other sectors should integrate care and services across the health continuum, including the adoption of models that provide comprehensive support for the whole person in a contextually informed manner, leveraging and connecting existing community resources wherever possible, with a focus on prevention.

Support Payment Reform to Allow for Upstream Investment

Payment structures have a profound impact on how resources are invested and the ability to address complex, interrelated causes of poor health using multisector approaches. In many sectors, payment remains tied to the delivery of a service rather than its success in achieving an intended outcome, creating incentives to focus on the processes of providing services and maximize the associated billing of those processes rather than on creating better health outcomes. Similarly, the regulatory structure that governs how funds flow within and across systems is a major impediment to both cross-sector work and the spread and scale of interventions or programs that are known to succeed. As noted earlier, nearly every major system or sector has its own regulatory and/or funding structure, which is primarily designed to ensure accountability to spending within that system; there are usually rules that ensure the money within a sector stays within that sector. Accountability policies can also discourage upstream investment. For example, in the education system, schools and districts are not held accountable for school outcomes until 3rd grade at the earliest, which creates disincentives for school leaders to invest in the early grades or before kindergarten.

Another strategy is to move to payment models that attach payment to the value of a provided service or its desired outcome rather than to the delivery of the service. Value-based structures promote efficiency and impact over quantity of services and encourage upstream investment to address root causes rather than downstream work to deliver services. Payment models that emphasize upstream investment have substantial focus on prevention in health care, ECE, and community services. In many cases, as documented in earlier chapters, the downstream payoff may come much later, sometimes years later.

Finally, there is a need to rethink budgeting and contracting to address the "success penalty" problem. For systems that contract with government, budget and contracting policies often set reimbursement rates or budgets by examining expenditures versus costs in previous years. When systems invest upstream and reduce costs, they risk being penalized by having their budgets reduced or rates cut the following year, thus dis-incentivizing success. Models that allow successful systems to reinvest some portion of saved dollars into scaling and spreading the approaches that helped them achieve that success will incentivize change.

> **Recommendation 8-7: Policy makers and leaders in the health care, public health, social service, criminal justice, early care and education/education, and other sectors should invest in programs that improve population health and in upstream programs that decrease long-term risk and poor health outcomes. These changes should be accompanied by accountability metrics to ensure that the spending is tangibly and demonstrably in service to the goals behind the original funding, but offer more flexibility in how those goals are achieved.**

Support Transdisciplinary Research on the Complex Pathways of Health Equity

As described in this report, a tremendous amount is known about what works to advance health equity in early development (and the life-long benefits of doing so), but there are still many unknowns in the area of implementing and scaling up interventions. Many interventions have shown promising results at small scale but have not been fully tested across multiple settings or in diverse communities and populations. Others have promising preliminary data but little high-quality evidence. The evidence around systems and policy changes—the work needed to address inequities with a multisector and systems-based approach—remains less certain than programmatic evidence in many cases precisely because it is complex and set in shifting environments that make it challenging to confidently attribute effects. There is also a relative dearth of research on heath equity produced through genuinely participatory methods that authentically engage the communities and populations most impacted by health inequities to help formulate, conduct, interpret, and disseminate results to community members, advocates, policy makers, and other decision makers.

The committee has identified important research needs in this report relevant to the chapter topics (see Recommendations 2-2, 4-1, 4-2, and 4-3); here, however, the committee recommends strategies focused on how to conduct research differently to help translate science to action across sectors, including needed data to inform subgroup analysis and to elucidate the complex causality related to health inequities to better target interventions across sectors. Recommendation 8-8 also identifies research needs that would support strategies identified throughout this report and relate to all systems that frequently interact with children and their families (e.g., research on addressing discrimination, structural racism, and implicit bias training), and calls for an increase in participatory methods that engage communities, especially historically marginalized or excluded communities, as partners in research on health equity.

An important caution, however, is that although more targeted research is needed, enough is already known to act now to advance health equity in the prenatal and early childhood periods—this has been made abundantly clear in the preceding chapters of this report. The research recommended below is important to continually improve efforts and increase impact, but this should not impede action at the federal, state, tribal, territorial, local, and community levels. Here, the committee provides guidance on charting the course for future research to better meet the needs of the nation's children in the future and, specifically, to advance health equity.

> **Recommendation 8-8: The National Institutes of Health, Agency for Healthcare Research and Quality, Centers for Disease Control and Prevention, Health Resources and Services Administration, Centers for Medicare & Medicaid Services, U.S. Department of Education, philanthropies, and other funders should support research that advances the state of the science in several critical ways to advance health equity. Specific actions and research to support include the following.**

Research Methods

- **Explore alternative methods to address complex causality.** Randomized controlled trials (RCTs) are often considered to be the gold standard for scientific evidence, and they remain a valuable tool (see Chapter 1 for more on their strengths and limitations). However, RCTs are not designed to assess the complex, interconnected causality that lies at the heart of health equity—if anything, they excel at reducing or controlling for complexity to isolate a single cause. It is necessary to embrace new approaches, including data science/data mining, multilevel modeling, integrated mixed methods, rapid-cycle analysis,[5] and other methods designed to employ a wide range of data and evidence to uncover

---

[5] For example, the Frontiers of Innovation platform at the Center on the Developing Child at Harvard University employs a "structured but flexible framework that facilitates idea generation, development, implementation, testing, evaluation, and rapid-cycle iteration" (see https://developingchild.harvard.edu/innovation-application/frontiers-of-innovation for more information [accessed July 1, 2019]).

the most effective approaches. Additionally, research needs to move beyond assessing cause and effect to explore the mediators and moderators of differential effectiveness—to identify not only what works, but what works for whom, and under what circumstances—to pursue a deeper understanding of causality that facilitates the ability to adapt promising and evidence-based models to optimally fit the needs and priorities of diverse populations.

- **Expand research into individual differences (heterogeneity) in response to adversity and treatment.** Many programs have shown some impact on important health outcomes; yet, in many cases, the effect sizes have been small to moderate. In part, this reflects the differential vulnerability and response to adversity and the differences in response to interventions. Studying heterogeneity in context and how it shapes responses to interventions and promising programs is a critical component of actionable research, but current knowledge to identify these differences is limited. Exploring and understanding these differences will enable more targeted and tailored interventions.

- **Promote scientific research that includes individuals and families from underrepresented communities.** Even programs with a good evidence base often rely on studies that were conducted in dominant culture settings or with communities that are not representative of the full range of diversity (see Chapter 4) of characteristics such as race and ethnicity, socioeconomic or immigrant status, or sexual minority parent status. Studies are needed that seek to not only understand what works but to move beyond top-line findings to explore variation in outcomes across populations, settings, and subgroups (see Chapter 4 for a discussion on subgroup variation)—what works for whom, and under what circumstances. The results can be used to target efforts to address inequities more precisely in contextually informed ways. This scientific work should be informed by appropriate theoretical frameworks that take into consideration the multifactorial nature of early childhood development in diverse populations. Members of these populations or scientists with extensive research and/or clinical experience working with these populations should be part of the investigative teams.

Research Content

- **Promote research that explicitly seeks to understand the interconnected mechanisms of health inequities.** Health equity has complex, interconnected root causes—factors that unfold across the distinct systems highlighted in this report—and also complex, interconnected mechanisms by which those factors shape health outcomes differentially across the life course. These mechanisms include biological development, social-psychological development, and differential opportunity structures and choice architectures that life presents people based on their circumstances. In addition, the biological and psychosocial responses to these mechanisms vary across the life course, with some developmental periods of high plasticity offering critical windows for establishing long-term trajectories for health outcomes. Understanding the *root causes* of inequities allows actions to be taken to prevent them; understanding the *mechanisms* by which root causes shape inequities helps promote more effective intervention when prevention is less than perfect, and understanding *variation in responsiveness* to those mechanisms across the life course will help ensure interventions are optimally targeted for maximum impact.

- **Support research that addresses discrimination and structural racism.** There is an urgent need for research on the structural roots of racism; how to stem the development of negative societal stereotypes, attitudes, and implicit biases; how to change those biases once they are formed; and how to develop applications of that knowledge that can help reduce discrimination. The impact of these forces—both the negative belief systems themselves and their structural and historical roots—on health and health outcomes are keenly felt, but there are few proven tools that allow for effective response.

- **Support research for trauma-informed care and implicit bias training.** As discussed in Recommendation 8-3, TIC and implicit bias training are critical tools for advancing health equity in the preconception through early childhood periods. However, that research base needs to be expanded further. Regarding research on structural racism and implicit bias, the 2017 National Academies report *Communities in Action: Pathways to Health Equity* provided the following recommendation on this topic, and the committee endorses it:

> *The committee recommends that research funders support research on (a) health disparities that examines the multiple effects of structural racism (e.g., segregation) and implicit and explicit bias across different categories of marginalized status on health and health care delivery; and (b) effective strategies to reduce and mitigate the effects of explicit and implicit bias.*

There have been promising developments in the search for interventions to address implicit bias, but more research is needed, and engaging community members in this and other aspects of research on health disparities is important for ethical and practical reasons. . . . In the context of implicit bias in [schools], workplaces and business settings, including individuals with relevant expertise in informing and conducting the research could also be helpful. Therefore, teams could be composed of such nontraditional participants as community members and local business leaders, in addition to academic researchers. (NASEM, 2017, p. 115)

- **Support systematic dissemination and implementation research.** In many sectors and increasingly across sectors, there are numerous well-tested examples of what works to help young families and improve outcomes. Enhancing and improving access to these programs will benefit from an extensive program of dissemination and implementation research to bring them to scale. Furthermore, a mechanism to capture what has been tested but does not work is needed.

Measuring Success

Disparities have been measured for a long time and show the *outcomes* of inequity. What is lacking are good tools for measuring the various systemic and personal factors that influence and interact in complex ways to shape health outcomes over the life course. In the absence of such measures, designing the right kinds of system change remains a challenge.

The committee has identified a number of measures and indicators that can currently be measured and are important for tracking progress within each of the systems that act as key leverage points for early childhood development. For example, measures for primary caregivers include maternal depression and stress, parental feelings of rejection or hostility to the child, and support for mothers/primary caregivers. For children, measures include infants born at low or very low birth weight, breastfeeding at 6 months, blood lead levels, social-emotional learning, meeting expectations in language development (e.g., measures of vocabulary), and kindergarten readiness. Measures for families include poverty (using the Supplemental Poverty Measure), food insecurity, homelessness, health care insurance coverage, and exposure to toxicants through the home or early care environments. Taken together, improvements in these key metrics would represent systems that are moving in the right direction to address early-life drivers of inequities. However, other measures will be needed that are not yet available; the following section outlines these.

The committee's conceptual model in Chapter 1 identifies two important dimensions to consider when exploring the early-life drivers of health inequities: the key systems that play the largest role in helping "set the odds" for healthy development and the interrelated mechanisms or pathways by which the influence of those systems are expressed into health outcomes over the life course (see Figure 8-1).

The model leads naturally to several important insights about measurement. First, the systems that set the trajectory for health are explicitly connected and nested in the model—a child's biological, psychological, and socio-behavioral development (innermost ring) is nested within family and caregiver social systems, but those systems exist within and are shaped by key institutional systems like health care or ECE, which in turn exist within and are shaped by structural inequities and other historical, political, or macroeconomic forces. This means it is not enough to just have a good measure of caregiver attachment or access to health care—it is necessary to have good measures of how those constructs *interact* to collectively set the odds of healthy early-life development and why systems present some populations with a greater or lesser probability of exposure to those constructs.

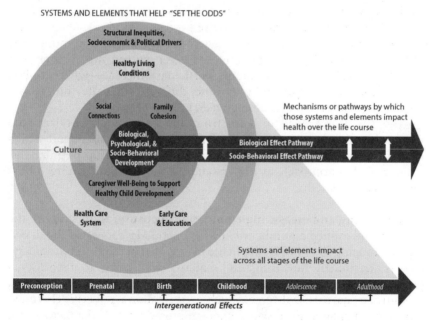

FIGURE 8-1 Leveraging early opportunities to achieve health equity across the life course: A conceptual framework.
NOTE: The elements and systems included in the nested circles impact every stage of the life course.

The mechanistic pathways by which those constructs act to shape health across the life course are also complex and interconnected. They might act via a biological pathway, whereby events or exposures that occur in childhood result in changes to key neurological or other biological systems that act over the years to enable or impede good health. They might also act via a socio-behavioral or psychological pathway, whereby events or exposures that occur in childhood change the likelihood that other events or exposures will occur later in life, alter the way people formulate their own identity or move through and react to key systems, or result in differences in the kinds of opportunities or choices that life ultimately presents to someone. Crucially, these pathways are far from mutually exclusive: things that happen in one may profoundly impact another in positive and/ or negative ways. This makes subgroup analyses based on the biological dynamics of the SDOH difficult.

None of this is deterministic. Rather, the committee conceptualizes health equity as a probabilistic challenge, with each element in the model contributing some adjustment to the odds of experiencing healthy development in early life and continued good health across the life course. Each factor contributes a probability that someone experiencing that factor will have good health outcomes; a person's overall odds of experiencing good health are a cumulative function of all of those probabilities. When populations experience different rates of exposure within systems for any reason, their cumulative odds will systematically differ. Even though the odds are not individually predictive—a given person may or may not "beat the odds" and experience any particular outcome—when applied to populations and expressed over time, different odds play out as systematically disparate outcomes between groups of people.

There is also a need to learn from and continuously collect data on both intervention successes and failures to better understand which program elements do or do not work for which subgroup populations. In light of this approach to understanding health equity, more robust measures are needed:

Understanding and measuring cumulative exposure. In this report, the committee identified a number of key factors that impact early-life development, ranging from influences in the microsocial or family environment, such as attachment, nurturing, and maternal well-being, to institutional levers, such as access to prenatal care or effective responses to trauma exposure, to macrosocial forces, such as racism and poverty. There are good tools available to measure exposure to some of these factors, but there are few methods for empirically understanding how exposures to risks or protective factors accumulate and combine over time to establish a cumulative overall risk profile. In the absence of a means to measure cumulative exposure, there is a lack of "math" for how to most effectively intervene when exposures occur.

Understanding the interaction among developmental pathways. Significant gains have been made in understanding how biological processes react to some contextual exposures—for instance, in the areas of science of trauma and toxic stress. However, there are few frameworks for understanding the multidirectional relationship between the biological, social-behavioral, and psychological development of young children. In particular, it is critical to understand how that interaction may vary across the life course in response to changing plasticity of biological systems, different stages of personal and cognitive development, and different life conditions and accumulated experiences in order to build a health equity strategy that puts the right responses in the right places at the right points of optimal potential impact.

Measuring interactions between systems. There are good methods for measuring how distinct elements of systems or policies impact health outcomes—for example, assessing whether systems with a given feature tend to produce better outcomes than systems without it. But understanding the dynamic interplay between systems—how a design decision in health care might interact with an economic policy or early learning curriculum to cumulatively shape the odds of good health—is not as developed. Models that can estimate "integrated risk" by combining key data from across the sectors where people live their lives are needed. Similarly, measures that examine results from cross-sector collaboration can help in documentation and accountability. As an example, school readiness at age 5 reflects both a child's health status and the family's access to basic income and housing, prevention of early adversity through support of maternal well-being, and community early education systems. Other measures, including variability in high school completion, 3rd-grade reading readiness, unemployment, or arrest rates, may hold similar multisector significance as a lens on equity, though more work is needed to understand how measures like these ripple through the health continuum to impact disparities measures within other connected systems.

Improving methods to assess complex causality. As outlined in Recommendation 8-8, perhaps the biggest challenge facing health equity research is that of complex causality. As noted, many of the preferred tools of science, such as RCTs, are designed to control for and isolate single causes rather than embrace complex, interrelated causality that may include multilevel, multidirectional, and nested effects. For example, there needs to be greater exploration of effective community-based intervention approaches that use existing resources (e.g., as in "natural experiments").

CONCLUSION

These measurement needs represent a significant barrier to advancing the understanding of the biological and social pathways by which early life experiences are translated into health inequities, and the committee calls for improved measurement and research methodologies that can advance the state of the science and better inform effective societal responses. However, as noted earlier, there is no reason to wait for the science to solve all of these challenges before taking action. There are systemic disparities in health outcomes between populations, and the groundwork is laid for those disparities in early life. There are many solutions available to start now (see Chapters 4–7 and the system-level recommendations in this chapter). Measuring progress and refining approaches needs to continue, but there is no reason not to deploy the tools that are already available. Chapter 9 summarizes these actions and the key principles discussed in this report that provide a roadmap to advance health equity in preconception through early childhood.

REFERENCES

IOM (Institute of Medicine). 2001. *Improving the quality of long-term care.* Washington, DC: National Academy Press.

Mongeon, M., J. Levi, and J. Heinrich. 2017. *Elements of Accountable Communities for Health: A review of the literature.* NAM Perspectives. Discussion Paper. National Academy of Medicine, Washington, DC. doi: 10.31478/201711a.

NASEM (National Academies of Sciences, Engineering, and Medicine). 2017. *Communities in action: Pathways to health equity.* Washington, DC: The National Academies Press.

Rudolph, L., J. Caplan, K. Ben-Moshe, and L. Dillon. 2013. *Health in All Policies: A guide for state and local governments.* http://www.phi.org/uploads/application/files/udt4vq0y712qpb1o4p62dexjlgxlnogpq15gr8pti3y7ckzysi.pdf (accessed July 12, 2019).

Spencer, A., and F. Bianca. 2016. *Advancing state innovation model goals through Accountable Communities for Health. Center for Healthcare Strategies.* https://www.chcs.org/media/SIM-ACH-Brief_101316_final.pdf (accessed July 12, 2019).

Teutsch, S. M., and M. L. Berger. 2005. Misaligned incentives in America's health: Who's minding the store? *Annals of Family Medicine* 3(6):485–487.

9

A Roadmap for Applying the Science of Early Development

This chapter highlights the main findings and concepts discussed throughout this report and summarizes the report's recommendations to lay out a roadmap for applying and advancing the science of early development. First, the chapter highlights the key big-picture findings gleaned from this report, followed by briefly reviewing the specific actions to be taken within each sector or area based on the report content.

OPPORTUNITIES FOR ACTION

Key Report Findings

The persistence of disparities between groups of people shows that there is more involved in producing them than individual behavioral choices (see Chapter 1 and NASEM, 2017). The factors that drive health disparities from the preconception period through early childhood are complex, interconnected, and systemic; they result from exposures and experiences that children and families encounter throughout their lives, as well as choices they make. These exposures add up over the life course to exert a cumulative effect on health that is probabilistic, not deterministic. That is, the odds of good health are never fixed; individual exposures, experiences, and choices help set and adjust them over time. While groups of people have varying rates of exposure to key adversities and experiences, their distinct contexts shape their choices and opportunities, and thus they have different odds of experiencing good or poor health outcomes over time. For any given child, these odds may or may not lead to a particular health outcome. Applied to groups or populations over time, however, they manifest as health disparities.

To understand how certain subsets of U.S. children (e.g., racial/ethnic minority and low-income children) have heightened risk of exposure to the key drivers of poor health outcomes, the systems in which lives are lived and organized need to be examined. If those systems present different opportunity structures and choices to some groups of children and families, intentionally or not, they may generate health disparities upstream (early in life) even as those same systems might be working to address disparities downstream. Reducing health disparities by addressing their systemic roots is foundational to advance health equity; although it is a substantial challenge, it cannot be ignored.

As discussed in Chapter 8, health equity is a systems challenge. Implementing programs aimed at people in crisis alone will not advance health equity—those programs are important for addressing immediate needs, but until the systemic roots of inequity are addressed, there will likely be another set of crises around the corner.

In assessing the state of the evidence on early-life factors that shape health inequities, the committee developed a conceptual model (see Chapter 1, Figure 1-9) that summarizes the complex considerations that need to be addressed to break this cycle. Inherent in the model are three insights that are foundational to an effective health equity strategy targeted at the early-life period (preconception to early childhood).

The Importance of Intervening Early

The preconception through early-life periods are foundational for healthy development across the life course. Biologically, a number of critical systems are developing, and humans have high plasticity during these life stages. Social-psychological and cognitive development are also important leverage points in the early years of life. Biological and social-psychological developmental pathways interact over the entire life course to set the trajectory for positive health outcomes, but the initial trajectories are established in early life. With the opportunity to play out across an entire life course, even small changes in initial health trajectories can result in large differences in long-term outcomes. Additionally, what happens early in life may impact not only initial health trajectories but how responsive those trajectories are to subsequent efforts to change them later in life—"resiliency" in the face of challenging circumstances. It is generally easier to change health trajectories for the better early on.

The Importance of Addressing Systemic and Structural Factors

This is critical because individual experiences, exposures, and choices are nested within and informed by those factors. The likelihood that a child or family will experience positive or adverse exposures is impacted by the systems they move through in their lives, including microsocial systems such as families or immediate social networks, larger institutional systems such as health care or education, and the cultural and historical forces that shape those institutional systems and experiences within them. In addition to affecting exposures to health-positive or health-negative factors, systems also impact how individuals *respond* to exposures or to interventions designed to mitigate the effects of negative exposures. Individual experiences within systems vary dramatically based on racial, cultural, or other personal characteristics. The effects of these systemic factors are by no means individually deterministic, but they do help set the odds, and when different odds play out over time and across groups of people, they generate systematically different health outcomes. A health equity approach requires systems to change in ways that improve opportunities for good experiences and reduce the odds of adverse exposures for populations that are currently experiencing disparate health outcomes.

The Interconnected Nature of Health Disparities

The systems that influence developmental and health trajectories are profoundly interconnected. The microsocial environment of children's daily lives—families and immediate social networks—is nested within and impacted by the key institutional systems that form the framework of society, and those institutional systems are nested within and impacted by cultural and historical forces that have shaped their essential character. The impact of any one of these systems will inevitably ripple across and shape what happens in others. In terms of the early-life drivers of health inequities, this means that there is no one-sector solution: the root causes are crosscutting, and improving outcomes in one sector is often interdependent on what happens in another. Poor outcomes in the early learning system may have roots in the family environment, which may in turn be shaped by the family's economic circumstances, and may also mean that the family is unable to access needed services in health care or other systems. Complex and interconnected root causes call for comprehensive and crosscutting solutions; one-dimensional strategies are not enough.

What Works?: The Key Elements of a Successful Strategy

The above insights are not meant to suggest that the work being done to improve health outcomes within individual settings is unimportant or somehow reflects inadequate thinking. In fact, a tremendous amount has been learned about what works and what actions need to be taken—enough to identify the key building blocks of a successful strategy for addressing health equity. In this report, the committee examined the evidence to identify "what works" in a number of different critical contexts.

What Works in the Family Environment (Chapter 4)

Supporting the well-being of children starts with supporting the well-being of their caregivers, and strategies designed to reduce children's potential exposure to maltreatment are particularly important. Strategies built to harness existing social resources within a family's environment or community are both cost effective and able to improve the continuity of support systems for caregivers. Context is important: culturally specific or experience-specific processes need to be considered to best respond to families' unique needs in ways that are most likely to engage them, and tiered approaches that recognize the different degrees of risk that families face and offer appropriate resources based on that assessment are more likely to succeed than a one-size-fits-all approach.

What Works in the Health Care System (Chapter 5)

Health care practice, especially in the preconception, prenatal, and pediatric arenas, has not yet caught up to the current science to encompass key advances, such as the life course perspective, the role of adversity, trauma, and the toxic stress response, and the integration of the social determinants of health (SDOH), to transform health care for young families into a system designed to facilitate health production. However, strengthening the content of health care alone will not advance health equity—access to health-enhancing services for all populations by expanding public coverage and addressing nonfinancial barriers to participation will be critical. Furthermore, holding health systems accountable for this shift through changes in equity-focused quality measures and aligned incentives that more comprehensively address health and the risks of poor health will be required. Other necessary actions include transforming the organization, payment, and delivery of health care services to allow for the adoption of integrated, whole-person care models that emphasize a life course approach and address upstream causes of poor health; facilitating the spread of multidisciplinary team-based care; developing trauma-informed systems that can respond effectively when a child is exposed to early-life adversity; and supporting cross-sector partnerships that intentionally connect health care services to the work of partners outside of the health system that are taking the lead to address the SDOH.

What Works in the Early Living Environment (Chapter 6)

It is critically important to provide predictability and security in the lives of children and their families by reducing childhood poverty, ensuring economic stability, and establishing a healthy and safe living environment. Money matters—having resources available to meet basic needs can improve health and reduce health and developmental disparities in early childhood, and public programs that provide resources to those families represent critical investments that "pay off" in the form of better outcomes for children as they enter school healthy and ready to learn and later move into adulthood. However, hinging these benefits on employment or earned income requirements that take caregivers from the home may be counterproductive for families if those requirements increase caregiver stress or hinder opportunities for developing healthy family relations, attachment between mother and child, or breastfeeding. Finally, the critical role of safe, stable, and affordable housing and food security are key determinants of childhood health, as are efforts to prevent and mitigate the impact of exposure to environmental toxicants during the preconception and early childhood periods.

What Works in Early Childhood Education (Chapter 7)

Early childhood education programs play a critical role in ensuring that children are healthy and ready for school life and beyond. It is necessary to incorporate health outcomes and health equity into a comprehensive approach to school readiness, including integrating it into the preparation and training of teachers. Educators—who are critically important caregivers to the children they work with—need adequate compensation and supports for their own health and well-being to ensure their effectiveness in the classroom or learning environment. Family support programs based in the home environment can provide valuable support when aligned with existing early childhood education systems. Last, there is a critical need to address access and affordability of promising models in early childhood education, especially for populations who have historically experienced health inequities.

Roadmap to Advance Health Equity Across the Life Course

In this report, the committee identified knowledge gaps that can be closed with greater investment in biological, behavioral, psychological, intervention, and implementation research. Each of these areas is equally important for addressing the gaps, and the committee recommends multidisciplinary research efforts to bring fresh, new ideas and practical approaches (such as innovative measurements and research methodologies) to advance efforts in tackling head on the serious challenges of health disparities to achieve health equity. The committee emphasized, however, that the great advances in knowledge since the release of *From Neurons to Neighborhoods* (NRC and IOM, 2000) make it very clear that policy makers, health providers, business leaders, and others in the public and private sectors do not need to wait any longer to take action. As the report brings to the fore, there are important opportunities to harness the many promising and evidence-based approaches that have come from advances in the understanding of how to address the neurobiological and socio-behavioral determinants of health disparities. In brief, the roadmap the committee has put forth includes the following key strategies (see Table 9-1):

- **Intervene early:** In most cases, early intervention programs are easier to implement, more effective, and less costly.
- **Support caregivers:** This includes both primary caregivers and caregivers in systems who frequently interact with children and their families.
- **Reform health care system services to promote healthy development:** Redesign the content of preconception, prenatal, postpartum, and pediatric care while ensuring ongoing access, quality, and coordination.
- **Create supportive and stable early living conditions:**
  o **Reduce child poverty and address economic and food security,**
  o **Provide stable and safe housing, and**
  o **Eliminate exposure to environmental toxicants.**
- **Maximize the potential of early care and education to promote health outcomes.**
- **Implement initiatives across systems to support children, families, other caregivers, and communities:** Ensure trauma-informed systems, build a diverse and supported workforce, and align strategies that work across sectors.
- **Integrate and coordinate resources across the education, social services, criminal justice, and health care systems, and make them available to translate science to action.**

It is the committee's hope that this roadmap will catalyze the steps that need to be taken across systems to close the health equity gap and improve the lives of the nation's children.

TABLE 9-1 Roadmap to Apply the Science of Early Development[a]

Roadmap	Specific Action	Who
Intervene early	Implement programs that ensure families have access to high-quality, cost-effective community programs, including interventions to foster strong attachments and group-based supports in communities (Recommendation 4-4)	Federal, state, tribal, territorial, and local policy makers; philanthropic organizations
	Routinely track levels of risk among mothers and children over time using periodic assessments (Recommendation 4-5)	Health care providers
Support caregivers	Strengthen and expand evidence-based home visiting programs (Recommendation 4-3)	Federal policy makers; HRSA; ACF; federal, state, territorial, tribal, and local agencies overseeing program implementation
	Implement paid parental leave (Recommendation 6-1)	Federal, state, tribal, territorial, and local policy makers
Reform health care system services to promote healthy development	Increase access to preconception, prenatal, postpartum, and pediatric health care (Recommendation 5-1)	HHS; Medicaid agencies; public and private payers; federal, state, local, tribal, and territorial policy makers
	Expand accountability and improve quality of preconception, prenatal, postpartum, and pediatric care (Recommendation 5-2)	Public and private payers; HRSA, CDC, CMS, perinatal and pediatric quality collaboratives, and health care–related workforce development entities
	Adopt policies and practices that improve the organization and integration of care systems from preconception through pediatric care and that focus on the caregiver and child together as the unit of care (Recommendation 5-3)	HHS; state Medicaid agencies; health systems leaders; federal, state, tribal, and territorial policy makers
	Transform preconception, prenatal, postpartum, and pediatric health care to address the root causes of poor health and well-being (Recommendation 5-4)	HHS; public and private payers; medical accreditation bodies; WPSI, Bright Futures, ACOG, AAP, AAFP, and others

continued

TABLE 9-1 Continued

Roadmap	Specific Action	Who
Create supportive and stable early living conditions • Address economic, food, and housing security • Eliminate exposure to environmental toxicants	Reduce barriers to participation to WIC and SNAP benefits; do not tie these benefits to parent employment for families with young children or for pregnant women (Recommendation 6-2)	Federal, state, tribal, territorial, and local policy makers
	Increase the supply of high-quality affordable housing that is available to families (Recommendation 6-3)	Federal, state, tribal, territorial, and local agencies
	Develop a comprehensive plan to ensure access to stable, affordable, and safe housing in the prenatal through early childhood periods (Recommendation 6-4)	Secretary of the HHS in collaboration with HUD and other relevant agencies
	Test new Medicaid payment models that engage providers and other community organizations in addressing housing safety concerns, especially those focused on young children (Recommendation 6-5)	Center for Medicare & Medicaid Innovation
	Address the critical gaps between family resources and family needs through a combination of benefits that have the best evidence of advancing health equity, such as SNAP benefits, increased housing assistance, and a basic allowance for young children (Recommendation 6-6)	Federal, state, tribal, and territorial policy makers
	Support and enforce efforts to prevent and mitigate the impact of environmental toxicants during the preconception through early childhood periods (Recommendations 6-7, 6-8, and 6-9)	Federal, state, territorial, tribal, and local governments; CDC, EPA, FDA, the U.S. Consumer Product Safety Commission; health care providers

TABLE 9-1 Continued

Roadmap	Specific Action	Who
Maximize the potential of ECE to promote health outcomes	Develop a comprehensive approach to school readiness that explicitly incorporates health outcomes and leverages ECE systems and programs, including home visiting (Recommendation 7-1)	Federal, state, local, tribal, and territorial governments and other public agencies (e.g., school districts, city governments, public–private partnerships); Office of Child Care and Office of Head Start; health and human service entities, the federal Early Learning Interagency Policy Board, state Early Childhood Advisory Councils, and federal, state, local, tribal, and territorial agencies; HHS; OPRE; ED
	Develop and strengthen coursework or practicums that focus on competencies of educators, principals, and ECE program directors that are critical to children's health, school readiness, and life success (Recommendation 7-2)	Degree granting institutions, professional preparation programs, providers of ongoing professional learning opportunities
	Develop and implement a strategic plan to (1) improve the quality of ECE programs by adopting health-promoting standards and (2) expand access to comprehensive, high-quality, and affordable ECE programs across multiple settings (Recommendation 7-3)	Federal, state, tribal, and territorial policy makers in coordination with HHS, the Office of Head Start, and Office of Child Care
Implement initiatives across systems to support children, families, and other caregivers	Develop cross-sector initiatives that align strategies to address barriers to data sharing and integration, cross-sector financing, and other challenges to cross-sector collaboration (Recommendation 8-1)	For all actions in this section: policy makers and leaders in the health care, public health, social service, criminal justice, ECE/education, and other sectors who frequently interact with children and their families
	Enhance detection of early-life adversity and improve response systems (Recommendation 8-2)	
	Develop trauma-informed systems (Recommendation 8-3)	
	Build a diverse, culturally informed workforce in all relevant systems (Recommendation 8-4)	

continued

TABLE 9-1 Continued

Roadmap	Specific Action	Who
	Improve access to programs and policies across systems that provide parental or caregiver supports and help build or promote family attachments and functioning. For families with intensive support needs, develop programs or initiatives designed to provide comprehensive wraparound services (Recommendation 8-5)	
	Integrate care and services across the health continuum, including the adoption of models that provide comprehensive support for the whole person by leveraging and connecting existing community resources (Recommendation 8-6)	
Resources need to be integrated and coordinated to translate science to action	Support payment reform to allow for upstream investment (Recommendation 8-7)	Policy makers and leaders in the health care, public health, social service, criminal justice, ECE/education, and other sectors who frequently interact with children and their families

NOTE: AAFP = American Academy of Family Physicians; AAP = American Academy of Pediatrics; ACF = Administration for Children and Families; ACOG = American College of Obstetricians and Gynecologists; CDC = Centers for Disease Control and Prevention; CMS = Centers for Medicare & Medicaid Services; ECE = early care and education; ED = U.S. Department of Education; EPA = U.S. Environmental Protection Agency; FDA = U.S. Food and Drug Administration; HHS = U.S. Department of Health and Human Services; HRSA = Health Resources and Services Administration; HUD = U.S. Department of Housing and Urban Development; OPRE = Office of Planning, Research & Evaluation; SNAP = Supplemental Nutrition Assistance Program; WIC = Special Supplemental Nutrition Program for Women, Infants, and Children; WPSI = Women's Preventative Services Initiative.

[a] Some of these actions fit in more than one category but are only listed once; this table does not include recommendations from this report that are solely research based.

REFERENCES

NASEM (National Academies of Sciences, Engineering, and Medicine). 2017. *Communities in action: Pathways to health equity.* Washington, DC: The National Academies Press.
NRC and IOM (National Research Council and Institute of Medicine). 2000. *From neurons to neighborhoods: The science of early childhood development.* Washington, DC: National Academy Press.

A

Criteria for Selecting Promising Models

The below criteria are adapted from the 2017 National Academies report *Communities in Action: Pathways to Health Equity* (NASEM, 2017) that this report is building from per the committee Statement of Task. The criteria were used to identify promising models from the prenatal through early childhood phases to highlight in this report. The committee did not evaluate the overall effectiveness of these efforts; rather, it used these promising models as examples throughout the report to highlight bright spots that have been able to use what is known from the science to advance health equity in the preconception through early childhood periods. Furthermore, "promising" does not imply that the model is new but rather that it is a program or intervention that met the committee's core criteria, and each promising model has a unique approach and is at a different phase of development: some have been around for more than 30 years and have changed based on evaluations or input from users, while others have emerged in the past few years. These examples are not blueprints, and exact replicas might not work with all populations or locations, but the lessons learned and approaches used are valuable to those working to create positive change toward health equity during the preconception through early childhood periods. See Chapter 1 for more details.

This report applied three sets of criteria:

1. **Core criteria:** These function like inclusion criteria (i.e., to be included for consideration, the examples need to meet each of the six core criteria).

2. **Aspirational criteria:** The examples need to meet at least one, and preferably more, of the aspirational criteria.
3. **Contextual criteria:** These criteria are applied to the examples that meet the six core criteria and a number of the aspirational criteria to ensure that the examples are diverse in terms of communities/populations, approaches to solutions, and other characteristics.

Set 1: Core Criteria

1. It focuses on preconception/prenatal and/or early childhood (whether intervention is focused on children or caregivers in their lives).
2. It is informed by findings from the neurobiological, closed-behavioral, and/or biological sciences.
3. It addresses at least one, preferably more, of the nine social determinants of health identified in the 2017 National Academies report (health systems and services, education, employment, the physical environment, the social environment, housing, income and wealth, public safety, and transportation) (NASEM, 2017).
4. It is designed to have or has evidence of having an impact on a group or population that experiences health inequities.
5. It is multisectoral (i.e., at least two sectors engaged).
6. It includes an assessment of evidence, including data or best available information, to
    a. identify a problem and
    b. develop a solution that has a measurable outcome that there are plans to measure.

Set 2: Aspirational Criteria

1. It includes nontraditional partners and/or nonhealth domains.
    Note: This is meant to be inclusive of nontraditional partners for communities to engage that may not necessarily be sectors (i.e., community organizers, parent–teacher association groups).
2. It is interdisciplinary.
    a. The solution draws on multiple sources, including practice-based experience and research from multiple disciplines.
3. It is multilevel—the intervention has multiple levels of influence, such as individual, family, organizational/institutional, or governmental.
    Note: This does not mean that a solution must target each of these levels.

4. It has a strong evaluation plan in place, including relevant measures to track the impact of the intervention.

5. It documents what it is trying to achieve, why that is important, how it plans to achieve the desired outcome (i.e., a theory of change), and/or the mechanisms being targeted based on scientific evidence.

6. It includes a plan for sustainability, including consideration of
   a. Long-term strategy and structure;
   b. Funding, operating costs, resources, etc.;
   c. Efficient use of resources;
   d. Potential cost savings realized or return on investment;
   e. Increased community capacity to shape outcomes;
   f. Building the next generation of leaders; and
   g. Clear policy solutions/changes at the local, state, or federal levels to support or scale a promising intervention or strategy.

7. It has transferable key elements[1] that could practically be applied or adapted to similar contexts in order to scale impact.

8. It incorporates the evidence required of proposed intervention(s):
   a. It addresses a significant health disparity (or disparities) based on data of a documented need or problem and data showing impact on at least one proximal or distal measure of a health disparity.
   b. The actual or projected health benefits are substantial/ meaningful to the population(s) and community as a whole (not just statistically significant).
   c. There is ongoing data collection of processes and outcomes (flexibility in terms of what type of data is generated and applied).
   d. There is one or more high- or moderate-quality impact study of the approach.
   Note: This includes health outcomes in a broad sense, related to social determinants (e.g., 3rd-grade reading level rates) that are strongly linked to health outcomes.

9. The implementation process is well documented, including
   a. The key elements and subtleties of how the solution is contributing to success (not referring to legal documents/individual health data);
   b. Performance measurement;

---

[1] Key elements are the functions or principles and activities of the solution that are necessary to achieve similar outcomes.

c. Particular practice (training, supervisory);
d. Funding;
e. Regulatory context; and
f. Political context.
10. It is community-driven or informed: engagement with the community is evident preintervention and incorporated in the solution or the solution is initiated by the community/a community group/local government.
11. The solution is freely available to the community and not a proprietary resource.

Set 3: Contextual Criteria

As a whole, the set of examples selected will

1. Address a range of the nine determinants of health identified in the 2017 National Academies report (health systems and services, education, employment, the physical environment, the social environment, housing, income and wealth, public safety, and transportation).
2. Reflect rural, suburban, and urban contexts.
3. Reflect diversity in several of the following population characteristics:
   a. Race,
   b. Ethnicity,
   c. Age,
   d. Gender identity,
   e. Sexual orientation status,
   f. Socioeconomic status,
   g. Disability status, or
   h. Other statuses (e.g., documentation status).
4. Include solutions that require changes in the systems or policies within which the solution was implemented and those that did not require changes in systems or policies to be effective.
5. Reflect various levels of political engagement.

REFERENCE

NASEM (National Academies of Sciences, Engineering, and Medicine). 2017. *Communities in action: Pathways to health equity*. Washington, DC: The National Academies Press.

B

Public Meeting Agendas

MEETING 1

Thursday, May 31, 2018
Keck Center of the National Academies,
500 Fifth Street, NW,
Washington, DC 20001

11:35 am–12:15 pm   **Presentation of the Statement of Task,**
                        Background, and Discussion
                        Dwayne Proctor, Ph.D., *Senior Adviser to the*
                        President, Robert Wood Johnson Foundation

12:15 pm   **ADJOURN**

MEETING 2

Monday, August 6, 2018
Keck Center of the National Academies,
500 Fifth Street, NW,
Washington, DC 20001

8:30 am   **Attendee Check-In Outside Room 100**

9:00–9:15 am   **Welcome and Opening Remarks**
                     Jennifer E. DeVoe, M.D., D.Phil. (*Chair*),
                     Oregon Health & Science University
                     Victor J. Dzau, M.D., *President, National
                     Academy of Medicine* (via video)

9:15–9:55 am   **Opening Presentation—Early Childhood Seen
                     Through a Health Equity Lens**
                     Paula Braveman, M.D., M.P.H., *University of
                     California, San Francisco*

                     Discussion
                     Moderator: Myra Parker, J.D., Ph.D.,
                     Committee member

9:55–10:55 am   **Panel 1: Translating Early Development
                     Science into Interventions and Policies
                     Gene–Environment Interactions: Role in
                     Susceptibility and Resilience**
                     Fernando Martinez, M.D., *University of
                     Arizona College of Medicine*

                     **Translating Scientific Knowledge into
                     Action on Early Childhood Development**
                     Phil Fisher, Ph.D., *University of Oregon*

                     Discussion
                     Moderator: Pat Levitt, Ph.D., *Committee member*

10:55–11:10 am   **BREAK**

11:10 am–12:45 pm   **Panel 2: Approaches to Promote Healthy
                     Development During the Prenatal and Early
                     Childhood Phases
                     Early Childhood Innovation Network:
                     Moving from Science to Action**
                     Sarah Barclay Hoffman, M.P.P.,
                     Early Childhood Innovation Network

                     **All Children Thrive: A Learning Network to
                     Promote Child Health Equity in Cincinnati**
                     Robert Kahn, M.D., M.P.H., *Cincinnati
                     Children's Hospital*

The First 1,000 Days on Medicaid Initiative: A Medicaid-Driven, Cross-Sector Approach to Improving Child Outcomes
Suzanne C. Brundage, M.S., *Children's Health Initiative, United Hospital Fund*

The MOMS® Partnership: Partnering with Communities to Use Neurobiological and Socio-Behavioral Sciences to Address Maternal Depression
Megan Smith, Dr.P.H., M.P.H., *MOMS Partnership, Yale School of Medicine*

Discussion
Moderator: Iheoma Iruka, Ph.D., *Committee member*
Discussant: Lee Beers, M.D., *Children's National Health System*

12:45–1:45 pm	**LUNCH** *(lunch is not provided but can be purchased in the cafeteria located on the third floor)*
1:45–2:55 pm	**Panel 3: Policy and Systems Changes for Prenatal–Early Childhood Development**

Leveraging the Science of Early Development: Creating Systems to Help Children Thrive
Neal Halfon, M.D., M.P.H., *University of California, Los Angeles, Fielding School of Public Health*

Social Determinants of Health Interventions, Fatherhood, and Reproductive Health
Milton Kotelchuck, Ph.D., *Harvard University Medical School*

Discussion
Moderator: Albert Wat, M.A., *Committee member*

2:55–3:35 pm	**Closing Presentation—The Next Step in Evidence-Based Policy: Implementing and Evaluating Universal Programs**

Ron Haskins, Ph.D., *The Brookings Institution*

Discussion
Moderator: Cynthia García Coll, Ph.D.,
Committee member

Public Comment

3:35–4:00 pm

Please add your name to the public comment sign-in sheet at the registration desk if you are interested in providing brief remarks to the committee.

4:00 pm   **ADJOURN**

MEETING 3

**Monday, October 1, 2018
Beckman Center of the National Academies,
100 Academy Way,
Irvine, CA 92617**

8:00–8:05 am   **Welcome and Opening Remarks**
Jennifer E. DeVoe, M.D., D.Phil. (*Chair*),
Oregon Health & Science University

8:05–9:05 am   **Panel 1: Translating Early Development Science into Interventions**
Greg Miller, Ph.D., M.A., *Northwestern University*
Greg Duncan, Ph.D., *University of California, Irvine*

Discussion

9:05–10:20 am   **Panel 2: Policy Perspectives on Prenatal and Early Childhood Development**
Representative Ruth Kagi, *Washington House of Representatives*
Senator Elizabeth Steiner Hayward,
Oregon Senate
Bobby Cagle, M.S.W., *Los Angeles County Department of Children and Family Services*
Senator David Wilson, *Alaska Senate*

Discussion

10:20–10:35 am	**BREAK**

10:35 am–12:00 pm **Panel 3: Approaches to Promote Healthy Development During the Prenatal and Early Childhood Phases**
Jessica Pizarek, M.A., *PolicyLink*
Helena Sabala, *Chula Vista Promise Neighborhood*
Anne Mauricio, Ph.D., M.A., *Family Check-up, Arizona State University*
Elisa Nicholas, M.D., M.S.P.H., *The Children's Clinic, Serving Children and Their Families*

12:00–1:00 pm **Panel 4: Caregiver Perspectives**
Ana De Jesus, *Caregiver*
Abraham Gomez, *Caregiver*
Shalice Gosey, *Caregiver*
Lori Hernandez, *Caregiver*
Yesenia Manzo-Meda, *Caregiver*
Maria Rodgers, *Caregiver*

Discussion
Discussants:
Patricia McKenna, *SHIELDS for Families*
Reggie Van Appelen, *SHIELDS for Families*
Jennifer Eich, *Western Youth Services*
Alexa Bach, *Network Anaheim*

1:00–1:15 pm **Public Comment**

1:15 pm **ADJOURN**

C

Committee Biographical Sketches

Jennifer E. DeVoe, M.D., D.Phil. (*Chair*), is chair of and Saultz Endowed Professor in the Department of Family Medicine at Oregon Health & Science University (OHSU). As a practicing family physician and doctorally trained health services researcher, Dr. DeVoe studies access to health care, disparities in care, and the impact of practice and policy interventions on vulnerable populations. Her research portfolio spans both OHSU Family Medicine and OCHIN, Inc., a national community health information network based in Portland, Oregon. Dr. DeVoe leads a multidisciplinary research team with expertise in informatics, sociology, epidemiology, biostatistics, economics, primary care, mental health, health services research, clinical medicine, health care disparities, and anthropology. Dr. DeVoe is the senior research advisor at OCHIN, where she previously served as chief research officer and executive director of its practice-based research network of community health centers from 2010 to 2016. Dr. DeVoe is a principal investigator (PI) or co-investigator on numerous research studies funded by the Patient-Centered Outcomes Research Institute; the Agency for Healthcare Research and Quality; the National Cancer Institute; and the National Heart, Lung, and Blood Institute with nearly $20 million in active grant funding. She also serves as co-PI of the ADVANCE Clinical Data Research Network, part of PCORnet, which is "horizontally" integrating electronic health record data, creating a unique community laboratory to include disadvantaged and vulnerable patients across the country. She holds joint appointments in the OHSU Department of Medical Informatics and Clinical

Epidemiology and the Kaiser Permanente Northwest Center for Health Research. She also serves on the National Core Team for Family Medicine for America's Health Board of Directors and is past president of the North American Primary Care Research Group. She was elected to the National Academy of Medicine (NAM) in 2014. Dr. DeVoe served as an NAM Puffer/American Board of Family Medicine anniversary fellow from 2012 to 2014, and she was on the National Academies' Committee on Accessible and Affordable Hearing Health Care for Adults from 2015 to 2016. Dr. DeVoe earned her M.D. from Harvard Medical School in 1999. Selected as a Rhodes Scholar in 1996, she also earned an M.Phil. and a D.Phil. from Oxford University in 1998 and 2001, respectively. She completed her family medicine residency at OHSU in 2004 and earned an M.C.R. from OHSU in 2010.

Cynthia García Coll, Ph.D., is currently an adjunct professor in the Pediatrics Department at the University of Puerto Rico Medical School and the Charles Pitts Robinson and John Palmer Barstow Professor Emerita at Brown University. Previously, Dr. García Coll was a professor in the clinical Ph.D. program and associate director of the Institutional Center for Scientific Research at Albizu University in San Juan, Puerto Rico. Prior to moving back to Puerto Rico, she spent 30 years at Brown University. Her research focuses on the interplay of sociocultural and biological influences on child development, with particular emphasis on at-risk and minority populations. She received her Ph.D. in personality and developmental psychology from Harvard University. Dr. García Coll has served on the editorial boards of many leading academic journals, including as the senior editor of *Child Development and Developmental Psychology*. She is a fellow of the American Psychological Association and the Association for Psychological Science. She has received awards from Tufts University and Brown University, the Erikson Institute, the Society for Developmental and Behavioral Pediatrics, the Society for Research in Child Development (SRCD), and Progreso Latino. She has been on the governing boards of the United Way of Rhode Island, Rhode Island Community Foundation, SRCD, Society for the Study of Human Development, and Foundation of Child Development. She also served as member and chair of the Young Scholars Program at the William T. Grant Foundation for 11 years. Her research has been funded by the National Institutes of Health, the McArthur Foundation, the William T. Grant Foundation, and the Spencer Foundation.

Elizabeth E. Davis, Ph.D., is a professor of applied economics at the University of Minnesota and recently served as a member of the National Academies' Committee on Financing Early Care and Education with a

Highly Qualified Workforce. Dr. Davis conducts research in economics and public policy related to low-income families, child care and early education, and low-wage and rural labor markets in the United States. Her recent research has focused on disparities in access to high-quality child care, including development of new measures of access that are family centered and take cost, proximity, and quality into account. Other studies on early childhood topics have examined the role of child care subsidies in families' decisions about employment and the type, quality, and stability of child care arrangements. In related work, she has examined the dynamics of participation in child care subsidy programs in Maryland, Minnesota, and Oregon and advised state and federal agencies on child care subsidy policy. Her other research has examined the impact of local competition on wages and job turnover in the retail food industry, income equality, and the relationship between local labor market conditions and employment outcomes for disadvantaged workers. Dr. Davis earned her Ph.D. and M.A. in economics from the University of Michigan, Ann Arbor.

Nadine Burke Harris, M.D., M.P.H., FAAP, is the first Surgeon General of California (appointed February 2019). Before her appointment, Dr. Burke Harris was the chief executive officer (CEO) of the Center for Youth Wellness. She is a pioneer in the field of medicine, dedicated to changing the way society responds to one of the most serious, expensive, and widespread public health crises of our time: childhood trauma. As founder and CEO of the Center, Dr. Burke Harris has brought this critical work to stages at the Mayo Clinic, American Academy of Pediatrics (AAP), The Aspen Institute, and Partnership for a Healthier America. Her TED Talk, "How Childhood Trauma Affects Health Across a Lifetime," has been viewed more than 3.8 million times. Her work has been profiled in best-selling books, including *How Children Succeed* by Paul Tough and *Hillbilly Elegy* by J. D. Vance, as well as in Jamie Redford's feature film *Resilience*. It has also been featured on CNN, NPR, and Fox News and in *USA Today* and *The New York Times*. Dr. Burke Harris wrote a book on the issue of childhood adversity and health called *The Deepest Well: Healing the Long-Term Effects of Childhood Adversity*, which released in January 2018. Dr. Burke Harris received the Arnold P. Gold Foundation Humanism in Medicine Award, presented by AAP, and the Heinz Award for the Human Condition. Additionally, she serves as an expert advisor to the Too Small to Fail initiative and as a member of AAP's National Advisory Board for Screening.

Iheoma U. Iruka, Ph.D., is the chief research innovation officer and director of the Center for Early Education Research and Evaluation at High-Scope Educational Research Foundation. Prior to joining HighScope, she was at the Buffet Early Childhood Institute at the University of Nebraska and the Frank Porter Graham Child Development Institute at the University of North Carolina at Chapel Hill. Dr. Iruka's research focuses on determining how early experiences impact the learning and development of low-income and ethnic minority children and the role of the family and education environments and systems. She is engaged in projects and initiatives focused on how evidence-informed policies, systems, and practices in early education can support the optimal development and experiences of low-income, ethnic minority, and immigrant children, such as through family engagement and support, quality rating and improvement systems, and early care and education systems and programs. She is co–principal investigator for the Institute of Education Sciences–funded Early Learning Network, Nebraska Site, a large-scale and far-reaching study aimed at identifying malleable factors that support early learning in preschool through 3rd grade that may be effective at closing the achievement gap for disadvantaged students. In particular, she has been engaged in addressing how to best ensure excellence for young diverse learners, especially black children, such as through development of a classroom observation measure, public policies, and publications geared toward early education practitioners and policy makers. She has served on numerous national boards and committees, including the National Academies' Committee on Supporting the Parents of Young Children and the National Research Conference on Early Childhood. Dr. Iruka has a B.A. in psychology from Temple University, an M.A. in psychology from Boston University, and a Ph.D. in applied developmental psychology from the University of Miami.

Pat R. Levitt, Ph.D., is the chief scientific officer, vice president, and director of the Saban Research Institute. He is also a professor of Pediatrics, the Simms/Mann Chair in Developmental Neurogenetics at Children's Hospital Los Angeles, and the W.M. Keck Provost Professor in Neurogenetics at the Keck School of Medicine of the University of Southern California. He is the chief scientific officer for Children's Hospital Los Angeles. Dr. Levitt has held leadership positions at the University of Pittsburgh, Vanderbilt University, and the University of Southern California. In 2013, Dr. Levitt was elected to the National Academy of Medicine. Named a McKnight Foundation Scholar in 2002, Dr. Levitt also was a MERIT awardee from the National Institute of Mental Health and served as a member of its National Advisory Mental Health Council. He is an elected fellow of the American Association for the Advancement of Science, serving as the Neuroscience Section Chair in 2014–2015, and an elected member of the Dana Alliance for Brain Initiatives. He is a senior fellow at the Center on the Developing Child at Harvard University and serves as co–scientific director of the National Scientific Council on the Developing Child, a policy council that brings the best research from child development and neuroscience to assist policy makers and business leaders in making wise program investment decisions. He is a member of scientific advisory boards for several foundations and university programs and currently serves as editor-in-chief of *Mind, Brain, and Education* and on several editorial boards. Dr. Levitt's research program includes basic and clinical studies to identify the genetic and environmental factors that ensure healthy development of the brain architecture that controls learning and emotional and social behavior. His clinical research studies address how toxic stress responses in infants and toddlers may be detected as early as possible to promote resilience and better prevention, and children with autism who also have co-occurring medical conditions, such as gastrointestinal disorders. Dr. Levitt has published 295 scientific papers and made hundreds of academic and public presentations. He received his B.A. in biological sciences from The University of Chicago and a Ph.D. in neuroscience from the University of California, San Diego. He completed a postdoctoral fellowship in neuroscience at Yale University.

Michael C. Lu, M.D., M.S., M.P.H., is the dean of the University of California (UC), Berkeley's School of Public Health (term began in July 2019). Before his appointment, Dr. Lu was a professor and the senior associate dean for academic, student, and faculty affairs at The George Washington (GW) University Milken Institute School of Public Health. Prior to joining GW, Dr. Lu was the director of the Maternal and Child Health Bureau for the U.S. Department of Health and Human Services from 2012 to 2017. During his tenure, Dr. Lu transformed key federal programs in maternal and child health, launched major initiatives to reduce maternal, infant, and child mortality in the United States, and received the prestigious Herbert H. Humphrey Award for Service to America. Dr. Lu joined the federal government from the UC Los Angeles Schools of Medicine and Public Health, where he held a joint faculty appointment in obstetrics-gynecology and community health sciences for nearly 15 years. He was best known for his research on racial/ethnic disparities in birth outcomes and his leadership in developing, testing, and translating a theory on the origins of maternal and child health disparities based on the life course perspective. Dr. Lu has served on two Institute of Medicine (IOM) committees: Committee to Reexamine IOM Pregnancy Weight Guidelines and Committee on Understanding Premature Birth and Assuring Healthy Outcomes. Dr. Lu received his B.A. in political science and human biology from Stanford University, an M.A. in health and medical sciences and public health from UC Berkeley, a medical degree from UC San Francisco, and his residency training in obstetrics and gynecology from UC Irvine.

Suniya S. Luthar, Ph.D., is a Foundation Professor of Psychology at Arizona State University and professor emerita at Columbia University's Teachers College. Dr. Luthar's research involves vulnerability and resilience among various populations, including youth in poverty, families affected by mental illness, mothers under stress, and teens in high-achieving, affluent communities (who reflect high rates of symptoms relative to national norms). Previously, she served on the faculty of the Department of Psychiatry and the Child Study Center at Yale University and then at Columbia University's Teachers College. Dr. Luthar is a fellow of the American Association for Psychological Science and American Psychological Association (APA) Divisions 7 and 37. She received the Boyd McCandless Young Scientist Award from APA, a Research Scientist Development (K) Award from the National Institutes of Health (NIH), an American Mensa Foundation Award for Excellence in Research on Intelligence, and an award for Integrity and Mentorship from the Society for Research in Child Development's Asian Caucus. Dr. Luthar's work is frequently cited in major news outlets in the United States, including *The New York Times, The Washington Post, The Wall Street Journal, The Atlantic,* NPR, PBS, and CNN, as well as overseas. Dr. Luthar has served as chair of a grant review study section at NIH and a member of the Governing Council of the Society for Research on Child Development. At APA, she served on the Committee on Socioeconomic Status and its Council of Representatives, and she is currently president of Division 7 (Developmental). Dr. Luthar received her B.S. and M.S. from Delhi University in 1978 and 1980, respectively, and her Ph.D. (Distinction) in developmental/clinical psychology from Yale University in 1990.

Amy Rohling McGee, M.S.W., has served as the president of the Health Policy Institute of Ohio, a nonpartisan, independent, nonprofit organization that provides information and analysis to state policy makers, since 2010. Her prior public-sector experience includes work in the executive branch of state government focused on policy related to issues such as health insurance, health system improvement, health information technology, and Medicaid. She served in the state legislature as a Legislative Service Commission intern in the mid-1990s. Her private-sector experience includes 5 years as the executive director of the Ohio Association of Free Clinics, representing health clinics that served the uninsured, primarily through volunteers, and several years in a management position at FIRSTLINK (now HandsOn Central Ohio). Ms. McGee earned her B.A. and M.A. from The Ohio State University. She has received the Business First "Forty under Forty" award and The Ohio State University Alumni Association William Oxley Thompson award.

Myra Parker, Ph.D., J.D. (Mandan-Hidatsa-Cree) is an assistant professor in the Center for the Studies of Health and Risk Behavior, Department of Psychiatry and Behavioral Sciences, University of Washington School of Medicine. She also works at the Indigenous Wellness Research Institute at the University of Washington School of Social Work. Dr. Parker has worked for more than 10 years on tribal public health program implementation and coordination with tribal communities in Arizona, Idaho, and Washington and tribal colleges and universities across the United States. She has more than 5 years of experience in tribal public health research. Prior to embarking on a career in research, Dr. Parker worked for 5 years in the policy arena within the Arizona state government, in tribal governments, and with tribal working groups at the state and national levels. Her research experience in public health involves community-based participatory research, cultural adaptation of evidence-based interventions, and disparities research. She received a Robert Wood Johnson Foundation New Connections Junior Investigator grant in 2011, 1 year into her postdoctoral fellowship. Dr. Parker's research on this project focused on alcohol-related fatalities and tribal cross-jurisdictional agreements with local non-Native communities. She has provided trainings to tribal health department staff, tribal research teams, and urban Indian service delivery teams. She has also provided indigenous health research training to University of Washington students, from undergraduates through Ph.D. students. As an enrolled member of the Mandan and Hidatsa tribes, she is aware of the historical health practices and misconduct perpetuated on tribes and other minority and disenfranchised populations in the United States. Her background in law and policy has informed a broader understanding of the principles of ethics and honed her skills in identifying methods to address the disparities in research control and access through the use of formalized agreements. She has experience in working with tribes in their ongoing efforts to balance the collective rights of communities and individuals. Dr. Parker received her B.A. in human biology from Stanford University. She received a J.D. from the James E. Rogers College of Law at the University of Arizona in 2001, with an emphasis in federal Indian law. She received her M.A. in public health from the Mel and Enid Zuckerman School of Public Health at the University of Arizona in 2002. Dr. Parker graduated with a Ph.D. in health services from the University of Washington School of Public Health in 2010.

James M. Perrin, M.D., is a professor of pediatrics at Harvard Medical School, the former director of the Division of General Pediatrics at the Massachusetts General Hospital (MGH) for Children, and the associate chair of pediatrics for research at MGH. His research has examined asthma, middle ear disease, children's hospitalization, health insurance, and childhood chronic illness and disabilities, with recent emphases on the epidemiology of childhood chronic illness and organization of services for the care of children and adolescents with chronic health conditions. Dr. Perrin holds the John C. Robinson, MD, Chair in Pediatrics; founded the MGH Center for Child and Adolescent Health Policy (a multidisciplinary research and training center with an active fellowship program in general pediatrics); and directed the center for more than 15 years. He is former president of the American Academy of Pediatrics, former chair of its Committee on Children with Disabilities, past president of the Ambulatory (Academic) Pediatric Association, and founding editor-in-chief of its journal, *Academic Pediatrics*. He also directed the Evidence Working Group reporting to the Maternal and Child Health Bureau for the Secretary's Advisory Committee on Heritable Disorders and Genetic Diseases in Newborns and Children. Dr. Perrin was elected to the National Academy of Medicine in 2016. He currently serves on the Board on Children, Youth, and Families and has previously served on the National Academies' Committee on Improving Health Outcomes for Children with Disabilities and Committee to Evaluate the Supplemental Security Income Disability Program for Children with Mental Disorders, as well as earlier committees on long-term care quality, disability in the United States, and the evaluation of federal health care quality activities. Dr. Perrin earned his A.B. from Harvard College and his M.D. from Case Western Reserve University School of Medicine. He had his residency and fellowship training at the University of Rochester.

Natalie Slopen, Sc.D., M.A., is an assistant professor in the Department of Epidemiology and Biostatistics at the University of Maryland, College Park, School of Public Health. Dr. Slopen's research focuses on social influences on health, health disparities, and psychological and biological mechanisms through which childhood experiences are embedded to increase risk for later chronic diseases. The overarching goal of her research is to identify processes and conditions that can be targeted by interventions in order to reduce health disparities and promote health over the life course. Dr. Slopen completed her Master of Arts in Social Sciences at The University of Chicago, her Doctorate of Science in Social Epidemiology at the Harvard T.H. Chan School of Public Health, and her postdoctoral fellowship training at the Center on the Developing Child at Harvard University.

Albert Wat, M.A., is a senior policy director at the Alliance for Early Success, where he supports the organization's strategy and goals for early education, including increasing access to high-quality pre-kindergarten (pre-K), improving the early learning workforce, and enhancing alignment with K–12 policies. Before joining the Alliance, Mr. Wat was a senior policy analyst in the Education Division of the National Governors Association (NGA) Center for Best Practices, where he helped governors' staff and advisors improve their early care and education policies from early childhood through 3rd grade. Prior to NGA, Mr. Wat was the research manager at Pre-K Now, an advocacy campaign at the Pew Center on the States, where he authored a number of policy reports, managed research activities for the initiative, and provided analysis and information about the latest pre-K and early education research and policy developments to Pre-K Now staff and its network of state partners. In 2014, Mr. Wat served on the Institute of Medicine and National Research Council's Committee on the Science of Children Birth to Age 8: Deepening and Broadening the Foundation for Success, which released the report *Transforming the Workforce for Children Birth Through Age 8: A Unifying Foundation* in April 2015. He also serves on the board of the Council for Professional Recognition. Mr. Wat has worked with schools, school reform nonprofits, and community-based organizations in the San Francisco Bay Area, southeastern Michigan, and Washington, DC. He holds a B.A. in psychology, an M.A. in education from Stanford University, and an M.A. in education policy from The George Washington University.

Bill J. Wright, Ph.D., is the director of the Center for Outcomes Research and Education, an organization devoted to conducting innovative health policy and health services research in support of health care transformation, with an emphasis on the social determinants of health. As a sociologist whose primary emphasis is on longitudinal survey research on vulnerable or underserved populations, Dr. Wright has led the design and implementation of numerous panel studies assessing the impacts of health systems and policy changes on historically underserved or excluded communities. Dr. Wright was a principal investigator on the Oregon Health Insurance Experiment, the first randomized trial assessing the impacts of health insurance expansion, and currently oversees a portfolio of research on the impact of social needs and adversity on health and health care outcomes in vulnerable populations. He received his Ph.D. in sociology from South Dakota State University.